Neurologic Athletic Head and Spine Injuries

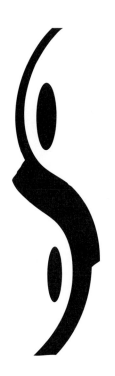

Neurologic Athletic Head and Spine Injuries

Robert C. Cantu, M.A., M.D., F.A.C.S., F.A.C.S.M.
Chief, Neurosurgery Service
Director, Service of Sports Medicine
Emerson Hospital
Concord, Massachusetts
Medical Director
National Center for Catastrophic
Sports Injury Research
Chapel Hill, North Carolina

W.B. SAUNDERS COMPANY
A Harcourt Health Sciences Company
Philadelphia   London   New York   St. Louis   Sydney   Toronto

W.B. SAUNDERS COMPANY
A Harcourt Health Sciences Company

The Curtis Center
Independence Square West
Philadelphia, Pennsylvania 19106

Library of Congress Cataloging-in-Publication Data

Neurologic athletic head and spine injuries / [edited by] Robert C. Cantu.

p.   cm.

ISBN 0-7216-8339-8

1. Brain—Wounds and injuries.   2. Spinal cord—Wounds and injuries.
   3. Sports injuries.   I. Cantu, Robert C. [DNLM: 1. Brain Injuries.
   2. Athletic Injuries.   3. Spinal Cord Injuries.   4. Sports Medicine—
   methods.   WL 354 N49426 2000]

RD594.N4686 2000   617.1′027—dc21

DNLM/DLC   99-057426

Editor: Richard H. Lampert
Editorial Assistant: Beth LoGiudice
Manuscript Editor: Jeffrey L. Scheib
Production Manager: Natalie Ware
Book Designer: Steven Stave

NEUROLOGIC ATHLETIC HEAD AND SPINE INJURIES   ISBN 0-7216-8339-8

Printed in the United States of America.

Last digit is the print number: 9   8   7   6   5   4   3   2   1

To my wife Tina, without whose support and tolerance
this book would not have been possible.

R.C.

Contributors

Julian E. Bailes, M.D.
Professor and Chairman, Department of Neurological Surgery; West Virginia University School of Medicine, Morgantown, West Virginia
On the Field Management of Athletic Head and Neck Injuries, Guidelines for Safe Return to Play After Athletic Head and Neck Injuries, Guidelines for Return to Contact or Collision Sport After a Cervical Spine Injury

Jeffrey T. Barth, Ph.D.
John Edward Fowler Professor, University of Virginia School of Medicine, Chief, Medical Psychology/Neuropsychology, University of Virginia Health Sciences Center, Charlottesville, Virginia
Outcome After Sports Concussion

Richard B. Birrer, M.D., M.P.H.
Associate Professor, Emergency Medicine, Albert Einstein College of Medicine; Associate Professor of Medicine, Cornell—Columbia, New York, New York; Professor of Family Medicine, State University of New York Health Sciences Center at Brooklyn, New York
Head and Spine Injuries in Martial Arts

W. H. Brooks, M.D.
Neurosurgical Associates, Lexington, Kentucky
Neurologic Injuries in Equestrian Sport

Charles J. Burke, III, M.D.
Assistant Professor of Orthopedics, Allegheny University Hospital; Orthopedic Surgeon, Director of Orthopedic Trauma, Allegheny General Hospital, Pittsburgh, Pennsylvania
Concussions in Ice Hockey: The National Hockey League Program

Robert C. Cantu, M.A., M.D., F.A.C.S., F.A.C.S.M.
Instructor, Pediatrics, Boston University School of Medicine; Chief, Neurosurgical Service, Director, Service of Sports Medicine, Emerson Hospital, Concord, Massachusetts; Medical Director, National Center for Catastrophic Sports Injury Research, Chapel Hill, North Carolina
Biomechanics of Head Injury, Guidelines for Safe Return to Play After Athletic Head and Neck Injuries, Overview of Concussion, Return to Play Guidelines After Concussion, Intracranial Hematoma, Malignant Brain Edema and Second Impact Syndrome, Return to Competition After Life Threatening Head Injury, Guidelines for Return to Contact or Collision Sport After a Cervical Spine Injury, Cervical Spinal Stenosis: Diagnosis and Return to Play Issues

Robert V. Cantu, M.D.
Resident, Department of Orthopedics, University of Massachusetts Medical Center, Worcester, Massachusetts
Epilepsy and Athletics

James D. Carson, M.D., Dip Sport Med., C.C.F.P.
Lecturer, Departments of Family & Community Medicine, and Surgery, University of Toronto; Staff Physician, Sport Care, Women's College Campus, Sunnybrook & Women's College Health Sciences Centre, Toronto, Ontario, Canada
Spinal Injuries in Canadian Ice Hockey Players, 1966–1996

Kenneth S. Clarke, Ph.D.
Sun City, California
The Epidemiology of Athletic Head Injuries, The Epidemiology of Athletic Spine Injuries

Robert Cushman, M.D., M.Sci., F.R.C.P.C.
Medical Officer of Health, Region of Ottawa—Carleton, Ottawa, Ontario, Canada
Spinal Injuries in Canadian Ice Hockey Players, 1966–1996

Phillip M. Davis, J.D. Law
Davis, White & Pettingell, Boston, Massachusetts
Medicolegal Considerations of Head or Spine Injury

Arthur L. Day, M.D.
Professor, Residency Program Director, Co-Chairman, Department of Neurological Surgery, Ebleu Scholar in Cerebrovascular Surgery, Department of Neurosurgery, University of Florida College of Medicine; Neurosurgical Consultant—University of Florida

Athletic Association, University of Florida, Gainesville, Florida
Thoracic and Lumbar Spine Injuries in Athletics

Robert J. Dimeff, M.D.
Assistant Clinical Professor of Family Medicine, Case Western Reserve University School of Medicine, Cleveland, Ohio; Associate Professor of Family Medicine, The Ohio State University College of Medicine, Columbus, Ohio; Vice Chairman, Department of Family Practice, Medical Director, Section of Sports Medicine, Department of Orthopaedic Surgery, The Cleveland Clinic Foundation, Cleveland, Ohio
Headaches in the Athlete

Mark A. Giovanini, M.D.
Neurosurgical Group, Pensacola, Florida
Thoracic and Lumbar Spine Injuries in Athletics

Christopher C. Giza, M.D.
Postgraduate Researcher, University of California, Los Angeles, UCLA School of Medicine, Los Angeles, California
Ionic and Metabolic Consequences of Concussion

John B. Harris, M.D., F.A.C.S.
Assistant Clinical Professor, Department of Neurological Surgery, University of California, Davis, School of Medicine, Davis, California; Director, Tahoe Neurosurgical Ski Safety Foundation, South Lake Tahoe, California
Neurologic Injuries in Alpine Skiing

Stanley A. Herring, M.D.
Clinical Professor, Department of Rehabilitation, Clinical Professor, Department of Orthopaedics, University of Washington School of Medicine; Puget Sound Sports and Spine Physicians; Team Physician, Seattle Seahawks, Professional Football Team, Seattle, Washington
Assessment and Rehabilitation of the Athlete With a Stinger

Edward G. Hixson, M.D.
General Surgeon, Adirondack Medical Center, Saranac Lake, New York; Expedition Physician, China–Everest '82 Expedition, 1983 Seven Summits Everest Expedition, China–Everest '84 Expedition
Mountaineering Head and Spine Injuries

Thomas Blaine Hoshizaki, Ph.D.
Associate Professor, University of Windsor, Windsor, Ontario, Canada
Engineering Head Protection

David A. Hovda, Ph.D.
Associate Professor, Departments of Molecular and Medical Pharmacology and Surgery, Division of Neurosurgery, University of California, Los Angeles, UCLA School of Medicine, Los Angeles, California
Ionic and Metabolic Consequences of Concussion

Barry D. Jordan, M.D., M.P.H.
Adjunct Clinical Assistant Professor of Neurology, The Weill Medical College at Cornell University, New York, New York; Director, Brain Injury Program, Burke Rehabilitation Hospital, White Plains, New York
Head and Spine Injuries in Martial Arts, Head and Spine Injuries in Boxing

Lauren M. Littlefield, Ph.D.
Assistant Professor of Psychology, Washington College, Chestertown, Maryland
Outcome After Sports Concussion

Mark R. Lovell, Ph.D.
Division Head, Neuropsychology, Henry Ford Health System—One Ford Place, Detroit, Michigan
Concussions in Ice Hockey: The National Hockey League Program

Stephen N. Macciocchi, Ph.D.
Adjunct Associate Professor, Department of Rehabilitation Medicine, Emory University School of Medicine; Director, Neuropsychology Division, Shepherd Center, Atlanta, Georgia
Outcome After Sports Concussion

Paul McCrory, M.B., B.S., F.R.A.C.P., F.A.C.S.M., F.A.S.M.F, F.R.S.M.
Clinical Fellow, Department of Neurology, University of Melbourne, Austin Repatriation Medical Centre, Melbourne, Australia; Director, Brain Injury Clinic, Department of

Neuroscience, Box Hill Hospital,
Victoria, Australia
*Convulsions in Contact and Collision
Sports, Stroke in Athletes*

Frederick O. Mueller, Ph.D.
Professor, Chair, Exercise and Sport
Science, University of North
Carolina at Chapel Hill; Director,
National Center for Catastrophic
Sports Injury Research, Chapel Hill,
North Carolina
*Fatalities from Brain and Cervical Spine
Injuries in Tackle Football: 54 Years'
Experience*

Harry Nafpliotis, Ph.D., P.T.
Director, Physical Therapy Center of
Teaneck, Teaneck, New Jersey;
President, New Jersey Hellenic
Health Professionals
Head, Neck, and Spine Soccer Injuries

Stephen E. Olvey, M.D.
Associate Professor of Neurological
Surgery, University of Miami School
of Medicine; Director, Neuroscience
Intensive Care Unit, UM/Jackson
Memorial Hospital; CART, Director
of Medical Affairs, Miami, Florida
Neurologic Injury in Motorsports

James C. Otis, Ph.D.
Associate Professor of Applied
Biomechanics in Orthopaedic
Surgery, The Weill Medical College
of Cornell University; Senior
Scientist, Department of
Biomechanics & Biomaterials, The
Hospital for Special Surgery, New
York, New York
Biomechanics of Spine Injuries

**Meheroz H. Rabadi, M.D.,
M.R.C.P.I.**
Fellow, Neurology and
Neurorehabilitation, The Weill
Medical College of Cornell
University, New York, New York;
Fellow, Neurology and
Neurorehabilitation, Burke
Rehabilitation Hospital, White
Plains, New York
Head and Spine Injuries in Martial Arts

**Alan T. Scher, M.B.Ch.B.(Cape
Town), D.M.R.D., R.C.P.(Lond),
R.C.S.(Eng.)**
Professor & Head, Department of
Radiology: Senior Lecturer,
University of Stellenbosch; Chair,
Department of Radiology, Tygerberg
Hospital, Tygerberg, South Africa
*Rugby Injuries to the Cervical Spine and
Spinal Cord*

Charles H. Tator, M.D., Ph.D.
Professor of Neurosurgery, University
of Toronto and Toronto Western
Hospital; President, ThinkFirst,
Canada, and SportSmart, Canada,
Toronto, Ontario, Canada
*Spinal Injuries in Canadian Ice Hockey
Players, 1966–1996*

W. Lee Warren, M.D.
Department of Neurosurgery,
Allegheny General Hospital,
Pittsburgh, Pennsylvania
*On the Field Management of Athletic
Head and Neck Injuries, Guidelines for
Safe Return to Play After Athletic Head
and Neck Injuries*

Stuart M. Weinstein, M.D.
Clinical Associate Professor,
Department of Rehabilitation
Medicine, University of Washington;
Private Practice, Puget Sound
Sports & Spine Physicians, P.S.;
Consultant—Sports Medicine
Program, University of Washington,
Seattle, Washington
*Assessment and Rehabilitation of the
Athlete With a Stinger*

Jack E. Wilberger, Jr., M.D.
Professor and Chairman, Department
of Neurosurgery; Allegheny General
Hospital, Pittsburgh, Pennsylvania;
Vice Dean, Medical College of
Pennsylvania Hahnemann School of
Medicine, Philadelphia,
Pennsylvania
*Athletic Cervical Spinal Cord and Spine
Injuries, Guidelines for Return to Contact
or Collision Sport After a Cervical Spine
Injury*

Foreword

I am pleased and honored to provide some opening words for this major work by Dr. Robert Cantu. Dr. Cantu has accumulated in these pages the insight of more than 30 international experts on neurologic athletic head and spine injuries. The result is a thoroughly comprehensive and scientifically impeccable treatment of this crucial area of sports medicine.

Certainly this is a timely undertaking. Organized sports participation and competition has increased worldwide at an unprecedented rate during the past 30 years. This phenomenon encompasses people of all ages, from children and adolescents through senior citizens. It also includes both genders, as women are now literally making great strides in athletic endeavours off-limits to them in previous generations—notably contact and collision sports, such as soccer, rugby, and wrestling.

The benefits of organized sports activity are well known. They include improved health, opportunities for socialization, and sheer enjoyment of competition and exercise. These benefits have increased merit at a time when other forms of recreation competing for people's time—notably, computer games and the internet—are sedentary, solitary, and bereft of the joy associated with vigorous physical activity.

Sports participation almost always yields positive results. One of the few downsides is injury. As to be expected, the growth in sports participation has precipitated an increase in sports injuries. Different injury patterns have emerged, with the potential, however rare, for serious and even life threatening injuries present in contact or collision sports and those activities where there is the possibility of striking surrounding obstacles at high speeds. Injuries to the head or spine are among the most common cause of such catastrophic injury and represent the worst nightmare for any parent or coach.

Thus, the responsibilities of the modern-day team physician are enormous, and perhaps nowhere more important than where it comes to managing head and spine injuries.

Today's team physician must be competent to perform an accurate initial assessment of a head and spine injury and arrange for safe immobilization and transport of the athlete to a secondary care center where accurate diagnosis and effective treatment are available. The team physician may actively participate in the rehabilitation of the injured athlete in preparation for return to play. Finally, the all-important decision as to return to play falls on the shoulders of the team physician—when and if this should occur, at what level or capacity, and with what type of protective equipment or limitations of play in place.

There is also the "big picture" contribution that sports medicine personnel can make to sports safety. Educating the public and parents about the relative risks of sports participation, particularly to the head and spine, as well as about risk factors and safety interventions that can reduce the occurrence or severity of these injuries are important responsibilities of medical personnel at any level of sports. The paramount importance of sports safety and its relationship to the epidemiologic study of sports injuries was one of the focal points of a recent joint pronouncement by the International Federation of Sports Medicine and the World Health Organization.[1] In this consensus statement, these venerable international organizations called for an emphasis on sports safety and sports education at the inception of any organized sports program, and particularly those involving children.

Dr. Cantu's book addresses these issues and more. The reader of this volume will be treated to the most in-depth and up-to-date assessment of head and spine injuries that has ever been made available to the sports medicine profession. As such, it has a place in the library or on the bookshelf of any researcher or physician, and will prove to be of particular benefit to active practitioners of sports medicine.

LYLE J. MICHELI
Harvard Medical School
Boston Children's Hospital
Past President, American
   College of Sports Medicine

---

[1]FIMS/WHO Ad Hoc Committee on Sports and Children (Micheli LJ [Chair], Armstrong N, Bar-Or O, Boreham C, Chan K, Eston R, Hills AP, Maffulli N, Malina RM, Nair NVK, Nevill A, Roland T, Sharp C, Stanish WD, Tanner S). Sports and children: Consensus statement on organized sports for children. Bull World Health Organ 1998;76:445–447.

Preface

The head and cervical spine are unique in that their contents, the brain and spinal cord, are largely incapable of regeneration. Thus, injury to the head and the neck takes on a singular importance. Although today many parts of the body can be replaced, either by artificial hardware or transplanted parts, the head and spine cannot because their contents cannot be transplanted.

Furthermore, neurologic injuries to the head, especially the subdural hematoma, malignant brain edema syndrome of children, second impact syndrome of adults, and neck quadriplegia, are the most frequent catastrophic athletic injuries. These same neurologic injuries are also the most common causes of *direct* (defined as due to the skills of the sport) athletic death.

This textbook focuses primarily on athletic head injuries of a neurologic nature and does not cover injuries to the scalp, eyes, ears, nose, and mouth. The neck section for the most part examines athletic injuries to the cervical spine or its contents, the vertebral arteries and spinal cord, rather than other neck structures, such as the larynx and trachea.

Given the morbidity and the mortality associated with neurologic athletic head and spine injuries, it is obvious that prevention of these types of injuries is of paramount importance. Prevention starts with an understanding of the epidemiology of these injuries as well as with correct on-the-field evaluation. Prevention is also enhanced by an accurate diagnosis, prompt proper treatment, including rehabilitation, and correct return to play decisions. Each of these areas is comprehensively covered. In addition, special issues of singular importance that all members of the sports medicine team must understand fully with respect to head injury (i.e., the second impact syndrome, epilepsy and athletics, and outcome from mild head injury), and cervical spine injury (i.e., the correct diagnosis of cervical spinal stenosis and brachial plexus and cervical nerve root injury) are covered in depth. A number of myths are discounted, such as that the football, baseball/softball, or lacrosse helmet protects the neck. These helmets are made to a NOCSAE standard to afford a significant degree of head protection, but they do not protect the neck.

This text is not written exclusively for neurologists, neurosurgeons, and orthopedic surgeons, who today increasingly function as sports medicine consultants, but equally for today's sports medicine primary care providers: general practitioners, pediatricians, hospital emergency department physicians, internists, athletic trainers, EMTs, physical therapists, and chiropractors.

Today no medical text on injuries would be complete without a section on medicolegal aspects, and this area is covered by a prominent attorney with decades of experience with the legal aspects of athletic head and spine injuries. This volume also includes a sports-specific section, which covers sports that have the greatest risk of neurologic head and spine injury, i.e., boxing, football, ice hockey, and rugby.

For me it has been a most stimulating, enlightening, and rewarding intellectual experience to work with the renowned experts contributing to this textbook, and I most sincerely hope you will feel the same after reading our effort.

ROBERT C. CANTU

Contents

PREVALENCE AND PROTECTION

1

Biomechanics of Head Injury

Robert C. Cantu

An understanding of three principles is necessary in order to comprehend how biomechanical forces produce skull and brain injury. First, a forceful blow to the resting movable head usually produces maximal brain injury beneath the point of cranial impact (coup injury). This is the situation when the head in a resting state is forcibly struck by another object, such as a left hook punch or an opponent's football helmet.[2] Second, a moving head colliding with a nonmoving object usually produces maximal brain injury opposite the site of cranial impact (contrecoup injury). An example is an individual falling over backward, striking the head on the ground at the instant of impact. Third, if a skull fracture is present, the first two dictums do not pertain, because the bone itself, either transiently (linear skull fracture) or permanently (depressed skull fracture), is displaced at the moment of impact and may directly injure the brain tissue.

An understanding of the mechanisms of brain injury further requires a realization that there are three distinct types of stresses that can be generated by a force applied to the head. The first two, namely compressive and tensile (the opposite of compressive and sometimes called negative pressure), are linear forces. These forces are also used synonymously with the term translational. In sports these types of forces are most commonly generated when the athlete's body and head, traveling at a given speed, strike a solid object, or when the stationary athlete's cranium is in turn struck by a moving object. Such forces usually produce focal injuries, such as brain contusions, or intracranial hematoma. It has been documented both experimentally and clinically that most focal injuries are associated with impact loading.[11]

The third type of force is a rotational or

shearing one (a force applied parallel to a surface). These forces usually lead to diffuse brain injury along a continuum from mild concussion to more severe concussion to diffuse axonal injury with profound shearing of white matter fiber tracts and disruption of axons, depending on the magnitude of the angular acceleration force imparted to the brain.[12, 21] Such diffuse injury is associated with impulsive loading conditions resulting from acceleration-deceleration phenomena.[11] With severe diffuse rotational injuries there is usually a period of coma. There is a significant chance of death, and for those who recover, severe cognitive and emotional deficits are common. A classic example of rotational angular forces being imparted to the head would be the left hook in boxing. Blows to the side of the head tend to produce greater angular acceleration forces than those to the face, whereas blows to the chin, which acts as a lever, produce maximal forces. It is generally believed that it is the rotational component of cranial impact that most directly leads to a loss of consciousness.

Thus, athletic head injuries may result from both linear and rotational forces being imparted to the brain. Although one or the other of these mechanisms usually predominates, it is not uncommon for both of these forces to be imparted by the same impact. Contact sports such as football, ice hockey, and boxing have a high degree of linear and acceleration forces being repetitively delivered to the brain during a single contest.

While most athletic head injuries occur from direct blows received by the head, it is possible to impart linear and even rotational forces indirectly to the brain. Examples of this would be violent hits to the chest that snap the head forward and violent hits to the posterior thorax that snap the head backward.

To protect against external forces, the brain has it own cushioning and protective shock absorber, the cerebrospinal fluid (CSF). The CSF essentially converts focally applied external stress to compressive stress because the fluid follows the contours of the sulci and gyri and distributes the force in a uniform fashion. Without CSF, compressive forces would be received by gyri crests but not in the depths of the sulci, thus potentiating a greater degree of the damaging shearing forces.

The CSF, however, does not totally prevent shearing forces from being imparted to the brain, especially when rotational forces are applied to the head. Shearing forces also occur at those sites where rotational gliding is hindered. Characteristically there are three such sites: (1) the dura mater–brain attachments that impede brain motion such as the midline falx cerebri and the tentorium cerebelli; (2) the rough, irregular surface contacts between the brain and the skull that hinder smooth movement and are especially prominent on the floor of the frontal and middle fossas; and (3) dissipation of CSF between the brain and the skull. The third condition explains the mechanisms of coup and contrecoup injuries. When the head is accelerated prior to impact, the brain lags toward the trailing surface, thus squeezing away the protective CSF and allowing excess CSF to accumulate on the opposite surface. This allows the shearing forces to be maximal at the site where CSF is thinnest and thus has its least cushioning effect, which is opposite the site of impact.

On the other hand, when the head is stationary prior to the impact, there is neither brain lag nor disproportionate distribution of CSF. In this situation, the shearing stresses are greatest at the site of cranial impact and explain the mechanism of the coup injury.

In understanding how acceleration forces are applied to the brain, it is important to keep in mind Newton's law: force = mass × acceleration, or, stated another way, force/mass = acceleration. An athlete's head can sustain far greater forces without injury if the neck muscles are tensed, such as when the athlete sees the collision coming. In the relaxed state, the mass of the head is essentially its own weight, whereas in the tensed state, the mass of the head takes on an approximation of the mass of the body. Therefore, as the mass of the head increases, the forces must also increase to produce the same amount of acceleration. The athlete is at greater risk for brain injury when the neck is limp, such as when one does not see the blow coming or when one is stunned (a boxer with concussion) and cannot maintain neck muscle rigidity.

Experimental primate studies by Gennarelli and colleagues[13] over the last 20 years have confirmed and extended the work of Russell and Denny-Brown at Oxford in the first years of World War II, when they showed that brain damage was more extensive when the head of a monkey was free to move when it was struck.[9] The findings of Gennarelli and coworkers also confirmed the predictions of the Oxford physicist Holbourn, who in the 1940s experimented with gelatin models of the brain and simulated the shearing lesion of white matter that is now called diffuse axonal injury (DAI). This was first described in detail by Strich, who dissected the brains of patients who had died after long periods with severe disability.[26, 27]

As a result of collaborative research by teams in Philadelphia and Glasgow, it appears that all the lesions found in humans can be reproduced experimentally in laboratory animals by varying the magnitude, duration, and direction of applied acceleration and deceleration forces.[1, 13] There now is no doubt that shearing forces acting on nerve fibers and blood vessels are the main mechanism for producing impact or primary damage. Thus primary damage that occurs at the moment of injury takes the form of surface contusion or laceration, diffuse axonal injury, and intracranial hemorrhage. These experiments have also shown that axonal damage in continuity can occur; whether this progresses to a permanent lesion may depend on factors that could be influenced by pharmacologic interventions. This has altered the philosophy of approach to the treatment of impact brain damage, which had been based on the assumption that damage is maximal at onset and is irreversible.

Today it is widely understood that significant secondary brain injury may occur owing to ischemic damage related to increased intracranial pressure, hypertension, and reduced cerebral blood flow as well as from the release of neurotoxic substances from injured brain. This secondary injury may not present clinically for a period of hours to days after the initial injury. A more in-depth discussion can be found in Chapter 9.

Intracranial hemorrhage, especially subdural hematoma, is the leading cause of death resulting directly from participation in the skills of a sport.[20] Overall in sports today the leading cause of death is indirect death from sudden cardiac arrhythmia (sudden death syndrome).[20] It also appears that the same biomechanical forces applied to a child's or adolescent's head can produce injuries different from those in an adult. With an incidence of 219 per 100,000 population, head injury is the most common cause of acquired brain damage resulting in either deficits of cognition, memory, attention, language, and psychosocial adaptation[5, 7, 8, 10, 14, 18, 19] or death[15] in children.

Moreover, in children it appears that the frontal and anterior temporal lobes are particularly vulnerable to contusion and hematoma injuries. Using volumetric measuring by magnetic resonance imaging (MRI), Berryhill and colleagues found that in children with head injury, even in the absence of focal brain injuries demonstrable by MRI, frontal lobe tissue especially was lost.[3] They postulated that the frontal lobes sustain diffuse injury, even in the absence of focal brain lesions detectable by MRI.[3] Thus it appears that the incidence of cognitive insults, even in the absence of injury demonstrable by MRI, is higher in children than in adults. Such findings raise concerns over children participating in sports where repetitive blows to the head occur, for example, boxing, soccer ("heading" the ball), and so forth.

Another head injury unique to the child or adolescent athlete is the malignant brain edema syndrome. This condition consists of rapid neurologic deterioration from an alert, conscious state to coma and sometimes death, minutes to several hours after head trauma.[22, 25] Although this sequence in adults almost always is caused by an intracranial clot, pathology studies in children show diffuse brain swelling with little or no brain injury.[25] Rather than true cerebral edema, Langfitt and colleagues have shown that the diffuse cerebral swelling is the result of true hyperemia or vascular engorgement.[16, 17] Prompt recognition is extremely important because there is little initial brain injury, and the serious or fatal neurologic outcome is secondary to raised intracranial pressure with herniation.

Prompt treatment with intubation, hyperventilation, and osmotic agents has helped to reduce the mortality.[4, 6] This condition, as well as the second impact syndrome[23, 24] that occurs especially in young adults, is discussed in greater detail in Chapter 14.

The forces that can be imparted to an athlete's head are multiple and may lead to initial focal or diffuse injury due to disruption of brain tissue; contusion, hematoma, or delayed ischemic injury; injury due to anoxia; hypotension; increased intracranial pressure caused by altered autoregulation of cerebral blood flow; and release of cytotoxic substances from injured brain tissue. Furthermore, it is apparent that the pediatric athlete is at greater risk of frontal lobe and anterior temporal lobe injury in particular, as compared with an adult. Children and adolescents are also uniquely at risk for the rare malignant brain edema syndrome. Thus it appears warranted to protect that age group with rules and protective equipment that will minimize the delivery of repetitive acceleration forces to their young brains.

References

1. Adams JH, Doyle D, Ford I, et al. Diffuse axonal injury in head injury: Definition, diagnosis and grading. Histopathology 1989;15:49–59.
2. Albright JP, McAuley E, Martin RK, et al. Head and neck injuries in college football: An eight year analysis. Am J Sports Med 1985;13:147–152.
3. Berryhill P, Lilly MA, Levin HS, et al. Frontal lobe changes after severe diffuse closed head injury in children: A volumetric study of magnetic resonance imaging. Neurosurgery 1995;37:393–399.
4. Bowers SA, Marchall LF. Outcome in 200 consecutive cases of severe head injury treated in San Diego County: A prospective analysis. Neurosurgery 1980;6:237.
5. Brown G, Chadwick O, Shaffer D, et al. A prospective study of children with head injuries: Psychiatric sequelae. Psychol Med 1981;11:63–78.
6. Bruce DA, Alavi A, Bilaniuk L, et al. Diffuse cerebral swelling following head injuries in children: The syndrome of malignant brain edema. J Neurosurg 1981;54:170–178.
7. Chadwick O, Rutter M, Brown G, et al. A prospective study of children with head injuries: Cognitive sequelae. Psychol Med 1981;11:49–61.
8. Chapman SB, Culhane KA, Levin HS, et al. Behavioral changes after closed head injury in children and adolescents. Brain Lang 1992;43:42–65.
9. Denny-Brown D, Russell WR. Experimental cerebral concussion. Brain 1941;64:93.
10. Fletcher JM, Ewing-Cobbs L, Miner ME, et al. Behavioral changes after closed head injury in children. J Consult Clin Psychol 1990;58:93–98.
11. Gennarelli TA, Thibault LE. Biomechanics of Head Injury. *In* Wilkins RH, Rengacinary SS (eds): Neuro-

surgery. New York, McGraw-Hill, 1985, pp 1531–1536.

12. Gennarelli TA, Sewawa H, Wald U, et al. Physiological Response to Angular Acceleration of the Head. *In* Grossman RG, Gildenbert PL (eds): Head Injury: Basic and Clinical Aspects. New York, Raven Press, 1982, pp 129–140.

13. Gennarelli TA, Thibault LE, Adams JH, et al. Diffuse axonal injury and traumatic coma in the primate. Ann Neurol 1982;12:564.

14. Kaufmann PN, Fletcher JM, Lewis HS, et al. Attentional disturbance after pediatric closed head injury. Child Neurol 1993;8:348–353.

15. Kalus JF, Rock A, Hemyari P. Brain injuries among infants, children, adolescents, and young adults. Am J Dis Child 1990;144:684–691.

16. Langfitt TW, Kassell NF. Cerebral vasodilations produced by brainstem stimulation: Neurogenic control vs autoregulation. Am J Physiol 1978;215:90.

17. Langfitt TW, Tannenbaum HM, Kassell NF. The etiology of acute brain swelling following experimental head injury. J Neurosurg 1966;24:47.

18. Levin HS, Culhane KA, Mendelsohn D, et al. Cognition in relation to magnetic resonance imaging in head-injured children and adolescents. Arch Neurol 1993;50:897–905.

19. Levin HS, High WM Jr, Ewing-Cobbs L, et al. Memory functioning during the first year after closed head injury in children and adolescents. Neurosurgery 1988;22:1043–1052.

20. Mueller FO, Cantu RC, VanCamp SP. Catastrophic injuries in high school and college sports. HK Sport Science Monograph Series, Champaign IL, 1996.

21. Peerless SJ, Rewcastle NB. Shear injuries of the brain. CMAJ 1967;96:577–582.

22. Pickles W. Acute general edema of the brain in children with head injuries. N Engl J Med 1950; 242:607.

23. Saunders RL, Haraugh RE. Second impact in catastrophic contact-sports head trauma. JAMA 1984; 252:538.

24. Schneider RC. Head and Neck Injuries in Football. Baltimore, Williams & Wilkins, 1973.

25. Schnitker MT. A syndrome of cerebral concussion in children. J Pediatr 1949;35:557.

26. Strich SJ. Shearing of nerve fibers as a cause of brain damage due to head injury. Lancet 1961; 2:443–448.

27. Strich SJ. Diffuse degeneration of cerebral white matter in severe dementia following head injury. J Neurol Neurosurg Psychiatry 1956;19:163–185.

2

Biomechanics of Spine Injuries

James C. Otis

The purpose of this chapter is to review the biomechanical aspects of cervical spine injuries. Cervical spine trauma results in catastrophic consequences to individuals who sustain spinal column injuries that compromise the spinal cord. In sports such as football, the neck is subjected to a variety of forces, yet rarely do these forces produce catastrophic injury to the cervical spine. In football, catastrophic neck injuries result from primary contact of the crown of the helmet during blocking and tackling activities. These spearing-type activities and the number of catastrophic injuries increased in the 1960s with the transition from leather helmets to the contemporary head-face protection systems that comprise a hard shell with a load-distributing suspension and a face guard. The increased protection provided a sense of invulnerability for the head and resulted in the use of the head in these high-risk activities that led to catastrophic cervical spine injuries.

MECHANISM OF ENERGY ABSORPTION

During routine contact sport activities, the head is subjected to numerous impacts that result in forces being applied to the cervical spine. Why is the spine able to sustain such trauma on a repeated basis yet survive catastrophic injury? What are the mechanisms that protect the spine from injury during these frequently applied forces? When energy is imparted to the body, it is essential that the energy be dissipated in a manner that the body can tolerate. Energy is the potential to apply a force over a distance in an amount equal to the product of the force multiplied by the distance and has units of newton-meters (Nm). It can be kinetic (moving) energy, which is equal to $\frac{1}{2} mv^2$,

where m is the mass of the moving object and v is its velocity; or it can be potential (static) energy, which is equal to mgh, where m is the mass of an object, g is the gravitational constant, and h is the height of the mass with respect to a reference, such as the ground. Potential energy can also be stored energy, such as that found in a spring that has a force applied to maintain it in a lengthened or shortened state. In contact sports the primary source of injury-producing energy is in the form of kinetic energy and is associated with players on the move.

Energy reflects the potential to do work, and work is the means by which energy is transferred from one object to another. Work is defined as a force applied over a distance. Accordingly, 10 Nm of energy can be utilized to do work over a 10-cm distance with a 100 newton (N) force, or over a 0.5-cm distance with a 2000 N force. When considering trauma to the body, it is desirable to maintain force at a minimum, or at least within the limits of tolerance to bodily injury. This would require the force to be applied over a relatively large distance in most cases. Unfortunately, we do not generally have the freedom to select these parameters as needed to prevent injury. Knowledge of the fundamentals of energy as it affects the human body will allow us to better educate those individuals involved in teaching and playing sports and provide a basis for the design of protective devices that will be effective in minimizing injury.

In the musculoskeletal system, the muscles are the primary elements for producing mechanical work, and they are also the primary elements for energy absorption. Muscle does positive work when a muscle generates force during a shortening contraction, as do the biceps when lifting an object with the hand, as in a curl. On the other hand, energy is absorbed about joints when muscles across the joints undergo eccentric, or lengthening, contractions. This is often referred to as negative work. The amount of energy absorbed depends on the force in the muscle and the amount of lengthening that occurs. This requires that there be range of motion available at the joint. The more limited is the range of motion, the lesser is the capacity to absorb energy.

How much energy is involved during sporting activities? An 80-kg athlete moving at 5 m/s has kinetic energy of $\frac{1}{2} \times (80 \text{ kg}) \times (1 \text{ N-s}^2/\text{kg-m}) \times (5 \text{ m/s})^2 = 1000$ Nm. One can appreciate the magnitude of this energy when one realizes that a femur is capable of absorbing on the order of 30 Nm of energy before failing. A cervical spine segment can withstand approximately 3 Nm of energy before failing. Thus, it can be appreciated that the level of energy generated during athletic activities far exceeds the capacity of the bony (and ligamentous) elements to absorb energy. Muscles, on the other hand, are capable of absorbing these high energy levels generated. For example, in landing after a jump from a height of 1 m, the velocity at ground contact is about 5 m/s (Figure 2–1). A significant portion of the energy is taken up by the knee extensors, which are capable of absorbing on the order of 10 Nm per degree of flexion, or 20 Nm per degree bilaterally. Consequently, if all of the energy were absorbed about the knees, the landing would require both knees to flex approximately 50 degrees to safely absorb the energy of the landing (50° × 20 Nm/° = 1000 Nm). If flexion at the hips also occurred, the hip extensors would share the burden and reduce the force requirements of the knee extensors and range of motion necessary. Thus, the human body has the capability to deal with these high levels of energy and to dissipate them in a safe manner when the energy is properly directed.

Does such a mechanism exist for the cervical spine? Consider the example illustrated in Figure 2–2. It can be seen that an impact to the anterior aspect of the head produces extension of the cervical spine. This extension results in elongation of the anterior neck muscles, which, during a controlled activity, would be activated in order to absorb the energy of the impact. If the neck begins in a more flexed position, there is more excursion available for the muscles to lengthen and a greater capacity to absorb energy. In addition, the greater the range of motion available in this situation, the greater is the likelihood that the head will be moved out of the path of the applied force, and the greater is the likelihood that the head and neck complex will not exceed its injury threshold. This chapter reviews the mechanisms during which the cervical

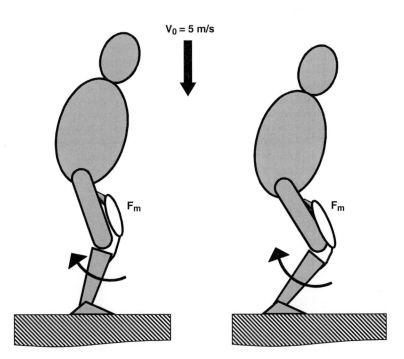

Figure 2–1. Upon landing, the kinetic energy associated with the vertical velocity of 5 m/s is absorbed to a great extent by the knee extensors as knee flexion occurs, causing lengthening of the actively contracting muscles.

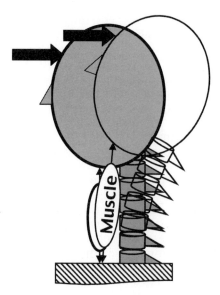

Figure 2–2. An impact to the head which produces bending of the cervical spine, extension in this example, generates lengthening of the active muscles resisting the movement and, thereby, absorbs energy.

spine is subjected to loads that are not capable of being absorbed by muscle and result in catastrophic injuries in sports and recreational activities.

History

It is essential to understand the mechanisms by which cervical spine injuries occur, because only then is it possible to determine methods for preventing such injuries. As discussed by Otis, Burstein, and Torg,[3] historically, two concepts have been put forth as being responsible for cervical spine injuries occurring in tackle football. One implicates the facemask as providing a lever by which the head and neck can be forced into hyperflexion, and the second purports that the back rim of the football helmet acts as a guillotine. Neither of these concepts, however, is supported by current scientific evidence.

A cineradiographic study was conducted by Virgin[11] to quantify the spatial relationship between the posterior rim of the football helmet relative to the cervical spine as the head moved from the fully flexed to the fully extended position for several loading conditions. Virgin studied 16 subjects with five different brands of football helmets. No contact was observed between the posterior rim of any of the helmets tested and the

spinous processes of the cervical column (Figure 2–3). Virgin concluded that the concept of the posterior rim and the helmet striking the cervical spine above the level of C7 was without basis.

Carter and Frankel[1a] performed a biomechanical analysis of cervical spine hyperextension using a static-free–body analysis. They calculated the forces imposed on the cervical spine with the face guard force acting in such a manner as to produce hyperextension of the cervical spine. They examined three different loading conditions, each associated with a different helmet design. The conditions consisted of a posterior rim that was cut high enough so that it did not impinge on the cervical spine, a posterior rim that would impact at the level of the fourth cervical vertebra, and a posterior rim that would impact the shoulder pads. Their analysis suggests that the condition with the posterior rim highest would result in the worst hyperextension situation and would lead to high forces and possibly to serious injury of the upper cervical spine. In their analysis the forces were reduced considerably with the mid-height condition of the posterior rim.

The results did not support the "guillotine" theory as the mechanism of injury. Clinical data dealing with the mechanisms of injury to the cervical spine do not support the concept of a hyperextension-guillotine mechanism of injury. It was noted by Torg and colleagues[9, 10] that only 3% of injuries that resulted in quadriplegia could be explained as being due to hyperextension, while 8% of those that resulted in fracture-dislocation without quadriplegia were consistent with this mechanism (Table 2–1).

According to the National Football Head and Neck Injury Registry,[10] 72% of cervical spine injuries resulting in quadriplegia in high school football between 1971 and 1975 were a result of tackling. In college football during the same interval, 78% of the quadriplegia were a result of tackling. At the high school level, defensive backs constituted 52% of the injured players, speciality teams 13%, and linebackers 10% of the injured players. At the college level, defensive backs comprised 73% of the players who were rendered quadriplegic. These data indicated that direct, head-on collisions with the crown of the helmet occurred in 52% of all the cervical spine quadriplegia from 1971 to 1975. Thus the defensive backs, linebackers,

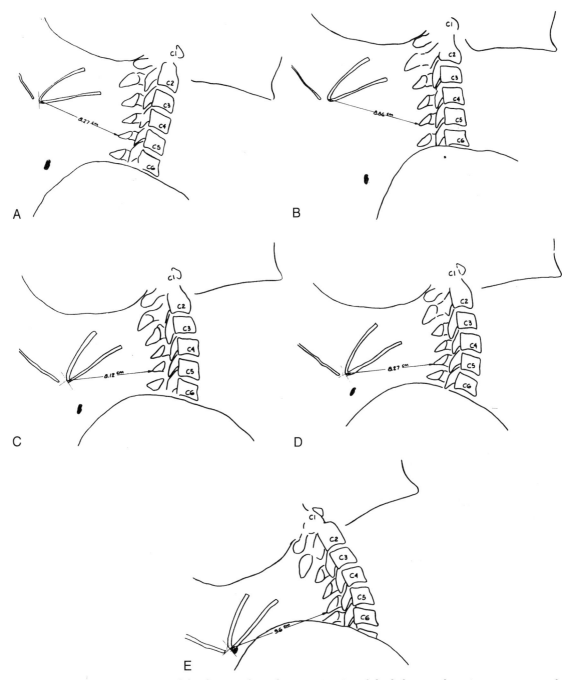

Figure 2–3. *A–E*, Measurements of the distance from the posterior rim of the helmet to the spinous processes of C5 from the neutral position to the point of impingement: $A = 8.27$ cm; $B = 8.06$ cm; $C = 8.12$ cm; $D = 8.27$ cm; and $E = 9.6$ cm. (From Virgin H. Cineradiographic study of football helmets and the cervical spine. Am J Sports Med 1980;8:310. Used with permission.)

and specialty team members who impact initially with the tops of their heads are at the greatest risk of sustaining these catastrophic cervical spine injuries.

Tator and coworkers[8] reviewed cervical spine injuries in hockey and concluded that the most frequent event that led to catastrophic spinal injury in ice hockey was a push or a check from behind. In general, the injured player was unaware of the impending impact and was hurled horizontally into the boards in such a manner that head

Table 2–1. Mechanism of Injury Resulting in Permanent Cervical Quadraplegia, 1971–1975

	Injuries Resulting in Quadraplegia (%) (n = 73)	Injuries Not Resulting in Quadraplegia (%) (n = 136)
Hyperflexion	10	11
Hyperextension	3	8
Vertical compression	52	39
Knee or thigh to head	15	17
Collision, pileup or ground contact	11	19
Tackled	7	7
Machine related	3	0
Face mask acting as a lever	0	0

(From Otis JC, Burstein AH, Torg JS. Mechanisms and Pathomechanics of Athletic Injuries to the Cervical Spine. *In* Torg JS [ed]: *Athletic Injuries to the Head, Neck, and Face.* St. Louis, Mosby–Year Book, 1991, pp 438–456. Used with permission.)

contact occurred, resulting in axial loading of the spine and catastrophic injury. They compared cervical spinal cord injuries sustained during two 3-year periods, 1988 to 1990 and 1991 to 1993. Of 12 cases of cervical spine injury in the earlier period, 7 resulted from a check from behind and had cord injury. During the more recent period, only 3 of 15 suffered cord injury. Of the 186 cases with documentation, 37% were due to a push or check from behind, 23% were pushed or checked but not from behind, 20% tripped on the ice, and 16% were due to sliding along the ice. The majority, 70% of documented injuries, occurred as the result of an impact with the boards, and 14% occurred as a result of impacts with other players. These authors commented that the more frequent collisions in smaller rinks and the lack of shock absorption of the boards in newer rinks are also possible causes of spinal injury. As will be discussed, the work of Nightingale and colleagues[6] does not support the contention that increased shock absorption of the boards would reduce the likelihood of spinal injury, and, to the contrary, suggests that padding the surface may subject the spine to increased risk of catastrophic injury.

The generally accepted injury mechanism responsible for fracture-dislocation of the cervical spine is believed to be failure of the spine owing to local flexion as a result of axial loading. The biomechanics of this injury mechanism are illustrated in Figure 2–4. With forward flexion of the neck, the cervical spine is straightened and can be modeled as a segmented column. Impacting the head results in axial loading F_1, which compresses the column as the energy absorbing structures take up load as the force increases to F_2. Because the force is axial and does not generate a bending moment to produce any type of flexion, the column reaches its limit with respect to axial compression, and acute local flexion occurs, with fracture, dislocation, or unilateral or bilateral facet dislocation.

Cadaver-Based Models

Nightingale and coworkers[4] developed a cadaver-based impact model that included the head and the spine through the second thoracic vertebra. They utilized the head and neck injury drop apparatus illustrated in Figure 2–5. A 16-kg mass was used to simulate the weight of the torso. The system permitted simulation of an impact at the top of the head with the body mass following. With this model they examined the relationships among the motion of the head, local deformation of the cervical spine, and the mechanisms of injury. Previously, the mechanism of injury to the cervical spine had been attributed to extension and flexion motions. They examined 11 specimens dropped in an inverted posture from a vertical height that would produce an impact velocity on the order of 3.2 m/s. They varied the angle of the impact surface and the surface padding. These investigators observed motion of the head that was not consistent with the mechanism of injury to the cervical spine. Furthermore, these experiments revealed that the injury occurred before noticeable motion of the head occurred.

The model allowed characterization of the local mechanism of injury. Nightingale and colleagues observed buckling of the cervical

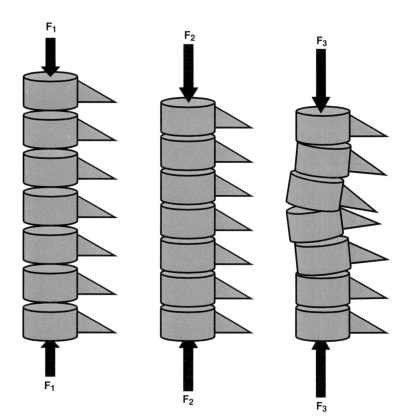

Figure 2–4. The segmented column illustrates the mechanism of axial loading of the cervical spine in which the spine is compressed and shortened until failure occurs in acute flexion, producing fracture, dislocation, or unilateral or bilateral facet dislocation.

spine that involved extension between the third and sixth vertebrae and flexion between the seventh and eighth vertebrae. They were able to conclude that the previous theories of flexion and extension of the head as the mechanism of injury could not be applied to a vertical impact of the head, and furthermore, that motion of the head was not a reliable indicator of the mechanism of injury. This point was quite apparent from their study in which flexion of the head occurred in 6 of 11 specimens with no flexion injury, but with four extension injuries of the cervical spine. Extension of the head occurred in 5 specimens with two flexion injuries, nine extension injuries, and three vertical compression injuries. Furthermore, regardless of the orientation of the impact plate or the type of padding on the impact surface, the cervical spine buckled. A distinct pattern of deformation was recorded that was consistent with the distribution of injuries. The pattern was characterized by extension of C3 through C6 and flexion of C7 and C8.

It is generally accepted that catastrophic cervical spine injuries occur because the neck is compressed axially between the head and the torso. If it is possible to move the head out of the way during the impact, the compressive load in the cervical spine can be avoided as the head and neck go into extension or flexion modes. Nightingale and colleagues[5] examined the inertial effects of the head and torso to determine whether the head mass is sufficient to constrain the head in a position that will allow axial loads to be generated in the cervical spine. Their experiments demonstrated that cervical spine motion can be constrained sufficiently by head inertia to allow compressive forces in the cervical spine. This was true for the unconstrained vertex impacts and the anterior impacts in which the major component was along the axis of the spine and only a minor component of force was available to accelerate the head and neck out of the path of the torso. Their experiments also documented cervical spine loading as a result of head rebound for conditions of padded impact surfaces. This phenomenon was consistent with the modeling study of Otis and coworkers,[3] in which the spring element associated with the helmet suspension resulted in a rebound of the head and additional loading of the cervical spine.

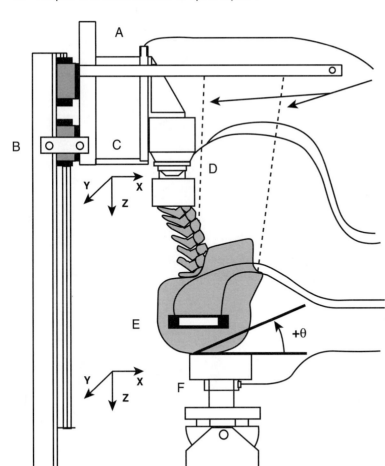

Figure 2–5. Diagram of test apparatus showing (C) the carriage, torso, and linear bearing sliders, (F) the impact surface and 3-axis load cell, (D) 6-axis load cell, and (E) the head accelerometer array. (From Nightingale RW, McElhaney JH, Richardson WJ, Meyers BS. Dynamic responses of the head and cervical spine to axial impact loading. J Biomech 1996;29:307–318. Used with permission.)

Nightingale and colleagues[6] examined the hypothesis that deformable impact surfaces pose a greater risk of cervical spine injury than do rigid surfaces. The results were quite surprising, considering the generally held belief that energy absorbing devices offer protection and reduce the risk of injury. In an earlier study[5] the results suggested that the inertia of the head was sufficient to constrain head motion and allow time for neck injury to occur, that is, the cervical spine remained in line with the impact force long enough to allow excessive compression to be developed along the long axis of the spine. In the present study the investigators considered the hypothesis that padded impact surfaces, by constraining motion of the head, will increase the risk and severity of injury to the cervical spine. A total of 18 drop tests were performed with six test combinations using variations of impact angle and impact surface padding. The impact angles were −15 degrees, 0 degrees, and +15 degrees, which resulted in a posterior impact, vertex impact, and anterior impact, respectively. The surface types consisted of a 3-mm sheet of lubricated Teflon or a 5-cm-thick, highly deformable, open-cell polyurethane.

With the anterior impacts, all three padded impacts produced unstable injuries. With the padded impacts, there was little or no head motion after impact, with the neck being virtually constrained between the head and the torso. Two of the rigid surface impacts produced injury, and posterior translation of the head occurred after the injury. In the one case of a rigid impact without injury, the posteriorly-directed forces were able to push the head into extension out of the way of the torso load before injury could occur.

The impacts to the vertex produced injury for all three padded impact conditions. The head and neck motions for these padded conditions were similar to those for these padded condition with the anterior impacts, that is, there was little motion of the head, and the neck was compressed between the torso and the head. All the rigid vertex impacts resulted in 5 degrees to 10 degrees of head extension followed by anterior translation of the head and, lastly, head and neck flexion. Again, all injuries occurred before there was consequential motion of the head.

When the impact was posterior, injury occurred with the padded condition in all three cases. However, none of the posterior impacts with the rigid surface produced injury. In both the padded and the rigid posterior impacts, these investigators observed a small amount of extension followed by anterior translation and flexion of the head and neck. The posterior impacts produced a component of velocity in the anterior direction relative to the impact surface, and, combined with the anteriorly-directed neck force, accelerated the head anteriorly. In the padded condition, however, the padding resisted the forward motion for a period of time sufficient enough for large forces to develop in the neck and for injury to occur.

In these experiments, injury occurred on average at 4.8 ms with rigid surfaces and at 18.3 ms with padded impacts. This does not allow sufficient time for reflex-mediated neck muscle forces to provide any protection to the head-neck complex. Furthermore, for the positions tested where the forces act primarily along the axis of the spine, the forces do not generate the bending moments necessary to cause elongation and energy absorption on the part of the muscles.

This well-controlled study also demonstrated differences in the axial neck impulses as a function of the impact angle. The posterior impact demonstrated the lowest impulse along the axis of the spine and is consistent with injury results. The data show a significantly greater frequency of injury with padded impacts than with rigid impacts. One message from this study clearly is that padded contact surfaces increase the likelihood of injury for a given impact condition, and, consequently, padded surfaces should be employed with caution in the sports environment.

This group also utilized a computational head-neck model to test the hypothesis that increases in friction between the head and the impact surface will increase injury risk.[1] The model results suggest that the most significant reductions in injury potential occur when coefficients of friction are decreased below 0.2. Clearly, this can be achieved experimentally, but reducing the coefficient of friction to such a low level in the real world remains a challenge.

With the increasing involvement of females in a variety of athletic activities, it is important to characterize the potential for injuries to the cervical spine with respect to gender in order to provide effective measures for prevention of injuries. Pintar and colleagues[7] used two statistical models to quantify the effect of age, gender, and loading rate on the force requirements necessary to produce failure in the cervical spine. They used human cadaveric head-neck specimens which included the second thoracic vertebra. The specimens were fixed inferiorly at T1–T2. The inferior portion was mounted to a load cell. Head posture was maintained using pulleys, and load was supplied to the crown of the head using the piston apparatus. Twenty-five specimens, 15 male and 10 female, ranging in age from 38 to 95 years, were tested. Axial load to failure was the measure chosen for cervical spine strength. The failure loads for the males were on average 600 N greater than those for the female specimens for all age groups and at all loading rates. The effect of loading rate was greater at the lower age groups. Age and loading rate were found to be interdependent variables. These results were consistent, with cervical spine strength between men and women being approximately the same when normalized to size. However, it should be appreciated that the force generated in the cervical spine during axial loading as a result of an impact at the crown of the head is more sensitive to velocity at impact and less affected by variations in torso mass.[3]

The structural response of the cervical spine under direct axial impact loading has been described by Yoganandan and coworkers.[13] Fresh adult human cadaver head-neck complexes that were isolated by transection at the T2–T3 intervertebral disk space were utilized. The distal ends of the specimens were potted and secured to a six-axis load cell and were rigidly attached to the platform of an electrohydraulic testing device via an x-y cross table. The experiments simulated cervical spine musculature through springs and static weights attached to a halo that was rigidly fixed to the skull. Dynamic loading was applied to the cranium at rates ranging from 5.3 m/s to 8.5 m/s. Peak dynamic forces ranging from 3300 N to 5600 N and compressive displacement ranging from 2.5 cm to 4.2 cm were recorded at the distal end of the preparation. The maximum acceleration at the C4 vertebral body ranged from 258 g to 526 g and was consistently less than that for the mastoid process, which ranged from 376 g to 546 g. It was evident from this study that the loads experienced by the more distal vertebral segments were less than those experienced by the proximal segments. Furthermore, the duration of loading was found to be longer in the more distal segment than in the proximal segments. The temporal localized kinematics of each vertebra along the length of the column were also documented. Documentation of the local kinematics allowed the observation that, despite the head-neck complex being subjected to external forces at a constant dynamic rate, the local kinematics of the spinal segments were quite different, even for adjacent segments. Such test results are invaluable to our understanding the biomechanics of cervical spine injury. Single segment testing, although providing useful data with respect to the segmental structural characteristics, do not allow inference of the behavior of the column during axial loading,

as do the cadaver-based studies of the head-neck complex reviewed in this section.

Anatomic Model–Impact Simulation

Cervical spine injuries resulting from an impact to the crown of the head occur over a very short duration of time, that is, between 5 ms and 20 ms. To better illustrate to the athletic community the phenomenon of the cervical spine being compressed between the torso and the head, Otis and co-workers reviewed the results of high-speed photography at 9000 frames per second to document the dynamics of a simulated spearing-type impact. To accomplish this, a plastic skeleton model of the head, neck, and torso was modified and swung on a double pendulum such that the crown of the head impacted a relatively stiff foam pad fixed to the wall (Figure 2–6). To the cranial and thoracic cavities of the skeleton were added 4.5-kg and 10-kg masses, respectively, resulting in a total mass of 29 kg for the model. The intervertebral disk spaces, interfaces of the skull and upper spine, the facet joint spaces, and the anterior and posterior longitudinal ligament locations were filled with silicone sealant. The head and cervical spine were maintained in a slightly flexed position (to remove the lordosis) until the sealant cured. During the test the head and neck orientation were maintained in align-

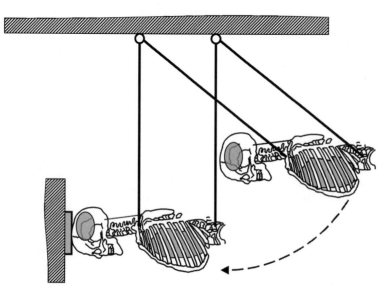

Figure 2–6. A plastic skeleton model of the head, neck, and torso was modified and swung on a double pendulum such that the crown of the head impacted a relatively stiff foam pad fixed to the wall. Masses of 4.5 kg and 10 kg, respectively, were added to the cranial and thoracic cavities of the skeleton, resulting in a total mass of 29 kg for the model.

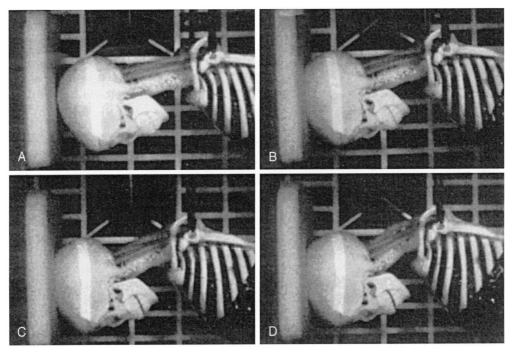

Figure 2–7. Selected frames from the high-speed photography demonstrate the greater forward displacement of the torso versus the head from the time of impact to the time of mechanical failure of the spine 22 ms later.

ment with the prone, horizontal torso by using stretched latex tubing to substitute for the neck extensor muscle forces. The speed at impact was approximately 3 m/s.

Selected frames from the high-speed photography (Figure 2–7) demonstrate the greater forward displacement of the torso versus the head from the time of impact to the time of mechanical failure of the spine 22 ms later. The failure was observed to occur locally at the midcervical spine as a result of buckling.

Analytic Model

The advantages of an analytic model to simulate the impact conditions include the following: the ability to explore the effects of varying parameters without requiring the time, effort, and expense of conducting experiments on cadaver specimens; the results of the simulation help to define experimental conditions for cadaver studies so that the greatest knowledge can be derived from more rigorous selection of cadaver experiments; and it allows insight into the interactions between the components of the system, that is, the helmet, head, neck, and torso.

The analytic model of Otis and colleagues[3] was used to simulate conditions resulting in axial loading of the cervical spine during football activities. Two- and three-degree of freedom models were developed to examine the effects of a helmeted player impacting a fixed object or being impacted by another player. The models were used to quantify the relative merits of different helmet designs with respect to their ability to absorb energy and lessen the force transmitted to the cervical spine, thereby quantifying the relative degree of neck protection. The model arose from the need to understand the roles that helmet suspension type, impact velocity, and body weight played in the production of these catastrophic injuries.

The components of the two degree of freedom model are the helmet, head, neck, and a portion of the trunk (Figure 2–8). The model assumes a motion along the horizontal, and that the helmet impacts a fixed, rigid barrier such that the reaction force of the impacted surface (which is equal and opposite to the helmet force) acts at the crown and is in line with a central axis through the cervical spine. The three degree of freedom model includes an additional mass to represent a portion of another moving player and allows

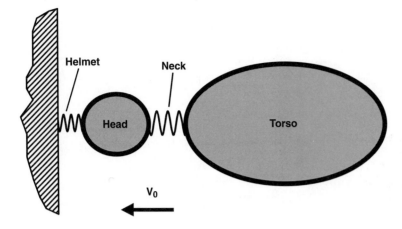

Figure 2–8. The two degree of freedom analytic model consisted of the trunk and head modeled as masses and the helmet and neck modeled as springs, all in series, with simulated impact into a fixed surface at an initial velocity v_0. The three degree of freedom model (not shown) replaces the fixed barrier with an additional mass.

the simulation of a two-player impact with one or both players moving.

The head mass was held constant, and the mass for the portion of the torso that was responsible for compressing the neck was varied. Full body mass of approximately 70 kg was not studied because it is unlikely that the full mass of the body would be aligned with the long axis of the cervical spine, and, furthermore, it was realized that the behavior of the model output was no different whether full or one-half body mass was employed. The helmet and cervical spine were modeled as massless, nonlinear springs. The spring properties of the helmet

were obtained for each helmet by placing them on a rigid headform and subjecting them to vertical loads at the crown of the helmet while recording the load versus displacement curves. Simulations were conducted to determine whether, for physically relevant parameters, the axial compressive force in the neck would develop to between 3340 N and 4450 N.

The results for a simulation with an impact velocity of 4.6 m/s (about one-half the maximum running speed for a conditioned athlete), a torso mass of 36 kg (about one-half body mass), and a Riddell PAC 3 football helmet are shown in Figure 2–9. The

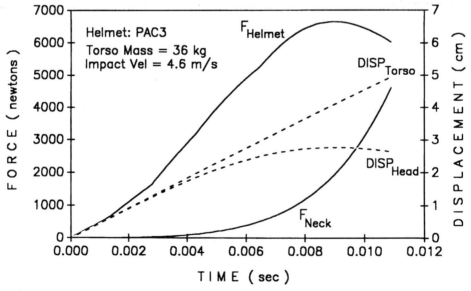

Figure 2–9. Force and displacement curves after impact with a fixed barrier demonstrate that the helmet force increased until a time at which the head rebounded. Torso displacement can be seen to continue at a nearly constant rate until the force limit was reached for the cervical spine. (From Otis JC, Burstein AH, Torg JS. Mechanisms and Pathomechanics of Athletic Injuries to the Cervical Spine. *In* Torg JS [ed]: Athletic Injuries to the Head, Neck, and Face. St. Louis, Mosby–Year Book, 1991, pp 438–456. Used with permission.)

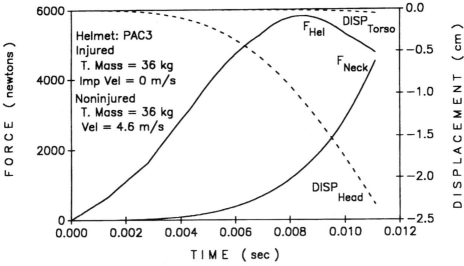

Figure 2–10. The force and displacement curves for a stationary injured player resulting from an impact by a moving opponent illustrate the rapid increase in force at the helmet as it is pushed toward the body of the injured player and the resulting head displacement against a nearly fixed torso, which results in an increase in neck force until failure occurs. (From Otis JC, Burstein AH, Torg JS. Mechanisms and Pathomechanics of Athletic Injuries to the Cervical Spine. *In* Torg JS [ed]: Athletic Injuries to the Head, Neck, and Face. St. Louis, Mosby–Year Book, 1991, pp 438–456. Used with permission.)

outputs of the simulated impact demonstrate a central point regarding the dynamics of this system, that is, the neck force achieves its upper limit of 4450 N in less than 11 ms. Moreover, at the time the failure load is achieved, neck force is observed to be increasing at an increasing rate, exhibiting the potential for injury even if neck strength were greater.

Note that although the helmet force peaks prior to 9 ms and then decreases, the neck force continues to increase. At first glance this may seem inconsistent; however, this force, which is compressing the helmet liner system, decreases as a result of the head rebounding. This reversal of velocity results in the head moving toward the torso to further add to the axial compression of the neck. This is evident when viewing the displacement curve for the head. It can be seen that head displacement reaches its peak at about 9 ms and reverses direction. The torso mass, on the other hand, displaces in a linear fashion and appears to be unaffected by the axial force that has been generated in the cervical spine at this time. The difference between the displacement curve for the torso and that for the head reflects the amount of compression of the cervical spine. It is apparent that this difference is minimal at 6 ms; however, between 6 ms

and 10 ms the cervical spine was quickly pushed to its limit as it rapidly compressed.

Utilizing the three degree of freedom model, the effect of a moving opponent impacting the crown of the helmet of the injured player was examined. In this simulation, the injured player wore the same helmet and had the same effective body mass as in the prior simulation; however, the injured player had a zero velocity, that is, he was stationary, as if in position at the line. The opposing player was modeled as a 36-kg mass traveling at a velocity of 4.6 m/s at the time of impact. As in the prior simulation, the neck failed at approximately 11 ms, and the force in the helmet peaked at around 9 ms (Fig. 2–10). The differences in the dynamics are apparent when considering the displacement curves for the head and torso of the injured player. As a result of the impact, the head is displaced in the direction of the torso approximately 2.5 cm. The torso displacement, on the other hand, is negligible, as its inertia resists any significant displacement within the first 10 ms. Thus, from the standpoint of the cervical spine, these two impact situations are essentially no different.

The effects of varying impact velocity and also of varying the portion of torso mass aligned with the neck were studied. Impact velocities of 2.3, 4.6, and 6.1 m/s, which encompass fast walking to about two thirds of maximum running speed, were compared while maintaining a torso mass of 36 kg and the PAC 3 helmet properties. It is evident in Figure 2–11 that the cervical spine reached failure load at each of the three velocities. The time at which the failure loads were reached, however, differed considerably. At 2.3 m/s it took twice as long for failure to occur as it did at 6.1 m/s. When the torso mass was varied using 36, 18, and 9 kg, the force-time histories for the neck were no different. These were conducted at the 4.6 m/s velocity and also utilized the properties of the PAC 3 helmet. The greater sensitivity when varying velocity, as compared with varying torso mass, clearly demonstrates the role of kinetic energy, which is proportional to velocity raised to the second power but to mass raised only to the first power.

The importance of energy is appreciated from Figure 2–12, which illustrates the kinetic energy of the two masses, the torso and the head, and also illustrates the amounts of energy absorbed by the helmet suspension and by the neck following impact. This is shown with an effective torso mass of 36 kg and impact velocity of 4.6 m/s. Note that prior to impact, all the energy is kinetic energy. Following impact, the kinetic energy of the head decreases as its energy is transferred to the helmet and stored as potential energy in the nonlinear spring properties of the liner as it is compressed. When the helmet reaches its energy absorbing limit, energy is then transferred to the neck. At that time, the neck force becomes significant enough to produce a noticeable slowing of the torso mass, and the torso energy is seen to decrease. It can be appreciated in Figure 2–12 that the amount of energy absorbed by the neck is minimal, and that only a small fraction of the torso energy is lost at the time of neck failure. The ability of the neck to absorb energy for the velocity and mass conditions used is essentially negligible compared with the available energy involved in impacts of the type studied.

It becomes apparent that the cervical spine was not designed to deal with the type of external loads that produce these injuries. During walking and running activities, the axial loads experienced by the neck as a result of inertial loading are due to the mass of the head as the external loads are applied to the lower extremities. Thus, building up neck strength through conditioning will not contribute to preventing these compression injuries. In other loading modes, that is,

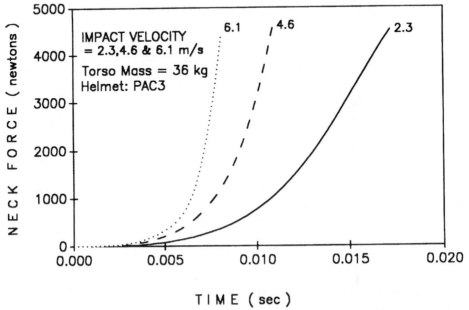

Figure 2–11. The neck force histories are illustrated for variations in impact velocity from 2.3 m/s to 6.1 m/s with a constant torso mass of 36 kg. (From Otis JC, Burstein AH, Torg JS. Mechanisms and Pathomechanics of Athletic Injuries to the Cervical Spine. *In* Torg JS [ed]: Athletic Injuries to the Head, Neck, and Face. St. Louis, Mosby–Year Book, 1991, pp 438–456. Used with permission.)

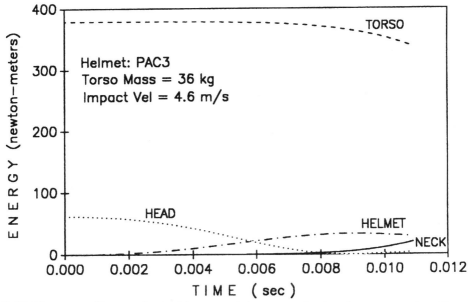

Figure 2–12. The curves illustrate the initial energy of the moving head and torso. Immediately after impact, kinetic energy of the head is first transferred to the helmet, which bottoms out, and, subsequently, the kinetic energy of the torso is transferred to the neck. Failure of the neck occurs with nearly all of the kinetic energy of the torso remaining. (From Otis JC, Burstein AH, Torg JS. Mechanisms and Pathomechanics of Athletic Injuries to the Cervical Spine. *In* Torg JS [ed]: Athletic Injuries to the Head, Neck, and Face. St. Louis, Mosby–Year Book, 1991, pp 438–456. Used with permission.)

flexion, extension, lateral bending, and axial rotation, the neck is capable of absorbing energy through elongation of its musculature. Enhancing the capacity of the neck musculature to absorb energy is beneficial under these loading conditions, which comprise the majority of the loads experienced by the neck during football and other contact sports.

METHODS OF NECK PROTECTION

Protection of the neck is indeed a challenging task. Clearly, since the 1970s the best approach to reducing catastrophic injury to the cervical spine has been through education. Otis and Burstein[2] reviewed some attempts at devices that will protect the neck during football. They also proposed a method for evaluating neck protection equipment. The motivation for the proposal arose from the pending development of two neck protection systems. One was an air bag collar that incorporated the technology used in automotive air bag systems, and the second was a double helmet system that was designed to transmit helmet loads over the

chest and back, while avoiding loads to the head and neck and also bypassing the shoulder. These authors cited the diversity between the two types of protective devices and the need for a method of equipment evaluation that can be applied to a spectrum of systems. They proposed the use of analytic screening methods that would determine whether a protection system meets basic, broadband requirements; avoids the need and cost of developing a spectrum of physical testing capabilities; and allows the protection system to be evaluated under simulated dynamic conditions.

The application of the analytic model as a method for screening was discussed, and an application of the model as an initial screening device for the air bag collar system was presented. The feasibility of using an air bag at the base of the helmet to transfer loads to the shoulders was examined using a modification of the analytic model. The parameters of the air bags, which can be varied in order to determine a possible solution, are (1) the time after impact at which the air bag was deployed, and (2) the amount of force the air bag generates. For the simulation, it was assumed that the bag would generate its maximum force instanta-

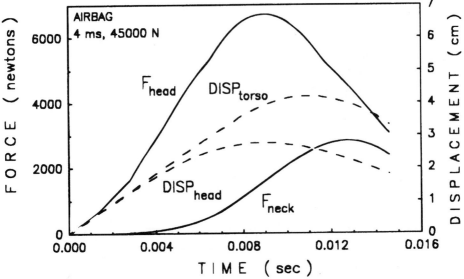

Figure 2–13. With a deployment delay time of 4 ms and the collar air bag maintained at 45,000 N, the simulation produces no fractured cervical spine. (From Otis JC, Burstein AH. A Proposed Method for Evaluating Neck Protection Equipment. *In* Hoerner EF [ed]: Safety in American Football. Vol. STP 1305, American Society for Testing and Materials, 1997, pp 75–82. Used with permission.)

neously at the time of deployment and maintain that force. The dynamics of the interaction with the head, neck, and torso are illustrated in Figure 2–13. After several iterations of varying the two parameters, it was determined that in order to prevent the neck force from exceeding its failure limits, it was necessary to deploy the air bag within 4 ms of the initial impact and to generate a force of 45,000 N with the air bag collar. With these values the torso displacement is observed to be retarded at about 8 ms and actually reverses direction at about 10 ms. The force in the neck reaches its peak at 12 ms, when the velocity of the torso in the reverse direction becomes greater than the rebounding velocity of the head such that the neck is being allowed to lengthen. The parameter values of 4 ms and 45,000 N were not attainable with the available technology at the time the simulation was conducted. If the technology were to become available, it would be necessary to devise a means by which the force of the collar on the shoulders and upper body can be assessed with respect to injury potential. In addition, it would be necessary to assess the potential for injury to the player impacted by the helmet when the air bag collar is activated. It is important to keep in mind that the analytical model is a first order of approximation that considers only the axial loading

mechanism, which is responsible for the most catastrophic injuries. Clearly there is a need for assessing and developing a system for reducing the risk of neck injuries in those cases that do not involve the spinal cord but that are more frequent, costly, and debilitating to the athlete. The evolution of standard guidelines for neck protection devices would be welcomed by the majority of those involved in the sport and those in the business of supplying football equipment. Manufacturers of such devices would welcome guidelines that would ensure some level of protection and help to clarify issues of liability when injuries occur.

CERVICAL SPINE INJURIES DURING OTHER ATHLETIC ACTIVITIES

With the exception of some discussion of injuries in hockey, the discussion of cervical spine injuries in sports has been largely with respect to football because of the greater frequency of these injuries in that sport, which has resulted in greater documentation and analysis. The mechanism of catastrophic cervical spine injury is often the same for other athletic activities, that is, the inertia of the torso applies load to the cervical spine after the head stops. Injuries during diving are a result of an impact of the head with the pool bottom or, when in bodies of fresh water, with the sandy or muddy base. The sand or dirt can have the same effect as a padded surface where the head, as it indents the sand, is held in position, unable to move out of the way of the torso mass as it continues toward the head and compresses the cervical spine. On the other hand, during activities such as gymnastics, catastrophic spine injuries occur under dynamically more complex conditions because they often involve a greater element of body rotation in conjunction with impacting the head.

References

1. Camacho DLA, Nightingale RW, Meyers BS. Surface friction in near-vertex head and neck impact increases risk of injury. J Biomech 1999;32:293–301.
1a. Carter DR, Frankel VH. Biomechanics of hyperextension injuries to the cervical spine in football. Am J Sports Med 8:302–309, 1980.
2. Otis JC, Burstein AH. A Proposed Method for Evaluating Neck Protection Equipment. In Hoerner EF (ed): Safety in American Football. Vol. STP 1305, American Society for Testing and Materials, 1997, pp 75–82.
3. Otis JC, Burstein AH, Torg JS. Mechanisms and Pathomechanics of Athletic Injuries to the Cervical Spine. In Torg JS (ed): Athletic Injuries to the Head, Neck, and Face. St. Louis, Mosby–Year Book, 1991, pp 438–456.
4. Nightingale RW, McElhaney JH, Richardson WJ, et al. Experimental impact injury to the cervical spine: Relating motion of the head and the mechanism of injury. J Bone Joint Surg 1996;78-A:412–421.
5. Nightingale RW, McElhaney JH, Richardson WJ, Meyers BS. Dynamic responses of the head and cervical spine to axial impact loading. J Biomech 1996;29:307–318.
6. Nightingale RW, Richardson WJ, Meyers BS. The effects of padded surfaces on the risk for cervical spine injury. Spine 1997;22:2380–2387.
7. Pintar FA, Yoganandan N, Voo L. Effect of age and loading rate on human cervical spine injury threshold. Spine 1998;23:1957–1962.
8. Tator CH, Carson JD, Edmonds VE. Spinal injuries in ice hockey. Clin Sports Med 1998;17:183–194.
9. Torg JS, Truex RC Jr, Marshall J, et al. Spinal injury at the level of the third and fourth cervical vertebrae from football. J Bone Joint Surg 1977;59-A:1015–1019.
10. Torg JS, Vegso JJ, Sennett B, Das M. The National Football Head and Neck Injury Registry: 14-year report on cervical quadriplegia, 1971–1984. JAMA 1985;254:3439–3443.
11. Virgin H. Cineradiographic study of football helmets and the cervical spine. Am J Sports Med 1980;8:310.
12. Yoganandan N, Pintar FA. Inertial loading of the human cervical spine. J Biomech Eng 1997;119:237–240.
13. Yoganandan N, Pintar FA, Sances A Jr, et al. Strength and kinematic response of dynamic cervical spine injuries. Spine 1991;16:S511–S517.

3

The Epidemiology of Athletic Head Injuries

Kenneth S. Clarke

SYNOPSIS

Although more common in collision sports, head injuries (for this chapter confined to cerebral neurotrauma) may occur in virtually any form of athletics. A few such injuries lead to death, especially the second impact syndrome and subdural hematoma. The so-called more minor cerebral injuries, concussions, are subject to widespread misunderstanding in definition and severity. These misunderstandings in the field have contributed to a paucity of reliable epidemiologic information about their actual frequency. The concerns accompanying cerebral insult are more discussed than studied, but much can be gained in principle from the history of attentions to concussions in football.

INTRODUCTION

The Nature of Epidemiology Attentions

Epidemiology characterizes the frequency of a given disease in a population, and athletic injury can be tracked epidemiologically as one does a disease. However, one needs to compare the discovered frequency with something else (e.g., the previous year, or another sport, or a different age group) to evaluate it. However, there may be fewer or more athletes at risk in the comparison group. As a result, rates of relative frequency are employed.

For example, the population size must be known or estimated to rationally depict the number of persons who could have experienced the disease or injury during the study period. For comparisons then, whether one

season to another or one sport to another, one must convert that frequency to rates that characterize the relative frequency of that occurrence in a standardized population, for example, 3 injuries per 100 athletes.

Rates can be made more sensitive if one can introduce an index of exposure as well, for example, 14 injuries per 1000 athlete-days (the number of athletes multiplied by the number of days in which the athletes participated that season, whether by practice or games).

Further, it is necessary for the sports practitioner to appreciate the difference between two basic kinds of rates used for different purposes. Incidence is the rate of new cases occurring in the study period (typically the annual season). Prevalence, on the other hand, is the rate of cases present (typically midpoint) during the study period. The annual incidence of permanent nonfatal brain damage, for example, has value for those with injury control responsibilities, whereas the value in knowing the annual prevalence of these cases is in the attentions to their medical and economic management.

Proportionate Data/Internal Patterns

The vast bulk of sports injury data available for review and use apply a different definition of relative frequency—that for internal patterns. These data essentially constitute percentages of frequencies within the total injuries experienced. They can be very strategic but should not be confused with rates. For example, 10% of youth baseball injuries may occur to batters, but one would need to include the population at risk to know, for example, whether this meant 50 of every 1000 players or .5 of every 1000 players were being injured as a batter. The value of proportionate data is finding the targets of attention that would reduce the relative frequency of injuries in that sport and population.

Decision Making in Sport

Any attempt to reduce the complexities of valid and reliable reporting of injuries in sport to meet the demands of epidemiologic surveillance of athletic injuries has many hurdles to overcome,[4] but when overcome, it reasonably provides knowledge for the decision makers in sport, where voids are filled with opinion.[5] As a result, most professional sharings on athletic injuries have concerned their clinical nature and significance according to the author's experience, often accompanied by case study data along with the author's resulting recommendations concerning the management and/or prevention of such injuries. This has served well for two needed outcomes on behalf of the participant in the communities across the United States: (1) more consistently implemented injury control measures of acceptable nature, and (2) more consistently available medical expertise on the immediate and long-term management of the injury that occurs.

Should experts disagree on matters of significance in this regard, however, few will find reasonably sound epidemiologic data for reference, unless the issue concerns catastrophic neurotrauma in football.

FOOTBALL FATALITIES

The Football Helmet Controversy

In 1962 the American Medical Association (AMA)'s newly established Committee on Medical Aspects of Sports hosted the National Conference on Head Protection for Athletes, which convened authorities of that era in what was emerging as sports medicine to discuss current issues within this concern.[13] Football was the focus, and the efficacy of the recent changes in the football helmet and the advent of the football facemask concerning catastrophic injury became the issue. "Catastrophic injury" meant neurotrauma.

Prompting the conference was the realization of a significant upward trend of head/neck deaths since the mid-1950s. In 1931 the annual Football Fatality Report was initiated under the aegis of the American Football Coaches Association with the endorsement of the organizations responsible for interscholastic and intercollegiate football.[14] This forerunner of today's efforts to track epidemiologically all catastrophic injuries in sport ironically was what led to the first nationally organized sports medicine action on a safety issue within sports. It was during the 1950s when football began adopting the new hard-shelled helmets being produced and then adding the new facemasks. By 1962 use of the new helmets was being shown as having resulted in an ever-increasing incidence of catastrophic injury among those at risk.

It is perhaps ironic that this initial major sports medicine conference demonstrated the functional value of ongoing epidemiology of significant injuries in sport. This was especially good for sports at that time. Sports had escaped scrutiny as to what was considered acceptable endemic rates of injury, and little research-worthy data accompanied any declaration of cause and solution of a problem that had been shared among the administrators and professional practitioners involved. Unfortunately, except for football and a few isolated registries for catastrophic injury, sport continues to escape epidemiologic attentions to cerebral injury.

The Applicability of Epidemiology to Sports Injury Issues

Epidemiology emerged from public health interests as the tool for learning the incidence of a given disease in a population and, for preventive efforts, the factors associated with that incidence. Incidence is the frequency of occurrence in a known population expressed as a rate, for example, 10 cases per 100,000 persons who could have experienced such an occurrence. Epidemiology, however, cannot be left to mere relative frequencies. Of concern are the factors associated with that frequency or with a change in that frequency (internal patterns of associated factors). Basic to applied epidemiology, therefore, is a universally understood definition of what is to be reported should it occur, a repository for receiving reported occurrences, and a reasonable estimate of the number of persons at risk (i.e., to whom it could have occurred).

What had been lacking in sport as well as society was the consideration of injury as a disease having the same host, cause, and environment trilogy of relationships that helped epidemiology characterize the infectious diseases in the early 20th century. Those with access to sports injury data often attempt to characterize such factors but must rely on the availability of information that is obtained with reasonable reliability. The United States Consumer Product Safety Commission (CPSC), for example, can project that head injuries constitute about 30% of all consumer-product related hospital emergency room visits, that about 15% of these head injuries were concussions or fractures (unfortunately including the cheek or nose), and that the overall hospitalization rate of a head injury is about 3%.[7] Although it did not provide a percentage that came from sport, the incidence (with the general population as a whole considered at risk) for respective sports showed the top five being basketball (258 per 100,000), bicycles (233 per 100,000), baseball (174 per 100,000), football (167 per 100,000), and playground equipment (102 per 100,000). Identification of the activity along with the person's age and sex constituted the accompanying factors that the CPSC was able to obtain.

It should be added, however, that if one looks at cerebral insult, invariably, including that provided by the CPSC above, the incidence is highest for those age 5 and younger.[7, 11]

It should be further added that this author purposely ignored discussion of brain injuries in boxing, principally because of the absence of epidemiologic studies that characterize by definition and reliable reporting the gradual onset of chronic brain damage from repeated blows.

Epidemiology must also concern itself with awareness and education. One would think, for example, that football and concussions would be a combined source of concern among parents of young football players. However, one study[10] has shown that only 7.7% of a set of parents studied in this regard mentioned concussions in free association with the injury concerns in that sport. Prompted, 83% agreed, yet only about a third were aware of the warning label about head and neck injuries that has been on helmets since the late 1970s.

Many more considerations are fundamental to the helpful use of epidemiology, including when applicable if the population being followed is only a sample of all who are at risk. The scenario of the 1962 AMA conference, however, enjoyed the basics from a natural perspective (even though it is most doubtful that epidemiology was even mentioned at the time). Conference participants were aware of the estimated combined number of high school and college football players at risk (681,690 in that era), that this was a national estimate (not a sampling), and that the incidence of head/neck fatalities had risen consistently from .73 per 100,000 in 1951 to 2.35 per 100,000 in 1961 (Table 3–1). The principal accompanying factor of change over that period was accepted as being the advent of the new hard-shelled helmet with facemask in the conduct of organized football. With relatively small actual numbers of annual occurrences being the case nationally in football (30 was the worst), fluctuations were apt to occur occasionally thanks to Murphy's Law; it was the year-to-year consistency in trends that must be examined.

Significance of the 1962 AMA Conference

The findings of the 1962 conference[6, 13] have been relived many times since then, in other sports[1, 3, 8] as well as in football— namely (1) that the advent of protective equipment requires performance standards that define that protective equipment for acceptability in use, and (2) that the advent of effective protective equipment can and will change the behavior of the protected athlete to create new targets of risk. In explanation:

The 1962 conferees agreed that the new protective head gear was necessary for the protection of the player, but that coaching and officiating attentions were needed to curb the players' tendency to consider themselves invulnerable to injury because of that protection and thus to lead with the helmet in creating contact with their opponents.

Table 3–1. College and High School Football Fatalities (Direct Only)

Year	Total	Rate*	Head Only	Rate* Head	% Head
1997	5	0.32	5	0.32	100
96	5	0.32	4	0.25	80
95	4	0.25	4	0.25	100
94	1	0.06	1	0.06	100
93	4	0.25	3	0.19	75
92	2	0.13	2	0.13	100
91	3	0.19	3	0.19	100
90	0	0.21	0	0.17	0
89	4	0.25	4	0.25	100
88	7	0.51	4	0.25	67
87	4	0.29	2	0.15	50
86	11	0.80	9	0.65	75
85	6	0.44	5	0.36	83
84	5	0.36	5	0.36	100
83	4	0.29	4	0.29	100
82	7	0.51	6	0.44	86
81	7	0.51	6	0.44	86
80	9	0.65	7	0.51	78
79	4	0.29	3	0.22	75
78	9	0.65	4	0.29	44
77	9	0.65	3	0.22	33
76	15	1.09	12	0.87	80
75	14	1.10	12	0.94	86
74	11	0.86	9	0.71	82
73	7	0.55	6	0.47	86
72	18	1.41	12	0.94	67
71	18	1.41	11	0.87	61
70	26	2.04	15	1.18	58
69	19	1.62	15	1.28	79
68	30	2.79	24	2.23	80
67	19	1.77	12	1.12	63
66	20	1.86	14	1.30	70
65	21	1.95	15	1.40	71
64	24	3.52	18	2.64	75
63	13	1.91	10	1.47	77
62	12	1.76	10	1.47	83
61	16	2.35	9	1.32	56
60	12	1.76	11	1.61	92
59	10	1.47	5	0.73	50
58	11	1.61	7	1.03	64
57	14	2.05	9	1.32	64
56	13	1.91	9	1.32	69
55	7	1.03	5	0.73	71
54	14	2.05	9	1.32	64
53	8	1.17	6	0.88	75
52	5	0.73	3	0.44	60
51	7	1.02	4	0.59	57
50	12	1.76	7	1.03	58

*Per 100,000 football players.

From: Annual Surveys of Football Fatalities: The American Football Coaches Association, The National Collegiate Athletic Association, and the National Federation of State High School Athletic Associations. (See Refs. 14 and 15.)

"Spearing" was labeled as the deliberate ramming of the helmet into the opponent, and allegations that it was done for the purpose of hurting that player as well as gaining a blocking or tackling advantage began to take root.

As the 1960s continued, sports medicine/safety speakers' warnings against spearing became prevalent at football coaches' meetings and the ever-increasing sports medicine conferences around the country. Yet, few if any coaches were teaching spearing, helmets were still being produced according to the theories of the competing manufacturers' engineers without the advantage of reference performance standards, and the incidence of head/neck fatalities continued to be high (compared with the past), rising to 3.52 per 100,000 in 1964 and still at 2.79 per 100,000 in 1968 (see Table 1) as the manufacturers tried to respond individually to the acknowledged need for a better protective design.

The Arrival of NOCSAE Standards

It was at this time that the football helmet manufacturers, school/college administrators, and researchers agreed to arrive at consensus standards for protective head gear. It took several years for the manufacturers to determine (1) that the ASTI Z–90 standard for motorcycle helmets was inadequate because it relied on a single-impact test, whereas the football helmet had to withstand multiple impacts every day of contact; (2) that the ASTM system for establishing consensus standards would be too time-consuming to rely upon for the earliest possible resolution of this problem; and (3) that they would organize a nonprofit organization, The National Operating Committee for Safety in Athletic Equipment (NOCSAE), including many members with American Society for Testing and Materials (ASTM) experience, for equivalent purposes. The manufacturers then contracted with Wayne State University for the research that would yield valid and reliable performance tests and the basis for consensus standards as to a threshold for acceptability of any football helmet of any engineering design.

The final results of this research were not available until 1973, but, interestingly, a decline in the incidence of head/neck fatalities in football had begun, presumably as a result of the renewed examination by the helmet manufacturers of the effectiveness of their particular engineering qualities and the anticipated nature of the forthcoming reference standards. The 1970 season was the last with a fatality rate above 2.0 per 100,000 (see Table 3–1). During the 1973–74 school year, high schools and colleges adopted NOCSAE standards as required of all football helmets to be worn after a given grace period (differing between high schools and colleges owing to the economics of helmet turnover), and also continued the antispearing warning but adding the necessity to fit the helmet to the player and to follow a course of helmet maintenance to preserve protective qualities. By 1976 the incidence had declined to and plateaued at about 1.1 per 100,000. By this juncture in the history of football epidemiology, refinements in attention had matured.

REFINEMENTS IN THE EPIDEMIOLOGY OF SPORTS NEUROTRAUMA

Separating the Head from Head/Neck

It was not until the mid-1970s that the tradition of considering football catastrophic injuries as head/neck was realized as disguising the respective and differing epidemiological patterns of catastrophic head and neck injuries. In 1966 Schneider, who was an active conferee in 1962, published his national survey of neurosurgeons as to the frequency and nature of football-related neurotrauma in their practice in 1959 through 1963.[16] With a 61% response rate but a tabular display style that did not warn readers that the same case could appear in several tables, the study was not as epidemiologically sound as intended. However, it reflected well the dominance of serious cerebral injuries over spinal cord injuries in frequency of occurrence in those years and the significance of concussions and subdural hemorrhaging in football. In 1968 the AMA published a booklet, *Standard Nomenclature of Athletic Injuries,*[17] with Schneider as a member of the subcommittee that produced it, that gave needed credence to the concept that a concussion need not be a knockout to be diagnosed a concussion and thereby a possible precursor to the life-threatening subdural hematoma.

The annual football fatality data were thus reworked to distinguish epidemiologically the head-related death from the neck-related death (Fig. 3–1). The incidence of head-related deaths for the years discussed previously as head/neck deaths was found to account for 2.64 per 100,000 in 1964; 2.23 per 100,000 in 1968; and 1.18 per 100,000 in 1970 (Table 3–1). Between 1955 and 1970, only one year, 1959, had an incidence of head deaths below 1 per 100,000.

The spike in incidence of football deaths over the 1960s was thus due essentially only to head deaths. As discussed in Chapter 4, neck deaths did not increase in the same

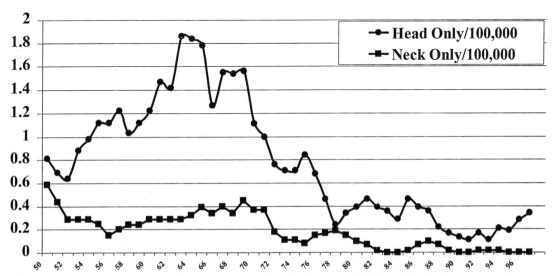

Figure 3–1. Head and Neck Fatalities in High School and College Football (Smoothed). Source: Annual Surveys of Football Fatalities: The American Football Coaches Association, The National Collegiate Athletic Association, and the National Federation of State High School Athletic Association. (See Refs. 14 and 15.)

manner, which both removed the helmet from direct relevance to the incidence of neck deaths and re-emphasized the relevance of attentions to the helmet in efforts to lower the incidence of serious cerebral neurotrauma.

The renewed emphasis on the helmet was further strengthened by the enacting of rules at both the high school and college levels in 1976 clarifying that *any* initial and intentional impact of the helmeted head when tackling or blocking (i.e., "butt blocking" and "face tackling" as well as spearing) was now illegal and therefore could not be taught. With less exposure to the helmeted head being the brunt of the initial impact of a hit, along with the continued use of helmets meeting NOCSAE standards, the incidence of head-related fatalities again dropped, now to a consistent level of .20 or so per 100,000 in and since 1977, exceeding .50 per 100,000 only twice through 1997 (see Table 3–1, Fig. 3–1).

Note: The year-to-year fluctuation in small number frequencies, mentioned earlier, is often softened for the sake of reviewing trends by the practice of smoothing the rates of interest. That is, the annual incidence of occurrence for a given year is derived by utilizing that year's data plus that for the year before and the year after. The result is a more easily observable trending of the occurrence of interest. Figure 3–1 was prepared in this way.

The Nonfatal Head-Related Catastrophic Injury (Football)

It was not until the late 1970s that the efforts of Torg to track quadriplegic injuries in football and of Mueller and Cantu[14, 15] to track football fatalities led to an organized approach to tracking nonfatal cerebral neurotrauma of permanently severe nature. Since 1986, two years after the beginnings of reported data, the trend line has been essentially flat, averaging about .3 per 100,000 for the incidence of permanent but nonfatal cerebral injury (Table 3–2 and Fig. 3–2).

Fatal and Nonfatal Head-Related Catastrophic Injury (Other High School and College Sports)

Table 3–3 was prepared from personal communications with Mueller concerning the summary data contained within the annual report from the National Center for Catastrophic Sports Injury Research.[15] What was thereby provided for perspective via this table was the incidence of head-related cases for each sport, presented in common manner epidemiologically for each in comparison with that known for football.

In Table 3–3, utilizing the terminologies and definitions of the source, "non-fatal cat-

Table 3–2. High School and College Football Cerebral Injuries (Permanent)

Year	High School Total*	High School Rate†/ 100,000	College Total†	College Rate†/ 100,000	Combined Total	Combined Rate/ 100,000
1997	7	0.47	1	1.33	8	0.51
96	5	0.33	0	0.00	5	0.32
95	2	0.13	0	0.00	2	0.13
94	4	0.27	1	1.33	5	0.32
93	5	0.33	0	0.00	5	0.32
92	4	0.27	0	0.00	4	0.25
91	3	0.20	1	1.33	4	0.25
90	2	0.13	0	0.00	2	0.13
89	6	0.40	0	0.00	6	0.38
88	4	0.31	0	0.00	4	0.29
87	2	0.15	0	0.00	2	0.15
86	2	0.15	0	0.00	2	0.15
85	4	0.31	1	1.33	5	0.36
84	5	0.38	2	2.67	7	0.51

*Obtained from the National Center for Catastrophic Sports Injury Research.
†Population size of high school and college football teams obtained from the American Football Coaches Association Annual Surveys of Football Fatalities.

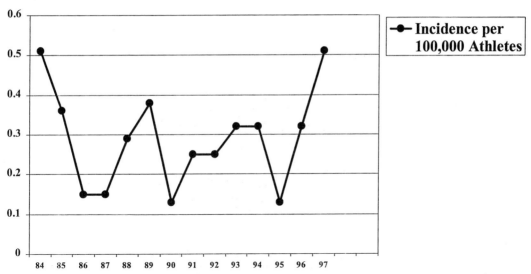

Figure 3–2. Nonfatal Cerebral Injuries in High School and College Football (Permanent). Source: The National Center for Catastrophic Sports Injury Research. (See Refs. 14 and 15.)

astrophic" (i.e., permanent brain damage) and "serious" (e.g., severe but not permanently disabling) were combined as companion totals to "fatal." It must be remembered that these data concern only organized interscholastic and intercollegiate sport, with the advantage being a reasonably known number of players at risk. It is clear from the data that the relatively small numbers of participants at the college level nationally can produce a sizeable jump in incidence from the experience of each occurrence.

Concussions

The vagaries of defining, observing, and reporting the concussion in football (as well as in any other activity of life) have stifled use of epidemiologic principles in learning the incidence of concussions. One 3-year study immediately after the adoption of NOCSAE standards, utilizing the definitions advocated by the AMA[17] plus the time-loss criterion of the National Athletic Injury/Illness Reporting System,[4] found an annual incidence of 5.4–6.2 per 100 players for all reported concussions and 0.6–0.7 per 100 players for "significant" concussions, "significant" being those keeping the athlete out of participation for at least one week.[5] Designed to examine the factor of the brand and type of helmet worn in that era (early NOCSAE), each of the 12 helmets being

worn with any frequency among the study group was associated with the same incidence of "significant concussion," that is, .1 per 1000 athlete exposures (one athlete exposure being a practice or game in which the athlete participated and thereby had an opportunity to be so injured while wearing that helmet). The rate for "reportable game-related concussions" (causing the player to be evaluated, whether returned to play or not), fluctuated from 3 to 7 occurrences per 1000 athlete-exposures, but such fluctuation was much tightened to 5.0–5.7 per 1000 athlete-exposures among the helmets in common use.

From the same database, limited to college football and extended for a total of 8 years, the factor of player and team activity accompanying concussion was studied in a multivariate manner.[2] Predominantly effected were those offensive and defensive players involved in a block on a rushing play.

Concussions as Precursors to Catastrophic Cerebral Neurotrauma

Of critical concern is now the frequency and nature of concussions that precede the onset of intracranial hemorrhaging and fatal or nonfatal brain damage.[12] Anecdotally, it is accepted that the vast majority if not all of the head-related fatalities in football did not arise initially from a blow on that given

Table 3–3. Head-Related Catastrophic Injuries in High School and College Sports, 1982–1995*

Sport	Fatalities	Nonfatalities	Total Cases/ Year	Annual Cases/ 100,000 Athletes
Football				
High School	43	56	7.6	0.88
College	5	6	0.8	2.25

Sport	Fatalities	Nonfatalities & Serious Injuries	Total Cases/ Year	Annual Cases/ 100,000 Athletes
Baseball				
High School	4	1	1.2	0.21
College	1	1	0.2	0.74
Basketball				
High School	0	1	0.1	0.17
College	0	1	0.1	0.56
Cheerleading				
High School	1	6	0.5	Unk
College	1	5	0.5	Unk
Cross Country				
High School & College	0	0	0.0	0.00
Gymnastics				
High School	1	0	0.1	0.43
College	0	0	0.0	0.00
Hockey (Ice)				
High School	0	1	0.1	0.34
College	0	1	0.1	1.95
Lacrosse				
High School & College	0	0	0.0	0.00
Skiing				
High School	0	0	0.0	0.00
College	1	0	0.2	15.11
Soccer				
High School	2	4	0.5	0.14
College	0	0	0.0	0.00
Softball				
High School	0	1	0.1	0.03
College	0	0	0.0	0.00
Swimming				
High School	0	1	0.1	0.10
College	0	0	0.0	0.00
Tennis				
High School & College	0	0	0.0	0.00
Track & Field				
High School	10	14	1.8	0.38
College	2	2	0.3	0.92
Wrestling				
High School & College	0	0	0.0	0.00

*Adapted from Mueller F, Cantu R. 13th Annual Report (Fall 1982–Spring 1995), National Center for Catastrophic Sports Injury Research, Chapel Hill, NC, 1996.

day, but from an exacerbation of an earlier concussive blow that had not healed. Since at least the mid-1970s, educational efforts have been made to encourage those who evaluate athletes with concussions to utilize methods of eliciting signs of intracranial bleeding or disruption before authorizing a return to play, as well as to encourage the athletes to disclose symptoms of such bleeding, for examples, headaches, dizziness, confusion, or nausea. Although the frequency of nonfatal cerebral neurotrauma of significance is as low as that for fatal cerebral neurotrauma, both can be effected by more reliable eliciting of both signs and symptoms of continued need for cerebral healing.

CONCLUSION

The incidence and patterns of cerebral injuries in sports is not well documented beyond the annual reporting of fatal and permanent nonfatal cerebral neurotrauma in football. Medical and on-field management of such injuries relies on existing standards for protective helmets, teaching of skills that minimize direct head impact even in contact sport, enforcement of relevant rules to minimize head injury mechanisms in the sport, and practical evaluation of even the so-called minor concussion. The advantages of following the incidence and patterns of cerebral neurotrauma of whatever nature, however, justify the commitment that one would have to bring to such opportunities so that the effects of various preventive interventions can be tracked as well as the occurrences themselves.

References

1. Biasca N, Simmen H, Bartolozzi, et al. Review of typical ice hockey injuries—Survey of the North American NHL and Hockey Canada versus European leagues. Unfallchirurg 1995;98:283–288.
2. Buckley W. Concussions in college football. Am J Sports Med 1988;16:51–56.
3. Chitnavis J, Gibbons C, Hirigoyen M, et al. Accidents with horses: What has changed in 20 years? Injury 1996;27:103–105.
4. Clarke K. Premises and pitfalls of athletic injury surveillance. J Sports Med 1975;3:292–295.
5. Clarke K, Powell J. Football helmets and neurotrauma—An epidemiological overview of three seasons. Med Sci Sports 1979;11:138–145.
6. Committee on the Medical Aspects of Sports. Heads and Helmets: Tips on Athletic Training V. American Medical Association, 1963, pp 1–2.
7. CPSC Directorate for Epidemiology, Head Injuries, NEISS Data Highlights, Consumer Product Safety Commission, 14 (Jan–Dec): 1990.
8. Finvers K, Strother R, Mohtadi N. The effect of bicycling helmets in preventing significant bicycle-related injuries in children. Clin J Sport Med 1996;6:102–107.
9. Gerberich S, Priest J, Graft J, et al. Injuries to the brain and spinal cord. Minn Med 1982 (Nov);691–696.
10. Goldhaber G. A national survey about parent awareness of the risk of severe brain injury from playing football. J Athl Training 1993;28:306–311.
11. Henry P, Hauber R, Rice M. Factors associated with closed head injury in a pediatric population. J Neurosci Nurs 1992;24:311–316.
12. Maroon J, Bailes J, Yates A, et al. Assessing closed head injuries. Phys Sportsmed 1992;20:37–38, 43–44.
13. Medical news: Hard-shelled helmets best for athletes, experts say. JAMA 1962;180:23–24.
14. Mueller F, Schindler R. Annual survey of football injury research, 1931–1997. National Collegiate Athletic Association, National Federation of State High School Athletic Associations, and the American Football Coaches Association, 1998.
15. Mueller F, Cantu R. Annual Survey of Catastrophic Football Injuries, 1977–1997, National Center for Catastrophic Sports Injury Research, University of North Carolina, 1998.
16. Schneider R: Serious and fatal neurosurgical football injuries. Clin Neurosurg 1965;12:226–236.
17. AMA Subcommittee on Classification of Sports Injuries. Standard Nomenclature of Athletic Injuries. Chicago, American Medical Association, 1966, p 20.

4

The Epidemiology of Athletic Spine Injuries

Kenneth S. Clarke

SYNOPSIS

Neck injuries in sport are common, typically debilitating, and in retrospect quite predictable by mechanism of injury as to one of four natures, sprains or strains, fractures, brachial plexus pinches or stretches, and spinal cord injury. Of these, the spinal cord injury, whether a concussion or contusion or physical disruption, is obviously the most severe. It also, ironically, is the best tracked of sports injuries because of its finality and notoriety when it is experienced. This chapter discusses the essence of what has been learned epidemiologically over recent decades since the advent of organized attention to spinal cord injuries among athletes.

INTRODUCTION

Chapter 3 attends to the principles underlying the presence and use of epidemiologic data in sports. In organized sports, the best of the available epidemiologic data concern serious spinal injuries, especially cervical spinal neurotrauma (quadriplegia). The better than usual attention given in sports to such injuries is due to (a) the infrequency of quadriplegia (enabling a single registry to capture national occurrences with reasonable reliability), (b) its finality (the permanence of quadriplegia or death is readily recognizable and definable with reasonable validity), and (c) its profundity (the sudden tragedy to a young, achieving human specimen produces a professional as well as a societal call for accountability).

NATIONAL OVERVIEW

Sport vs. Non-Sport

From 1973 through 1981, the United States had a central repository for all spinal cord injuries, supported principally by the Department of Education's Rehabilitation Services Administration.[29] Until it was closed from cessation of federal funds, reports were submitted by regional spinal cord injury centers to the National Spinal Cord Injury Data Research Center (National Center) and there compiled for viewing internal patterns of frequency.

It was acknowledged that what was received were a minority of spinal cord injuries experienced nationally, but it was hoped that those cases were representative of what was being experienced. The aggregate of the National Center's final database, for example, revealed that "Sport" produced 15% of the spinal cord injuries reported and 25% of quadriplegia cases. Spinal cord injury meant quadriplegia in 95% of the sport-related cases.[29]

Within "sport-related," 70% of these quadriplegia cases came from diving. However, this finding requires a reminder that the definition of "sport-related" in this repository did not distinguish competitive from recreational or organized from informal. As a result, "diving" in the context of this report was an activity instead of a sport. U.S. Diving is the national governing body for the sport of diving, and it is unaware of any spinal cord injury ever having occurred to a U.S. competitive diver, in practice or competition (personal communication, T. Smith, U.S. Diving). This problem has been confined to recreational settings with, for example, most hotels or motels responding by removing swimming pool diving boards and posting warning signs as well as highlighting pool depths.

Interestingly, at about the same time, a review of spinal cord injuries in Canadian sport and recreation at two Ontario spinal cord injury centers (for the years 1948–1983) also found the activity of diving to constitute 69% of their database.[25]

Within Sports

Table 4–1 lists the relative frequency of cases associated with all sports identified in the National Center's report. Only diving and "Sport, Other" had been identifiable in the categories distinguishing paraplegia (from thoracic or lumbar spinal injury) from quadriplegia (from cervical spinal injury). To this information, the National Center director has added that sport-related cases reported over all the years of the center's existence principally affected young people, that is, having an average age of 21, with one fourth being 16 or younger.[30]

In 1979 and until it closed, the author served as a consultant to the National Center concerning sports-related cases.[8, 30] Table

4–2 provides a consequent list of frequency of the sports-related cases reported as occurring in 1980 and 1981, when more detail was being obtained by special supplemental inquiry.

Of special interest is (a) the consistency in proportionate data by sport between this sampling and that found over all the years (Table 4–1), (b) the identification of the sports from the "Sports/Other" category that produced paraplegics (snow sports, cycling, equestrian, and hang gliding), and (c) the reality that even Frisbee has produced a quadriplegic injury (from chasing the disk downhill and tumbling).[9]

Receiving special attention were the aquatic cases. Body surfing (7%) and water skiing (4%) were the aquatic activities that accompanied diving. Of the diving cases, home pools contributed 29%, community pools 17%, and lakes or rivers the majority. All of the community pool cases were recreational in nature, and half of both home and community pool cases occurred in depths exceeding 4 feet. Anecdotally, alcohol was an accompanying factor in many cases.

Within Intercollegiate/ Interscholastic Sports

In 1975, with an eye on an anecdotal awareness of a seemingly increasing frequency of quadriplegia injuries in high school and college football and on the paucity of any spinal cord injury information in any sport, Clarke[6] conducted a retrospective national survey covering the 1973–1975 school years of schools and colleges reporting permanently disabling spinal cord injuries in their sports or physical education programs. The cooperation and encouragement of the principal sports governing bodies for interscholastic and intercollegiate sport caused no need for sampling, but 6 affiliates of the 51 associated with the National Federation of State High School Associations chose not to distribute the forms to their school members. The study's acceptance of strict confidentiality as to the source of data precluded any attempt to identify the missing schools within the cooperating affiliates and thereby to augment returns by follow-up procedures.

With a greater than 40% return nationally, the results showed not only an expected upward trend of permanent neurotrauma in

Table 4–1. Frequency of Spinal Cord Injuries by Sport, 1973–1981

Activity	Cases	Percent All Cases	Percent Sport Cases
Aquatics	598	10	69
Football	63	1	7
Gymnastics	50	1	6
Snow sports	45	1	5
Wrestling	23	*	3
Air sports	22	*	3
Equestrian	16	*	2
Field sports	10	*	1
Rodeo	9	*	1
Basketball	6	*	1
Baseball	5	*	1
Track & Field	2	*	*
Skateboard	1	*	*
Other sports	16	*	2
Nonsport	5148	86	—
Unknown	10	*	—
TOTAL—All	6014	99	—
—Sports	866	14	101†

*Less than .5% but greater than 0.

†Percent total does not equal 100% owing to small number rounding.

Adapted from Young J, Burns P, Bowen A, et al. Spinal Cord Injury Statistics: Experience of the Regional Spinal Cord Injury Systems. Phoenix, AZ, Good Samaritan Medical Center, 1982.

Table 4–2. Frequency and Selected Characteristics of Spinal Cord Injuries by Sport, 1980–1981

Activity	Cases #	Cases %	Age Mean	Age Range	Percent Male	Percent White	Percent Quadriplegia	Percent Recreation*	Percent Skilled†
Aquatics	97	66	21	13–47	90	91	99	100	52
Snow sports	9	6	27	17–54	89	89	33	89	50
Football	9	6	20	14–37	100	100	100	67	22
Gymnastics	8	5	18	13–21	88	100	100	88	25
Cycling	7	4	24	14–57	100	100	43	86	43
Equestrian	5	3	28	19–42	100	80	60	60	80
Hang gliding	4	3	38	21–64	75	100	25	100	75
Wrestling	3	2	20	17–22	100	100	100	100	0
Rugby	2	1	21	20–22	100	100	100	0	100
Track & Field	1	1	18	—	100	100	100	0	100
Lacrosse	1	1	17	—	100	100	100	100	100
Ice skating	1	1	22	—	100	100	100	100	100
Frisbee	1	1	Unk	—	100	100	100	100	Unk
TOTAL	148	100							
Average			22	16–41	92	93	91	92	50
w/o Aquatics	51	34	23	14–64	94	96	96	78	46

*Not a participant in an organized class or team when injured.
†Adept in the skills of the sport in which injured.
　Adapted from Clarke K. Sport-Related Permanent Spinal Cord Injuries, 1980–1982: A Report to the National Spinal Cord Injury Data Research Center, Phoenix AZ, 1983.

competitive football, but also the clear presence of this injury in gymnastics and wrestling. In all, nine sports were represented, but only in gymnastics were females among the injured. Table 4–3 shows the incidence of the cases as reported.

In 1982 the National Center for Catastrophic Sports Injury Research (NCCSIR) was established to bring focal continuity of professional attention to catastrophic injuries in organized sport.[19] Although it principally registers fatal and nonfatal catastrophic injuries in high school and college

football,[20] the center also tracks and comments annually on trends in incidence and major preventive efforts for all sports having injuries of relevance, including cheerleading. It continues to be the sole source repository of such data (Tables 4–4 and 4–5).

TRAMPOLINE

Historical Perspective

In the National Center's report, 32 of the 50 gymnastics cases reported over those

Table 4–3. Average Annual Incidence of Permanent Spinal Cord Injuries by Varsity/ Subvarsity Sport, 1973–1975

Group	Football	Wrestling	Gymnastics (male)	Gymnastics (female)	Baseball	Basketball
High School						
Cases/100 programs	0.2	0.1	0.2	0.1	0	0.0*
Cases/1000 athletes	0.0*	0.0*	0.1	0.0*	0	0.0*
2–year College						
Cases/100 programs	0.7	0	0	0	0.2	0
Cases/1000 athletes	0.1	0	0	0	0.1	0
4–year College						
Cases/100 programs	0.7	0	1.4	0.3	0.1	0
Cases/1000 athletes	0.1	0	0.8	0.3	0.1	0
Total						
Athletes/case	28,000	62,000	7,000	24,000	177,000	793,000
Programs/case	403	1781	281	1113	6254	23,024

*Less than .5 but greater than 0.
　Adapted from Clarke K. A survey of sports-related spinal cord injuries in schools and colleges, 1973–1975. J Safety Res 1977;9:140–146.

Table 4–4. High School and College Football Quadriplegia

Year	High School Total*	High School Rate†/ 100,000	College Total*	College Rate†/ 100,000	Combined Total	Combined Rate/ 100,000
1997	7	0.47	1	1.33	8	0.51
96	6	0.40	3	4.00	9	0.57
95	7	0.47	1	1.33	8	0.51
94	1	0.07	1	1.33	2	0.13
93	8	0.53	0	0.00	8	0.51
92	6	0.40	0	0.00	3	0.38
91	1	0.07	0	0.00	1	0.06
90	11	0.73	2	2.67	13	0.83
89	12	0.80	2	2.67	14	0.89
88	10	0.77	1	1.33	11	0.85
87	9	0.69	0	0.00	7	0.51
86	4	0.31	0	0.00	4	0.29
85	6	0.47	3	4.00	9	0.65
84	5	0.39	0	0.00	5	0.37
83	11	0.85	1	1.33	12	0.87
82	7	0.54	2	2.67	9	0.65
81	7	0.54	2	2.67	9	0.65
80	13	1.00	2	2.67	15	1.09
79	8	0.62	4	5.33	12	0.87
78	14	1.08	0	0.00	14	1.02
77	14	1.08	2	2.67	16	1.16
76	25	1.92	8	10.67	33	2.40
75	21	1.75	6	8.00	27	2.12
74	14	1.17	5	6.67	19	1.49
73	18	1.50	1	1.33	19	1.49
72	7	0.58	1	1.33	8	0.63
71	10	0.83	1	1.33	11	0.86
61						1.03‡

*Obtained from the National Football Head and Neck Injury Registry (1971–1987) and the National Center for Catastrophic Sports Injury Research (1988–1997).

†Population size of high school and college football teams obtained from the American Football Coaches Association Annual Surveys of Football Fatalities.

‡Estimated from Schneider R. Serious and Fatal Neurosurgical Football Injuries. Clin Neurosurg 1965;13:226–236.

nine years came from trampoline accidents.[29] It is not known whether these arose from home use, physical education, or competition. National attention was brought to the risks of this apparatus for serious neck injuries in 1960 by Ellis and colleagues[15] with a report of five cases involving trampolines in school, at home, and at commercial amusement centers, three of which resulted in quadriplegia and all but one identified with an incorrectly attempted somersault.

By the mid 1970s, in-depth professional attention to this source of spinal cord injury returned, based on an increasing anecdotal collection of neurotraumas resulting from this apparatus and from the advent of the minitramp as well.[16, 21, 22, 28]

American Academy of Pediatrics

In 1977, based on the review and recommendations of its accident prevention committee, the American Academy of Pediatrics (AAP) took a formal and public stand to ban the use of the trampoline in schools and colleges as an avoidable source of quadriplegia.[10] Use of the minitramp and of the backyard family trampoline was not mentioned. Cited in the brief position statement were the results of Clarke's 1973–1975 survey of spinal cord injuries in schools and colleges[6] from which the AAP determined, "Next to football, trampolines were found to be the highest cause of permanent paralysis." Up to then, concerns over the frequency of such injuries were accompanied by recommendations for better injury control measures.[21] Clarke had found in his survey that trampoline quadriplegia resulted from "on-apparatus" injuries, which indicated the necessity of competent teaching and control of the advanced maneuvers.

A flurry of professional activity resulted at both the physical education and organized sport levels. In spring 1978, the American

Table 4–5. College and High School Football Fatalities (Direct Only)

Year	Total	Rate*	Neck Only	Rate* Neck	% Neck
1997	5	0.32	0	0.00	0
96	5	0.32	0	0.00	0
95	4	0.25	0	0.00	0
94	1	0.06	0	0.00	0
93	4	0.25	1	0.06	25
92	2	0.13	0	0.00	0
91	3	0.19	0	0.00	0
90	0	0.00	0	0.00	0
89	4	0.25	0	0.00	0
88	7	0.51	1	0.06	17
87	4	0.29	2	0.15	50
86	11	0.80	1	0.07	8
85	6	0.44	0	0.00	0
84	5	0.36	0	0.00	0
83	4	0.29	0	0.00	0
82	7	0.51	0	0.00	0
81	7	0.51	1	0.07	14
80	9	0.65	2	0.15	22
79	4	0.29	1	0.07	25
78	9	0.65	3	0.22	33
77	9	0.65	4	0.29	44
76	15	1.09	0	0.00	0
75	14	1.10	2	0.16	14
74	11	0.86	1	0.08	9
73	7	0.55	1	0.08	14
72	18	1.41	2	0.16	11
71	18	1.41	4	0.31	22
70	26	2.04	8	0.63	31
69	19	1.62	2	0.17	11
68	30	2.79	6	0.56	20
67	19	1.77	3	0.28	16
66	20	1.86	4	0.37	20
65	21	1.95	4	0.37	19
64	24	3.52	3	0.44	13
63	13	1.91	1	0.15	8
62	12	1.76	2	0.29	17
61	16	2.35	3	0.44	19
60	12	1.76	1	0.15	9
59	10	1.47	2	0.29	20
58	11	1.61	2	0.29	18
57	14	2.05	1	0.15	7
56	13	1.91	1	0.15	8
55	7	1.03	1	0.15	14
54	14	2.05	3	0.44	21
53	8	1.17	2	0.29	25
52	5	0.73	1	0.15	20
51	7	1.02	3	0.44	43
50	12	1.76	5	0.73	42

*Per 100,000 football players.

Data from Annual Surveys of Football Fatalities: The American Football Coaches Association, the National Collegiate Athletic Association, and the National Federation of State High School Athletic Associations. National Center for Catastrophic Sports Injury Research, Chapel Hill, NC.

Alliance for Health, Physical Education, and Recreation held national hearings on a draft set of guidelines for the controlled use of the trampoline and minitramp. With minor editing and broad support, the organization then adopted the guidelines as an official position.[3] Principal among the guidelines was the prohibition of any somersault in basic physical education programs (as well as securing the apparatus from use when unattended).

Shortly afterwards, the safety committee of the National Collegiate Athletic Association (NCAA) adopted these guidelines for the controlled use of the trampoline for the development of competitive skills.[12] Ironically, among divers and gymnasts, the trampoline was considered an injury prevention device that, with the use of a safety belt, better enabled the athlete to learn advanced skills involving the inverted position than other alternatives. There was no competitive trampolining in schools and colleges.

A national registry for catastrophic injuries in the breadth of gymnastics was initiated the following year, which continued for four years,[5] when the previously mentioned NCCSIR was established. By that time, the AAP, upon the continued review and recommendations of its accident prevention committee and its physical fitness and sport committee as well, rescinded its ban on the use of the trampoline and emphasized the need for supervisory controls.[11]

FOOTBALL

Historical Perspective

Chapter 3 describes how the advent of the modern helmet led to a significant rise in the frequency of head-related football fatalities, how helmet standards began to be addressed, and, later, how rules were changed to lessen the frequency of the helmeted head receiving the brunt of the initial impact of a block or tackle. With such a focus, it took longer for football programs to turn to and realize that nonfatal catastrophic neck injuries were on an upward climb, but based on a more subtle mechanism of injury.

Schneider was certainly aware of catastrophic neck-related injuries in football, and included them in his landmark survey of fellow neurosurgeons.[23] However, with the dominance of cerebral neurotrauma over spinal cord injuries within sports medicine of that era,[13, 18] and neck-related fatalities staying relatively flat during the 1960s,[20] he gave little attention to the spinal cord injuries reported in the survey and instead a few years later perpetuated a belief of that era, that the mechanism of injury for quadriplegia was hyperextension, a "karate chop."[24]

By the late 1960s, anecdotal awareness of an apparent increase in nonfatal neck injuries began to cause concern. "Spearing" had been condemned much earlier, but the American Medical Association's Committee on Medical Aspects of Sports took a position that the new and better helmets were now being accompanied by a new coaching technique, "face into the numbers." By teaching players to place the facemask on the numbers while blocking and tackling, coaches were teaching "heads up," not spearing, and it was easier for the player to go left or right with the opponent. However, the committee warned that when players failed to execute the maneuver as taught, they would be in a very hazardous position.[14]

It took until early 1976 for the rules of football to include that warning and, in effect, to forbid the continued use of the heads up technique. It also had taken until 1975 for football to have a clinical study of the subtle changes to the cervical spine among young football players who had been leading with their heads in the customary manner of the times,[2] and to take into account epidemiologic data from two coincidental sources that revealed the concurrently rising magnitude of quadriplegic injuries.[6, 26] While Clarke's 1973–1975 survey had obtained data from schools and colleges, Torg had utilized Schneider's model of surveying

neurosurgeons for the frequency of this injury in sport, and then established an ongoing registry of the same.[27] Their independently derived data found essentially the same incidence and internal patterns by position and activity at the time of injury, and organized sport made special efforts to have educational activities accompany these major rule changes.

Interestingly, it was at that time that "axial loading," as the biomechanic mechanism of the football quadriplegic injury, became defined and accepted to explain why "so few" injuries of this nature were being experienced. Fortunately the posture of having the cervical spine straightened out *and* striking one's opponent in the same plane *at that moment* with the crown of the helmet is a rare occurrence. By making it even rarer by minimizing the opportunity for the inadvertent spear, that is, by players "sliding off" with their heads to the side should they duck their heads for any reason, the occasions did indeed drop. Figure 4–1 demonstrates the instant and dramatic drop in incidence of football quadriplegia, which declined to a handful per year in the mid-1980s. Interestingly, a coincidentally concurrent tracking of the brachial plexus injuries in football (among all injuries experienced) before and after the 1976 change in the rules found no increase in incidence, a tradeoff for quadriplegia that would have been acceptable.[7]

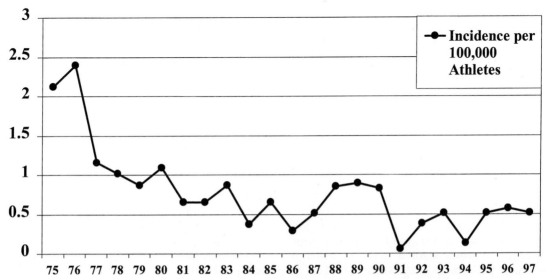

Figure 4–1. Quadriplegia in High School and College Football. Source: National Football Head and Neck Injury Registry (1971–1987) and the National Center for Catastrophic Sports Injury Research (1988–1997).

By 1988 the NCCSIR absorbed the registry of nonfatal catastrophic football injuries initiated by Torg and colleagues.[27]

It was then that football experienced what is not uncommon in other areas of interest in public health. With the long-term absence of a consciousness of a problem and of a behavioral solution, people can revert to an earlier behavior (or be so new at the activity as not to know better). One film-analysis study documented in 1990 that the number of helmet contacts in play (defined by the author as unintentional and intentional spearing) was the same as it had been in 1975.[17] The return of the frequency of quadriplegia to double digits in 1990 for the third consecutive season also was experienced, which prompted educational action at both high school and college levels of play (personal communication, R. Schindler, National Federation of State High School Associations). The NCAA also modified its rules to make the facemask explicitly part of the helmet and thereby explicitly relevant to what had been understood but implied since 1976.[1] The result was again dramatic; the national frequency of quadriplegia injuries dropped to but one case in 1991 and has remained essentially a handful annually through 1997.

ICE HOCKEY

Historical Perspective

Tator's review of spinal cord injuries in Canadian sport from 1948 through 1983 recorded the first case in hockey in 1976, with 27 more occurring by the study's completion.[25] In the United States as well as in Canada, the recent introduction of this risk into hockey accompanied the advent of the protective helmet and, as in football, the resulting tendency of the helmeted player to let the head take the hit (in this instance, typically, into the boards).

Also as in American football with the advent of a better helmet, the commitment to keep the helmet in the sport for its intended purposes (protecting the head and, by the attached faceguard, the face as well) prevailed but was accompanied by admonitions and rule changes against certain observed behavior patterns to address the problem of serious neck injuries. In hockey it was "checking" from behind, in which the checked player had less opportunity to avoid inadvertent spearing of the boards.

USA Hockey and "Heads Up Hockey"

By the end of the 1980s, the rule providing for a major penalty for checking from behind was in place, and the anecdotal frequency of quadriplegia of one to three a season dropped. With most hockey played in the U.S. being in other than interscholastic and intercollegiate programs, however, the NCCSIR data were not representative of the national toll. By the mid-1990s, it became apparent not only that the rule against checking from behind needed the fullest of support, and got it, but also that spinal cord injuries were occurring from other causes that led to hitting the boards with the helmeted head, for example, missing a check. As a result, a comprehensive educational program was developed by the medical/safety committee of USA Hockey, the governing body for amateur hockey in the U.S., entitled "Heads Up Hockey," which in effect is intended to keep coaches and players of all ages conscious of the threat of quadriplegia the moment players let their heads take a hit in the downward position, whatever the play at the time.[4]

SWIMMING

Data are not in hand, but anecdotally, it is well accepted that a new cause of quadriplegia in aquatic sport emerged in the mid-1980s, stemming from the "pike" racing dive made popular by a few swimmers at the 1984 Olympic Games. A swimmer skilled in the pike was said to gain a few milliseconds by this form of entry into the water. Executed by a swimmer unskilled in this technique, especially in the shallow pools of older design, the pike led to head contact with the pool bottom at entry, resulting in another form of inadvertent spearing. Eventually, it became apparent to those responsible for the sport that these occurrences were indeed a pattern of a defined mechanism, and guidelines emerged that dealt with the height of the blocks and the depth of the pool in both training and competition.

BASEBALL

The data on baseball quadriplegia is limited, but it does demonstrate that it can happen, and that the pattern is one of head-first sliding in which the hands separate, allowing the crown of the head to inadvertently spear the shin of the baseman or catcher.[19]

RUGBY

The mechanism of spinal cord injury in rugby differs from that in football, hockey, and baseball. Instead of an acute impact of a head against a player or barrier while in a vulnerable axial loading position, the mechanism for rugby players was being slowly "scrunched" against the ground. The typical scenario was during a scrum when the front row began to collapse, and the player found himself inverted as the collapse continued. As a result, based on the pragmatics of "anecdotal epidemiology," most rugby leagues now permit the official to stop play when the scrum begins to break down.

CONCLUSION

Quadriplegia, the permanent loss of sensory and motor pathways below the cervical spine, is a devastating injury, is now well known as a possible occurrence in virtually any sport, and receives due attention when patterns of occurrences become observed. The discipline and tools of epidemiology assist these attentions by tracking their relative frequency and accompanying associated factors continuously, by providing a sensitivity to change, and by enabling one to see the validity of contentions as to the extent, cause, and/or solution of the problem of interest. Athletes in several major sports have now benefited from the continuum of awareness of the problem, remedial efforts, and awareness of the effects of these efforts, both direct and indirect. Of major significance is that the epidemiology of neck injuries in sport has shown that sports behavior can be changed by educational methods.

References

1. Adams J (ed). Points of Emphasis. *In* NCAA Football Rules & Interpretation. National Collegiate Athletic Association, 1993.
2. Albright J, Feldick H. Nonfatal cervical spine injuries in interscholastic football. JAMA 1976;236:1243–1245.
3. American Alliance for Health, Physical Education, and Recreation. The Use of Trampolines and Minitramps in Physical Education. Author, 1978.
4. Ashare A, Smart M. On the Safe Side. American Hockey Magazine 1996(Jan):160.
5. Christensen C, Clarke K. Fourth Annual National Gymnastic Catastrophic Injury Report. Washington, DC, U.S. Gymnastics Safety Association, 1983.
6. Clarke K. A survey of sports-related spinal cord injuries in schools and colleges, 1973–75. J Safety Res 1977;9:140–146.
7. Clarke K, Powell J. Football helmets and neurotrauma—An epidemiological overview of three seasons. Med Sci Sports 1979;11:138–145.
8. Clarke K. Spinal cord injuries in organized sports. SCI Digest 1980(Summer):16.
9. Clarke K. Sport-Related Permanent Spinal Cord Injuries, 1980–1982: A Report to the National Spinal Cord Injury Data Research Center, Phoenix, AZ 1983.
10. American Academy of Pediatrics, Committee on Accident and Poison Prevention. Trampolines. Author, 1977.
11. Committee on Accident and Poison Prevention and Committee on Pediatric Aspects of Physical Fitness, Recreation, and Sports. Trampolines II. Pediatrics 1981;67:438.
12. Committee on Competitive Safeguards and Medical Aspects of Sports. Use of the Trampoline for the Development of Competitive Skills. National Collegiate Athletic Association, 1978.
13. Committee on the Medical Aspects of Sports. Heads and Helmets: Tips on Athletic Training V. American Medical Association, 1963, pp 1–2.
14. Committee on the Medical Aspects of Sports. Spearing in Football: Tips on Athletic Training X, American Medical Association, 1968, pp 1–2.
15. Ellis W, Green D, Holzaepfel, et al. The trampoline and serious neurological injuries, JAMA, 1960;174:1673–1676.
16. Hay J. Survey of Trampoline Injuries Statistics: A Report for the Nissen Corporation, 1974, 27 pp.
17. Heck J: The incidence of spearing during a high school's 1975 and 1990 football seasons. J Athl Training 1996;31:31–37.
18. Medical News. Hard-shelled helmets best for athletes, experts say. JAMA 1962;180:23–24.
19. Mueller F, Cantu R, Van Camp S. Catastrophic Injuries in High School and College Sports. Human Kinetics Sports Science Monograph Series 8. 1996, p 114.
20. Mueller F, Schindler R. Annual Survey of Football Injury Research 1931–1997. National Collegiate Athletic Association, National Federation of State High School Athletic Associations, and the American Football Coaches Association, 1998.
21. Rapp G, Nicely P. Trampoline injuries. Am J Sports Med 1978;6:269–271.
22. Schields C, Fox J, Stauffer E. Cervical cord injuries in sports. Phys Sportsmed 1978;6:71–76.
23. Schneider R. Serious and fatal neurosurgical football injuries. Clin Neurosurg 1965;12:226–236.
24. Schneider R. Head and Neck Injuries in Football. Baltimore, William & Wilkins, 1973.

25. Tator C, Edmonds V. Sports and recreation are a rising cause of spinal cord injury. Phys Sportsmed 1986;14:157–160, 165–167.
26. Torg J, Quedenfeld T, Moyer R, et al. Severe and catastrophic neck injuries resulting from tackle football. J Am Coll Health Assoc 1977;25:224–226.
27. Torg J, Truex R, Quedenfeld T. The national football head and neck injury registry—Report and conclusions. JAMA 1979;241:1477–1479.
28. Torg J, Das M. Trampoline-related quadriplegia: Review of the literature and reflections on the American Academy of Pediatrics' position statement. Pediatrics 1984;74:804–812.
29. Young J, Burns P, Bowen A, et al. Spinal Cord Injury Statistics: Experience of the Regional Spinal Cord Injury Systems. Phoenix, AZ, Good Samaritan Medical Center, 1982, p 1.
30. Young J. From the data bank. SCI Digest 1980(Summer):45–46.

5

Engineering Head Protection

Thomas Blaine Hoshizaki

Head and brain trauma has, unfortunately, become an integral part of many athletic endeavors, especially those activities involving body contact at high speeds. While brain injuries are recognized as the result of participating in these activities, they are seldom accepted as part of the game. Subsequently, participants look toward the scientific and medical communities to take a leadership role in establishing rules and developing products that lessen the likelihood of serious injuries. To suggest that it is possible to eliminate head and brain injuries in athletic activities is simply not reasonable; however, the opportunity to mitigate these injuries is a realistic goal. The challenge lies in providing a safer environment without dramatic change to the nature of the game. In sports such as motor racing, where the use of crash helmets is commonplace, head protection has a very attractive benefit–to–performance-interference ratio. If the helmet begins to compete with the athlete's performance, or the likelihood of an injury is so remote the athlete places a low priority on the protection, helmet use drops off dramatically. The scientific and medical communities face the challenge of providing head protection that is safe yet meets the performance needs of the athlete.

The types of head injuries addressed in this chapter involve blunt trauma to the skull resulting in impact injuries. While laceration and bruising injuries are a concern for helmet designers, by far the most common and often problematic injuries arise from impacts. The types of impact injuries include skull depression injuries, skull fractures, and concussions, with concussions by far the most common. It is important to make the distinction between different levels of both concussion and fracture injuries to the skull and brain, as design solutions used to protect the brain from a Grade 3 concussion may not involve the same strategy used to protect against Grade 1 injuries.

MEASURING HEAD AND BRAIN TRAUMA

In order to evaluate protective devices, certain fundamental information concerning the level of energy resulting in concussive effects was needed. Gurdjian and coworkers[5] provide intracranial pressure–time tolerance curve data collected using anesthetized dogs. The data provided the basis for establishing the relationship between intracranial pressure over time and severe concussions (Fig. 5–1).

Although the data from Gurdjian and coworkers provided an understanding of the principle underlying the relationship between intracranial pressure and time related to brain injury, it was impractical to measure. Acceleration of the head was thought to be more expedient to work with, and data collected on human cadavers provided a similar-shaped acceleration–time curve, as shown in Figure 5–2.[4] That tolerance curve was based on the correlation between the appearance of a linear skull fracture and a moderate to severe concussion. The authors argued that a moderate to severe concussion was the level of injury or tolerance acceptable in defining the performance of a safety helmet. This was followed by the development and publication of the Wayne State University (WSU) Tolerance Curve.[4] Subsequently, this curve is considered the benchmark for use by standards committees who set tolerance levels for protection against head impacts. Standards committees are charged with the responsibility to set helmet safety performance requirements using the best knowledge available. The acceptance of the preceding two relationships as appro-

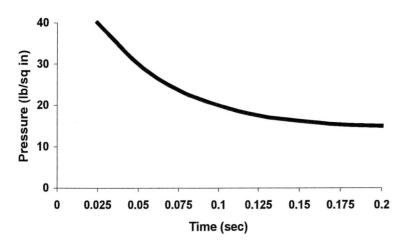

Figure 5–1. Pressure and time relationships in cases of severe concussions. From Gurdjian ES, Webster JE, Lissner HR. Observations on the mechanism of the brain concussion, contusion, and laceration. Surg Gynec Obstet 1955;101:680–690.

priate led to an accepted peak acceleration during an impact of 275–300 g. It should be noted that the above criteria for defining the level of performance for safety helmets were accepted only after a great deal of debate reflecting many different opinions.[6]

In order to establish injury criteria, it was necessary for the committee to agree on what constitutes an unacceptable injury and what the helmet should be expected to protect against. For example, should a helmet be expected to protect against all forms of head injury? A concussion can begin with a Grade 1 concussion that has been estimated to result from impacts producing as low as 80 peak g^{13} right up to when the skull fractures (expected at approximately 275 to 300 g^4). Clearly no one expects a helmet to protect against all forms of head injuries; however, the consumer has the right to be informed of the protection limits of the product.

Acceleration–Time

The relationship of acceleration and time to injury is not accounted for by acceleration

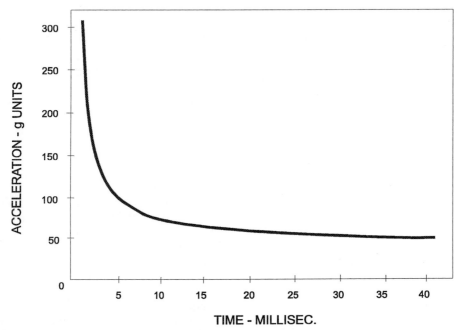

Figure 5–2. Tolerance curve for the human head (acceleration in gravity units, time in milliseconds). From Gurdjian ES, Roberts VL, Thomas LM. Tolerance curves of accelerations and intracranial pressure and protective index in experimental head injury. J Trauma 1966;6:600–604.

alone, so a number of formulas were developed including both acceleration and time. The Gadd Severity Index[1] (GSI) = ∫a(t)2.5 dt(1000) is the most commonly applied of these measures. Acceleration-time pulses that integrate to a GSI of 1000 equate to the original Wayne State University curve. The values in the Wayne State curve were based on short duration impulses and on results obtained from cadaver skull fractures. The data were collected using a rigid, flat-surface impact on the forehead.[9] Gadd, the originator of the GSI, has pointed out many instances of distributed impact (nonfracturing) in which volunteers experienced a much higher GSI without a concussion.[2] Accordingly, he has recommended a GSI of 1500 for distributed impacts in which the fracture hazard is absent.[7] The percentage of a normal population that can expect a severe

brain injury when receiving a blow resulting in a GSI of 1500 (Head Injury Criteria [HIC] 1750) is about 70% (Fig. 5–3).[10] Figure 5–3 provides an estimation of the probability of serious head injury in a normal population using the Abbreviated Injury Scale (AIS).[15] Setting a level of tolerance for head injury that is acceptable to the public at large is an enormous challenge. The unpredictable nature of head and brain injuries makes the task extremely precarious. Serious head injuries and even death have resulted from what seemed by observers to be very minor blows to the head, yet in other incidences what seemed to be severe impacts have resulted in no observable injury. In addition, the importance of the brain in maintaining quality of life adds yet another dimension for consideration in setting safe levels of tolerance when evaluating head protection.

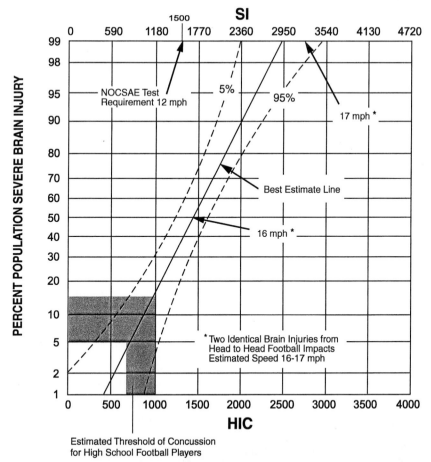

Figure 5–3. Percentage of population expected to experience a serious brain injury for a given impact as defined by HIC. From Mertz HJ, Weber DA. Interpretations of the impact responses of a three year old child dummy relative to child injury potential. *In* Proceedings of the 9th International Technical Conference of Experimental Safety Vehicles, Kyoto, Japan, 1982.

HEAD PROTECTION

The objective of the helmet is to reduce the relative velocity between the head and the impactor to zero without damaging the brain. The distance through which the velocity changes has to be sufficient to limit the acceleration and to keep the force values below injury thresholds.[12] Helmets designed to protect at high-energy impacts are typically efficient at protecting the wearer from skull fractures at 40 to 60 J impacts but are not necessarily effective at preventing concussions. Helmets designed to work efficiently at lower energy impacts generally do not perform efficiently at higher energy impacts. In Figure 5–4[11] the relationship between force and material is charted for three different types of helmet materials. The force curves provide an illustration of how materials labeled strong compare with a weak material in managing force created by an impact. It is obvious from this figure that if the absorbing material for a helmet is too strong, the amount of energy to be absorbed can quickly exceed a safe level of force. If the absorbing material is too weak, the deformation of the material is too great, resulting in a bottoming-out phenomenon, and again the force will exceed a safe limit. It is essential that the material used in the helmet be chosen in light of its proposed function. The advantage of hard shell helmets is that they employ two primary elements to manage the impact. The hard shell distributes the load over a greater surface and also increases the amount of the liner material involved in absorbing the energy.

An obvious answer to the preceding dilemma is to increase the thickness of a softer (weak) material to allow the liner to manage both high-and low-energy impacts. The curves in Figure 5–5 use a simple formula to depict the theoretical distance required to manage impacts of a head traveling at 10, 15, and 20 mph.[11] Theoretically, at 10 mph (16 kph) a liner of 1 cm is capable of attenuating enough energy to prevent concussion. However, at 20 mph (32 kph) a helmet of at least 5 cm is needed to prevent concussion-level accelerations. The curves presented in Figure 5–5 are theoretical and exist only in an ideal state. It is obvious that designing helmets to protect the head from both high-and low-impact energies without resulting in an unacceptably large helmet is a challenge.

Hodgson[8] produced Figure 5–6 to demonstrate the limits of helmets in protecting the brain from concussions. It is clear from this figure that in order to prevent concussions at velocities encountered during most sport activities, helmets need to be greater than 5 cm thick. A helmet with a 2-in (5.08 cm) energy attenuation liner would dramatically increase the overall size of the helmet.

Angular Accelerations

Hodgson[8] and Newman[11] cautioned against using stiff materials to meet higher energy limits set by standards organizations. Hodgson went on to state that materials that are effective at managing high-energy impacts may be too stiff to be effective in pro-

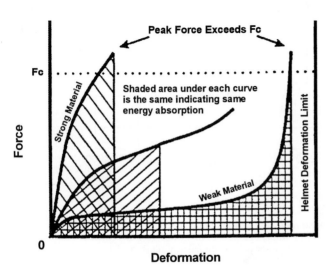

Figure 5–4. Effect of padding strength when the same energy is absorbed. From Newman JA. Biomechanics of Human Trauma: Head Protection. *In* Nahum AM, Melvin JW (eds): Accidental Injury Biomechanics and Prevention. New York, Springer Verlag, 1993.

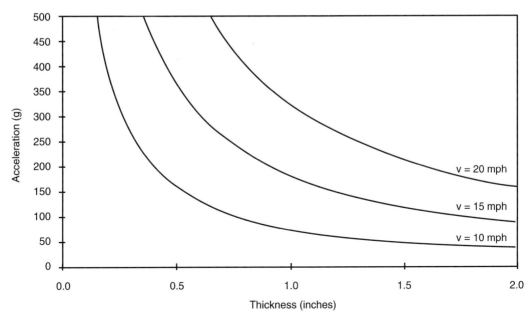

Figure 5–5. Minimum acceleration achievable for a given thickness. From Newman JA. Biomechanics of Human Trauma: Head Protection. *In* Nahum AM, Melvin JW (eds): Accidental Injury Biomechanics and Prevention. New York, Springer Verlag, 1993.

tecting against concussions even at lower-energy impacts. To this caution may be added the concerns presented by Sano and coworkers[14] demonstrated in Figure 5–7*A* and *B,* the potential dangers of angular acceleration injuries. The larger the helmet, the greater is the risk of creating larger angular accelerations. Sano impacted the head forms with ice hockey helmets at two velocities (v1 = 15 ft/sec, v2 = 18 ft/sec) and used the WSU tolerance curve to indicate the performance of the helmet. In Figure 5–7*A* the helmets proved effective in protecting the head from concussions resulting from linear accelerations. However, when the angular accelerations were measured under the same conditions, Figure 5–7*B* revealed that the helmets did not protect the brain. The study supported concerns of researchers that the lack of methods for measuring angular accelerations has limited our knowledge in the effectiveness of helmets in mitigating head injuries caused by rotational accelerations. As a result, helmet innovation has largely ignored the influence of helmet design on managing rotational accelerations.

Present helmets are not designed to manage rotational accelerations, nor are the standards designed to measure these criteria. As a result, designers have to be cautious in designing helmets that are larger than ex-

isting helmets. Doing so may result in creating an environment that increases head injuries from rotational accelerations. A fine balance is required to provide adequate distance to manage linear impact energies without dramatically increasing the likelihood of angular accelerations.

Helmet Design

Hodgson[8] produced the following four load (in kN) by displacement (in cm) curves for a skateboard helmet, an ice hockey helmet, a crash helmet, and an American football helmet (Fig. 5–8). He included a concussion threshold range as a reference. The lower limit was set at 8.9 kN, with the upper range set at 10 kN. This was calculated by using 200 and 225 *g* of acceleration as the limits, correlating with a GSI of 1500 with a 44 N head form. The concussion threshold defined on this graph provides a realistic if not an absolutely accurate value to compare the performance of the four types of helmets tested. Three distinct protection design strategies are clearly identified by the data. The first is the least effective and reflects the performance of the skateboard helmet. It does not have a great deal of energy absorbing capacity and quickly "bottoms out";

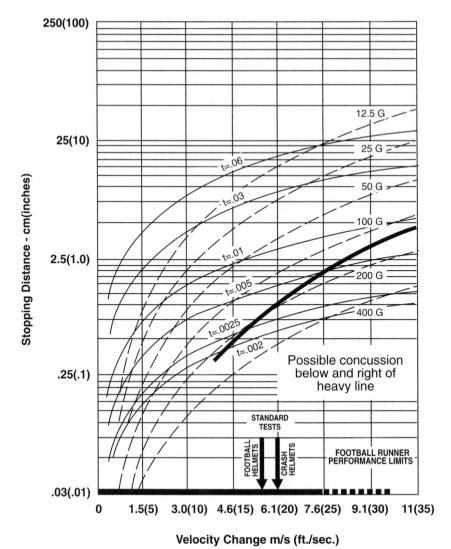

Figure 5–6. The relationship between absorption distance and impact velocity. From Hodgson V. A Standard for Protective Equipment. *In* Torg JS (ed): Athletic Injuries to the Head, Neck and Face. Philadelphia, Lea & Febiger, 1982, pp 27–35.

after a short .5 cm displacement, the force curve increases above the concussion threshold almost immediately. It is obvious this type of helmet is able to manage only the smallest energy impacts (5.8 J). Skateboard helmets are usually made with a rigid shell and a soft, open-cell foam liner. While the force curve of the crash helmet rises quickly to the concussion threshold, the crash helmet is able to manage a great deal of total impact energy (area under the curve). However, a large amount of the energy absorbed by the helmet occurred above the defined concussion threshold. The crash helmet absorbed only 44 J of energy below the concussion threshold while absorbing a total of 193 J. This provides an important understanding of the protective strategy a crash helmet employs. The helmet is designed to protect against catastrophic injuries during very high energy impacts. Of course, as reflected in the curve, it does provide some protection from concussion at lower energy impacts. Crash helmets are intended to be used in situations in which an impact to the head is a rare, unplanned, accidental occurrence. As a result, the athletes are thankful to be alive, and if a concussion is the only head injury sustained, they consider themselves lucky.

Ice hockey and football helmets use a similar strategy in managing impact energies.

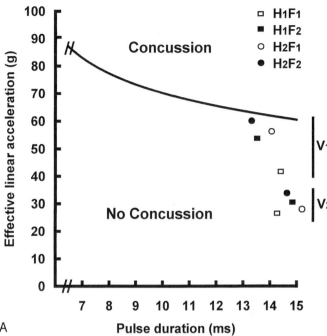

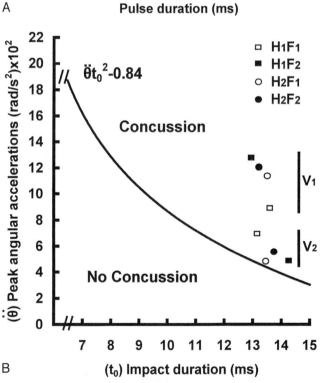

Figure 5–7. *A,* Plot of translational accelerations on WSU Tolerance Curve. *B,* Plot of rotational accelerations on WSU Tolerance Curve. From Sano K, Nakamura N, Hirakawa K, Hashizuma K. Correlative studies of dynamics and pathology in whiplash and head injuries. Scand J Rehabil Med 1972;4:47–54.

Because both of these games include body contact as an integral part of the sport, a helmet must be able to manage energies from multiple incidental impacts so as to avoid concussions. The football helmet is designed using a smooth, round, very hard shell and a thick (3 cm) liner of vinyl nitrile foam. The shell distributes the impact over a larger surface in addition to effectively involving more of the energy-absorbing liner. In this manner the designers are able to use a softer, less dense liner, thereby increasing the comfort and fit of the helmet. The curve in Figure 5–8 demonstrates the

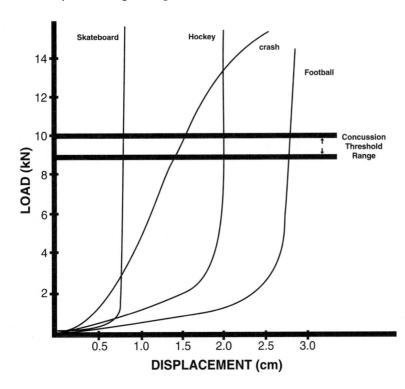

Figure 5-8. Comparison of static load-deflection curves of four helmet types. From Hodgson VR. Approaches and Evaluation Techniques for Helmets: A Symposium on Biomechanics Assessments of Sports Protective Equipment. 9th Congress of the International Society of Biomechanics, Waterloo, Ontario, Canada, 1983, pp 23–28.

effectiveness of this type of helmet in managing energy below the concussion threshold (34 J) with 88 J of total energy absorbed. The ice hockey helmet is designed using a semi-rigid geometric shell designed to absorb and distribute impact energy. A vinyl nitrile-type liner that is capable of managing multiple impacts is also used to absorb energy. The combination of the shell and liner absorbs a total of 26 J of energy below the concussion threshold.

The four curves in Figure 5–8 provide an interesting comparison of at least three, possibly four, strategies for protecting the head. The figure also provides the reader with an understanding of the differences in how energy is managed in helmets used for different activities. A helmet designed to manage high-impact energies effectively may in fact be very poor at protecting the head from concussions during low-energy impacts. As well, strategies used to design head protection against low-energy impacts and concussion may be limited in managing high-energy impacts. Observations of many of the original researchers in head protection concerning the need to design helmets that are specific to the activity seem well founded in light of the preceding data.

Historically, helmet designers have employed design strategies and materials

unique to the needs of each sport. Minimum performance requirements of the safety standards for each sport reflected this approach. Recently there has been a trend to employ similar design strategies across a variety of sport helmets. Expanded bead technology, including expanded polystyrene (EPS), expanded polypropylene (EPP), and expanded polyethylene (EPE), have allowed designers to pass multiple impact certification standards using what was strictly a crash helmet material. A multiple impact-type helmet must be evaluated beyond the ability of the helmet to pass a number of impacts at a single impact energy. How it manages the impacts in light of the type of injury it is intended to avoid must be considered. Expanded bead technology was developed in the helmet industry as a liner that absorbs energy by crushing or destroying the structures (beads). Expanded bead liners constructed using elastic materials allow helmet designers the opportunity to pass helmet certification standards that do not take into account the acceleration or force curves at different impact energies. As long as the helmet designs are able to pass impact tests at a single impact energy level, the helmet is deemed safe. How successfully the helmet handles low-impact energies and the influence of $80+$ g allowable acceleration of the skull resulting in a concussion is not considered.

SUMMARY

Helmet design should not be simply a matter of meeting the performance requirements set in certification standards. Understanding the principles governing what the measurement criteria reflect and what acceptable threshold limits are intended to protect against is the foundation of safe helmet design. Knowing the limits of both the science and the art involved in helmet design technology is fundamental in designing a safe helmet.

Careful consideration must be made before increasing impact energies in search of a safer standard. Ignoring the resulting effect of denser material on performance at lower-energy impacts may prove to increase the incidence of concussion injuries. A similar caution must be given when employing a greater energy absorbing distance in order to meet high-energy certification requirements. Helmet designers must be well schooled in the scientific foundation from which the original performance criteria were established or risk the chance of designing unsafe helmets. In sports the head may have to be protected against low-, intermediate-, or high-velocity impact blows. In football accidents, low-velocity blows are quite common. However, in sports like ice hockey, medium- to high-velocity impacts occur. Helmets must be designed specifically for the unique conditions of each sport. All conceivable conditions should be considered and taken into account in helmet design. In this way helmet designers can achieve compromises in their designs to provide maximum protection for the environment of interest.[3]

References

1. Gadd CW. Use of a Weighted Impulse Criterion for Estimating Injury Hazard. Paper No. 660793, Proc. Tenth Conference, Society of Automotive Engineers, Inc., New York, 1966, pp 164–174.
2. Gadd CW. Tolerable severity index in whole-head, nonmechanical impact. *In* Fifteenth Stapp Car Crash Conference Proceedings. New York, Society of Automotive Engineers, Inc. 1971, pp 809–816.
3. Gurdjian ES, Hodgson VR, Hardy WG, et al. Evaluation of the protection characteristics of helmets in sports. J Trauma 1964;4:309–324.
4. Gurdjian ES, Roberts VL, Thomas LM. Tolerance curves of accelerations and intracranial pressure and protective index in experimental head injury. J Trauma 1966;6:600–604.
5. Gurdjian ES, Webster JE, Lissner HR. Observations on the mechanism of the brain concussion, contusion and laceration. Surg Gynec Obstet 1955; 101:680–690.
6. Hirsh AE. Current Problems in Head Protection. *In* Caveness WF, Walker AE (eds): Head Injury Conference Proceedings. Philadelphia, JB Lippincott, 1966, pp 37–40.
7. Hodgson V. A Standard for Protective Equipment. *In* Torg JS (ed): Athletic Injuries to the Head, Neck and Face. Philadelphia, Lea & Febiger, 1982, pp 27–35.
8. Hodgson VR. Approaches and Evaluation Techniques for Helmets: A Symposium on Biomechanics Assessments of Sports Protective Equipment. 9th Congress of the International Society of Biomechanics, Waterloo, Canada, 1983, pp 23–28.
9. King AI. Survey of the State of the Art of Human Biodynamic Response. *In* Saczalski K, Singley GT III, Pilkey WD, et al. (eds): Aircraft Crashworthiness. Charlottesville, VA, University Press of Virginia, 1975, pp 83–120.
10. Mertz HJ, Weber DA. Interpretations of the Impact Responses of a Three Year Old Child Dummy Relative to Child Injury Potential. *In* Proceedings of the 9th International Technical Conference of Experimental Safety Vehicles, Kyoto, Japan, 1982.
11. Newman JA. Biomechanics of Human Trauma: Head Protection. *In* Nahum AM, Melvin JW (eds): Accidental Injury Biomechanics and Prevention. New York, Springer Verlag, 1993, pp 292–310.
12. Patrick LM. Head Impact Protection. *In* Caveness WF, Walker AE (eds): Head Injury Conference Proceedings. Philadelphia, JB Lippincott, 1966, pp 41–48.
13. Patrick LM, Grime G. Applications of Human Tolerance Data to Protective Systems: Requirements for Soft Tissue, Bone and Organ Protective Devices. *In* Impact Injury and Crash Protection. 1969, pp 444–473.
14. Sano K, Nakamura N, Hirakawa K, Hashizuma K. Correlative studies of dynamics and pathology in whiplash and head injuries. Scand J Rehabil Med 1972;4:47–54.
15. The Abbreviated Injury Scale (1980). American Association for Automotive Medicine, 1997.

ON THE FIELD EVALUATION

6

On the Field Management of Athletic Head and Neck Injuries

W. Lee Warren and Julian E. Bailes

Contact sports carry an inherent risk of injury to their participants. The athletes involved in these events are susceptible to head and cervical spine injuries, which can be career or life threatening. Although organized sports are becoming safer through rule changes, player education, improved conditioning, equipment, and techniques, a significant number of devastating injuries still occur each year in the United States.

Team trainers, coaches, and physicians have a responsibility to understand the various types of head and neck injury that athletes may sustain in order to properly handle and treat them. An asymptomatic athlete who is rendered unconscious may have only a mild concussion and be safe to return to play, whereas an awake, symptomatic athlete may have a developing subdudral hematoma or other intracranial process that will evolve into an emergency. In addition, a player with an unstable cervical spine injury who is initially neurologically intact can suffer iatrogenic spinal cord injury if improperly handled. The medical team members must accurately and thoroughly assess the injured player and have a plan for dealing with these injuries in an organized way when they occur.

The purpose of this chapter is to discuss the spectrum of athletic head and neck injuries, and to review the guidelines for the evaluation and management of these injuries on the field of play. Only organized sporting events will be discussed, as it is exceedingly difficult to affect the incidence of neurologic athletic injury in recreational sports owing to the lack of equipment and supervision.

ATHLETIC HEAD INJURY

The American athlete most likely to suffer a head injury is the teenage male football player.[22, 63] Other sports accounting for the majority of athletic head injuries are high-impact activities such as boxing, rugby, and ice hockey.[38, 49, 50, 60, 61] Head injury has also been reported in other sports, including soccer, baseball, and figure skating.[2, 7, 13, 17, 30, 35, 44, 46, 47, 67] Annually in the United States, approximately eight deaths occur as a result of head injuries sustained while playing football.[39] Acute subdural hematoma (ASDH) is the most common cause of death in these athletes.[2, 39] Up to 20% of football players suffer minor head injuries each season, with the total number of these injuries exceeding 200,000 annually.[9, 16, 64] A player who sustains one concussion is at fourfold risk to sustain another.[64]

Devastating head injuries are usually easy to identify. However, some pathologic entities such as ASDH and epidural hematoma (EDH) can develop over time, and a player may initially seem unharmed only to deteriorate later. Mild head injury, on the other hand, is difficult to assess in terms of its permanent effect on the athlete. It is known that athletes may develop significant long-term neuropsychologic problems from repeated minor head injuries.[11, 12, 22, 54, 64] This information has generated much interest in the detection of minor head injuries and in rule changes that affect which and when athletes may return to competition after minor head injury.[21] Athletes without gross external signs of injury, those without neurologic deficits, or those who quickly regain consciousness are often rushed back into play without proper evaluation. This is evidenced by the fact that 70% of American football players who are "knocked out" during a game return to play in the same game.[2] In addition, it was found that in ice hockey, 72% of players with knee injuries saw a physician, whereas only 8% of players with athletic brain injuries saw a physician.[2] In the light of data implicating minor head injury as a significant problem for the future of these young athletes, these statistics must change.

Types of Athletic Head Injuries

Athletic head injuries involve the same spectrum of pathology as is seen in nonathletic injuries.[29, 38] Epidural hematoma, subdural hematoma, intracerebral hematoma, diffuse axonal injury, subarachnoid hemorrhage, cerebral contusion, and cerebral concussion are all seen occasionally in head-injured athletes. The major difference in athletic and nonathletic head injuries is the frequently preventable nature of the injuries to athletes.[30, 31] In some cases, relatively minor head trauma can result in severe neurologic injury as a result of brain swelling from a previous injury. This is known as second impact syndrome[45] and will be discussed later.

The most common sports-related head injury is the "mild" or "minor" variety, which is also known as concussion. The athlete with a minor head injury has a Glasgow Coma Scale (GCS) score of 13 to 15 (Table 6–1). Cerebral concussion represents the mildest of a spectrum of closed head inju-

ries ranging from very brief periods of neurologic dysfunction, such as confusion and posttraumatic amnesia, to severe global brain injury producing coma.[42] The most severe of these injuries are comprised by a category known as diffuse axonal injury (DAI). The typical mechanism producing closed head injury is sudden deceleration of the head or a blow that sharply deforms the skull. Both of these mechanisms have been shown to produce sudden dysfunction in the neurons of the brain stem reticular activating system. Experimental models of cerebral concussion have shown transient cerebral ischemia, edema, widespread neuronal depolarization from acetylcholine release, and shearing of neurons and fibers as potential mechanisms for the alteration in mental status seen after closed head injury. Although no consistent neuropathologic finding has been demonstrated in experimental concussion models, scattered capillary damage and disruption of multiple neurons in the brain stem reticular system have been seen.[23]

Several authors have developed classification schemes to define the various degrees of brain dysfunction in cerebral concussion (Table 6–2).[3, 21, 28] At its simplest, concussion is any traumatically induced alteration in mental status with or without loss of consciousness. Hallmarks of concussion are confusion, amnesia, easy distractibility, and poor vigilance.[27, 36, 37] The athlete with a concussion may be unable to maintain a stream of coherent thought or carry out a sequence of goal-directed actions. The confusion and memory disturbance can be of immediate or delayed onset, necessitating close observation of the potentially head-injured athlete.

Athletes with concussions may have a blank stare, exhibit delayed verbal responses, or be easily distracted. He or she may be disoriented, or have slurred or incomprehensible speech, or gross motor coordination problems. Finally, the athlete suffering a concussion may be emotionally labile or have short-term memory deficits following the injury.[28]

Severe closed head injuries are relatively rare in organized sporting events. Just as in nonathletic-related head injury, however, these injuries can result in serious consequences. Contact sports can involve tremendous force transfers between players, which can occasionally produce massive structural damage to the brain. Severe head injuries

---

Table 6–1. The Glasgow Coma Scale

Eye Opening	
Spontaneous	E4
To speech	3
To pain	2
None	1
Verbal Responses	
Oriented	V5
Confused	4
Inappropriate	3
Incomprehensible	2
No sounds	1
Intubated	1T
Motor Responses	
Follows commands	M6
Localizes	5
Withdraws	4
Flexor posturing	3
Extensor posturing	2
No movement	1

Coma Score = E + V + M = 3–15

Intubated Patient = 3T–11T

Table 6–2. Classification Schemes for Cerebral Concussion

	Grade I/Mild	Ia	II/Moderate	III/Severe	IV
AAN	No LOC Symptoms <15 minutes	N/A	No LOC Symptoms >15 minutes	Any LOC	N/A
VNI	Short LOC, PTA <1 hour, GCS 15	Short LOC, PTA 1–24 hours, GCS 15	LOC <5 minutes, PTA 24 hours, GCS <15 for <5 minutes	LOC <5 minutes, PTA N/A, 12 <GCS <15 for <1 hour	GCS <12 for >5 minutes or <15 for >1 hour
Torg	(Grade I–II) No LOC or amnesia (except PTA)	N/A	(Grade III–IV) LOC < "few minutes" PTA or retrograde amnesia	(Grade V–VI) LOC/coma, confusion, amnesia	N/A
Colorado Consortium	No LOC Confusion without amnesia	N/A	No LOC Confusion + amnesia	Any LOC	N/A
Cantu	No LOC or PTA <30 min	N/A	LOC <5 minutes PTA 30 min–24 hours	LOC >5 minutes PTA >24 hours	N/A

AAN, American Academy of Neurology; VNI, Virginia Neurological Institute; LOC, loss of consciousness; N/A, not applicable; PTA, posttraumatic amnesia; GCS, Glasgow Coma Score.

usually manifest themselves in prolonged loss of consciousness or frank coma, and are defined as any head injury producing a GCS of less than or equal to 8.[24]

Diffuse axonal injury (DAI) (Fig. 6–1) is most common in victims of motor vehicle accidents, but is occasionally seen in severe athletic-related head trauma. Severe DAI un-

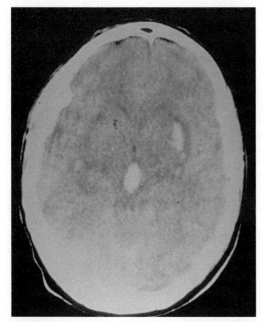

Figure 6–1. CT scan demonstrates diffuse axonal injury. Punctate hemorrhagic lesions and intraventricular hemorrhage are seen.

accompanied by a mass-producing lesion occurs in almost half of patients with a severe head injury and accounts for one third of all head injury–related deaths.[23] DAI is the most frequent cause of persistent vegetative state and significant disability following head injury. Pathophysiologically, DAI is the shearing of multiple axons due to rotational forces. This explains the other common name for DAI, that is, shear injury. DAI, like cerebral concussion, represents a spectrum of severity ranging from mild to severe forms. The severe cases have three characteristic features on computed tomography (CT) scans, which appear in varying degrees among the less severe forms of DAI. First, there are focal lesions in the corpus callosum. These are sometimes associated with intraventricular hemorrhage. Next, focal lesions are seen in the dorsolateral rostral brain stem. Finally, punctate hemorrhages are seen diffusely throughout the white matter of the cerebrum.[23]

Some athletes harboring cerebral contusion (Fig. 6–2) or traumatic intracerebral hematoma will have never demonstrated loss of consciousness or focal neurologic deficit. These players may have persistent headache or periods of confusion after their head injury, as well as posttraumatic amnesia. Failure of the athlete's mental status to rapidly clear should lead to CT scanning, which will reveal the intracranial pathology. Contusion and intracerebral hematoma require

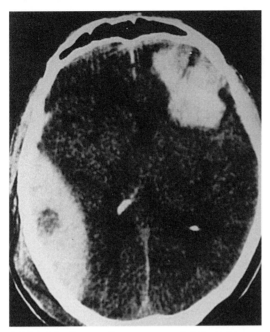

Figure 6–2. CT scan demonstrates a left frontal hemorrhagic contusion, along with a right epidural hematoma.

close observation, as they frequently lead to the development of significant mass effect or hydrocephalus and may require surgical evacuation.[8]

Skull fractures that cross the bony grooves harboring meningeal vessels can cause disruption of the vessels and lead to the formation of an epidural hematoma. The bleeding is usually arterial and fails to tamponade prior to causing serious brain compression and neurologic injury. The most frequently involved vessels are the middle meningeal artery and vein. Especially in children, the bony edges can also be a source of significant bleeding.

Classically, the patient with epidural hematoma will have transient loss of consciousness at the time of the injury, secondary to the force of the impact. This is followed by a brief period of arousal in which the patient may appear quite normal (lucid interval). The patient then exhibits a declining level of consciousness as the volume of the clot expands and produces increasing mass effect on the brain, and usually has a dilated pupil unilaterally (ipsilateral to the clot). If left without surgical evacuation, the clot will expand and produce decerebrate posturing and contralateral weakness, and ultimately death from brain stem compression. The classic presentation

of the lucid interval is seen in only about one third of patients with epidural hematoma.[8]

Acute subdural hematoma (ASDH) (Fig. 6–3) is approximately three times more common in head-injured athletes than is epidural hematoma. The ASDH in athletes, however, frequently differs from the typical clot seen in the elderly. Brain atrophy from aging creates a favorable environment for the development of a large collection of blood in the subdural space, causing mass effect on the brain. This is the case in most ASDH in adults, associated with a varying degree of underlying brain injury.[23] Conversely, the athlete with ASDH frequently has a small collection with underlying brain contusion and hemispheric swelling. This is due to the lack of atrophy, and therefore a smaller subdural space, in the young brain. Undoubtedly, some of the neurologic compromise seen in association with acute subdural hematoma is related to the underlying brain injury, as opposed to mass effect from the clot.[8] Although the underlying injury may not be improved by surgery, evacuation provides an opportunity to decompress whatever mass effect is being produced by the clot, as well as to stop any active bleeding on the cortical surface. Obviously, decisions regarding whether sur-

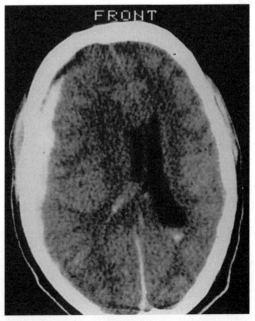

Figure 6–3. CT scan demonstrates a right side acute subdural hematoma with midline shift. This is the most frequently fatal type of head injury among athletes.

gery is indicated in the athlete with ASDH must be made by a neurosurgeon.

The athlete with ASDH is typically unconscious with or without a history of deterioration. Focal neurologic findings, such as pupillary asymmetry or decerebrate posturing, are often seen. These patients should be immediately transported to a facility with neurosurgical services, where a CT scan can be obtained.

A syndrome of massive cerebral edema and death in athletes who sustain relatively minor head injuries shortly after previous similar head injuries is well known.[45] The athlete is usually still symptomatic from the first injury, such as a player who sustains a minor concussion and returns to play prior to completely clearing his sensorium. This syndrome has been termed second impact syndrome, and is thought to result from cerebral vascular sensitivity from the first injury. The second injury then leads to cerebral autoregulatory dysfunction, vascular congestion, and subsequent intracranial hypertension. This can lead to the precipitous death of the victim, and has occurred in athletes with mild head injury without loss of consciousness.[45, 60]

On the Field Evaluation and Management of the Head-Injured Athlete

The team medical staff frequently includes trainers, coaches, physical therapists, and physicians. These individuals assume responsibility for the evaluation and treatment of the players. It is imperative that these individuals understand the various presentations of athletes with head injuries as well as the fact that severe head injuries can often initially look very benign. In addition, mild head injury can present with dramatic neurologic symptoms. Thus, extreme caution and prudence are required in all aspects of managing the athlete with suspected head injury.[57]

The adequate evaluation of the potentially head injured athlete involves three requirements. First, there must be recognition that a head injury has potentially occurred. Second, there must be accurate assessment of which athletes require transport to a medical facility for further work-up and treatment. Finally, a decision must be made regarding when the athlete may return to competition.[55] Detection of a potentially life threatening or neurologically devastating injury is of paramount importance. In light of the possibility of second impact syndrome, those athletes with mild head injuries must be cautiously observed and returned to play only when they are symptom free.

Any athlete who receives a blow to the head or any significant acceleration-deceleration–type force to the head should be suspected of having a possible head injury and thoroughly evaluated. The athlete should be evaluated for level of consciousness, steadiness of gait, orientation, posttraumatic amnesia, and retrograde amnesia. Those players with Grade 1 concussions should be observed for 15 to 20 minutes. If the sensorium totally clears, and there are no residual symptoms, the athlete may be allowed to return to the game. Any persistent symptoms, such as headache, dizziness, or confusion, necessitate removal from competition and evaluation by a physician.[55] An athlete with a Grade 2 concussion should be removed from the game. Evaluation by a physician is suggested in most cases. In Grade 3 concussion, there is prolonged or severe alteration in the athlete's level of consciousness or orientation, or other neurologic deficit. Transport to a hospital for emergency evaluation of the player by a neurosurgeon and diagnostic neuroimaging should be immediately undertaken.[26] A very important point is that the head-injured athlete with any alteration in level of consciousness should be assumed to have an injured spine and managed as such until proven otherwise. A cervical collar and long spine board should be used to prevent any secondary injury to the player until spinal involvement can be definitely excluded.[1]

The unconscious athlete must be treated as any other unconscious patient. The airway must be secured and adequate breathing ensured. The protection of the airway may occasionally require emergent intubation. Hemodynamic monitoring should ensure adequate circulation. If there are any focal neurologic changes such as posturing or a dilated pupil, moderate hyperventilation can be undertaken. After the airway is secured, the spine is protected and the patient is rapidly transported to a trauma center for assessment.[1] If the injured athlete is helmeted, the helmet should not be removed until the integrity of the cervical spine is ensured, provided adequate protection of the airway is possible with the helmet in place. If helmet removal is necessary, the shoulder pads and helmet should be removed as a unit in order to maintain neutral spine alignment.[40]

Treatment of Athletic Head Injuries

The treatment of head-injured athletes and those individuals with nonathletic head injuries does not differ. Comprehensive guidelines for management of severe head injury have been published elsewhere.[24] Severe diffuse axonal injury can be neurologically devastating and places the athlete who survives in need of long-term care and rehabilitation. Epidural hematoma and significant subdural hematoma are typically managed surgically, as are very large intracerebral hematomas that cause mass effect. Although many patients with epidural hematoma recover well, acute subdural hematoma requiring surgery is associated with a very high mortality rate, up to 60% in some series.[8]

Conclusion

Contact sports carry certain risks. One of these is the risk to the players of sustaining head injuries. Although for years the player sustaining a mild head injury was considered to have had his "bell rung," it is now apparent that significant neuropsychologic and cognitive problems can result from even the minor injuries. Rarely, a player may even die after multiple mild injuries from changes in cerebral vascular autoregulation[45] (the so-called second impact syndrome). For these reasons, the team medical staff, coaches, and trainers must diligently and thoroughly evaluate players with suspected head injury. Those athletes allowed to play again must be completely symptom free. The team medical staff must also be able to recognize which players require further testing or treatment for more ominous forms of head injury.

The only difference in head injury among athletes and nonathletes is the preventable nature of athletic head injury. The same spectrum of injury occurs, and initial management, treatment, and outcomes are no different. The major issue then becomes the judgment regarding which player can return to competition and risk further injury. Some players who sustain concussion may safely return to play again, whereas others should be counseled to avoid further risk. It is the task of the team medical staff to make the right decisions for the players' well being, not in the context of pressure to return athletes to the team.[11, 18, 41]

ATHLETIC NECK INJURY

Among survivable traumatic injuries, spinal cord injury is perhaps the most devastating. In the United States, 2% to 3% of sports injuries involve the spinal cord, bony vertebral column, or its supporting ligamentous structures.[4] Mild cervical ligamentous sprain injuries are also very common. These injuries produce effects ranging from missed competition to chronic pain, functional disability, and permanent neurologic deficit.

Just as in sports-related head injuries, American football is the organized activity most commonly associated with cervical spine injuries[4] (Fig. 6–4). Among the recreational sports, cevical spine injuries occur most commonly in diving.[4] Ice skating, hockey, rugby, snow skiing, baseball, gymnastics (Fig. 6–5), soccer, and other activities also occasionally lead to spine injuries.[4, 6, 10, 25, 49] The most common sports associated with vertebral column injury in the United States are football and wrestling (with C5 being the most commonly injured level). Football, wrestling, and gymnastics are the most common activities resulting in neurologic deficit from cervical spine trauma.[5]

Owing to limited organization, protective equipment, rules, and supervision, it is very difficult to affect the incidence of spinal injury in recreational athletic activities. Organized sporting activity, however, can be policed in such a way as to reduce the number of spinal injuries. For example, the National Collegiate Athletic Association (NCAA) successfully lowered the incidence of cervical injury among college football players in the 1970s. After studying the biomechanics and mechanisms of football-related spinal injury, rule changes were made to decrease the use of certain playing techniques that had been determined to carry high risk of cervical spine injury.[10, 51, 53, 66]

In spite of much work done to characterize athletic spinal injury, determine its etio-

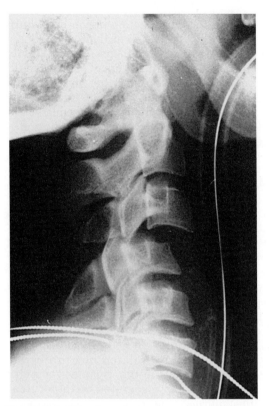

Figure 6–4. Lateral cervical spine radiograph demonstrates facet fracture and subluxation between C3 and C4 in a college football player.

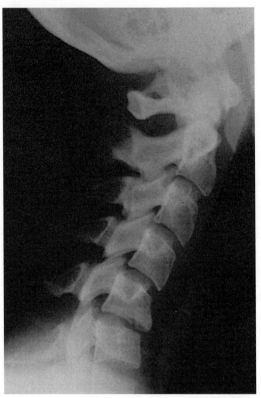

Figure 6–5. Lateral cervical spine radiograph demonstrates facet dislocation between C5 and C6 in a teenage gymnast. This is a common injury and is produced by the hyperflexion mechanism.

logic factors, and institute prevention programs, there remain the unfortunate few athletes annually who sustain this potentially devastating blow. Coaches, trainers, and team medical personnel must have a plan for dealing with these injuries in an organized way when they occur. Although the effects of primary neurologic injury usually are irreparable, secondary neurologic injury must be avoided by proper and rapid stabilization, evaluation, transport, and treatment of athletes who sustain cervical spine injuries on the playing fields of various sports.

Types of Athletic Neck Injuries

Before the management of cervical spine injuries can be adequately discussed, it is necessary to review the spectrum of injuries that occur. Team medical personnel responsible for the on-field management of these injuries must be aware of the conditions they would presume to treat. The various types of cervical spine injuries that occur in

athletics have been previously classified[32, 58] by the authors (Table 6–3). Type I injuries are those in which the athlete sustains permanent spinal cord injury. This includes both immediate, complete paralysis and incomplete spinal cord injury syndromes. The incomplete injuries are of four types:

Table 6–3. Types of Cervical Spine Injuries

Neurologic Injury

Type I (permanent injury)
Type II (transient injury)

Radiographic Abnormality (Type III Injury)

Fractures
Stable
Unstable
Spinal stenosis
Ligamentous instability
Posterior ligamentous compromise
Congenital fusion
Degenerative disease
Spear tackler's spine
Disk disease

Brown-Séquard syndrome, anterior spinal syndrome, central cord syndrome, and mixed types. The Brown-Séquard injury involves motor and contralateral sensory deficits below the level of the lesion. Anterior spinal syndrome patients have only posterior column function preserved, resulting in functional loss of movement and pain and temperature sensations. Central cord syndrome involves weakness of the upper extremities in excess of lower extremity findings secondary to selective damage to fibers in the central portion of the spinal cord that subserve arm and hand function. Various mixed types of spinal cord injury also occur, such as the finding of crossed motor and sensory deficits with upper extremities more prominently involved, which the authors consider a central cord/Brown-Séquard variant. Occasionally, the neurologic injury may be relatively minor, but is associated with demonstrable spinal cord pathology on imaging studies. For example, a high intensity lesion within the spinal cord seen on magnetic resonance imaging documents a spinal cord contusion (Fig. 6–6). Either clinical or radiographic evidence of spinal cord involvement essentially precludes further participation in contact sports.

The Type II injury is a transient neurologic deficit after trauma occurring in individuals with normal radiographic studies. These deficits completely resolve within minutes to hours, and eventually the athlete has a normal neurologic examination. An example of the type II injury is the "burning hands syndrome" described by Maroon.[34] This syndrome is characterized by burning dysesthesias of the hands and associated weakness in the hands and arms. It is thought to be a variant of the central cord syndrome. The majority of these patients have normal radiographic studies, and their symptoms completely resolve within about 24 hours.

The return of an athlete with a Type II injury to competition must be evaluated on a case by case basis. Those with no residual deficit who truly have a normal radiographic spine, including the absence of congenital conditions that yield a propensity for injury (e.g., spinal canal stenosis), may often return. However, athletes with repeated transient neurologic injury from sports should be considered at high risk for permanent injury and counseled to cease their participation in competitive sports.

Those individuals who have solely radiographic abnormalities comprise the Type III athletic spinal injuries. This category includes fractures, fracture-dislocations, pure ligamentous and soft tissue injuries, and herniated intervertebral disks. The multiple types of injury, along with the varying degrees of severity associated with a given bony or soft tissue vertebral column injury, make determination of future playing status

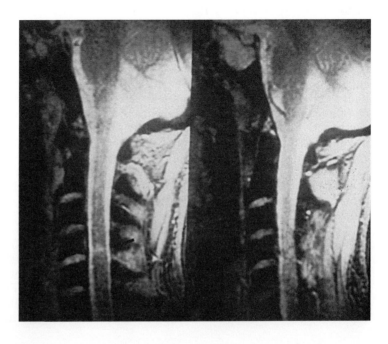

Figure 6–6. Mid-sagittal T_2-weighted magnetic resonance imaging scan reveals a high-intensity lesion at the C4–C5 level, representing a cervical spinal cord contusion *(arrow)*.

difficult. Some determination must be made as to the stability of the injury with and without treatment. Biomechanical considerations come heavily into play when discussing stability,[62] but the difficulty in athletes arises owing to the large forces to which athletes are subjected. Stability is traditionally defined in terms of normal physiologic loads,[62] and even a surgically repaired injury that is healed and stable for normal activities may be insufficient to sustain sports-related trauma safely.[52] Therefore, determination of whether an athlete can return to play another day may only be handled in a diligent, case-specific manner.

Torg and his colleagues[53] described a group of athletes who are at particularly high risk for the development of cervical spinal cord injuries because of a collection of congenital cervical spine features they termed the spear tackler's spine. This study demonstrated that football players with congenital cervical stenosis, straightened or reversed cervical lordosis, radiographic evidence of pre-existing cervical spine abnormalities, or a history of using spear tackling techniques are predisposed to cervical spine injuries from axial loading. When the congenitally narrow cervical spine is straightened, impact at the top of the helmet causes the neck to buckle as the head stops its motion while the trunk continues forward. The athletes Torg described were habitual users of the spear tackle and had radiographic evidence of previous injuries, such as healed compression fractures, intervertebral disk bulging or herniation, or ligamentous instability. Four of the 15 patients in the series who were investigated because of symptoms referable to the cervical spinal cord or brachial plexus sustained permanent neurologic injuries. Torg and his associates recommended that those players with the syndrome of spear tackler's spine not be allowed to participate in contact sports unless spearing techniques were adjusted and the cervical lordosis regained.

In addition to the previously mentioned types of spinal injuries, the medical team must be aware of the "burner" or "stinger" injury. This is characterized by burning dysesthesias usually beginning in the shoulder and radiating unilaterally into the arm and hand. There is occasionally associated weakness or numbness in a C5 and C6 nerve root distribution. This is a common injury, reported to occur in about half of college level football players in a given season.[15, 59] The stinger usually resolves in minutes, but sometimes the symptoms persist for days to a few weeks, including most commonly numbness or weakness. However, there is no lasting neurologic deficit in most cases. The stinger is thought to result from traction on the upper trunk of the brachial plexus that happens as force is directed onto the ipsilateral shoulder while the neck is in contralateral lateral flexion.[43] Another mechanism is impingement on the nerve root within the neural foramen ipsilaterally as the spinal column is briefly compressed in the axial direction. The clue that this is not a spinal cord injury is the unilaterality, brevity of the symptoms, and pain-free range of cervical motion. The determination of whether an injury is related to the spinal cord or merely a stinger should be made with caution because the answer to that question has great implications for the initial management of the athlete and his or her playing status.[32] When the player is pain and symptom free, can demonstrate full pain-free cervical range of motion, and has full muscle strength in the involved upper extremity, return to the playing field is allowed.[55]

On-field Evaluation and Management of the Athlete With a Neck Injury

When one is dealing with potentially injured athletes, it is vital to remember that an unstable spine injury can be easily converted into an injury with permanent neurologic deficit if the athlete is mishandled. Vegso[55] has pointed out that because severe athletic injuries are relatively rare, the experience of the on-site medical staff is usually limited. Thus, everyone who shares responsibility for managing spine-injured athletes should be adequately trained and frequently refreshed in the care of any situation that may arise. Prior preparation should ensure that all of the proper equipment, such as a spine board, cervical collars or immobilization devices, and stretcher, is available. There should be a clear hierarchy among the medical staff, with one member designated as the "captain" who directs the efforts of the team (Fig. 6–7). In addition, arrangements should be made in advance to have emergency medical services on site or close

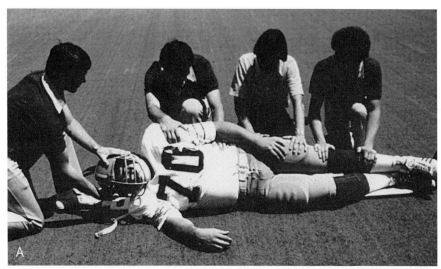

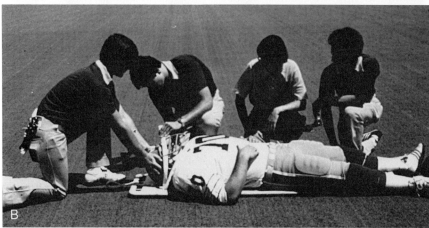

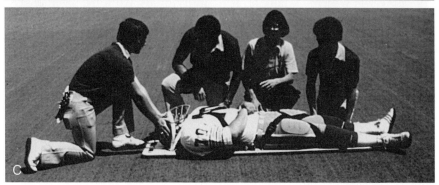

Figure 6–7. The proper technique is shown for moving the athlete believed to have a cervical spine injury. *A,* The medical team log-rolls the player onto a long spine board, with one member of the team solely responsible for the immobilization and neutral alignment of the player's head and neck. *B,* One medical team member continues to provide in-line immobilization of the player's head while another member secures the head to the board. *C,* The player is now ready for transport. Note that unless the airway is compromised, the helmet and facemask are left in place.

at hand. Preparation allays discomfort among providers and fosters efficiency and good decision making on behalf of the injured participant.[30] Finally, those who would manage injured athletes must be aware of the relevant medicolegal concerns.[19, 41]

Primary neurologic injury is that sustained at the time of impact. The severity of the primary injury is assessed once the player reaches a medical facility, and measures are undertaken to prevent secondary injury. Secondary neurologic injury is sustained after the occurrence of the primary injury, and results from a biochemical cascade of events such as hemorrhage, release of vasoactive amines, and edema formation.[65] As previously discussed, the prevailing goal among the medical team members should be the prevention of secondary neurologic injury due to improper handling of the fallen athlete. Cervical spine injury should be suspected and the athlete managed as if the injury were present whenever the mechanism of injury involves forced movement of the head and neck,[30] even in the absence of neurologic deficit. The head and neck of the player should be immediately immobilized in a neutral position. As in any resuscitation, assessment of airway, breathing, and circulation should proceed, as well as evaluation of the athlete's level of consciousness. Unless the player is unconscious or airway considerations exist, he or she should not be repositioned until safe transferral onto a spine board can be accomplished. If the player is wearing a helmet, it should be left in place until adequate immobilization of the head and neck can be instituted. Then the helmet can be gently removed in line with the neck without flexion or extension, but only in conjunction with simultaneous shoulder pad removal.[48, 56] The occiput should be firmly supported during and after helmet removal.[55] It is ordinarily not necessary to remove the helmet for airway access.[56]

If athletes are unconscious, they are usually best managed by log-rolling them into a supine position, removing the mouthpiece (if present), and evaluating the breathing pattern. If no breathing is present, any type of facemask worn by the player must be removed to facilitate rescue breathing. The techniques of rescue breathing follow general guidelines as taught in cardiopulmonary resuscitation courses. However, it should be kept in mind that significant structural and/or neurologic injury could occur with an injured cervical spine because of improper rescue breathing and subsequent intubation. Thus, any unconscious athlete should be treated as though a significant cervical spine injury exists until proven otherwise.[55]

As soon as the adequate airway, breathing, and circulation of the player are ensured, a thorough neurologic examination should be undertaken. Level of consciousness, pupillary response, response to pain, abnormal movements or posturing, as well as flaccidity or rigidity should be noted[55] as obvious indicators of head or spinal injury. Often, however, the team physician or trainer must actively seek clues to spine or spinal cord injury,[33] as the findings may be very subtle. Neck pain, numbness, dysesthetic pain, or weakness imply cervical spine or spinal cord injury. Especially foreboding is bilateral involvement of the upper extremities or the presence of neurologic deficits in both the arms and the legs.

The athlete with any signs or symptoms of bony or neural element cervical injury must be completely immobilized until radiographic studies and further assessment can be completed. A cervical collar should be placed to immobilize the cervical spine. Once the equipment and personnel are available to transport the player off the field, the log-roll technique may be employed to safely place the athlete onto a spine board. This is ordinarily accomplished with four individuals working together. One member of the medical team should apply gentle in-line immobilization of the cervical spine. This person counts and directs the movement of the athlete, functioning as the leader of the team. Another person is responsible for the torso, pelvis, and hips, and a third team member for the pelvis and legs. A fourth individual moves the spine board into place.[1] Teamwork, prior rehearsal, and coordination are essential. Circumstances surrounding the downed athlete with cervical injury often are fraught with fear, excitement, and confusion, making the medical teamwork's synergy of utmost importance.

The leader of the team maintains immobilization of the head and neck while the others grasp the side of the injured player opposite from themselves. On the count of the leader, the assistants gently and slowly roll the patient toward themselves, maintaining the spine in a straight line. The degree of roll should be as minimal as possible to allow the fourth assistant to slide the spine board under the player. Caution must be exercised at all times to avoid excessive movement and maintain the neutral position of the spine. Once the player is on the board, straps and pads are used to secure the position to avoid movement. To avoid the development of pressure sores, the player should be removed from the board as soon as possible.[1] After immobilization and placement on the spine board, the athlete is transported to a hospital where radiographic and clinical assessment can define the injury and appropriate therapy can be instituted.

Treatment of Athletic Neck Injuries

The treatment of the various forms of cervical spine injury has been previously summarized by the authors[5] and others[52] and follows established guidelines. As mentioned, the emphasis must be on preventing secondary or further neurologic injury through suboptimal management. Proper management begins with immobilization of the spine and withdrawal of the player from competition until the exact nature of the injury is delineated. When a vertebral column or a neurologic injury is identified, the athlete must be transferred promptly to a facility for definitive management.[33]

The initial caregivers of the spine and spinal cord–injured athlete must be aware of the potential for respiratory failure and hemodynamic instability. In addition, associated lesions such as head injuries may affect the timing and order of needed treatments.[4, 5, 10, 33] Owing to these concerns, patients with acute neurologic deficit from spinal cord injuries are initially managed in an intensive care environment. In the presence of neurologic deficits from spinal cord injury, methylprednisolone has been clearly shown to be beneficial if given in the first 8 hours from the time of injury.[20]

After initial resuscitation and radiographic evaluation of the player has been accomplished, informed decisions concerning management of the specific injuries can be made. Some body injuries, such as spinous process fractures or unilateral laminar fractures, may require no treatment or only immobilization in a cervical collar. Others, such as the bilateral pars interarticularis fracture of C2 (hangman's fracture), often may be treated with a cervical collar, or, in some cases, halo vest immobilization. Unstable injuries should initially be reduced and temporarily stabilized with cervical traction using Gardner-Wells tongs or a halo ring device. Contrast-enhanced CT scan or magnetic resonance imaging of the cervical spine oftentimes should be obtained prior to fracture reduction to rule out the presence of retropulsed intervertebral disk material. Unrecognized retropulsed disk material has been implicated in the sudden neurologic deterioration of patients undergoing reduction of their cervical fractures.[14] Surgical treatment may subsequently be required for severe vertebral body fractures, unstable posterior element fractures, Type II odontoid fractures, incomplete spinal cord injuries with canal or cord compromise, and in those patients with progression of their neurologic deficit to higher levels of spinal cord function.[33]

Conclusion

Spinal cord injury is devastating for the victim and the victim's family. The nature of contact sports ensures that there will be the occasional spine or spinal cord injury. When this unfortunate event occurs, it is the role of the team physician and trainers to rapidly assess the situation, immobilize the spine, and prepare the athlete for transport to a facility where definitive diagnosis and treatment can be performed. Most importantly, the medical staff must do nothing that places the athlete in any danger of further injury. Nowhere is the adage *primum non nocere* more applicable than in dealing with neurologic injury, and athletic endeavors are no exception.

Prevention of sports-related spinal injuries is far more satisfying than any management scheme. Through improved equipment, coaching, education of players, and rules changes, much to that end has been recently accomplished. However, for those unfortunate athletes who still suffer from spine or spinal cord injury, the team medical staff must be ready to act rapidly and correctly.

SUMMARY

Athletes engage in their sports with little awareness of the risks involved. Team medical personnel must be vigilant to teach and enforce principles that will help to decrease the incidence of serious injury to the players. As a result of rule and equipment changes over the years, most organized sports are much safer for their participants. However, the inherent nature of contact and high-impact sports ensures that there will continue to be those unfortunate athletes who suffer head and neck injuries on the field of play. When these injuries occur, the team physicians, trainers, and coaches must be ready to manage them safely, effectively, and quickly. The rapid evaluation and treatment or transport of the neurologically injured athlete is the mission of the medical team. If this mission is carried out properly, the player will have the maximum chance of recovery and prevention of secondary injuries.

References

1. Advanced Trauma Life Support Manual. American College of Surgeons, Chicago, 1993.
2. Alves WM, Polin RS. Sports-Related Head Injury. In Narayan RK, Wilberger JE, Povlishock JT (eds): Neurotrauma. New York, McGraw-Hill, 1996, p 913.
3. American Academy of Neurology. Practice parameter. Neurology 1997;48:581–585.
4. Bailes JE. Spinal Injuries in Athletes. In Menezes AH, Sonntag VKH (eds): Principles of Spinal Surgery. New York, McGraw-Hill, 1996, p 465.
5. Bailes JE, Hadley MN, Quigley MR, et al. Management of athletic injuries of the cervical spine and spinal cord. Neurosurgery 1991;29:4.
6. Bailes JE, Herman JM, Quigley MR, et al. Diving injuries of the cervical spine. Surg Neurol 1990;34:155–158.
7. Boden BP, Kirkendall DT, Garrett WE. Concussion incidence in elite college soccer players. Am J Sports Med 1998;26:238–241.
8. Bruno LA, Gennarelli TA, Torg JS: Management guidelines for head injuries in athletics. Clin Sports Med 1987;6:1.
9. Buckley WE: Concussions in college football. Am J Sports Med 1988;16:1.
10. Cantu R, Cantu RC, Wilberger JE Jr. Sports-Related Spinal Cord Injury. In Narayan RK, Wilberger JE Jr., Povlishock JT (eds): Neurotrauma. New York, McGraw-Hill, 1996, p 1301.
11. Cantu RC. When to return to contact sports after a cerebral concussion. Sports Med Digest 1988; 10:1–2.
12. Carlsson GS, Svardsuud K, Welin L. Long-term effects of head injuries sustained during life in three male populations. J Neurosurg 1987;67:197–205.
13. Cattermole HR: Injuries from hovercraft racing. Injury 1997;28:25–27.
14. Chesnut RM. Emergency Management of Spinal Cord Injury. In Narayan RK, Wilberger JE Jr., Povlishock JT (eds): Neurotrauma. New York, McGraw-Hill, 1996, p 1121.
15. Clancy WG, Brand RL, Bergfield JA. Upper trunk brachial plexus injuries in contact sports. Am J Sports Med 1977;5:209–216.
16. Clarke KS. Epidemiology of athletic head injury. Clin Sports Med 1998;17:1–12.
17. Clemett RS, Fairhurst SM. Head injuries from squash: A prospective study. N Z Med J 1980; 92:663.
18. Davis PM, McKelvey MK. Medicolegal aspects of athletic head injury. Clin Sports Med 1998;17:71–82.
19. Davis PM, McKelvey MK. Medicolegal aspects of athletic cervical spine injury. Clin Sports Med 1998;17:147–154.
20. Faden AI. Pharmacological Treatment Approaches for Brain and Spinal Cord Trauma. In Narayan RK, Wilberger JE Jr., Povlishock JT (eds): Neurotrauma. New York, McGraw-Hill, 1996, p 1481.
21. Fick DS. Management of concussion in collision sports. Postgrad Med 1995;97:2.
22. Gerberich SG, Priest JD, Boen JR, et al. Concussion incidences and severity in secondary school varsity football players. Am J Public Health 1983;73:12.
23. Graham DI. Neuropathology of Head Injury. In Narayan RK, Wilberger JE Jr., Povlishock JT (eds): Neurotrauma. New York, McGraw-Hill, 1996, pp 46–47.
24. Guidelines for the Management of Severe Head Injury. Brain Trauma Foundation, 1995.
25. Hodge B. Common spinal injuries in athletes. Sports Nurs 1991;26:1.
26. Jaffe R. Sports medicine emergencies. Primary Care 1986;13:1.
27. Kelly JP, Nichols JS, Filley CM, et al. Concussion in sports. JAMA 1991;266:20.
28. Kelly JP, Rosenberg JH. Diagnosis and management of concussion in sports. Neurology 1997;48:575–580.
29. Lehman LB, Ravich SJ. Closed head injuries in athletes. Clin Sports Med 1990;9:2.
30. Lehman LB. Preventing and anticipating neurologic injuries in sports. Am Fam Physician 1988;38:4.
31. Lindsay KW, McLatchie G, Jennett B. Serious head injury in sport. BMJ 1980;281:20.
32. Bailes JE, Maroon JC. Spinal cord injuries in athletes. N Y State J Med 1991;91:44–45.
33. Maroon JC, Bailes JE. Athletes with cervical spine injury. Spine 1996;21:19.
34. Maroon JC. "Burning hands" in football spinal cord injuries. JAMA 1977;238:2031–49.
35. McAbee GN, Ciminera PF. Intracranial hematoma in experienced teenage equestrians. Pediatr Neurol 1996;15:235–236.
36. McCrea M, Kelly JP, Kluge J, et al. Standardized assessment of concussion in football players. Neurology 1997;48:586–588.
37. McCrory PR. Were you knocked out? A team physician's approach to initial concussion management. Med Sci Sports Exerc 1997;29(Suppl):S207–S212.
38. McLatchie G, Jennett B. Head injury in sport. BMJ 1994;308:1624–27.
39. Mueller FO. Fatalities from head and cervical spine injuries occurring in tackle football: 50 years' experience. Clin Sports Med 1998;17:169–182.

40. Palumbo MA, Hulstyn MJ, Fadale PD, et al. The effect of protective football equipment on alignment of the injured cervical spine. Am J Sports Med 1996;24:446–453.

41. Patterson D. Legal aspects of athletic injuries to the head and cervical spine. Clin Sports Med 1987;6:1.

42. Plum F, Posner JB. Supratentorial Lesions Causing Coma. *In* The Diagnosis of Stupor and Coma, 3rd ed. Philadelphia, F.A. Davis Co. 1982, p 119.

43. Poindexter DP, Johnson EW. Football shoulder and neck injury: A study of the "stinger." Arch Phys Med Rehabil 1984;65:601–602.

44. Rivara FP, Thompson DC, Thompson RS. Epidemiology of bicycle injuries and risk factors for serious injury. Inj Prev 1997;3:110–114.

45. Saunders RL, Harbaugh RE. The second impact in catastrophic contact-sports trauma. JAMA 1984; 252:4.

46. Scher AT. Rugby injuries to the cervical spine and spinal cord: A 10-year review. Clin Sports Med 1998;17:195–206.

47. Sonzogni JJ, Gross ML. Assessment and treatment of basketball injuries. Clin Sports Med 1993;12:2.

48. Swenson TM, Lauerman WC, Blanc RO, et al. Cervical spine alignment in the immobilized football player. Am J Sports Med 1997;25:226–230.

49. Tator CH, Edmonds VE: National Survey of Spinal Injuries in Hockey Players. CMAJ 1984;130:875–880.

50. Tegner Y, Lorentzon R. Concussion among Swedish elite ice hockey players. Br J Sports Med 1996; 30:251–255.

51. Torg JS, Vegso JJ, Sennett B, et al. The National Football Head and Neck Injury Registry. JAMA 1985;254:24.

52. Torg JS. Management guidelines for athletic injuries to the cervical spine. Clin Sports Med 1987;6:1.

53. Torg JS, Sennett B, Pavlov H, et al. Spear tackler's spine. Am J Sports Med 1993;21:640–649.

54. Tysvaer AT, Storli OV. Soccer injuries to the brain. Am J Sports Med 1989;17:4.

55. Vegso JJ, Lehman RC. Field evaluation and management of head and neck injuries. Clin Sports Med 1987;6:1.

56. Waniger KN. On-field management of potential cervical spine injury in helmeted football players: Leave the helmet on! Clin J Sport Med 1998;8:124–129.

57. Warren WL, Bailes JE. On the field evaluation of athletic head injuries. Clin Sports Med 1998;17:13–26.

58. Warren WL, Bailes JE. On the field evaluation of athletic neck injury. Clin Sports Med 1998;17:99–110.

59. Weinstein SM. Assessment and rehabilitation of the athlete with a "stinger." Clin Sports Med 1998;17:127–135.

60. Wekesa M, Asembo WW, Njororai WS: Injury surveillance in a rugby tournament. Br J Sports Med 1996;30:61–63.

61. Wetzler MJ, Akpata T, Laughlin W, Levy AS. Occurrence of cervical spine injuries during the rugby scrum. Am J Sports Med 1998;26:177–180.

62. White AA, Johnson RM, Panjabi MM, Southwick WO. Biomechanical analysis of clinical stability in the cervical spine. Clin Orthop 1979;109:85–96.

63. Wilberger JE, Maroon JM. Head injuries in athletes. Clin Sports Med 1989;8:1.

64. Wilberger JE. Minor head injuries in American football. Sports Med 1993;15:5.

65. Wilberger JE. Pharmacological Resuscitation for Spinal Cord Injury. *In* Narayan RK, Wilberger JE Jr., Povlishock JT (eds): Neurotrauma. New York, McGraw-Hill, 1996, pp 1219–1228.

66. Winkelstein BA, Myers BS. The biomechanics of cervical spine injury and implications for injury prevention. Med Sci Sports Exerc 1997; 29(Suppl):S246–S255.

67. Zetner J, Franken H, Löbbecke G. Head injuries from bicycle accidents. Clin Neurol Neurosurg 1996;98:281–285.

7

Guidelines for Safe Return to Play After Athletic Head and Neck Injuries

W. Lee Warren, Julian E. Bailes, and Robert C. Cantu

Physicians and medical personnel charged with the on-field care of athletes bear a serious responsibility. Their task requires awareness of the various types of injury that may occur during participation in a given sport as well as the skills to diagnose and properly manage these injuries. Physicians caring for injured athletes, in addition, must make the frequently difficult decision of whether or when the player may return safely to play after an injury. These decisions are much more difficult when the player has suffered a head, cervical spine, or spinal cord injury, as these injuries pose a threat to the future of the player in many ways.

Athletes with mild head injury are at risk for malignant brain edema and death if they return to play before their brain injury is completely resolved. This is known as the second impact syndrome.[23] Certain athletes, furthermore, will harbor anatomic characteristics in their cervical spines predisposing them to permanent neurologic injury if they return to play after seemingly minor injuries.[10] These extremes illustrate the spectrum of potential danger lurking for the athlete with neurologic or bony cervical spine injuries, and underline the importance of proper decision making on the part of the team health care providers. Peer and coach pressures frequently render athletes incapable of making good decisions regarding their own health. Thus, the team medical staff should have well defined guidelines to make these decisions using the player's best interest as the only underlying motive.

This chapter discusses guidelines for the rational determination of when or if an athlete with a head, cervical spine, or spinal cord injury may return to the field of play. The on-field management of athletic head and neck injuries is discussed in a previous chapter.

ATHLETIC HEAD INJURY

Athletes who die of an injury related to their sport most commonly do so as a result of head injury, particularly acute subdural hematoma[11] (ASDH). Although many sports have been linked to head injuries, the athlete who most frequently suffers a head injury is the American football player.[30] Boxing, rugby, and soccer are other team sports in which head injuries are common.

The devastation to the quality of life of a player who survives a severe head injury is obvious. However, a far more prevalent problem is the mild head injury, or concussion. Football, for example, is estimated to have more than 1.5 million participants annually in the United States. Approximately 20% of these athletes, or up to 250,000 players, suffer a concussion each year.[5, 30] While the concussion has often been considered a minor injury, it is now clear that some repeated mild head injuries portend long-term neuropsychologic sequels for their victims.[9, 15, 17, 22, 24, 30]

Assessment of the Athlete With a Head Injury

Any player who suffers a loss of consciousness or any alteration of his or her mental status, regardless of the brevity of the alteration, is considered to have a head injury.[2] In the unconscious athlete, the team medical staff must assume the presence of an associated neck injury, and proper precautions must be taken to ensure the immobilization of the cervical spine. If the player is awake, the level of consciousness or alertness is the most reliable finding for both the initial assessment of the head injury and for follow-up.[7] Orientation to time, place, and person should also be evaluated. The presence or absence of posttraumatic amnesia should be determined, along with the player's ability to retain new information (recalling the names of four objects after 2 minutes, repeating play assignments, etc.). Other neurologic symptoms should also be sought, such as headache, dizziness, incoordination, sensory disturbances, or motor deficits.[7]

The Glasgow Coma Scale (GCS, Table 7–1) should be used for any athlete with an altered level of consciousness, and is defined in the on-field management chapter. The GCS score is useful in the determination of severity of the player's injury, as well as in the reliable communication of injury severity to other health care providers. A severe head injury is one in which the postresuscitation GCS is 8 or less.[16] The GCS is also useful in predicting the outcome of an injury and in assessing the worsening or improvement of an injured player.

Table 7–1. The Glasgow Coma Scale

Eye Opening	
Spontaneous	E4
To speech	3
To pain	2
None	1
Verbal Responses	
Oriented	V5
Confused	4
Inappropriate	3
Incomprehensible	2
No sounds	1
Intubated	1T
Motor Responses	
Follows commands	M6
Localizes	5
Withdraws	4
Flexor posturing	3
Extensor posturing	2
No movement	1

Coma Score = E + V + M = 3–15

Intubated Patient = 3T–11T

The medical team must be aware of the various types of injury that may occur in athletes and be prepared to manage these injuries appropriately. The spectrum of head injuries athletes are susceptible to includes intracerebral hemorrhage, brain contusion, diffuse axonal injury, subdural hematoma, epidural hematoma, cerebral concussion, and second impact syndrome.

Life-Threatening Head Injuries

Epidural hematoma (EDH) is the most survivable hemorrhagic head injury if promptly recognized and appropriately managed.[1] EDH is usually produced when a skull fracture (typically the temporal bone) tears a meningeal artery, causing hemorrhage. Less frequently, the injured vessel is a vein, producing slower bleeding that most often is self-limiting. Classically, the patient with EDH will have transient loss of consciousness at the time of the injury, secondary to the force of the impact. This is followed by a "lucid interval," a brief period of arousal in which the patient may appear quite normal. As the volume of the clot expands and produces increasing mass effect on the brain, the patient then exhibits a declining level of consciousness and usually has an ipsilaterally dilated pupil. Unless evacuated surgically, the clot will frequently expand and produce decerebrate posturing, contralateral weakness, and ultimately death from brain stem compression.

Approximately one third of patients with EDH will demonstrate the lucid interval; a more common presentation is the player who does not initially lose consciousness, but who develops headache and declining level of alertness over time following the injury.[1] Some patients, conversely, will lose consciousness immediately following the injury and never awaken. EDH is usually associated with mild or absent underlying injury to the brain. Thus, if the clot is rapidly evacuated, patients frequently make a complete neurologic recovery.

ASDH is much more common in athletes than is EDH. Whereas EDH is associated with good outcome in many of its victims, ASDH carries an approximately 40% mortality rate.[4, 7] The athlete with ASDH is typically unconscious with or without a history of deterioration. Focal neurologic findings, such as pupillary asymmetry or decerebrate posturing, are often seen. These patients should be immediately transported to a facility with neurosurgical services where a CT scan can be obtained. Occasionally, a player may develop ASDH over several hours following the concussion. For this reason, all players who remain symptomatic from the initial injury for more than 24 hours should have a thorough neurologic evaluation, and computed tomography (CT) should be performed.[7]

Athletes harboring cerebral contusion or traumatic intracerebral hematoma most commonly have loss of consciousness or focal neurologic deficit. Those players without loss of consciousness may have persistent headache or periods of confusion after their head injury, as well as posttraumatic amnesia. Failure of the athlete's mental status to clear rapidly should lead the team physician to send the player for a CT scan, which will reveal the hemorrhage. Contusion and intracerebral hematoma require close observation, as they frequently lead to the development of significant mass effect or hydrocephalus and may require surgical evacuation.[1]

Diffuse axonal injury (DAI), or shear injury, is the shearing of multiple axons due to rotational forces. DAI is most commonly related to motor vehicle accidents, but occasionally it occurs in severe athletic-related head trauma. It is the most frequent cause of persistent vegetative state and significant disability following head injury. Athletes with DAI will usually have significant alterations in their level of consciousness.[7] Traumatic subarachnoid hemorrhage (TSAH) is infrequent in athletes with head injuries. When present, it is usually seen in association with DAI and is a consequence of significant force having been applied to the head.

A syndrome of massive cerebral edema and death in athletes who sustain relatively minor head injuries shortly after previous similar head injuries is well known.[6] The athlete, such as a player who sustains a minor concussion, is still symptomatic from the first injury, but returns to play without completely clearing his sensorium. This syndrome has been termed "second impact syndrome" and is thought to result from cerebral vascular sensitivity from the first injury. The second injury then leads to cerebral autoregulatory dysfunction, vascular congestion, and subsequent intracranial hy-

pertension. This can lead to the precipitous death of the victim, and has occurred in athletes with mild head injury without loss of consciousness. This subject is also covered in greater detail in Chapter 14.

Return to Play After a Life-Threatening Head Injury

An athlete suffering permanent neurologic morbidity from a head injury is precluded from further competition. However, the return to play decisions affecting those athletes making a complete recovery must be individualized. In general, if the athlete has been neurologically normal for more than 1 year, the potential for safe return exists. These decisions require good judgment and diligence on the part of the team physician and frank discussions of the potential risks with the player and his or her family.[7]

Return to collision sports after a hemorrhagic brain injury requiring surgery is not allowed. The altered intracranial dynamics created by scarring in the subarachnoid space would seem to eliminate much of the normal cushioning provided by the cerebrospinal fluid, creating a high propensity for repeat injuries. In the absence of data showing safe return to play in this patient population, prohibiting return seems most prudent. The only exception to this would be the EDH in which the underlying brain is normal and the player makes a complete recovery. These players may potentially return if asymptomatic for at least 1 year. Players in low-impact or noncontact sports must have individualized approaches to return.[7]

Concussion

Cerebral concussion, or minor head injury, has long been thought to be as simple as the symptoms and signs exhibited by its sufferers. Once the player with a concussion was asymptomatic, he or she was assumed to be "over" the concussion. Unfortunately, it is now clear that the residual effects of minor head injuries may be significant, especially in those athletes who experience multiple concussions.[9, 15, 17, 22, 24, 30] Some players demonstrate poor information processing and other significant neuropsychologic deficits that are cumulative in proportion to the number and severity of their concussions.

An athlete who suffers one concussion is four times more likely to suffer another than a player who has never had a concussion.[30] In the light of data concerning cumulative neuropsychologic deficits in victims of multiple concussions, this statistical relationship is quite concerning to those making return to play decisions.[18, 19] Also dangerous for the player with a concussion is the possibility of second impact syndrome if the athlete is returned to play prior to becoming completely asymptomatic.[6]

Return to Play Following a Concussion

Cantu has devised a grading scale to accurately describe the categories that most concussions will fit into, and return to play guidelines to go along with the classification system (Table 7–2). The information presented here will follow his guidelines. This subject is also covered in greater detail in Chapter 12.

Because of the possibility of second impact syndrome, no player should return to the field until he or she is completely asymptomatic. Many athletes with mild head injuries will develop posttraumatic symptoms such as headache, irritability, fatigue, dizziness, double vision, impairments in memory and concentration, or behavior problems. Any of these symptoms should preclude competition until evaluation by a neurologist or neurosurgeon is performed.

A player who sustains a mild concussion may return to play after 1 week if he or she is symptom free. A second mild concussion in the same season should sideline the player for at least 2 weeks and should prompt CT scanning to evaluate the athlete for intracranial pathology. If the CT is normal and the athlete is asymptomatic, the player may compete the next week. A third mild concussion in the same season should prompt the termination of that individual's season.

An athlete suffering a Grade 2 concussion should be prevented from competition for at least 2 weeks. If a second moderate concussion occurs in the same season, 1 month off and a normal CT scan should be required prior to return to the playing field. A third should end the season and possibly the career for the player.

A single severe concussion should sideline the player with a normal CT scan for at least 1 month. A second severe concussion should finish the player's season and likely the career in that sport. It is well established that multiple mild head injuries can lead to significant long-term neurobehavioral and cognitive problems. Those individuals susceptible to repeated head injuries should be strongly encouraged to consider withdrawal from the sport to prevent long term morbidity.

Conclusion

The athlete with a head injury must be managed diligently in order to prevent fur-

Table 7–2. Cantu Classification and Return to Play Guidelines for Sports-Related Concussions

	Grade I/Mild	Grade II/Moderate	Grade III/Severe
Description	No LOC or PTA <30 min	LOC <5 minutes PTA 30 min–24 hours	LOC >5 minutes PTA >24 hours
1st Concussion	May return to play if asymptomatic for 1 week	Return to play after asymptomatic for 1 week	Minimum of 1 month; may then return to play if asymptomatic for 1 week
2nd Concussion	Return in 2 weeks if asymptomatic for 1 week	Minimum of 1 month; may return then if asymptomatic for 1 week; consider terminating season	Terminate season; may return next season if asymptomatic
3rd Concussion	Minimum of 1 month; may return then if asymptomatic for 1 week	Terminate season; may return next season if asymptomatic	

LOC, Loss of Consciousness; PTA, post-traumatic amnesia.
Asymptomatic = No headache, dizziness, impaired orientation, impaired concentration, or memory loss at rest or during exertion.

ther neurologic injury, and to maximize the chance of recovery. Those who survive and recover, however, face, a second challenge. They must now decide whether to return to play their sport. It is the team physician's task to perform thorough neurologic examinations, and to provide the player and family with accurate information regarding the risks of returning to play. In those situations in which the player is permanently neurologically injured, or is believed to be at high risk for repeat injury, the team doctor must inform the player of these facts very clearly.

The decision to return a player to competition is in some ways a double-edged sword. Medicolegal concerns encourage caution in returning the athlete to competition.[13] On the other hand, the players, coaches, and families involved can exert tremendous pressure on the team physicians to clear a player to play. No motivation other than the long-term health and neurologic status of the patient should influence the return to play decision making process. The wishes of the parents, the player, coaches, and teammates must be secondary to the prevention of long-term neurologic morbidity for the injured player.

ATHLETIC NECK INJURY

Spinal cord injury is devastating for the victim and the victim's family.[21, 25] The nature of contact sports ensures that there will be the occasional spine or spinal cord injury. When injury happens, the team physician and trainers must be ready to rapidly assess the situation, immobilize the spine, and prepare the athlete for transport to a facility where definitive diagnosis and treatment can be performed. More importantly, they must do nothing that places the athlete in any danger of further injury.

Once the athlete has been treated for and recovered from his or her spine or spinal cord injury, the question of when or whether the player may return to competition arises. To properly answer this question, the team physician must understand the spectrum of injuries that occur, and must be familiar with their individual natural histories and outcomes. The authors have previously published a classification scheme for these injuries, and guidelines for their management[3, 8, 21] (Figure 7–1).

Types of Athletic Cervical Spine Injuries and Return to Play Guidelines

Injuries producing complete paralysis, along with the incomplete spinal cord injury syndromes, comprise Type I injuries. The four types of incomplete injuries are Brown-Séquard syndrome, anterior spinal syndrome, central cord syndrome, and mixed types. The Brown-Séquard syndrome usually occurs with penetrating injury mechanisms, but can occur in athletes with fractures or herniated intervertebral disks. The syndrome involves motor and sensory deficits on opposite sides of the body, below the level of the lesion. The anterior spinal syndrome exists if the player has lost function that is referable to the neural tracts in the anterior two thirds of the spinal cord, preserving only posterior column function. This results in functional loss of movement and loss of pain and temperature sensations. Weakness or sensory loss (pain, temperature, or sharp-versus-dull discrimination) of the upper extremities in excess of lower extremity findings defines the central cord syndrome. This distribution of deficits is thought to be secondary to selective damage to fibers in the central portion of the spinal cord that subserve arm and hand function. Several types of mixed spinal cord injury also occur. For example, some patients demonstrate crossed motor and sensory deficits with upper extremities more prominently involved, which we consider a central cord/Brown-Séquard variant. Finally, some athletes will have relatively minor neurologic injury but magnetic resonance imaging (MRI) will demonstrate spinal cord contusions or other abnormalities. Clinical or radiographic evidence of spinal cord involvement essentially precludes further participation in contact sports.

When a transient posttraumatic neurologic deficit occurs in individuals with normal radiographic studies, a Type II injury exists. Within minutes to hours, these deficits completely resolve, and eventually the athlete has a normal neurologic examination. Maroon described a syndrome of burning dysesthesias of the hands and associated weakness in the hands and arms.[20] This example of a Type II injury is known as the "burning hands syndrome," and is thought to be a variant of the central cord syndrome.

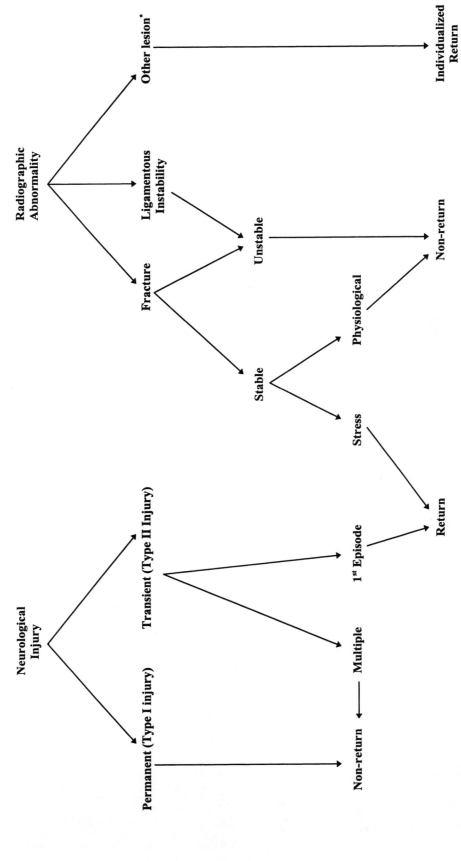

Figure 7-1. Classification and management algorithm for athletic neck injury. * = Posterior ligamentous compromise, congenital fusion, degenerative disease, herniated disk, spear tackler's spine, spinal stenosis, etc.

These patients usually have normal radiographic studies, and their symptoms completely resolve within about 24 hours.

Those athletes with a Type II injury who have no residual deficit, and who have a radiographically normal spine, including the absence of congenital conditions that yield a propensity for injury (e.g., spinal canal stenosis), may often return to play. However, athletes with repeated transient neurologic injury from sports should be considered at high risk for permanent injury and counseled to cease their participation in competitive sports.

Type III athletic spinal injuries are those in which the athletes have solely radiographic abnormalities. These injuries include fractures, fracture-dislocations, pure ligamentous and soft tissue injuries, and herniated intervertebral discs. Because it is often difficult to assess the severity of soft tissue injuries, and because of the many types of injury included in the Type III category, determination of future playing status is very difficult. The stability of the injury with and without treatment must be determined. Since stability is traditionally defined in terms of normal physiologic loads,[28, 29] a conservatively managed or surgically repaired injury that is healed may lack the biomechanical stability to safely sustain the forces associated with sports related trauma. Thus, return to play decisions in this group must be highly individualized.

Those athletes possessing the radiographic characteristics of "spear tackler's spine" (Table 7–3) are predisposed to cervical spine injuries from axial loading. When the congenitally narrow cervical spine is straightened, impact at the top of the helmet causes the neck to buckle as the head stops its motion while the trunk continues forward. Players with spear tackler's spine should not be allowed to participate in contact sports, unless spearing techniques are

adjusted and the cervical lordosis regained.[26]

Burning dysesthesias, beginning in the shoulder and radiating unilaterally into the arm and hand, are known as "burners" or "stingers."[12] There is occasionally associated weakness or numbness in a C5 and C6 nerve root distribution. This is a common injury, reported to occur in about half of college level football players in a given season. When the pain and symptoms have completely resolved, and the athlete has full, pain free cervical range of motion and normal muscle strength in the involved upper extremity, return to the play is permitted.[8, 27, 28]

Conclusion

The long-term health of and prevention of secondary neurologic injury to the athlete are the prevailing interests of the team physician. No other interest should influence the decision making process regarding the timing or permission of a player to return to competition. Since every athlete is different, return to play decisions often cannot be made according to a protocol. However, most injuries will fit within the framework presented here. Just as in head injuries, medicolegal action has been taken against team physicians for improperly allowing a player to return.[14] Therefore, the team medical staff must use good judgment with the best interest of the injured player in mind as these decisions are made.

Table 7–3. Constellation of Findings Defining "Spear Tackler's Spine"

Findings on lateral cervical spine radiograph:
1. Developmental narrowing of cervical spinal canal
2. Straightening or reversal of normal lordotic curve
3. Pre-existing evidence of post-traumatic cervical spine abnormalities

Plus, history of using spear tackling techniques

References

1. Alves WM, Polin RS. Sports-Related Head Injury. *In* Narayan RK, Wilberger JE Jr., Povlishock JT (eds): Neurotrauma. New York, McGraw-Hill, 1996, p 913.
2. American Academy of Neurology. Practice parameter. Neurology 1997;48:581–585.
3. Bailes JE, Hadley MN, Quigley MR, et al. Management of athletic injuries of the cervical spine and spinal cord. Neurosurgery 1991;29:4.
4. Bruno LA, Gennarelli TA, Torg JS. Management guidelines for head injuries in athletics. Clin Sports Med 1987;6:1.
5. Buckley WE. Concussions in college football. Am J Sports Med 1988;16:1.
6. Cantu RC: Second impact syndrome. Clin Sports Med 1998;17:37–44.
7. Cantu RC: Return to play guidelines after a head injury. Clin Sports Med 1998;17:45–60.
8. Cantu RC, Bailes JE, Wilberger JE. Guidelines for

return to contact or collision sport after a cervical spine injury. Clin Sports Med 1998;17:137–146.

9. Cantu RC. Reflections on head injury in sport and the concussion controversy. Clin J Sport Med 1997;7:83–84.
10. Cantu RC. Sports medicine aspects of cervical spinal stenosis. Exerc Sport Sci Rev 1999;23:399–409.
11. Cantu RC, Mueller F. Catastrophic spine injury in football, 1977–1989. J Spinal Disord 1990;3:227–231.
12. Clancy WG, Brand RL, Bergfield JA. Upper trunk brachial plexus injuries in contact sports. Am J Sports Med 1977;5:209–216.
13. Davis PM, McKelvey MK. Medicolegal aspects of athletic head injury. Clin Sports Med 1998;17:71–82.
14. Davis PM, McKelvey MK. Medicolegal aspects of athletic cervical spine injury. Clin Sports Med 1998;17:147–154.
15. Geddes JF, Vowles GH, Robinson SFD, Sutcliffe JC. Neurofibrillary tangles, but not Alzheimer-type pathology, in a young boxer. Neuropathol Appl Neurobiol 1996;22:12–16.
16. Guidelines for the Management of Severe Head Injury. Brain Trauma Foundation, 1995.
17. Hinton-Bayre AD, Geffen G, McFarland K. Mild head injury and speed of information processing: A prospective study of professional rugby players. J Clin Exp Neuropsychol 1997;19:275–289.
18. Kelly JP, Rosenberg JH. Diagnosis and management of concussion in sports. Neurology 1997;48:575–580.
19. LeBlanc KE. Concussions in athletics: Guidelines for return to sport. J La State Med Soc 1998;150:312–317.
20. Maroon JC. "Burning hands" in football spinal cord injuries. JAMA 1977;238:2031–2049.
21. Maroon JC, Bailes JE. Athletes with cervical spine injury. Spine 1996;21:19.
22. McCrea M, Kelly JP, Kluge J, et al. Standardized assessment of concussion in football players. Neurology 1997;48:586–588.
23. McCrory PR, Berkovic SF. Second impact syndrome. Neurology 1998;50:677–683.
24. Mendez MF. The neuropsychiatric aspects of boxing. Int J Psychiatry Med 1995;23:249–262.
25. Mueller FO. Fatalities from head and cervical spine injuries occurring in tackle football: 50 years' experience. Clin Sports Med 1998;17:169–182.
26. Torg JS, Ramsey-Emrhein JA. Management guidelines for participation in collision activities with congenital, developmental, or postinjury lesions involving the cervical spine. Clin J Sport Med 1997;7:273–291.
27. Torg JS, Corcoran TA, Thibault LE, et al. Cervical cord neurapraxia: Classification, pathomechanics, morbidity, and management guidelines. J Neurosurg 1997;87:843–850.
28. Weinstein SM. Assessment and rehabilitation of the athlete with a "stinger." Clin Sports Med 1998;17:127–135.
29. White AA, Johnson RM, Panjabi MM, Southwick WO. Biomechanical analysis of clinical stability in the cervical spine. Clin Orthop Res 1975;109:85–96.
30. Wilberger JE. Minor head injuries in American football. Sports Med 1993;15:5.

CONCUSSION

8

Overview of Concussion

Robert C. Cantu

Concussion is derived from the Latin concussus, which means *"to shake* violently." Initially it was thought to produce only a temporary disturbance of brain function caused by neuronal, chemical, or neuroelectrical changes without gross structural change. We now know that structural damage with loss of brain cells does occur with some concussions. In the last several years, the neurobiology of cerebral concussion has been advanced predominantly in animal studies but also in studies in humans as well. It has become clear that in the minutes to days following concussive brain injury, brain cells that are not irreversibly destroyed remain alive but in a vulnerable state. These cells are particularly vulnerable to minor changes in cerebral blood flow and/or increases in intracranial pressure and especially anoxia. Animal studies have shown that during this period of vulnerability, which may last as long as a week with a minor concussion, a minor reduction in cerebral blood flow that would normally be well tolerated actually produces extensive neuronal cell loss.[3, 4, 8, 9, 14] This vulnerability appears to be caused by an uncoupling of the demand for glucose, which is increased after injury, while cerebral blood flow is reduced. Although the precise mechanisms of this dysfunction are still in the process of being fully explained, it is now clear that although concussion in and of itself may not produce extensive neuronal damage, the surviving cells are in a state of vulnerability

characterized by a metabolic dysfunction that can be thought of as a breakdown between energy demand and production. Precisely how long this period of metabolic dysfunction lasts is not yet fully understood. Unfortunately, at present, there are no neuroanatomic or physiologic measurements that can be used to precisely determine the extent of injury with concussion, nor the severity of metabolic dysfunction, nor precisely when the concussion has cleared. It is precisely this fact that makes return to play decisions after a concussion a clinical judgment.

There is no more challenging problem faced by team physicians, athletic trainers, and other medical personnel responsible for the medical care of athletes than the recognition and management of concussion. Indeed, such injuries have captured many headlines in recent years and have spurred studies both within the National Football League and the National Hockey League. In discussions of concussion, it must be realized that there is no universal agreement on the definition and grading of concussion.[1, 7, 10, 13] Tables 8–1 to 8–8 present eight different attempts at grading concussion. As can be seen, all of the tables tend to focus on loss or retention of consciousness and on amnesia as hallmarks in the grading schemes. Furthermore, they perhaps tend to downplay the other signs and symptoms of concussion. As is commonly known, with concussion any combination of the following

---

Table 8–1. Cantu Grading System for Concussion[1]

Grade 1. No loss of consciousness; posttraumatic amnesia less than 30 minutes
Grade 2. Loss of consciousness less than 5 minutes in duration or posttraumatic amnesia lasting longer than 30 minutes but less than 24 hours in duration
Grade 3. Loss of consciousness for more than 5 minutes or posttraumatic amnesia for more than 24 hours

---

From Cantu RC. Guidelines for return to contact sports after a cerebral concussion. Phys Sportsmed 1986;14:76–79. Used with permission of McGraw-Hill, Inc.

Table 8–2. Colorado Medical Society Grading System for Concussion[12]

Grade 1.	Confusion without amnesia; no loss of consciousness
Grade 2.	Confusion with amnesia; no loss of consciousness
Grade 3.	Loss of consciousness

From Report of the Sports Medicine Committee. Guidelines for the management of concussion in sports. Colorado Medical Society, 1990 (revised May 1991). Class III.

Table 8–3. AAN Practice Parameter (Kelly and Rosenberg) Grading System for Concussion[7]

Grade 1.	Transient confusion; no loss of consciousness; concussion symptoms or mental status abnormalities on examination resolve in less than 15 minutes.
Grade 2.	Transient confusion; no loss of consciousness; concussion symptoms or mental status abnormalities on examination last more than 15 minutes.
Grade 3.	Any loss of consciousness, either brief (seconds) or prolonged (minutes).

From Kelly JP, Rosenberg JM. The diagnosis and management of concussion in sports. Neurology 1997;48:575–580.

Table 8–4. Jordan Grading System for Concussion[5]

Grade 1.	Confusion without amnesia; no loss of consciousness
Grade 2.	Confusion with amnesia lasting less than 24 hours; no loss of consciousness
Grade 3.	Loss of consciousness with an altered level of consciousness not exceeding 2–3 minutes; posttraumatic amnesia lasting more than 24 hours
Grade 4.	Loss of consciousness with an altered level of consciousness exceeding 2–3 minutes

From Jordan BJ, Tsairis PT, Warren RF (eds): Head Injury in Sports. In Sports Neurology. Aspen Publishers, 1989, p 227.

Table 8–5. Ommaya Grading System for Concussion[11]

Grade 1.	Confusion without amnesia (stunned)
Grade 2.	Amnesia without coma
Grade 3.	Coma lasting less than 6 hours (includes classic cerebral concussion, minor and moderate head injuries)
Grade 4.	Coma lasting 6–24 hours (severe head injuries)
Grade 5.	Coma lasting more than 24 hours (severe head injuries)
Grade 6.	Coma, death within 24 hours (fatal head injuries)

From Ommaya AK. Biomechanics of Head Injury: Experimental Aspects. In Nahum AM, Melvin J (eds): Biomechanics of Trauma. Appleton & Lange, 1985, pp 245–269.

Table 8–6. Nelson Grading System for Concussion[10]

Grade 0.	Head struck or moved rapidly; not stunned or dazed initially; subsequently complains of headache and difficulty in concentrating.
Grade 1.	Stunned or dazed initially; no loss of consciousness or amnesia; sensorium clears in less than 1 minute.
Grade 2.	Headache; cloudy sensorium longer than 1 minute in duration; no loss of consciousness; may have tinnitus or amnesia; may be irritable, hyperexcitable, confused, or dizzy.
Grade 3.	Loss of consciousness less than 1 minute in duration; no coma (arousable with noxious stimuli); demonstrates Grade 2 symptoms during recovery.
Grade 4.	Loss of consciousness for more than 1 minute; not comatose; demonstrates Grade 2 symptoms during recovery.

From Nelson WE, Jane JA, Gieck JH. Minor head injury in sports: A new classification and management. Phys Sportsmed 1984;12:103–107. Used with permission of McGraw-Hill, Inc.

Table 8–7. Roberts Grading System for Concussion[13]

Bell Ringer.	No loss of consciousness; no posttraumatic amnesia; symptoms less than 10 minutes
Grade 1.	No loss of consciousness; posttraumatic amnesia less than 30 minutes; symptoms greater than 10 minutes
Grade 2.	Loss of consciousness less than 5 minutes; posttraumatic amnesia greater than 30 minutes
Grade 3.	Loss of consciousness greater than 5 minutes; posttraumatic amnesia greater than 24 hours

From Roberts WO. Who plays? Who sits? Managing concussions on the sidelines. Phys Sportsmed 1992;20:66–76. Used with permission of McGraw-Hill, Inc.

Table 8–8. Torg Grading System for Concussion[16]

Grade 1.	"Bell rung"; short-term confusion; unsteady gait; dazed appearance; no amnesia
Grade 2.	Posttraumatic amnesia only; vertigo; no loss of consciousness
Grade 3.	Posttraumatic retrograde amnesia; no loss of consciousness; vertigo
Grade 4.	Immediate transient loss of consciousness
Grade 5.	Paralytic coma; cardiorespiratory arrest
Grade 6.	Death

From Torg JS. Athletic Injuries to the Head, Neck and Face. St. Louis, Mosby–Year Book, 1991, p 226.

signs and symptoms may be encountered: a feeling of being stunned or seeing bright lights, a brief loss of consciousness, light-headedness, vertigo, loss of balance, headaches, cognitive and memory dysfunction, tinnitus, blurred vision, difficulty concentrating, lethargy, fatigue, personality changes, inability to perform daily activities, sleep disturbance, and motor or sensory symptoms.

The lack of a universal definition or grading scheme for concussion renders the evaluation of epidemiologic data extremely difficult. As a neurosurgeon and team physician, I have evaluated many football players who have suffered a concussion. Most of these injuries were mild and were associated with retrograde amnesia, which is helpful in making the diagnosis, especially in mild cases. I have developed a practical scheme for grading the severity of a concussion based on the duration of unconsciousness and/or posttraumatic amnesia, which has worked well for me on the field and sidelines (see Table 8–1). The most mild concussion (Grade 1) occurs without loss of consciousness, and the only neurologic deficit is a brief period of confusion or posttraumatic amnesia which, by definition, when present lasts less than 30 minutes.

With the moderate (Grade 2) concussion, there is usually a brief period of unconsciousness, by definition not exceeding 5 minutes. Less commonly, there is no loss of consciousness but only a protracted period of posttraumatic amnesia lasting over 30 minutes but less than 24 hours.

Severe (Grade 3) concussion occurs with a more protracted period of unconsciousness lasting more than 5 minutes. Rarely, it may occur with a shorter period of unconsciousness but with a very protracted period of posttraumatic amnesia lasting more than 24 hours.

In 1991 Kelly and coworkers[6] proposed another guideline regarding the severity of

concussion in which the most mild concussion (Grade 1) had no loss of consciousness and no posttraumatic amnesia, but rather just a brief period of disorientation or confusion. A Grade 2 or moderate concussion was one in which there was no loss of consciousness but posttraumatic amnesia was present. This essentially split my Grade 1 into two grades depending on whether amnesia was present. In their guideline, all athletes rendered unconscious were placed in the Grade 3, or severe, category. This guideline essentially has been adopted by the American Academy of Neurology and has been subsequently published by that organization. While it can be debated that posttraumatic amnesia of more than 24 hours may reflect a more severe brain insult than does 30 seconds of unconsciousness, both guidelines will prevent the second impact syndrome, as no athlete still symptomatic from a prior head injury is allowed to return to competition.

Today, it is recognized that after concussion the ability to process information may be reduced,[2] and the functional impairments may be greater with repeated concussion, suggesting that the damaging effects of concussion may be cumulative.[2, 15] Furthermore, it is in proportion to the degree the head is accelerated and such forces are imparted to the brain, that concussion may produce a shearing injury to nerve fibers and neurons. Fortunately, in the vast majority of concussions, clinical recovery is complete.

References

1. Cantu RC. Guidelines for return to contact sports after a cerebral concussion. Phys Sportsmed 1986;14:76–79.
2. Gronwell D, Wrightson P. Delayed recovery of intellectual function after minor head injury. Lancet 1974;ii:605.
3. Jenkins LW, Marmarou A, Lewelt W, Becker DP. Increased vulnerability of the traumatized brain to

early ischemia. *In* Baethmann A, Go GK, Unterberg A (eds): 1986, pp 273–282.

4. Jenkins LW, Moszynski K, Lyeth BG, et al. Increased vulnerability of the mildly traumatized rat brain to cerebral ischemia: The use of controlled secondary ischemia as a research tool to identify common or different mechanisms contributing to mechanical and ischemic brain injury. Brain Res 1989;477:211–224.

5. Jordan BJ, Tsairis PT, Warren RF (eds). Head Injury in Sports. *In* Sports Neurology. Aspen Publishers, 1989, p 227.

6. Kelly JP, Nichols JS, Filley CM, et al. Concussion in sports: Guidelines for the prevention of catastrophic outcome. JAMA 1991;266:2867–2869.

7. Kelly JP, Rosenberg JH. The diagnosis and management of concussion in sports. Neurology 1997;48:575–580.

8. Lee SM, Lifshitz J, Hovda DA, Becker DP. Focal cortical-impact injury produces immediate and persistent deficits in metabolic autoregulation. J Cereb Blood Flow Metab 1995;15:S722 (abstract).

9. Lifshitz J, Pinanong P, Le HM, et al. Regional uncoupling of cerebral blood flow and metabolism in degenerating cortical areas following a lateral cortical contusion. J Neurotrauma 1995;12:129 (abstract).

10. Nelson WE, Jane JA, Gieck JH. Minor head injury in sport: A new classification and management. Phys Sportsmed 1984;12:103–107.

11. Ommaya AK. Biomechanics of Head Injury: Experimental Aspects. *In* Nahum AM, Melvin J (eds): Biomechanics of Trauma. Appleton & Lange, 1985, pp 245–269.

12. Report of the Sports Medicine Committee. Guidelines for the management of concussion in sports. Colorado Medical Society, 1990 (revised May 1991). Class III.

13. Roberts WO. Who plays? Who sits? Managing concussions on the sidelines. Phys Sportsmed 1992;20:66–76.

14. Sutton RL, Hovda DA, Adelson PD, et al. Metabolic changes following cortical contusion: Relationships to edema and morphological changes. Acta Neurochir [Suppl] 1994;60:446–448.

15. Symonds C. Concussion and its sequelae. Lancet 1962;I:1.

16. Torg JS. Athletic Injuries to the Head, Neck and Face. St. Louis, Mosby–Year Book, 1991, p 226.

9

Ionic and Metabolic Consequences of Concussion

Christopher C. Giza and David A. Hovda

INTRODUCTION

Definition

Concussive brain injury has traditionally been defined as traumatically induced neurologic dysfunction, manifested primarily by transient alterations in consciousness and cognition. Recently, it is becoming accepted that concussive brain injury may occur without an overt loss of consciousness, and that the sequelae of this injury may be remarkably persistent.[1-3] This ambiguity in the definition of concussion is caused by a lack of objective neuroanatomic or physiologic measures with which to characterize this clinical phenomenon. However, as the systematic study of traumatic brain injury has progressed, it has become apparent that specific physiologic and metabolic patterns are associated with cerebral concussion. Better understanding of these patterns will allow more accurate prediction of the outcome for a given injury and for rational development of therapeutic interventions.

Three distinctive characteristics of concussive injury are the diffuse nature of the injury, the delivery of biomechanical forces to the brain, and a relative paucity of overt histologic damage. Much of the clinical dysfunction associated with concussion may be related to transient ionic and metabolic derangements that are not easily detectable with current neuroimaging techniques. Fortunately, at least in milder injuries, these perturbations can resolve fully without permanent sequelae. Nonetheless, these temporary neurometabolic alterations may signal a period of increased vulnerability to further insults (i.e., repeated concussion) that may then result in long-lasting deficits and structural damage.

This chapter first addresses the cellular cascades associated with posttraumatic changes in potassium, calcium, and magnesium, and the subsequent alteration of glucose utilization and energy production. Secondly, acute and chronic axonal injury mechanisms and clinical correlations are discussed. Finally, several special scenarios particularly relevant to athletic concussive injury are reviewed, including the following: (1) concussion, secondary injury, and repeated concussion; (2) use-dependent neuronal damage due to premature activation of the injured brain; and (3) concussion in the developing brain.

Fluid Percussion Model of Concussive Brain Injury

The vast majority of mechanistic data regarding ionic and metabolic changes after purely concussive brain injury comes from animal experiments utilizing a fluid percussion model.[4-7] In this paradigm, a plastic injury cap overlying the cortex (unilateral parietal or midline) is attached to a fluid-filled piston, which delivers a brief pressure pulse to the epidural space. By altering the magnitude of the pressure pulse, varying severities of concussive injury may be simulated. In the mildest cases, there may be only a few seconds of unresponsiveness and no histologic damage, whereas in the most severe cases, prolonged apnea, cerebral contusion, and even death may result.

The derangements seen in experimental animals have also been reported in brain-injured humans,[8, 9] lending merit to the use of these animal models for studying human traumatic brain injury (TBI). The general lack of morphologic damage after mild experimental fluid percussion is corroborated by countless negative computed tomographic (CT) scans performed on patients and players after concussion. However, this lack of readily visible anatomic damage does not necessarily indicate the absence of injury. Indeed, alterations in ionic fluxes, cerebral blood flow (CBF), and cerebral glucose metabolism have all been documented in brain-injured patients.[9, 10] Microdialysis probes can detect ionic disturbances, radio-isotope studies and transcranial Doppler imaging are used to follow changes in CBF, and positron emission tomography (PET) scans can measure and help quantitate alterations in cerebral glucose metabolism in humans after TBI. Mechanisms explaining chronic posttraumatic symptoms and deficits in the absence of obvious structural changes rely on demonstrating lasting alterations in cellular metabolism, subtle morphologic abnormalities, or persistent derangements in neurotransmission.

Cascade Overview

Traumatic brain injury (TBI) triggers a complex and interwoven sequence of ionic and metabolic events from which damaged cells may eventually recover or, in certain circumstances, degenerate and die (Fig. 9–1). These events are briefly summarized here, then discussed in greater detail and referenced in later sections. After concussion, there is a significant K^+ efflux from cells, owing to mechanical membrane disruption, axonal stretch, and opening of voltage-dependent K^+ channels. Nonspecific depolarization of neurons leads to release of the excitatory neurotransmitter glutamate, which compounds the K^+ flux by activating N-methyl-D-aspartate (NMDA) and D-amino-3-hydroxy-5-methyl-4-isoxazole-propionic acid (AMPA) receptors. In an attempt to restore the membrane potential, the Na^+,K^+-ATPase works overtime, consuming increasing amounts of ATP. To meet these elevated ATP requirements, there is a marked upregulation of cellular glycolysis, which occurs within minutes after TBI. During this period of hyperglycolysis, there is a commensurate increase in lactate production.

In addition to K^+ efflux, NMDA receptor activation permits a rapid and sustained influx of Ca^{2+}. Elevated intracellular Ca^{2+} can be sequestered in mitochondria, eventually leading to dysfunction of oxidative metabolism and further increasing the cell's dependence on glycolysis-generated ATP. Calcium accumulation may also activate proteases that eventually lead to cell damage or death, and, in axons, excess Ca^{2+} can lead to dys-

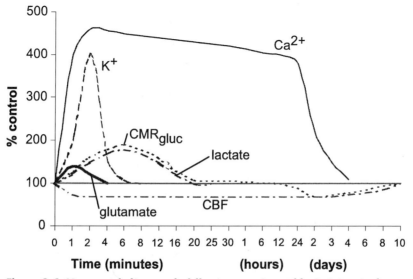

Metabolic cascade following traumatic brain injury

Figure 9–1. Neurometabolic cascade following experimental brain injury in the rat.

function and breakdown of neurofilaments and microtubules.

These ionic shifts and acute alterations in cellular energy metabolism occur in a posttraumatic setting where cerebral blood flow (CBF) is diminished, although not to ischemic levels. Rather, it is the mismatch between glucose delivery and glucose consumption that may predispose to secondary injury. CBF may remain depressed for several days after TBI, possibly limiting the ability of the brain to respond adequately to subsequent perturbations in energy demand.

After the initial period of profound postinjury ionic disturbance and resultant increase in glucose metabolism, the local cerebral metabolic rate for glucose ($lCMR_{gluc}$) decreases significantly below baseline, as does oxidative metabolism. In the rat, this period of diminished glucose metabolism is seen in the cerebral cortex ipsilateral to injury as early as 6 hours after fluid percussion and does not normalize until between 5 and 10 days later. Ipsilateral hypometabolism may also be seen in regions of the hippocampus at 6 hours postinjury, generally normalizing by 24 hours. The precise mechanism of this phenomenon is as yet unknown. It is currently uncertain as to whether this period of diminished cerebral metabolism is protective or whether it represents a second potential period of vulnerability.

POSTTRAUMATIC CELLULAR METABOLIC CASCADES

The immediate effects of TBI include ionic perturbations, changes in cerebral blood flow, and altered glucose metabolism. Derangements in neuronal ionic balance require massive expenditure of energy in an attempt to restore electrophysiologic equilibrium. Simultaneously, decreases in blood flow and substrate delivery may push metabolism to the breaking point. The magnitude of this "energy crisis" has important implications for cellular recovery and for increased vulnerability to secondary insults.

Potassium Cascade

Ionic Flux and "Spreading Depression"

Following TBI, the initial ionic response is an abrupt, marked elevation of extracellular potassium.[11, 12] Several mechanisms have been proposed to account for this efflux (Fig. 9–2). First, nonspecific breakdown of the plasma membrane may lead to K^+ leakage, particularly in the vicinity of contusions or hemorrhage.[11, 12] However, significant elevations of K^+ occur after concussive brain injury even in the absence of gross pathologic changes.[11, 13] This may be attributed to the diffuse mechanical force associated with brain trauma; indeed, deformation alone may induce depolarization and neuronal firing.[14] Some of this K^+ flux also seems to occur via voltage-gated K^+ channels.[13]

Another mechanism for posttraumatic increases in K^+ is through ligand-gated ion channels opened by indiscriminate release of excitatory neurotransmitters, particularly glutamate.[13, 15–17] Activation of kainate and AMPA receptors by excitatory amino acids (EAAs) allows the flow of both sodium and potassium ions across the cell membrane. EAAs also trigger NMDA receptors, which open channels permeable to Ca^{2+} in addition to Na^+ and K^+. Increased postinjury glutamate levels have been shown to correlate with increased K^+ levels, and treatment with the EAA blocker kynurenic acid greatly attenuates this posttraumatic elevation of K^+.[13]

In the normal brain, excess extracellular K^+ is subject to reuptake by surrounding glial cells.[18–20] This compensatory mechanism can maintain physiologic extracellular K^+ levels even after mild concussion or ongoing seizure activity.[21, 22] Larger insults, such as more severe concussive brain injury or ischemia, however, will overcome this glial safety valve.[23–25] Initially there is a slow rise in K^+, presumably owing to impaired glial reuptake. As the physiologic ceiling for K^+ balance is overcome, an abrupt increase occurs, leading to depolarization, release of EAAs, and further massive K^+ flux through EAA/ligand-gated ion channels. In the wake of this wave of excitation is a subsequent wave of hyperpolarization and relative suppression of neuronal activity.[26–30] This phenomenon is termed "spreading depression" and is a potential mechanism for movement of neurologic dysfunction across the cortical surface in clinical settings such as seizure propagation and migraine aura. In both seizures and migraine, the initial excitatory symptoms are followed by a postictal depression. One important difference between classic "spreading depression" and postconcussive K^+ release is that TBI affects wide

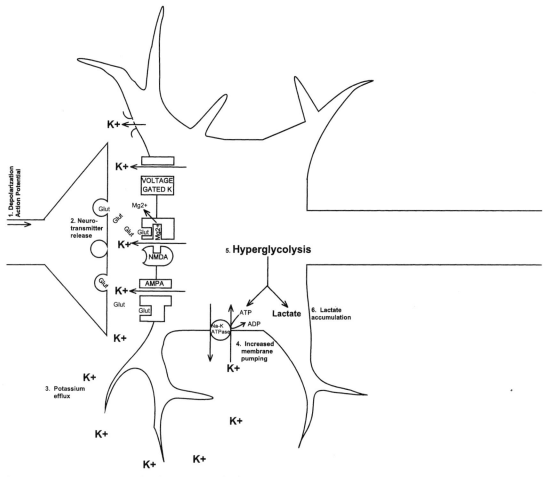

Figure 9–2. Potassium cascade after traumatic brain injury. (1) Mechanical stresses trigger membrane depolarization and action potential propogation. (2) Excitatory neurotransmitters are released. (3) Potassium exits the neuron via membrane disruption, voltage-gated K^+ channels, AMPA receptors, and NMDA receptors. The latter two are activated by the excitatory neurotransmitter glutamate. (4) Na^+,K^+-ATPase activity increases in an attempt to restore membrane potential. This creates a significant energy demand. (5) Glycolysis is increased to meet the elevated ATP requirements. (6) Lactate accumulates as a product of glycolysis.

areas of the brain simultaneously. Thus, loss of consciousness, amnesia, and cognitive impairment may be clinical correlations to post-TBI K^+ release and a "spreading depression-like" state.

Hyperglycolysis and Lactate Production

In response to pertubations of transmembrane ionic gradients, cells respond with an activation of energy-requiring ionic pumps[31–33] to attempt to restore the normal membrane potential. This results in an increase in glucose utilization. It is now well established that concussive injury to the brain also triggers dramatic increases in the $lCMR_{gluc}$.[34–36] Using 2-deoxyglucose autora-

diography in rats, $lCMR_{gluc}$ rose as much as 81% in cortex ipsilateral to injury. These elevations are seen immediately and persist up to 30 minutes after fluid percussion injury (Fig. 9–3[36]), and up to 4 hours after cortical contusion injury (in areas distant from the actual contusion core).[37] Increases in $lCMR_{gluc}$ are also seen over the same time course in ipsilateral hippocampus. It has been speculated that these changes are the result of increased energy needs in damaged cells attempting to restore ionic equilibrium. Given that cerebral oxidative metabolism normally runs near maximal capacity, it follows that acute increases in energy demand would necessarily require increases in glycolysis.[38, 39]

Acutely, there is some evidence that traumatic brain injury briefly disrupts oxidative

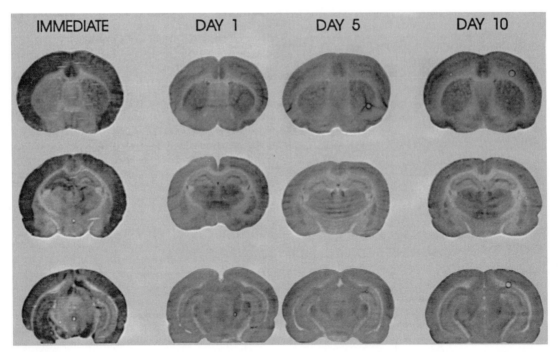

Figure 9–3. ^{14}C-2-deoxyglucose (2DG) autoradiograph time course after left lateral fluid percussion injury in the adult rat. Note the initial period of increased 2DG uptake followed by a relative decrease, returning to baseline by postinjury day 10. From Yoshino A, Hovda DA, Kawamata T, et al. Dynamic changes in local cerebral glucose utilization following cerebral concussion in rats: Evidence of a hyper- and subsequent hypometabolic state. Brain Res 1991;561:106–119 with permission from Elsevier Science.

metabolism. Following an impact accelera-tion injury, ADP levels in the brain stem were increased at 1 and 4 minutes,[40] as was oxygen utilization.[41] This transient defect in oxidative metabolism was hypothesized as due to mitochondrial dysfunction. Another study measured mitochondrial oxidative phosphorylation in rats after fluid percus-sion injury and found no clear evidence of impaired oxidative metabolism.[42] Specifi-cally, no significant changes in ADP per oxy-gen consumption ratio or in state 3 respira-tory rate were reported. Thus, traumatic brain injury does not lead to any apparent uncoupling between respiration and ATP synthesis, an important distinction from brain ischemia.

Lactate accumulation in the brain occurs after injuries leading to neuronal damage, such as ischemia,[43–45] and also after insults that do not cause overt morphologic change, such as concussion.[40, 46–50] Lactate levels may increase owing to either decreased metabo-lism or increased production. In ischemia, oxidative phosphorylation is impaired, and increases in lactate are likely as a result of decreased metabolism. Oxidative metabo-lism does not appear significantly impaired

immediately after concussive brain injury, while there is convincing evidence of an acute hyperglycolytic state after brain trauma.[34–36] The accumulation of lactate after concussive injury thus appears to be the result of increased lactate production, and is therefore fundamentally different from that seen in ischemia.

This hypothesis is supported by a study that showed that microdialysis infusion of glycolysis inhibitor 2-deoxyglucose-6-phos-phate attenuates lactate accumulation in vivo.[51] In addition, it is known that levels of cerebral hyperglycolysis correlate with in-jury severity, and posttraumatic measure-ments of extracellular lactate also demon-strate severity-dependent increases.[52, 53] Other studies demonstrated that by blocking the energy-requiring Na^+/K^+ pump with ouabain prior to injury, the postinjury lac-tate elevation was also significantly sup-pressed.[54] Unable to activate the Na^+,K^+-ATPase to restore ionic balance, there was no increase in energy demand or glycolysis, and hence, no increase in lactate. Elimina-tion of glial "safety valve" reuptake by infu-sion of barium placed greater reliance on the energy-dependent Na^+/K^+ pump, exacerbating posttraumatic hyperglycolysis and excess lactate production.[54] Finally, microdialysis perfusion of the broad-spectrum EAA antagonist kynurenic acid preinjury blunted the lactate response to injury,[54] presumably by diminishing the concussion-induced ionic flux and, hence, the need for energy-intense ion pumping.

Increased lactate levels post-TBI are the result of increased glycolysis and not due to significantly impaired lactate metabolism. Elevated lactate has been implicated in neuronal dysfunction by inducing acidosis, membrane damage, altered blood brain barrier permeability, and cerebral edema.[55–60] In TBI models, excess lactate appears to leave the affected cells more vulnerable to secondary ischemic injury.[61–63] It remains to be seen whether this relationship holds for trauma-induced lactate accumulation.

Relationship Between Potassium Efflux and Hyperglycolysis

Posttraumatic hyperglycolysis was connected with posttraumatic K^+ release by studies that examined the effects of EAA antagonists (which diminish K^+ flux) or a Ca^{2+} channel blocker on post-TBI glucose metabolism. The EAA antagonists used were APV, which selectively blocks the NMDA receptor, and CNQX, which acts only on non-NMDA receptors. Both EAA antagonists were effective in attenuating the posttraumatic hyperglycolysis,[64] while the Ca^{2+} channel blocker cobalt had no significant effect.[65] Among the EAA antagonists, APV had a more robust effect, suggesting that the NMDA receptor, rather than the AMPA receptor, plays the more prominent role in injury-induced hyperglycolysis. Further evidence of the importance of glutamatergic input in posttraumatic hyperglycolysis comes from a study where hippocampal CA3 lesions removed glutamatergic innervation to the CA1 region.[66] In CA3-lesioned animals after lateral FPI, the expected increase in $lCMR_{gluc}$ was seen in cerebral cortex, but no increase was seen in CA1 when compared with controls.

It appears that the primary ionic change seen postconcussion, that is, efflux of K^+, is significantly mediated through the NMDA receptor ionophore. This release of K^+ leads to increased metabolic demand as the injured cells attempt to restore normal membrane potential. Elevated energy requirements lead to hyperglycolysis and, in turn, accumulation of lactate. By blocking K^+ flux either with NMDA receptor antagonists or by lesioning glutamatergic inputs, posttraumatic hyperglycolysis can be attenuated. Diminution of post-TBI glycolysis proportionately alleviates increases in lactate.

Uncoupling of Cerebral Blood Flow and Glucose Metabolism

Alterations in cerebral blood flow (CBF) have been well documented in acute head trauma. Experimentally, fluid percussion injury may precipitate an almost immediate reduction of up to 50% in cerebral blood flow[67–70]; however, this reduction does not approach the levels associated with frank ischemia (85% reduction[71]). Clinically, human brain injury may also demonstrate decreases in CBF. Ischemia is not a major component of isolated concussive brain injury, although it may become a factor in the setting of severe cerebral edema, hemorrhage, or vasospasm.

Normally, cerebral blood flow is tightly coupled to cerebral glucose metabolism. Although posttraumatic decreases in CBF do not lead to overt ischemia, the injured brain may dramatically increase ATP utilization, requiring increased delivery of substrate to power cellular recovery mechanisms. In this setting of greater demand, impaired supply of metabolites may become an important factor in delayed injury or increased vulnerability to further insults.

This period of hyperglycolysis can be clinically significant for several reasons. First, it may serve as an acute marker for injury severity, with greater injury leading to larger K^+ efflux and concomitant increases in glucose metabolism. Second, hyperglycolysis may represent a period of increased vulnerability to a second insult. Although it lasts only a few hours in rats, in humans the period of increased glucose metabolism may be significantly longer. If the cellular systems are already overtaxed in terms of ATP generation, any further derangement in ionic balance may exceed the ability of these compensatory mechanisms and result in relative energy failure and permanent damage. Finally, the true determinant of injury severity and prognosis may be a factor that considers both the elevation in glucose metabolism and the decline in CBF. This would make CBF maintenance of paramount importance during the hyperglycolytic period. Careful monitoring of cerebral glucose and oxidative metabolism may provide the clinician with critical information regarding injury severity, vulnerability to further insults, and timing of recovery.

Calcium Cascade

Traumatic Brain Injury and Calcium Influx

After TBI, in addition to the K^+ efflux described above, there is a rapid and sustained influx of Ca^{2+}.[72-75] Neuronal depolarization and nonspecific membrane disruption after trauma lead to release of EAAs that, in turn, activate NMDA receptors. The activated NMDA receptor creates an open channel through which Ca^{2+} can enter the cell (Fig. 9–4). Calcium has been shown to accumulate in cerebral ischemia,[76-81] spinal cord contusion,[82-85] or concussive brain injury.[73, 86] The time course of calcium flux after fluid percussion injury has been well characterized, with an immediate increase in radiolabeled $^{45}Ca^{2+}$ accumulation, particularly in the cerebral cortex, dorsal hippocampus, and striatum ipsilateral to the injury. This elevation persists for at least 48 hours without resulting in significant morphologic damage, with the level returning to normal by 4 days postinjury. Administration of an N-type Ca^{2+} channel blocker diminishes the level and duration of posttraumatic $^{45}Ca^{2+}$ accumulation.[87, 88]

Inhibition of Oxidative Metabolism

When faced with excessive increases of intracellular Ca^{2+}, the cell may sequester calcium in mitochondria.[89, 90] Increases in mitochondrial Ca^{2+} can lead to metabolic dysfunction and, eventually, energy failure. Cytochrome oxidase (CO) histochemistry has been used to detect long-term changes in oxidative metabolism in many brain injury models.[91] In ipsilateral cerebral cortex, relative reductions in CO activity were detected 1 day after fluid percussion injury. This reduction in oxidative metabolism recovered on day 2 and was reinstated on day 3, becoming most pronounced 5 days after injury.

By 10 days, cortical CO activity recovered to normal levels. Lesser but more persistent changes were seen in ipsilateral hippocampus, with decreased CO activity evident up to 10 days postinjury in some regions. Other injury models in which diminished oxidative metabolism is seen include cortical contusion and ablation.

This reduction of oxidative metabolism occurs in the setting of a delayed posttraumatic decline in glycolysis, which is first evident as early as 24 hours after experimental FPI in the rat (Fig. 9–3). Diffuse postinjury impairment of glucose metabolism measured by 2-deoxyglucose autoradiography has also been reported after ischemia,[92-94] cortical freezing lesions,[95, 96] tumors,[93, 97] and neocortical ablations.[98, 99] Again, these posttraumatic changes in glucose metabolism may last significantly longer in humans. Overall decreased cerebral glucose metabolism may account for post-TBI impairments in consciousness, memory, and cognition. What is not clear is whether this hypometabolism is somehow protecting the injured brain from the detrimental effects of acute CBF/glucose metabolism mismatch or whether this represents a period during which the brain is metabolically unable to rise to the challenge of increased ATP demands. If the latter is true, this would be important for several reasons. One would be that a second ionic derangement, such as a second concussion, would be less rapidly compensated owing to insufficient energy to drive increases in Na^+,K^+-ATPase activity. The second consequence of an obligatory period of post-TBI metabolic depression might be that the brain is less able to be activated in response to stimuli, which has already been demonstrated experimentally in animals.[100, 101] In an athlete, an impairment of cerebral activation in response to stimuli might manifest as decreased performance, which in some sports would predispose the individual to a greater risk for a second injury. Similarly, the acquisition of new skills could be impaired during this period of metabolic depression. A final consideration would be that forced attempts to activate hypometabolic cortex may actually be damaging, a form of secondary injury. These ideas will be revisited later in this chapter in the section dealing with specific clinical scenarios relevant to athletic head injury.

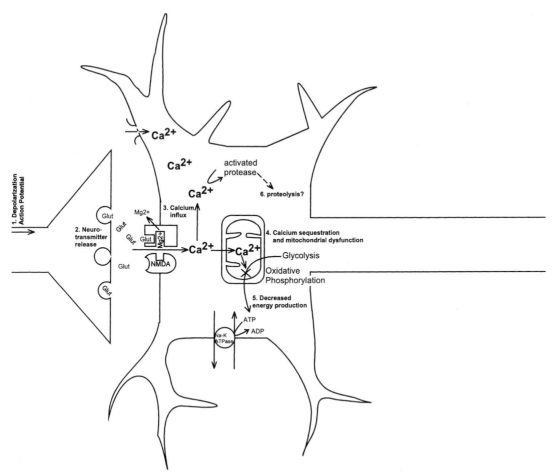

Figure 9–4. Calcium cascade after traumatic brain injury. (1, 2) Mechanical stresses trigger membrane depolarization, action potential propagation, and excitatory neurotransmitter release, as in Figure 9–2. (3) Activation of the NMDA receptor channel allows entry of calcium. (4) Excess intracellular calcium is sequestered in the mitochondria and can lead to metabolic dysfunction. (5) Impairment of mitochondrial oxidative metabolism results in decreased ATP production, with less energy to drive the Na^+,K^+-ATPase. (6) Additionally, intracellular calcium may activate proteases that degrade cellular proteins.

Delayed Cell Death and Secondary Degeneration

Intracellular accumulation of Ca^{2+} is of great importance given the well described role of Ca^{2+} in secondary cell death[102, 103]; however, the presence of increased Ca^{2+} postconcussion does not inevitably lead to detectable levels of neuronal loss. After mild and moderate experimental concussive injuries, Ca^{2+} accumulation peaks in 2 days and resolves, without significant cell loss, in 4 days.[73, 86] In animals sustaining more severe injuries and demonstrating morphologic damage, the elevation of $^{45}Ca^{2+}$ at the injury site persists beyond 4 days.[73] This suggests that there is a threshold of injury or Ca^{2+} accumulation, beyond which anatomic changes can be seen after concussive brain injury. However, these findings may also mean that there is a window of intervention for the reduction of post-TBI Ca^{2+} influx that may be neuroprotective.

Magnesium Cascade

After experimental traumatic brain injury, intracellular levels of Mg^{2+} have been shown to decrease significantly and remain depressed for up to 4 days.[104–107] This decrease in Mg^{2+} has been correlated with posttraumatic neurologic deficits in rats.[108] Using $MgCl_2$ or $MgSO_4$ the postinjury depression of Mg^{2+} has been partially alleviated, with concomitant improvements in neurologic motor performance.

There are many postulated mechanisms as to how decreased Mg^{2+} leads to neuronal dysfunction after brain injury (Fig. 9–5). Magnesium is so tightly woven into the fabric of cellular energy metabolism that a decrease in intracellular Mg^{2+} may have a multitude of detrimental effects.[109–111] Generation of ATP is impaired in both glycolysis and oxidative phosphorylation. Magnesium is also necessary for initiation of protein synthesis and maintenance of the cellular membrane potential.

In addition, the voltage gate of the NMDA receptor ionophore is dependent on the presence of Mg^{2+}. At rest, a Mg^{2+} ion obstructs the channel and is only dislodged by depolarization; in a stage of Mg^{2+} depletion, this voltage block may be overcome more easily, leading to greater influx of Ca^{2+} and its myriad of potentially dangerous intracellular sequelae.

DIFFUSE AXONAL INJURY

Originally, it was thought that the predominant form of traumatic axonal injury was due to mechanical disruption of axons owing to tensile forces at the time of injury. However, it now appears that a metabolic cascade also affects the integrity of axons, leading to a state of increased vulnerability[112, 113] from which the axons may either recover or degenerate (Fig. 9–6).

Acute Axolemmal Dysfunction

Acutely, stretch injury to axons leads to altered membrane potential and even depolarization. Changes in membrane permeability may be demonstrated up to 6 hours postinjury by horseradish peroxidase techniques.[114, 115] This increased axolemmal

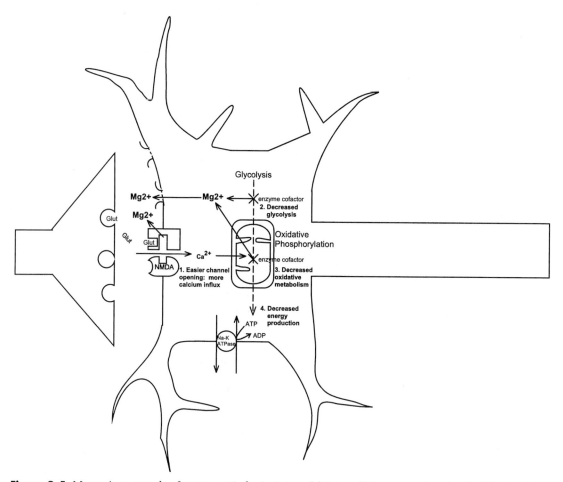

Figure 9–5. Magnesium cascade after traumatic brain injury. (1) Intracellular magnesium levels fall after injury, resulting in loss of the voltage block on the NMDA receptor channel, allowing greater calcium influx. (2, 3) Magnesium is a necessary cofactor for glycolytic and oxidative enzymes, and a decrease in the available magnesium inhibits both glycolysis and oxidative phosphorylation. (4) In turn, there is a decrease in the production of ATP and an overall reduction in the cell's bioenergetic state.

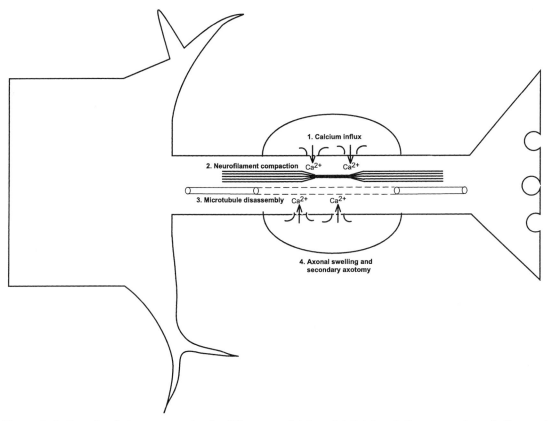

Figure 9–6. Cascade of changes occuring in diffuse axonal injury. (1) Calcium influx occurs through disrupted axolemma. (2) Neurofilaments compact due to either sidearm cleavage by proteases or conformational change mediated by changes in phosphorylation. (3) Microtubules depolymerize due to calcium alone or calcium-calmodulin. (4) Normally functioning axonal transport adjacent to the injured area continues to deliver organelles and substrates, creating an area of axonal swelling at the injury site. The myelin sheath loosens and the area of swelling develops a constriction, which ultimately divides the axon (secondary axotomy).

permeability appears to lead to axonal Ca^{2+} influx and mitochondrial swelling, which has been seen after primary axotomy following crush injury[116] and has more recently been reported after stretch injury without primary axotomy.[117]

Changes in the myelin sheath may be seen as early as 15 minutes following tensile axonal injury.[117] Loosening of the myelin sheath became more prominent over time, with myelin intrusions evident at 1 and 4 hours postinjury. Areas of abnormal myelination were associated with loss of ecto-Ca-ATPase activity and presumed elevations of free Ca^{2+} based on pyroantimonate precipitation.[117]

Microtubule Disassembly and Neurofilament Compaction

Axonal microtubules may be affected by Ca^{2+} influx in several ways. One subtype of microtubule, dubbed cold-labile, is exquisitely sensitive to Ca^{2+}, and rapidly broken down in the presence of elevated Ca^{2+}. Cold-stable microtubules, on the other hand, are more resistant to Ca^{2+}; however, when Ca^{2+} interacts with calmodulin, they, too, may undergo disassembly. Loss of microtubules appears most pronounced at the nodes of Ranvier, and may occur 6–24 hours after initial axonal injury, depending on the model.[118, 119]

Neurofilaments also undergo structural changes after axonal tensile injury. Starting as early as 5 minutes and lasting up to 6 hours after injury, neurofilaments may undergo compaction.[118] This decrease in interneurofilament distance is hypothesized to be caused by alterations in neurofilament sidearms, possibly by collapse or cleavage. Changes in phosphorylation may affect neurofilament structural stability or conformation.[120–122] Alternately, activation of calpain may lead to sidearm proteolysis and neurofilament collapse.[123]

Secondary Axotomy

Acutely after injury, structural changes in axonal microtubules and neurofilaments are seen, possibly in response to injury-induced Ca^{2+} influx. These disruptions lead to foci of impaired axonal transport. However, axonal transport continues to function in adjacent intact axonal segments. Thus, membranous organelles moving along the axon will accumulate in areas of cytoskeletal abnormality, leading to focal axonal swelling.[124] Over time, neurofilament compaction worsens, axolemmal-myelin connections are disrupted, and evidence of a constriction appears in the center of the area of axonal swelling.[125] This constriction ultimately leads to secondary axotomy with resultant formation of axonal bulbs. The earliest signs of secondary axonal disconnection are seen beginning 4 hours postinjury, but may continue to evolve over many days or even weeks in humans.[126]

SPECIAL SCENARIOS OF PARTICULAR RELEVANCE TO ATHLETIC CONCUSSIVE INJURY

Concussion, Secondary Injury, and Repeated Concussion

Concussive brain injury has been shown to elicit a neurometabolic cascade of acute ionic changes, metabolic perturbations, and axonal dysfunction. Longer term derangements that follow brain trauma include calcium accumulation, elevations in lactate, decreased glucose metabolism, decreased cerebral blood flow, axonal disconnection, and neurotransmitter disturbances. It is during this postinjury period, when energy metabolism may already be stretched to its limits, that the cell is most vulnerable to further insults.[127] Clinically, much of the management of the head-injured patient focuses on preventing delayed neuronal damage by maintaining cerebral perfusion, restoring electrolyte balance, providing adequate oxygenation, and minimizing excessive cerebral metabolic demands.

Hypoxia-Ischemia

Hypoxic-ischemic injury can occur in combination with concussive brain injury in the setting of an acute loss of consciousness with an inability to maintain airway patency, or after upper cervical spine injury with resultant respiratory paralysis. In either case, hypoxia may significantly exacerbate neuronal injury due to concussion and lead to neurocognitive sequelae in excess of that seen after concussion or hypoxia alone.

A study undertaken to describe the cumulative effects of mild fluid percussion brain injury and incomplete transient ischemia demonstrated no overt neuronal loss in the hippocampus after either injury alone. Silver staining for axonal swelling or retraction bulbs did not reveal evidence of diffuse axonal injury, and no significant macroscopic or histologic hemorrhage was reported. However, in the group subjected to mild concussive injury followed 24 hours later by transient ischemia, extensive neuron loss was detected in the CA1 region of the hippocampus as well as the subiculum.[62] The mild nature of the initial concussion should be emphasized, with unconsciousness times lasting less than 60 seconds, impaired motor functioning for less than 5 minutes, and no prolonged behavioral deficits. These findings would suggest that even after a brain injury unlikely to come to clinical attention, the brain is in a state of altered metabolism rendering it more vulnerable to ischemic damage. Other investigations with more severe TBI have also demonstrated the detrimental effects of concomitant hypoxia-ischemia.[128, 129]

Potential Mechanisms of Increased Vulnerability to Secondary Ischemic Injury

Concussive brain injury results in receptor mediated excitotoxicity, which is apparently mediated through both NMDA receptors and muscarinic acetylcholine receptors. Studies utilizing pharmacologic blockade of glutamate neurotransmission with phencyclidine palmitate (PCP) and cholinergic neurotransmission with scopolamine were conducted to determine the contributions of these systems to posttraumatic ischemic vulnerability. When given simultaneously 15 minutes prior to a midline fluid percussion injury, PCP and scopolamine significantly attenuated the loss of CA1 pyramidal cells seen 1 week after the double traumatic/ischemic insult.[130]

Another investigation demonstrated that mild closed head injury triggered transient (15 minute) increases in microdialysis-detectable glutamate, and 30 minutes in a hypoxia chamber did not. Combined closed head injury followed by immediate hypoxia precipitated glutamate increases of equal magnitude to closed head injury alone, but with a duration of up to 60 minutes. Pretreatment with the noncompetitive NMDA receptor antagonist MK-801 abolished the prolonged elevation of glutamate induced by the addition of hypoxic injury.[131]

These studies suggest that inhibition of increases in NMDA receptor activity provides some protection against secondary ischemic injury. One hypothesis is that the initial trauma leads to NMDA receptor activation and resultant Ca^{2+} influx. Increases in Ca^{2+} are known to persist for up to 2 days after experimental concussive brain injury.[73, 86] A cell already partially loaded with excess Ca^{2+} may be particularly vulnerable to a second Ca^{2+} increase, which triggers protease activation and then the cascade leading to cell death. Rescue of at-risk neurons by pretreatment with an NMDA antagonist supports this idea.

Another possibility is that the initial traumatic insult leaves the cell metabolically vulnerable. The previously described postconcussive increases in glycolytic metabolism may be necessary for rapid restoration of cerebral ionic balance. However, immediate postinjury hypoxia may trigger a crisis of increased energy demand and impaired substrate delivery, with the end result of energy failure, inability to restore membrane potential, and cell death. Alternately, an ischemic event 24 hours after trauma falls upon a brain that is metabolically depressed, and that may be incapable of the hyperglycolysis necessary to adequately respond to and recover from a second ionic pertubation.

Metabolic Periods of Potential Posttraumatic Vulnerability to a Second Concussion

One practical issue concerning athletic head injury is the appropriate time to refrain from sporting activity after a concussion. Understanding postinjury metabolic changes may suggest a time frame for increased vulnerability to repeated brain concussion.

First, the period of glucose metabolism–cerebral blood flow uncoupling may represent a time of increased danger for the injured brain. In the rat cortex, this period begins immediately after concussion and appears to last for at least 30 minutes.[36] At a time of metabolic stress (increased glucose need and decreased delivery), the brain may be less tolerant of further increases in metabolic demand in response to a second injury. Thus, neurons that are transiently dysfunctional after an initial injury may become irreversibly damaged after a recurrent injury.

Second, the accumulation of intracellular Ca^{2+} that occurs postinjury may leave cells in a perilous situation when faced with repeated Ca^{2+} influx. High levels of intracellular Ca^{2+} lead to mitochondrial dysfunction, impairing metabolism at a time when the cell can least tolerate it. Increased Ca^{2+} may also activate proteases that begin the cascade leading to cell death. In rats, the period of posttraumatic Ca^{2+} accumulation appears to last 2–4 days.[73, 86]

Last, postinjury derangements in neurotransmission are another potential mechanism by which a repeated concussive injury may lead to long-term deficits. A number of studies have implicated brain injury with subacute changes in glutamatergic,[132] adrenergic,[98, 133] and cholinergic[134] neurotransmission. A consequence of brain injury is the eventual down-regulation of excitatory neurotransmitter receptor function, which can last up to 2 weeks, depending on the receptor. A second injury during this period may trigger further diminution of receptor activity, leading to more severe or longer duration neurocognitive problems. Particularly in sports, where a player may be back in the game before full functional recovery, subtle impairments in cognition will likely place the individual at greater risk for recurrent injury.

Each of these trauma-induced physiologic changes (hyperglycolysis, Ca^{2+} accumulation, excitatory neurotransmitter downregulation) has its own particular time frame. Preliminary studies with a double concussion model demonstrate comparable increases in morphologic injury and prolonged metabolic depression when the two concussions were separated by 1, 2, or 5 hours.[135] In another study, double-concussed rats (1–2 hours between injuries) showed significantly increased glial fibrillary acidic protein (GFAP, a marker for gliosis/scarring) immunostaining and evidence of cell loss when compared with rats receiving only a single fluid percussion injury (Fig. 9–7[136]). In rats, therefore, it appears the time period of vulnerability to second concussion is at least 5 hours. It remains to be seen how this translates into the human condition. In general, the time frame for events in rats is significantly shorter than analogous periods in humans, so it would not be surprising if the duration of increased vulnerability in humans is actually much longer than in rat experimental models. Additionally, injury severity clearly has effects on the magnitude and duration of postconcussive metabolic dysfunction, and is likely another important variable to consider when developing back-to-play guidelines.

Other Considerations With Repeat Concussive Injury

Second impact syndrome is a very rare but catastrophic occurrence where a rela-tively minor second trauma superimposed on a brain recovering from an initial injury leads to rapid neurologic deterioration, cerebral edema, and death.[137] While diagnostic criteria for the syndrome are still undergoing debate, initial reports suggest a strong predilection for children and adolescents.[138–142] Children and adults respond to brain injury differently, with children seemingly more vulnerable to cerebral swelling and subdural hematomas after mild injury. One proposed mechanism for second impact syndrome suggests that impaired autoregulation in the traumatized developing brain leads to hyperemia and edema.[143, 144]

Another important issue is the possibility of permanent brain dysfunction or damage after multiple concussions. It may well be that the window of vulnerability to a second brain injury has two components, an acute period, where the brain is more susceptible to ionic and metabolic derangements that can lead to cell death, and a more chronic phase, where recovering neurotransmitter systems are at risk for developing permanent dysfunction through aberrant connections, with or without cell loss.

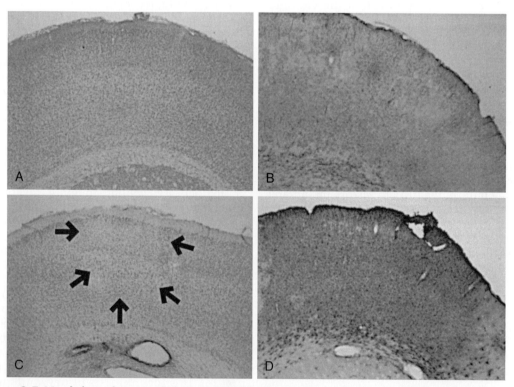

Figure 9–7. Morphologic changes and changes in glial fibrillary acidic protein (GFAP) after single and double fluid percussion injury (FPI). *A*, Cresyl violet stained cortex after single FPI. *B*, Cresyl violet stained cortex after double FPI (note cell loss in the circumscribed area). *C*, GFAP immunostained cortex after single FPI. *D*, GFAP immunostained cortex after double FPI (note marked increase in GFAP staining).

Overuse Injury

After many sports-related injuries, there is often significant pressure for the athlete to return to practice and competition as soon as physically possible. In general, there is an increasing awareness of the potential danger from rapid return to competitive play after cerebral concussion, particularly in regard to vulnerability to a second brain injury. On the other hand, return to vigorous practice might appear to be a safe alternative and a reasonable method for maintaining physical performance and conditioning until the athlete is ready to return to play.

Experimental studies with unilateral rat cortical injury have demonstrated the importance of limb use in restoration of function after brain lesioning.[145] After unilateral forelimb somatosensory cortex lesions, there is an overgrowth of dendrites in the homotopic cortical region of the uninjured hemisphere that is dependent on continued use of the uninjured forelimb. In unilaterally injured rats, immobilization of the intact forelimb not only impaired cortical dendritic growth but also resulted in more severe and long-lasting behavioral deficits. Perhaps even more concerning was the finding that this immobilization, and, hence, overuse of the injured limb, led to a marked increase in the lesion size in the injured cortex.[146] This suggests that increased functional demand placed upon the damaged cortex acutely may actually exacerbate the deficit, both anatomically and behaviorally. While there is no doubt that rehabilitative efforts are beneficial after brain injury, these findings would seem to indicate that, at least shortly after brain injury, it is possible to get "too much of a good thing."

A follow-up to the forced overuse study above demonstrated that when immobilization of the intact forelimb occurred within the first 7 days after cortical injury, there was both an impairment of functional recovery and a greater loss of brain tissue at the injury site. If the forced overuse was initiated longer than a week after cortical injury, there was still a delay in functional recovery, but the increase in the lesion size was not seen.[147] Thus, there appear to be post–brain injury windows of vulnerability, not only to a second injury as described in the previous section, but also possibly to excessive behavioral stimulation in the immediate postinjury period. It is not clear whether this postinjury sensitivity to overuse occurs in humans and if so, what its duration may be. At the very least, further studies are warranted in this area, and it may be prudent to limit extreme post-TBI behavioral rehabilitation or return to practice to a period somewhat after the acute injury, particularly after severe concussion or repeated concussions.

Concussion in the Developing Brain

Athletic brain injury is of particular concern in children, who tend to participate in sports putting them at risk for head trauma and in whom neurologic development is ongoing. Positron emission tomography (PET) studies of cerebral glucose metabolism in children up to age 15 years demonstrate clear differences in levels of $lCMR_{gluc}$ when compared with adults.[148] It is not unreasonable to assume that a severe diffuse injury might have lasting effects upon the complex neurochemical and anatomic events that occur during brain development. It is also important to realize that, although signs of overt neurologic dysfunction may not necessarily be prominent after juvenile brain injury, it is difficult to assess the possibility of lost cognitive potential, which may only be demonstrable at a later developmental period or under specific circumstances. Conversely, not all developmental difficulties that arise in a child postinjury are necessarily a result of the injury, as many brain-injured children have pre-existing neurologic abnormalities.

Age-Specific Vulnerability

Clinical experience suggests that, in general, the young brain may recover more rapidly and more completely from injury than the mature brain. This improvement in outcome has been attributed to greater plasticity in the developing brain. Immature rats subjected to moderate lateral fluid percussion injury show no evidence of neurologic or pathologic deficits posttrauma.[7, 149, 150] In a weight drop model, posttraumatic deficits are only seen at levels of injury where mortality in unventilated rats approaches 75%.[151] Spatial learning as assessed by Morris Water Maze performance is impaired by moderate concussive injury in adult rats, but not in postnatal day-17 rat pups.[149] Posttraumatic hyperglycolysis is also seen in immature rats, with levels of glucose utilization generally higher than that seen in adults after injury. Delayed hypometabolism of glucose is evident bilaterally 1 day after concussion, is milder than in adults, and resolves completely by 3 days.

However, there is also sufficient evidence to suggest that there are periods of developmental vulnerability when the immature brain is more sensitive to injury. Mortality after pediatric brain injury is higher in young children when compared with adolescents. Some series report an increased incidence of severe cerebral edema in head injured young children as a possible factor for this higher mortality.[141] In an experimental model of developmental fluid percussion injury, immature rats became hypotensive after concussion of all severities and tended to have longer apnea times than adults after mild injuries; in addition, mortality among immature rats subjected to severe levels of fluid percussion approached 100%.[7]

Age-dependent neurotransmitter sensitivities may also impact on the severity of traumatic brain injury. Neuronal excitotoxicity, mediated through the NMDA receptor, is more severe in neonatal rats. Direct injection of EAA agonists into neonatal brain regions leads to more severe neuronal necrosis than that seen in adults.[152] Hypoxic-ischemic insults also produce age-dependent brain injury that peaks at postnatal day 6 and gradually decreases with maturation.[153] Conversely, neonatal blockade of NMDA receptors triggers widespread neuronal apoptosis.[154] Developmental alterations in NMDA receptor number and subunit composition are known to occur[155, 156] and may be one mechanism through which age-specific neuronal vulnerability is manifested. NMDA receptor numbers increase after birth, peaking around postnatal day 28 in the young rat.[157] Perhaps more importantly, NMDA receptor subunit expression changes dramatically during cerebral maturation. Of the four regulatory subunits of the NMDA receptor (NR2A-D), the most sensitive subunit (NR2D) is expressed diffusely in rat brain during embryogenesis up to postnatal day 7,[156] mirroring the period of increased susceptibility to excitotoxic injury in the rat. By postnatal day 14, NR2D expression is negligible. Thus, it appears that a fine balance of excitatory neurotransmitter activity is necessary to maintain normal development and that either excess or diminution of NMDA receptor activity during this critical window may lead to permanent morphologic changes.

Developmental Plasticity and Traumatic Brain Injury

Developmental deficits after childhood brain trauma are difficult to assess as a result of variations in injury severity, location, and disruption of normal childhood activities resulting from hospitalization and corresponding rehabilitation. Long-term follow-up studies demonstrate persistent neurocognitive deficits in 23.7% of brain-injured children at 5 years.[158] In a study of visual and verbal memory function one year after closed head injury in three pediatric age ranges, injury severity was related to severity of posttraumatic visual memory deficits in all groups, consistent with the fact that visual memory functions were already well established in even the earliest age group. Verbal memory, which was rapidly expanding in adolescents but not well developed in younger children, demonstrated a relationship with injury severity only in adolescents. This is one example of how injury at a particular developmental time point may manifest age-dependent sequelae.[159]

Environment enrichment is an experimental model of developmental plasticity wherein rats reared as a group in a cage with multiple objects, toys, and tunnels demonstrate neuroanatomic changes and improved cognitive performance. Characteristic anatomic features of enrichment include increased cortical thickness and cortical weight, owing to increased neuronal size, more elaborate dendritic arborization, more synapses, and more glial cells.[160–162] When tested for spatial learning capacity with the Morris Water Maze, rats reared in the enriched environment consistently outperform their littermates reared in standard laboratory cages.[163] Although enrichment may occur at any age, it is usually most robust in young preweanling rats,[164] becoming more difficult to elicit with increasing age.

When postnatal day-20 rat pups were subjected to moderate lateral fluid percussion injury, they demonstrated no overt neurologic deficits or alterations in open field activity. Morris Water Maze testing showed no difference between injured and uninjured rat pups, and histologic evaluation revealed no structural lesions or cell loss. However, when these brain-injured young rats were reared in an enriched environment, they failed to develop the typical anatomic changes described above, and their performance in the Morris Water Maze was equivalent to unenriched rats (Fig. 9–8[150]). Thus, in this model, brain concussion led to a defect in developmental plasticity in the absence of detectable baseline morphologic and behavioral abnormalities. It remains to be seen if this impairment of normal development is permanent or if there is a window of dysfunction after which the animal may regain the ability for neural reorganization.

SUMMARY

Concussion is the result of a biomechanical injury to the brain, resulting in reversible, but occasionally persistent, neurologic dysfunction, manifested primarily by some or all of the following symptoms: alterations in consciousness, amnesia, visual disturbances, concentration problems, headache, nausea/vomiting, cognitive impairment, vertigo, and balance disturbance. In addition to these symptoms, chronic problems with sleep, fatigue, depression, and personality changes may occur.

The acute pathophysiology of concussion centers on injury-induced depolarization which triggers release of excitatory neurotransmitters. This, in turn, precipitates further opening of NMDA receptor–associated channels. Ionic derangements are countered by increased activity of the Na^+/K^+ pump, which triggers hyperglycolysis in an attempt to generate the required ATP for restoration of the membrane potential. Calcium influx via the NMDA receptor channel may lead to persistent mitochondrial dysfunction and a period of decreased glucose metabolism lasting days after injury. This same Ca^{2+} influx may set forth a degenerative cascade of axonal cytoskeletal components.

These initial posttraumatic derangements in cellular function leave the nervous system in a state of enhanced vulnerability for some time. Increased intracellular Ca^{2+}, suppressed glycolysis, impaired oxidative phosphorylation, and dysfunctional axonal transport put the injured cell on a metabolic tightrope from which it may either recover or plunge to its demise. Interventions aimed at diverting the course of this physiologic cascade may limit the degree of impairment or vulnerability, resulting in improved outcomes.

In the course of traumatic brain injury, every effort must be made to protect the damaged neurons from secondary injury by aggressively maintaining cerebral perfusion, providing adequate oxygenation, balancing fluids and electrolytes, and suppressing unnecessary cellular energy use. It is of great importance to adequately assess cerebral function on the sidelines after any sports-related concussion, regardless of how minor

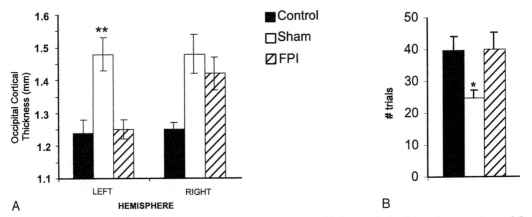

Figure 9–8. Loss of enriched environment (EE)-induced anatomic and behavioral plasticity after experimental fluid percussion injury (FPI). *A,* Control group shows cortical thickness of unenriched rats. Sham surgery rats demonstrated increased cortical thickness after EE. FPI rats housed in EE did not fully develop increased cortical thickness. *B,* The number of trials to reach criterion in the Morris Water Maze was significantly fewer in the rats showing increased cortical thickness after EE. Unenriched controls and rats housed in EE after concussive injury took a greater number of trials to reach criterion.

it may initially appear. Many postconcussive symptoms are subtle, such as mild cognitive problems, emotional changes, or subjective complaints of pain; they must be regarded as evidence of continuing cerebral dysfunction and allowed to resolve prior to the resumption of play or practice. Persistent postconcussive symptoms may be indicative of ongoing neuronal vulnerability; the risk of multiple, superimposed brain injuries should be seriously considered in the decision to return to sports-related activities. Current return to play guidelines rightfully call for careful neurologic and mental status testing to appropriately triage athletic head injuries.

Athletic brain injuries in childhood are relatively common, and children are certainly at risk for repeated concussion. Although such injuries usually resolve completely, they warrant close follow-up, as the neurobiologic effects of concussion on normal cerebral maturation are not yet fully understood.

ACKNOWLEDGMENTS

This work was supported by NS27544, NS30308, and the Lind Lawrence Foundation.

References

1. Cantu R. Guidelines for return to contact sports after a cerebral concussion. Phys Sportsmed 1986;14:75–83.
2. Guidelines for the Management of Concussion in Sports. Report of the Sports Medicine Committee. Colorado Medical Society, 1990 (revised 1991).
3. Practice parameter: The management of concussion in sports (summary statement). Report of the Quality Standards Subcommittee, Neurology, 1997;48:581–585.
4. Sullivan HG, Martinez J, Becker DP, et al. Fluid-percussion model of mechanical brain injury in the cat. J Neurosurg 1976;45:521–534.
5. McIntosh TK, Vink R, Noble L, et al. Traumatic brain injury in the rat: Characterization of a lateral fluid-percussion model. Neuroscience 1989; 28:233–244.
6. Dixon CE, Lyeth BG, Povlishock JT, et al. A fluid percussion model of experimental brain injury in the rat. J Neurosurg 1987;67:110–119.
7. Prins ML, Lee SM, Cheng CL, et al. Fluid percussion brain injury in the developing and adult rat: A comparative study of mortality, morphology, intracranial pressure and mean arterial blood pressure. Brain Res Dev Brain Res 1996;95:272–282.
8. Hovda DA, Lee SM, Smith ML, et al. The neurochemical and metabolic cascade following brain injury: Moving from animal models to man. Neurotrauma 1995;12:903–906.
9. Bergsneider M, Hovda DA, Shalmon E, et al. Cerebral hyperglycolysis following severe traumatic brain injury in humans: A positron emission tomography study [see comments]. J Neurosurg 1997;86:241–251.
10. Martin NA, Patwardhan RV, Alexander MJ, et al. Characterization of cerebral hemodynamic phases following severe head trauma: Hypoperfusion, hyperemia, and vasospasm. J Neurosurg 1997;87:9–19.
11. Takahashi H, Manaka S, Sano K. Changes in extracellular potassium concentration in cortex and brain stem during the acute phase of experimental closed head injury. J Neurosurg 1981;55:708–717.
12. Hubschmann OR, Kornhauser D. Effects of intraparenchymal hemorrhage on extracellular cortical potassium in experimental head trauma. J Neurosurg 1983;59:289–293.
13. Katayama Y, Becker DP, Tamura T, Hovda DA. Massive increases in extracellular potassium and the indiscriminate release of glutamate following concussive brain injury. J Neurosurg 1990;73:889–900.
14. Julian F, Goldman D. The effects of mechanical stimulation on some electrical properties of axons. J Gen Physiol 1962;46:297–313.
15. Hablitz JJ, Langmoen IA. Excitation of hippocampal pyramidal cells by glutamate in the guinea pig and rat. J Physiol (Lond) 1982;325:317–331.
16. Cotman C, Iverson L. Excitatory amino acids in the brain—Focus on NMDA receptors. Trends Neurosci 1987;10:263–265.
17. Mayer ML, Westbrook GL. Cellular mechanisms underlying excitotoxicity. Trends Neurosci 1987;10:59–61.
18. Ballanyi K, Grafe P, ten Bruggencate G. Ion activities and potassium uptake mechanisms of glial cells in guinea pig olfactory cortex slices. J Physiol (Lond) 1987;382:159–174.
19. Kuffler SW. Neuroglial cells: physiological properties and a potassium mediated effect of neuronal activity on the glial membrane potential. Proc R Soc Lond B Biol Sci 1967;168:1–21.
20. Paulson OB, Newman EA. Does the release of potassium from astrocyte endfeet regulate cerebral blood flow? Science 1987;237:896–898.
21. Moody WJ, Futamachi KJ, Prince DA. Extracellular potassium activity during epileptogenesis. Exp Neurol 1974;42:248–263.
22. Sypert GW, Ward AA, Jr. Changes in extracellular potassium activity during neocortical propagated seizures. Exp Neurol 1974;45:19–41.
23. Astrup J, Rehncrona S, Siesjö BK. The increase in extracellular potassium concentration in the ischemic brain in relation to the preischemic functional activity and cerebral metabolic rate. Brain Res 1980;199:161–174.
24. Hansen AJ. Extracellular potassium concentration in juvenile and adult rat brain cortex during anoxia. Acta Physiol Scand 1977;99:412–420.
25. Hansen AJ. The extracellular potassium concentration in brain cortex following ischemia in hypo- and hyperglycemic rats. Acta Physiol Scand 1978;102:324–329.
26. Nicholson C, Kraig RP. The Behavior of Extracel-

lular Ions During Spreading Depression. *In* Zeuthen T (ed): The Application of Ion-Selective Electrodes. New York, Elsevier, North-Holland, 1981, pp 217–238.

27. Prince DA, Lux HD, Neher E. Measurement of extracellular potassium activity in cat cortex. Brain Res 1973;50:489–495.

28. Sugaya E, Takato M, Noda Y. Neuronal and glial activity during spreading depression in cerebral cortex of cat. J Neurophysiol 1975;38:822–841.

29. Van Harreveld A. Two mechanisms for spreading depression in the chicken retina. J Neurobiol 1978;9:419–431.

30. Somjen GG, Giacchino JL. Potassium and calcium concentrations in interstitial fluid of hippocampal formation during paroxysmal responses. J Neurophysiol 1985;53:1098–1108.

31. Bull RJ, Cummins JT. Influence of potassium on the steady-state redox potential of the electron transport chain in slices of rat cerebral cortex and the effect of ouabain. J Neurochem 1973;21:923–937.

32. Mayevsky A, Chance B. Repetitive patterns of metabolic changes during cortical spreading depression of the awake rat. Brain Res 1974;65:529–533.

33. Rosenthal M, LaManna J, Yamada S, et al. Oxidative metabolism, extracellular potassium and sustained potential shifts in cat spinal cord in situ. Brain Res 1979;162:113–127.

34. Shah KR, West M. The effect of concussion on cerebral uptake of 2-deoxy-D-glucose in rat. Neurosci Lett 1983;40:287–291.

35. Sunami K, Nakamura T, Ozawa Y, et al. Hypermetabolic state following experimental head injury. Neurosurg Rev 1989;12(Suppl 1):400–411.

36. Yoshino A, Hovda DA, Kawamata T, et al. Dynamic changes in local cerebral glucose utilization following cerebral concussion in rats: Evidence of a hyper- and subsequent hypometabolic state. Brain Res 1991;561:106–119.

37. Samii A, Hovda DA. Delayed increases in glucose utilization following cortical impact injury. Society for Neuroscience (abst) 1998;24:738.

38. Ackermann RF, Lear JL. Glycolysis-induced discordance between glucose metabolic rates measured with radiolabeled fluorodeoxyglucose and glucose. J Cereb Blood Flow Metab 1989;9:774–785.

39. Lear JL, Ackermann RF. Why the deoxyglucose method has proven so useful in cerebral activation studies: The unappreciated prevalence of stimulation-induced glycolysis. J Cereb Blood Flow Metab 1989;9:911–913.

40. Nilsson B, Pontén U. Experimental head injury in the rat. Part 2: Regional brain energy metabolism in concussive trauma. J Neurosurg 1977;47:252–261.

41. Nilsson B, Nordström CH. Experimental head injury in the rat. Part 3: Cerebral blood flow and oxygen consumption after concussive impact acceleration. J Neurosurg 1977;47:262–273.

42. Vink R, Head VA, Rogers PJ, et al. Mitochondrial metabolism following traumatic brain injury in rats. J Neurotrauma 1990;7:21–27.

43. Corbett RJ, Laptook AR, Nunnally RL, et al. Intracellular pH, lactate, and energy metabolism in neonatal brain during partial ischemia measured in vivo by 31P and 1H nuclear magnetic reso-

nance spectroscopy. Neurochem 1988;51:1501–1509.

44. Biros MH, Dimlich RV. Brain lactate during partial global ischemia and reperfusion: Effect of pretreatment with dichloroacetate in a rat model. Am J Emer Med 1987;5:271–277.

45. Richards TL, Keniry MA, Weinstein PR, et al. Measurement of lactate accumulation by in vivo proton NMR spectroscopy during global cerebral ischemia in rats. Magn Reson Med 1987;5:353–557.

46. Yang MS, DeWitt DS, Becker DP, Hayes RL. Regional brain metabolite levels following mild experimental head injury in the cat. J Neurosurg 1985;63:617–621.

47. DeWitt DS, Jenkins LW, Wei EP, et al. Effects of fluid-percussion brain injury on regional cerebral blood flow and pial arteriolar diameter. J Neurosurg 1986;64:787–794.

48. Meyer JS, Kondo A, Nomura F, et al. Cerebral hemodynamics and metabolism following experimental head injury. J Neurosurg 1970;32:304–319.

49. Nelson SR, Lowry OH, Passonneau JV. Changes in energy reserves in mouse brain associated with compressive head injury. *In* Caveness WF, Walker AE (eds): Head Injury. Philadelphia, JB Lippincott, 1966, pp 444–447.

50. Nilsson B, Nordström CH. Rate of cerebral energy consumption in concussive head injury in the rat. J Neurosurg 1977;47:274–281.

51. Kuhr WG, Korf J. Extracellular lactic acid as an indicator of brain metabolism: Continuous on-line measurement in conscious, freely moving rats with intrastriatal dialysis. J Cereb Blood Flow Metab 1988;8:130–137.

52. Nilsson P, Hillered L, Pontén U, Ungerstedt U. Changes in cortical extracellular levels of energy-related metabolites and amino acids following concussive brain injury in rats. J Cereb Blood Flow Metab 1990;10:631–637.

53. Inao S, Marmarou A, Clarke GD, et al. Production and clearance of lactate from brain tissue, cerebrospinal fluid, and serum following experimental brain injury. J Neurosurg 1988;69:736–744.

54. Kawamata T, Katayama Y, Hovda DA, et al. Lactate accumulation following concussive brain injury: The role of ionic fluxes induced by excitatory amino acids. Brain Res 1995;674:196–204.

55. Friede RL, Van Houten WH. Relations between post mortem alterations and glycolytic metabolism in the brain. Exp Neurol 1961;4:197–204.

56. Gardiner M, Smith ML, Kågström E, et al. Influence of blood glucose concentration on brain lactate accumulation during severe hypoxia and subsequent recovery of brain energy metabolism. J Cereb Blood Flow Metab 1982;2:429–438.

57. Kalimo H, Rehncrona S, Söderfeldt B. The role of lactic acidosis in the ischemic nerve cell injury. Acta Neuropathol Berl (Suppl) 1981;7:20–22.

58. Kalimo H, Rehncrona S, Söderfeldt B, et al. Brain lactic acidosis and ischemic cell damage: 2. Histopathology. J Cereb Blood Flow Metab 1981;1:313–327.

59. Myers RE. A unitary theory of causation of anoxic and hypoxic brain pathology. Adv Neurol 1979;26:195–213.

60. Siemkowicz E, Hansen AJ. Clinical restitution following cerebral ischemia in hypo-, normo- and hyperglycemic rats. Acta Neurol Scand 1978;58:1–8.

61. Becker DP, Jenkins LW, Rabow L. The pathophysiology of head trauma. *In* Miller TA, Rowlands B, (eds): The Physiological Basis of Modern Surgical Care. St. Louis, Mosby, 1987, pp 763–788.

62. Jenkins LW, Moszynski K, Lyeth BG, et al. Increased vulnerability of the mildly traumatized rat brain to cerebral ischemia: The use of controlled secondary ischemia as a research tool to identify common or different mechanisms contributing to mechanical and ischemic brain injury. Brain Res 1989;477:211–224.

63. Ishige N, Pitts LH, Berry I, et al. The effects of hypovolemic hypotension on high-energy phosphate metabolism of traumatized brain in rats. J Neurosurg 1988;68:129–136.

64. Kawamata T, Katayama Y, Hovda DA, et al. Administration of excitatory amino acid antagonists via microdialysis attenuates the increase in glucose utilization seen following concussive brain injury. J Cereb Blood Flow Metab 1992;12:12–24.

65. Kawamata T, Hovda DA, Yoshino A, et al. Administration of excitatory amino acid antagonists vis microdialysis prevents the increase in glucose utilization seen immediately following concussive brain injury. Society for Neuroscience (abst) 1990;16:778.

66. Yoshino A, Hovda DA, Katayama Y, et al. Hippocampal CA3 lesion prevents postconcussive metabolic dysfunction in CA1. J Cereb Blood Flow Metab 1992;12:996–1006.

67. Yuan XQ, Prough DS, Smith TL, Dewitt DS. The effects of traumatic brain injury on regional cerebral blood flow in rats. J Neurotrauma 1988;5:289–301.

68. Yamakami I, McIntosh TK. Effects of traumatic brain injury on regional cerebral blood flow in rats as measured with radiolabeled microspheres. J Cereb Blood Flow Metab 1989;9:117–124.

69. Velarde F, Fisher DT, Hovda DA, et al. Fluid percussion injury induces prolonged changes in cerebral blood flow. J Neurotrauma (abst) 1992;9:402.

70. Doberstein C, Velarde F, Badie H, et al. Changes in local cerebral blood flow following concussive brain injury. Society for Neuroscience (abst) 1992;18:175.

71. Duckrow RB, LaManna JC, Rosenthal M, et al. Oxidative metabolic activity of cerebral cortex after fluid-percussion head injury in the cat. J Neurosurg 1981;54:607–614.

72. Cortez SC, McIntosh TK, Noble LJ. Experimental fluid percussion brain injury: Vascular disruption and neuronal and glial alterations. Brain Res 1989;482:271–282.

73. Fineman I, Hovda DA, Smith M, et al. Concussive brain injury is associated with a prolonged accumulation of calcium: A 45Ca autoradiographic study. Brain Res 1993;624:94–102.

74. McIntosh TK. Novel pharmacologic therapies in the treatment of experimental traumatic brain injury: A review. J Neurotrauma 1993;10:215–261.

75. Nilsson P, Hillered L, Olsson Y, et al. Regional changes in interstitial K+ and Ca2+ levels following cortical compression contusion trauma in rats. J Cereb Blood Flow Metab 1993;13:183–192.

76. Choi DW. Calcium-mediated neurotoxicity: Relationship to specific channel types and role in ischemic damage. Trends Neurosci 1988;11:465–469.

77. Dienel GA. Regional accumulation of calcium in postischemic rat brain. J Neurochem 1984;43:913–925.

78. Kato H, Kogure K, Nakano S. Neuronal damage following repeated brief ischemia in the gerbil. Brain Res 1989;479:366–370.

79. Sakamoto N, Kogure K, Kato H, Ohtomo H. Disturbed Ca2+ homeostasis in the gerbil hippocampus following brief transient ischemia. Brain Res 1986;364:372–376.

80. Rappaport ZH, Young W, Flamm ES. Regional brain calcium changes in the rat middle cerebral artery occlusion model of ischemia. Stroke 1987;18:760–764.

81. Deshpande JK, Siesjö BK, Wieloch T. Calcium accumulation and neuronal damage in the rat hippocampus following cerebral ischemia. J Cereb Blood Flow Metab 1987;7:89–95.

82. Stokes BT, Fox P, Hollinden G. Extracellular calcium activity in the injured spinal cord. Exp Neurol 1983;80:561–572.

83. Young W, Yen V, Blight A. Extracellular calcium ionic activity in experimental spinal cord contusion. Brain Res 1982;253:105–113.

84. Young W, Koreh I. Potassium and calcium changes in injured spinal cords. Brain Res 1986;365:42–53.

85. Happel RD, Smith KP, Banik NL, et al. Ca2+-accumulation in experimental spinal cord trauma. Brain Res 1981;211:476–479.

86. Prins ML, Osteen C, Moore AH, Hovda DA. Lateral fluid percussion injury in the developing rat: No evidence for an enduring calcium accumulation. Society for Neuroscience (abst) 1998;24:737.

87. Badie H, Smith ML, Hovda DA, et al. Omegaconopeptide reduces the extent of calcium accumulation following traumatic brain injury. Society for Neuroscience (abst) 1993;19:1485.

88. Hovda DA, Fu K, Badie H, et al. Administration of an omega-conopeptide one hour following traumatic brain injury reduces 45calcium accumulation. Acta Neurochir Suppl (Wien) 1994;60:521–523.

89. Verweij BH, Muizelaar JP, Vinas FC, et al. Mitochondrial dysfunction after experimental and human brain injury and its possible reversal with a selective N-type calcium channel antagonist (SNX-111). Neurol Res 1997;19:334–339.

90. Xiong Y, Gu Q, Peterson PL, et al. Mitochondrial dysfunction and calcium pertubation induced by traumatic brain injury. J Neurotrauma 1997;14:23–34.

91. Hovda DA, Yoshino A, Kawamata T, et al. Diffuse prolonged depression of cerebral oxidative metabolism following concussive brain injury in the rat: A cytochrome oxidase histochemistry study. Brain Res 1991;567:1–10.

92. Nedergaard M, Jakobsen J, Diemer NH. Autoradiographic determination of cerebral glucose content, blood flow, and glucose utilization in focal ischemia of the rat brain: Influence of the plasma glucose concentration. J Cereb Blood Flow Metab 1988;8:100–108.

93. Kushner M, Alavi A, Reivich M, et al. Contralateral cerebellar hypometabolism following cerebral insult: A positron emission tomographic study. Ann Neurol 1984;15:425–434.

94. Shiraishi K, Sharp FR, Simon RP. Sequential metabolic changes in rat brain following middle cerebral artery occlusion: A 2-deoxyglucose study. J Cereb Blood Flow Metab 1989;9:765–773.

95. Pappius HM. Dexamethasone and local cerebral glucose utilization in freeze-traumatized rat brain. Ann Neurol 1982;12:157–162.

96. Colle LM, Holmes LJ, Pappius HM. Correlation between behavioral status and cerebral glucose utilization in rats following freezing lesion. Brain Res 1986;397:27–36.

97. Patronas NJ, Di Chiro G, Smith BH, et al. Depressed cerebellar glucose metabolism in supratentorial tumors. Brain Res 1984;291:93–101.

98. Feeney DM, Sutton RL, Boyeson MG, et al. The locus coeruleus and cerebral metabolism: Recovery of function after cortical injury. Physiol Psych 1985;13:197–203.

99. Sutton RL, Hovda DA, Chugani HT. Time course of local cerebral glucose utilization (LCGU) alteration after motor cortex ablation in the rat. Society for Neuroscience (abst) 1989;15:128.

100. Dietrich WD, Alonso O, Busto R, Ginsberg MD. Widespread metabolic depression and reduced somatosensory circuit activation following traumatic brain injury in rats. J Neurotrauma 1994;11:629–640.

101. D'Ambrosio R, Maris DO, Grady MS, et al. Selective loss of hippocampal long-term potentiation, but not depression, following fluid percussion injury. Brain Res 1998;786:64–79.

102. Schanne FA, Kane AB, Young EE, Farber JL. Calcium dependence of toxic cell death: A final common pathway. Science 1979;206:700–702.

103. Choi DW. Ionic dependence of glutamate neurotoxicity. J Neurosci 1987;7:369–379.

104. Vink R, McIntosh TK, Demediuk P, Faden AI. Decrease in total and free magnesium concentration following traumatic brain injury in rats. Biochem Biophys Res Commun 1987;149:594–599.

105. Vink R, McIntosh TK, Weiner MW, Faden AI. Effects of traumatic brain injury on cerebral high-energy phosphates and pH: A 31P magnetic resonance spectroscopy study. J Cereb Blood Flow Metab 1987;7:563–571.

106. Vink R, Faden AI, McIntosh TK. Changes in cellular bioenergetic state following graded traumatic brain injury in rats: Determination by phosphorus 31 magnetic resonance spectroscopy. J Neurotrauma 1988;5:315–330.

107. Vink R, McIntosh TK. Pharmacological and physiological effects of magnesium on experimental traumatic brain injury. Magnes Res 1990;3:163–169.

108. McIntosh TK, Faden AI, Yamakami I, Vink R. Magnesium deficiency exacerbates and pretreatment improves outcome following traumatic brain injury in rats: 31P magnetic resonance spectroscopy and behavioral studies. J Neurotrauma 1988;5:17–31.

109. Garfinkel L, Garfinkel D. Magnesium regulation of the glycolytic pathway and the enzymes involved. Magnesium 1985;4:60–72.

110. Ebel H, Günther T. Magnesium metabolism: A review. J Clin Chem Clin Biochem 1980;18:257–70.

111. Aikawa JK. Magnesium: Its Biologic Significance. Boca Raton, FL, CRC Press, 1981, pp 21–29.

112. Povlishock JT, Becker DP, Cheng CL, Vaughan GW. Axonal change in minor head injury. J Neuropathol Exp Neurol 1983;42:225–242.

113. Povlishock JT. Traumatically induced axonal injury: Pathogenesis and pathobiological implications. Brain Pathol 1992;2:1–12.

114. Pettus EH, Christman CW, Giebel ML, Povlishock JT. Traumatically induced altered membrane permeability: Its relationship to traumatically induced reactive axonal change. J Neurotrauma 1994;11:507–522.

115. Povlishock JT, Pettus EH. Traumatically induced axonal damage: Evidence for enduring changes in axolemmal permeability with associated cytoskeletal change. Acta Neurochir Suppl (Wien) 1996;66:81–86.

116. Mata M, Staple J, Fink DJ. Changes in intra-axonal calcium distribution following nerve crush. J Neurobiol 1986;17:449–467.

117. Maxwell WL, McCreath BJ, Graham DI, Gennarelli TA. Cytochemical evidence for redistribution of membrane pump calcium-ATPase and ecto-Ca-ATPase activity, and calcium influx in myelinated nerve fibres of the optic nerve after stretch injury. J Neurocytol 1995;24:925–942.

118. Pettus EH, Povlishock JT. Characterization of a distinct set of intra-axonal ultrastructural changes associated with traumatically induced alteration in axolemmal permeability. Brain Res 1996;722:1–11.

119. Maxwell WL, Graham DI. Loss of axonal microtubules and neurofilaments after stretch-injury to guinea pig optic nerve fibers. J Neurotrauma 1997;14:603–614.

120. Sternberger LA, Sternberger NH. Monoclonal antibodies distinguish phosphorylated and nonphosphorylated forms of neurofilaments in situ. Proc Natl Acad Sci USA 1983;80:6126–6130.

121. Nakamura Y, Takeda M, Angelides KJ, et al. Effect of phosphorylation on 68 KDa neurofilament subunit protein assembly by the cyclic AMP dependent protein kinase in vitro. Biochem Biophys Res Commun 1990;169:744–750.

122. Nixon RA. The regulation of neurofilament protein dynamics by phosphorylation: Clues to neurofibrillary pathobiology. Brain Pathol 1993;3:29–38.

123. Johnson GV, Greenwood JA, Costello AC, Troncoso JC. The regulatory role of calmodulin in the proteolysis of individual neurofilament proteins by calpain. Neurochem Res 1991;16:869–873.

124. Maxwell WL, Povlishock JT, Graham DL. A mechanistic analysis of nondisruptive axonal injury: A review. J Neurotrauma 1997;14:419–440 [published erratum appears in J Neurotrauma 1997;14:755].

125. Povlishock JT, Christman CW. The pathobiology of traumatically induced axonal injury in animals and humans: A review of current thoughts. J Neurotrauma 1995;12:555–564.

126. Blumbergs PC, Scott G, Manavis J, et al. Staining of amyloid precursor protein to study axonal damage in mild head injury. Lancet 1994;344:1055–1056.

127. Jenkins LW, Marmarou A, Lewelt W, Becker DP. Increased Vulnerability of the Traumatized Brain to Early Ischemia. In Baethmann A, Go GK, Unterberg A (eds): Mechanisms of Secondary Brain Damage. New York, Plenum Press, 1986, pp 273–282.

128. Ishige N, Pitts LH, Hashimoto T, et al. Effect of hypoxia on traumatic brain injury in rats: Part 1. Changes in neurological function, electroencephalograms, and histopathology. Neurosurgery 1987;20:848–853.

129. Bardt TF, Unterberg AW, Härtl R, et al. Monitoring of brain tissue Po_2 in traumatic brain injury: Effect of cerebral hypoxia on outcome. Acta Neurochir Suppl (Wien) 1998;71:153–156.

130. Jenkins LW, Lu Y, Johnston WE, et al. Combined therapy affects outcomes differentially after mild traumatic brain injury and secondary forebrain ischemia in rats. Brain Res 1999;817:132–144.

131. Katoh H, Sima K, Nawashiro H, et al. The effect of MK-801 on extracellular neuroactive amino acids in hippocampus after closed head injury followed by hypoxia in rats. Brain Res 1997;758:153–162.

132. Miller LP, Lyeth BG, Jenkins LW, et al. Excitatory amino acid receptor subtype binding following traumatic brain injury. Brain Res 1990;526:103–107.

133. Pappius HM. Significance of biogenic amines in functional disturbances resulting from brain injury. Metab Brain Dis 1988;3:303–310.

134. Gorman LK, Fu K, Hovda DA, et al. Effects of traumatic brain injury on the cholinergic system in the rat. J Neurotrauma 1996;13:457–463.

135. Fu K, Smith M, Thomas S, et al. Cerebral concussion produces a state of vulnerability lasting for as long as 5 hours. J Neurotrauma (abst) 1992;9:59.

136. Badie H, Hovda DA, Becker DP. Glial fibrillary acidic protein (GFAP) expression following concussive brain injury: A quantitative study of the effects of a second insult. J Neurotrauma (abst) 1992;9:56.

137. Cantu RC, Voy R. Second impact syndrome: A risk in any contact sport. Phys Sportsmed 1995;23:27–34.

138. Pickles W. Acute general edema of the brain in children with head injuries. N Engl J Med 1950;242:607–611.

139. Bruce DA, Alavi A, Bilaniuk L, et al. Diffuse cerebral swelling following head injuries in children: The syndrome of "malignant brain edema." J Neurosurg 1981;54:170–178.

140. Bruce DA. Delayed deterioration of consciousness after trivial head injury in childhood [editorial]. BMJ 1984;289:715–716.

141. Aldrich EF, Eisenberg HM, Saydjari C, et al. Diffuse brain swelling in severely head-injured children: A report from the NIH Traumatic Coma Data Bank. J Neurosurg 1992;76:450–454.

142. Sports related recurrent brain injuries—United States. MMWR Morb Mortal Wkly Rep 1997;46:224–227.

143. Lobato RD, Rivas JJ, Gomez PA, et al. Head-injured patients who talk and deteriorate into coma: Analysis of 211 cases studied with computerized tomography [see comments]. J Neurosurg 1991;75:256–261.

144. Snoek JW, Minderhoud JM, Wilmink JT. Delayed deterioration following mild head injury in children. Brain 1984;107:15–36.

145. Schallert T, Kozlowski DA, Humm JL, Cocke RR. Use-dependent structural events in recovery of function. Adv Neurol 1997;73:229–238.

146. Kozlowski DA, James DC, Schallert T. Use-dependent exaggeration of neuronal injury after unilateral sensorimotor cortex lesions. J Neurosci 1996;16:4776–4786.

147. Humm JL, Kozlowski DA, James DC, et al. Use-dependent exacerbation of brain damage occurs during an early post-lesion vulnerable period. Brain Res 1998;783:286–292.

148. Chugani HT, Phelps ME, Mazziotta JC. Positron emission tomography study of human brain functional development. Ann Neurol 1987;22:487–497.

149. Prins ML, Hovda DA. Traumatic brain injury in the developing rat: Effects of maturation on Morris water maze acquisition. J Neurotrauma 1998;15:799–811.

150. Fineman I, Giza CC, Nahed BV, et al. Inhibition of neocortical plasticity during development by a moderate concussive brain injury. Submitted 1999.

151. Adelson PD, Dixon CE, Robichaud P, Kochanek PM. Motor and cognitive functional deficits following diffuse traumatic brain injury in the immature rat. J Neurotrauma 1997;14:99–108.

152. McDonald JW, Silverstein FS, Johnston MV. Neurotoxicity of N-methyl-D-aspartate is markedly enhanced in developing rat central nervous system. Brain Res 1988;459:200–203.

153. Ikonomidou C, Mosinger JL, Salles KS, et al. Sensitivity of the developing rat brain to hypobaric/ischemic damage parallels sensitivity to N-methyl-aspartate neurotoxicity. J Neurosci 1989;9:2809–2818.

154. Ikonomidou C, Bosch F, Miksa M, et al. Blockade of NMDA receptors and apoptotic neurodegeneration in the developing brain. Science 1999;283:70–74.

155. Wenzel A, Fritschy JM, Mohler H, Benke D. NMDA receptor heterogeneity during postnatal development of the rat brain: Differential expression of the NR2A, NR2B, and NR2C subunit proteins. J Neurochem 1997;68:469–478.

156. Scheetz AJ, Constantine-Paton M. Modulation of NMDA receptor function: Implications for vertebrate neural development. FASEB J 1994;8:745–752.

157. Insel TR, Miller LP, Gelhard RE. The ontogeny of excitatory amino acid receptors in rat forebrain—I. N-methyl-D-aspartate and quisqualate receptors. Neuroscience 1990;35:31–43.

158. Klonoff H, Low MD, Clark C. Head injuries in children: A prospective five year follow-up. J Neurol Neurosurg Psychiatry 1977;40:1211–1219.

159. Levin HS, Eisenberg HM, Wigg NR, Kobayashi K. Memory and intellectual ability after head injury in children and adolescents. Neurosurgery 1982;11:668–673.

160. Rosenzweig MR, Bennett EL. Psychobiology of plasticity: Effects of training and experience on brain and behavior. Behav Brain Res 1996;78:57–65.

161. Bennett EL, Diamond MC, Krech D, Rosenzweig MR. Chemical and anatomical plasticity of the brain. Science 1964;164:610–619.

162. Greenough WT, Volkmar FRR. Pattern of dendritic branching in occipital cortex of rats reared in complex environments. Exp Neurol 1973;40:491–504.

163. Tees RC, Buhrmann K, Hanley J. The effect of early experience on water maze spatial learning and memory in rats. Dev Psychobiol 1990;23:427–439.

164. Venable N, Pinto-Hamuy T, Arraztoa JA, et al. Greater efficacy of preweaning than postweaning environmental enrichment on maze learning in adult rats. Behav Brain Res 1988;31:89–92.

10

Outcome After Sports Concussion

Stephen N. Macciocchi, Jeffrey T. Barth, and Lauren M. Littlefield

In general clinical populations, symptoms such as impaired memory, attention and concentration, information processing speed, new problem-solving, abstract reasoning, and judgment, as well as complaints of headache, dizziness, nausea, fatigue, and emotional lability, have been observed following mild head injury.[3, 12, 17, 18, 39, 51] The vast majority of individuals who sustain mild head injury have few symptoms and make very rapid recoveries; however, a small subset of these patients continue to suffer multiple symptoms for extended periods of time.[3, 5, 6, 14, 20, 26–28, 39, 41, 42] The variability in postconcussion symptom presentation has generated considerable debate on the cause of neuropsychologic deficits noted in some patients following mild cerebral trauma. Factors such as diffuse and focal axonal injury, pain, substance abuse, previous psychiatric or neurologic history, pending litigation, and malingering and malingering-like disorders are presumed to play at least some part in determining symptom severity and duration.[4, 15, 27] Despite these speculations, researchers have failed to discover strong relationships between some of these variables and the presence of extended postconcussion symptoms.[1]

Controversy regarding the causes of symptoms following mild head injury (postconcussion syndrome) has been exacerbated by methodologic variability and limitations among scientific studies. Most studies of mild head injury suffer from some form of threat to internal and external validity, in-cluding imprecise injury definition, selection bias, subject attrition, reliance on self-report measures, lack of baseline neuropsychologic data for comparison, diverse outcome measures, variable test time sequences, and limited documentation or control of potentially influential subject factors.[15]

Although interest in the study of mild head trauma has increased significantly in the past decade, few well-controlled prospective studies have found their way to the literature. Consequently, much of our knowledge in this area has accumulated through retrospective investigations of selected populations, which imposes limits on generalizability and conclusive statements regarding outcome. Although quasi-experimental retrospective or selected nonequivalent control comparisons have an important place in research, using these paradigms to generate population-based predictions of outcome is problematic. Not surprisingly, there are even fewer controlled, prospective studies focused on sports-related mild head injuries.[1, 15]

Despite the limitations of existing research, a number of issues believed to influence outcome following sports-related concussion will be reviewed, including injury mechanism and pathophysiology, measurement of severity, frequency, complications and vulnerability factors, and clinical management. Although we will report research findings from several sports, boxing will not be one of our focuses, since the biomechanics of injury in that sport, and its objective (rendering an opponent unconscious), make it fundamentally unique.[40, 44] This chapter will emphasize well-controlled studies, and internal and external validity will be discussed within each context. Since

This chapter is a revision of Macciocchi SN, Barth JT, Littlefield LM. Outcome after mild head injury. *In* Cantu RC (ed): Neurologic Athletic Head and Neck Injuries, *Clinics in Sports Medicine.* Philadelphia, WB Saunders, 1998, pp 27–36.

clinical populations likely differ in many ways from young athletes, generalizations from the former to the latter may not be justified. As such, findings from general clinical and sports studies will be discussed independently.

MECHANISM OF INJURY AND PATHOPHYSIOLOGY

Biomechanical models of mild head injury and concussion have been proposed based on animal and cadaver experiments and observations. This work appears to have relevance to sports-related concussion because skull deformations are limited in mild head injury, and acceleration and impact injuries are generally viewed as equivalent.[35] In addition, both translational (straight line) and rotational (axial) forces are important as mechanical determinants of injury severity.[16, 35] Although a narrow range of injury response is observed in mild head injury, interacting translational and rotational forces may have relevance with regard to outcome in sports-related concussion.

Few studies have systematically documented injury mechanics in anything but an observational/descriptive manner.[2, 46, 48] Most studies have reported observed head and body trauma (i.e., hockey players body checking and boarding) and inferred mechanical forces that are likely to have affected the central nervous system.[44, 46] Studying injury mechanics requires an understanding of speed of acceleration, mass, and distance/time for deceleration, as well as vectors of physical forces, and to date such factors have not been measured adequately in sports concussion research models.[16, 35, 49] For this reason, the relationship between biomechanics of injury and outcome remains unclear.

Changes in neurophysiology following mild acceleration-deceleration injuries in primates have included axonal damage (shear-strain), principally found to be in the pons and midbrain.[21] These findings are generally consistent with human autopsy and cadaver studies, which have revealed diffuse axonal injury. Since mild head injury lesions are histologic (microscopic in origin) and are only likely to be revealed by the most sensitive neuroradiologic procedures,[41] those studying sports concussion must rely on the presence of postconcussion symptoms, neuropsychologic impairment, and evidence of pathophysiology.

Few controlled prospective studies of neuropsychologic functioning in sports populations have been completed to date. The University of Virginia College Football Study[2, 30] found 195 mildly concussed players with evidence of time limited neuropsychologic impairment, which was similar to controlled clinical studies in nonathletic populations.[27] These investigations of concussed college football players and general clinical populations, as well as other animal, clinical, and sports-related mild head injury research studies, suggest that there may be a pathologic base for some symptoms following mild closed head injury.[13, 16, 27, 30, 33, 35, 41] Unfortunately the precise relationship with specific pathophysiologic parameters in outcome is unknown.

MEASUREMENT OF SEVERITY OF INJURY

Clinical and animal studies clearly show that head injury severity and outcome are strongly related across the spectrum of head trauma[16, 35]; however, identifying poor outcomes within the range of mild concussions is problematic. To address this issue within the sports setting, a number of concussion or mild head injury severity scales have been published (Table 10–1).[10, 22, 25, 37, 47] Each scale defines severity by indexing duration of loss of consciousness (LOC) or confusion, and posttraumatic amnesia (PTA) or retrograde amnesia. In some scales, injuries range from mild (Grade 1) to severe (Grade 3),[10, 25, 37] or Grade 1 to Grade 4.[22, 47]

A number of factors can interact and confound injury severity on a case by case basis. For example, players may have a history of one or more documented head injuries. In addition, clinical indexing of injuries is most often based on report of symptoms and does not take into account specific pathophysiologic mechanisms underlying those symptoms.[33] Consequently, injuries with different pathophysiologies may be similar in initial presentation but have different outcomes. For example, in the University of Virginia Football Study, Grade 1 injuries rarely produced prolonged symptoms (beyond 5 to 10 days), but a very small percentage of football players were still symptomatic the following season. Surprisingly,

Table 10–1. Severity of Sports Concussion Scales

	Grade 1 (Mild)	Grade 2 (Moderate)	Grade 3 (Severe)	Grade 4
Cantu Severity Scales (R. C. Cantu, 1991)	No loss of consciousness and posttraumatic amnesia <30 minutes	Loss of consciousness <5 minutes or posttraumatic amnesia of 30 minutes to 24 hours	Loss of consciousness >5 minutes or posttraumatic amnesia >24 hours	
Colorado Severity Scales (J. Kelly, 1991)	Confusion without amnesia; no loss of consciousness	Confusion with amnesia; no loss of consciousness	Loss of consciousness	
Practice Parameters Severity Scales, 1997	Transient confusion, no loss of consciousness, concussion symptoms <15 minutes	Transient confusion, no loss of consciousness, concussion symptoms >15 minutes	Any loss of consciousness, brief or prolonged	
Torg Severity Scales (J. S. Torg, 1982)	Transient confusion	Transient confusion, posttraumatic amnesia	Transient confusion, posttraumatic amnesia and retrograde amnesia	Loss of consciousness
Jordan Severity Scales (B. D. Jordan, 1994)	Confusion without amnesia, no loss of consciousness	Confusion with amnesia <24 hours, no loss of consciousness	Loss of consciousness w/altered level of consciousness <2–3 minutes	Loss of consciousness w/altered level of consciousness >2–3 minutes

athletes with persistent symptoms did not experience greater periods of posttraumatic disorientation or confusion, which could indicate an equivalent injury by clinical standards, but outcome following injury in these players is clearly different.[30] Another descriptive study found similar extended postconcussion symptoms.[50]

In a very small number of cases, it appears that catastrophic injury can result from seemingly trivial multiple concussions. These cases, referred to as second impact syndrome, theoretically involve a loss of cerebral autoregulatory capacity, which leads to elevated intracranial pressure and vascular congestion. Athletes may be susceptible to catastrophic consequences (including mortality) from a second mild head injury (Grade 1) if it follows closely on the heels of a first mild concussion (typically 4 to 5 days).[43] There have also been reports of catastrophic outcomes following mild concussion in players who have subsequently been found to have infectious disease such as encephalitis or mononucleosis.[36, 47]

In summary, the effect of injury severity and associated variables on outcome after mild concussion has not been studied adequately in either general clinical or sports populations. Injury severity is typically established by clinical symptoms, which may or may not be directly reflective of underlying pathophysiology.[33] Even with measurement limitations, attempts to reliably define,

record, and study injury severity may lead to a more adequate understanding of the relationship between clinically indexed severity and outcomes.

FREQUENCY OF INJURY

A few case reports and descriptive group studies implicate multiple mild head injuries in poor outcomes.[38, 48] In one of these studies, soccer players who experienced numerous mild head injuries had observable neuropsychologic impairment; however, these deficits were evaluated only after the final injury. In contrast to this finding, a recent unpublished study of football players revealed no reliable differences in cognitive functioning or symptoms in players with two mild head injuries (Grade 1) compared with players with a single mild injury.[29] Most players in this study, however, sustained mild concussions in successive years rather than the same year. Two other studies of Australian Rules football players also revealed no cumulative effects of repeated mild head injuries.[24, 31]

Common sense suggests that multiple mild head injuries should negatively influence outcome, yet the results of existing studies are not consistent. These inconsistencies in the literature are likely due to methodologic variability among studies. For example, one investigation reporting cumulative effects of mild head injury in a clinical population included patients with multiple injuries consistent with Grade 3 severity, and sometimes in relatively close temporal proximity.[19] Other studies have failed to document time between injuries or the relative severity of these traumas.[48] Until studies document and control for injury severity and timing, and follow these patients/athletes over time, it will be difficult to draw definitive conclusions regarding the effects of multiple mild concussions on outcome.

MEDICAL, NEUROLOGIC, AND PSYCHOLOGIC COMPLICATIONS

Single case studies have documented significant effects of premorbid medical or neurologic disorders (i.e., previous mild head injuries) on injury outcomes in athletes; however, these cases usually involve catastrophic consequences.[43, 47] The more subtle effect of medical, neurologic, and psychologic factors on outcome has not been systematically studied. The vast majority of existing studies have made limited attempts to document these variables, when it is clear that previous head injury and systemic infection may have a significant influence on outcome. Psychologic factors may influence outcome by altering the threshold for reporting or denying symptoms, since it is reasoned that many athletes may not report postconcussion symptoms when they do exist, since they are concerned about losing playing time if they complain. Other athletes may be overly concerned with the effects of injury and report multiple symptoms without regard for cause.[38] This picture is further clouded by the fact that a 1993 study has shown that many symptoms of mild head injury are commonly observed at high base rates in the normal population.[15] Therefore, without experimental controls, reporting symptoms such as headaches, memory problems, and dizziness may have little meaning and cannot be viewed as definitive evidence of postconcussive disorder. Prospective documentation of all relevant medical, neurologic, and psychologic variables across longitudinal studies, preseason baseline neuropsychologic assessments, and use of control subjects will be essential to future research efforts to document the effects of these complicating factors.

RETURN TO PLAY CRITERIA

Return to play algorithms following single concussions are based upon injury severity and reported symptoms. Guidelines for return to play vary, but they generally rely upon self-reported symptoms to determine when athletes should return to play. Existing guidelines for clinical practice clearly assume that more severe and more frequent injuries should preclude rapid return to play (Tables 10–2 and 10–3).[7–11, 22, 25, 36, 37] Despite these recommended guidelines, clinical practice (on the field or at the school) may vary substantially. The clinical and research communities have recommended considering additional assessment procedures, including the Standardized Assessment of Concussion (SAC),[32] cardiovascular stress (challenge),[38] and neuropsychologic assessment to determine readiness for return to play.[27, 45] Thus far, there are limited data on the association between clinical management strategies (guidelines for return to play) and outcome. Nevertheless, it is logical to assume that premature return to play may increase morbidity associated with the initial injury or predispose players to increased risk for second, and perhaps more dangerous, injury.[7, 8] Clinical management decisions may effect outcome, even if catastrophic consequences like second impact syndrome do not occur. The team physician, trainer, or other clinician who is responsible for clinical management is in a difficult position, since data are not available for addressing the issue of optimal circumstances for return to play. It is recommended that conservative management decisions still rule the day, since the athlete's present and future health must be the clinician's primary concern. Evaluation of how clinical management strategies influence outcome would be a welcome addition to the literature of mild head injury in sports.

OUTCOME ASSESSMENT

The good news so far is that there are many sports concussion outcome studies in progress today; however, to date there is only one study that has prospectively examined the neurocognitive effects of mild head injury in sports in a comprehensive manner.[2, 30] In this study of 2350 football players, pre-injury medical, neurologic, and neuro-

Table 10–2. Guidelines for Return to Play: One Concussion

	Grade 1	Grade 2	Grade 3	Grade 4
Cantu Return Guidelines (R.C. Cantu, 1991)	May return to play if asymptomatic for 1 week.	May return to play if asymptomatic for 1 week.	Should not be allowed to play for at least 1 month; may then return if asymptomatic for 1 week.	
Colorado Return Guidelines (J. Kelly, 1991)	Remove from contest, examine immediately and every 5 minutes for amnesia or postconcussive symptoms at rest and with exertion. May return to play if no symptoms for 20 minutes and no amnesia.	Remove from contest and disallow return. Examine frequently for signs of evolving intracranial pathology. Re-examine the next day. May return to practice only after 1 full week without symptoms.	Transport from field by ambulance (w/cervical spine immobilization if indicated) to nearest hospital. Thorough neurologic evaluation. Hospital confinement if signs of pathology. If findings are normal, instructions to family for overnight observation. Return to practice in 2 weeks if no symptoms.	
Practice Parameters Return Guidelines, 1997	May return to play if symptoms resolve in <15 minutes.	If second Grade 1 concussion occurs on same day, player should be removed from play until asymptomatic for 1 week.	Remove from play 1 week if LOC is brief; 2 weeks if prolonged. If second Grade 3, player should be removed until asymptomatic for 1 month. If positive CT, MRI, or other findings, further participation should be discouraged.	
Torg Return Guidelines (J.S. Torg, 1992)	Return to play if asymptomatic.	Return to play not permitted on day of injury. Participation precluded as long as symptoms are present.	Return to play not permitted on day of injury. Participation precluded as long as symptoms are present.	Return to play not permitted on day of injury. Participation precluded as long as symptoms are present.
Jordan Return Guidelines (B.D. Jordan, 1994)	Return to play if asymptomatic at rest and after exertion after at least 20 minutes of observation.	Return to play if asymptomatic for 1 week.	Should not be allowed to play for at least 1 month. May then return to play if asymptomatic for 1 week.	Should not be allowed to play for at least 1 month. May then return to play if asymptomatic for 2 weeks.

psychologic data were collected, and athletes were assessed utilizing standardized neurocognitive tests at several intervals following injury. At the same time, red-shirted football players and student controls were assessed and utilized for comparison purposes. Contrary to case reports and some descriptive studies, this research revealed that most college football-related concussions are Grade 1 with few persistent symp-

Table 10–3. Cantu Guidelines for Return to Play After Single and Multiple Concussions

	Grade 1 (Mild)	Grade 2 (Moderate)	Grade 3 (Severe)
First Concussion	Return to play if asymptomatic for 1 week	Return to play if asymptomatic for 1 week	Minimum of 1 month; may return to play if asymptomatic
Second Concussion	Return to play in 2 weeks if asymptomatic for 1 week	Minimum of 1 month; return to play if asymptomatic for 1 week; consider terminating season	Terminate season; may return to play if asymptomatic
Third Concussion	Terminate season; may return to play next season if asymptomatic	Terminate season; may return to play if asymptomatic	

toms.[30] This study went on to reveal that recovery of neurocognitive function in relationship to pre-injury assessment and control subjects occurred within 5 to 10 days postinjury. These findings have had an obvious effect on the return to play criteria noted in the previous section.

Despite the methodologic strengths of this study, many questions remain unanswered. Fortunately, present research programs at the high school, college, and professional levels of sports are beginning to utilize stronger research methodologies similar to the above study, and such methodologic precision will undoubtedly provide us with better understanding of sports concussion severity and outcome, and with better return to play decision trees.

Although more rigorous research designs and pooling of outcome data will be necessary in order to make progress in protecting the athlete, a more comprehensive view of outcome is needed. Most existing studies have examined short-term symptoms or neuropsychologic functioning with minimal regard for more extensive or broad aspects of outcome. For example, no studies have addressed quality of life, academic performance, general psychologic well-being, or for that matter, athletic or job performance. These components of outcome will likely become critical in establishing morbidity following mild concussion. Continuing to focus on short-term outcomes may also ignore the long-term deleterious effects of repeated mild head injuries.[23, 34, 45] The solid economic foundation of athletics in our society suggests that well designed, comprehensive, and long-term outcome studies can be a reality.

SUMMARY AND CONCLUSIONS

Although concern about mild sports head injury has significantly increased in the 1990s, few well controlled studies exist. As such, we are not able to specify the effects of injury biomechanics, severity, frequency, and complications at outcome until more definitive research is completed. Management of mild head injury and return to play will necessarily be based on clinical judgment rather than empiric fact.

Despite present research limitations, several tentative conclusions are offered: (1)

Mild head injury is likely a frequent occurrence in sports. (2) The overwhelming majority of single, Grade 1 injuries have few persisting symptoms, and morbidity in the short-term appears limited. (3) Multiple mild head injuries, especially Grade 2 or 3, may have catastrophic and long-term, irreversible consequences. (4) It appears that athletes with apparently equivalent injuries by clinical standards may have different outcomes. Finally, outcome following sports concussion must receive increased research attention, and some symmetry and coordination of efforts in both short-term and long-term studies should be encouraged.

References

1. Alves MA, Macciocchi SN, Barth JT. Postconcussive symptoms after mild head injury. J Head Trauma Rehabil 1993;3:45–59.
2. Barth JT, Alves WA, Ryan T, et al. Mild head injury in sports: Neuropsychological sequelae and recovery of function. In Levin HS, Eisenberg, HM, Benton AR (eds): Mild Head Injury. New York, Oxford University Press, 1989, pp 257–275.
3. Barth JT, Macciocchi SN, Giordani B, et al. Neuropsychological sequelae of minor head injury. Neurosurgery 1983;13:529–533.
4. Binder LM. Malingering following mild head trauma. Clin Neuropsychol 1990;4:25–36.
5. Bohnen N, Jolles J, Twijnstra A. Neuropsychological deficits in patients with persistent symptoms six months after mild head injury. Neurosurgery 1992;30:692–695.
6. Bohnen N, Twijnstra A, Wijnen G, et al. Recovery from visual and acoustic hyperaesthesia after mild head injury in relation to patterns of behavioral dysfunction. J Neurol Neurosurg Psychiatry 1992;55:222–224.
7. Cantu RC. Cerebral concussion in sport: Management and prevention. Sports Med 1992;14:64–74.
8. Cantu RC. Head and spine injuries in youth sports. Clin Sports Med 1995;14:517–532.
9. Cantu RC. Head injuries in sport. Br J Sports Med 1996;30:289–296.
10. Cantu RC. Minor Head Injuries in Sports. In Dyment PG (ed): Adolescent Medicine: State of the Art Reviews. Philadelphia, Hanley & Belfus, 1991;2:17–30.
11. Cantu RC. When to return to contact sports after a cerebral concussion. Sports Med Digest 1998; 10:1–2.
12. Coonley-Hoganson RC, Sachs N, Desai BT, et al. Sequelae associated with head injuries in patients who are not hospitalized. A follow-up survey. Neurosurgery 1984;14:315–317.
13. Cremona-Meteyord SL, Geffen GM. Persistent visuospatial attention deficits following mild head injury in Australian rules football players. Neuropsychologia 1994;6:649–692.
14. Dikmen S, McLean A, Temkin N. Neuropsychological and psychosocial consequences of mild head

injury. J Neurol Neurosurg Psychiatry 1986;49:227–232.

15. Dikmen S, Levin HS. Methodological issues in the study of mild head injury. J Head Trauma Rehabil 1993;3:30–47.

16. Elson LM, Ward CC. Mechanisms and pathophysiology of mild head injury. Semin Neurol 1994;14:8–18.

17. Ettlin TM, Kischka U, Reichmann S. Cerebral symptoms after whiplash injury of the neck: A prospective clinical and neuropsychological study of whiplash injury. J Neurol Neurosurg Psychiatry Philadelphia 1992;55:945–948.

18. Gentili M, Nichelli P, Schoenhuber R. Neuropsychological evaluation of mild head injury. J Neurol Neurosurg Psychiatry 1985;48:137–140.

19. Gronwall D, Wrighton P. Cumulative effects of concussion. Lancet 1975;2:995–997.

20. Hugenholtz H, Stuss DT, Stethem LL, et al. How long does it take to recover from mild concussion? Neurosurgery 1988;22:853–858.

21. Jane JA, Steward O, Gennarelli T. Axonal degeneration induced by experimental noninvasive minor head injury. J Neurosurg 1985;62:96–100.

22. Jordan BD. Sports injuries. In National Athletic Trainers Association Research and Education Foundation. Proceedings: Mild Brain Injury in Sports Summit. Washington, D.C., 1994.

23. Jordan BD, Relkin NR, Ravin LD, et al. Apolipoprotein E ε4 associated with chronic brain injury in boxing. JAMA 1997;278:136–140.

24. Jordan SE, Green GA, Galanty HL, et al. Acute and chronic brain injury in United States national team soccer players. Am J Sports Med 1996;24:205–210.

25. Kelly JP, Nichols JS, Filley CM, et al. Concussion in sports: Guidelines for the prevention of catastrophic outcome. JAMA 1991;266:2867–2869.

26. Leininger BE, Gramling SE, Farrell AD, et al. Neuropsychological deficits in symptomatic minor head injury patients after concussion and mild concussion. J Neurol Neurosurg Psychiatry 1990;53:293–296.

27. Levin HS, Mattis S, Ruff RN, et al. Neurobehavioral outcome following minor head injury: A three-center study. J Neurosurg 1987;66:234–243.

28. Levin HS, Williams DH, Eisenberg HM, et al. Serial MRI and neurobehavioral findings after mild to moderate closed head injury. J Neurol Neurosurg Psychiatry 1992;55:255–262.

29. Macciocchi SN, Barth JT, Alves WM, et al. Multiple mild head injury in college athletes. Neurosurgery (in review).

30. Macciocchi SN, Barth JT, Alves WM, et al. Neuropsychological functioning and recovery after mild head injury in collegiate athletes. Neurosurgery 1996;39:510.

31. Maddocks DL, Saling M, Dicker GD. A note on normative data for a test sensitive to concussion in Australian rules footballers. Aust Psychol 1995;30:125–127.

32. McCrea M, Kelly JP, Kluge J, et al. Standardized assessment of concussion (SAC): On-site mental status evaluation of the athlete. J Head Trauma Rehabil 1998;13:27–35.

33. Mittl RL, Grossoman RI, Heihle JF, et al. Prevalence of MR evidence of diffuse axonal injury in patients with mild head injury and normal CT findings. AJNR Am J Neuroradiol 1994;15:1583–1589.

34. Mortimer JA, French LR, Hutton JT, et al. Head injury as a risk factor for Alzheimer's disease. Neurology 1985;35:264–266.

35. Ommaya AK. Head injury mechanisms and the concept of preventive management: A review of critical synthesis. J Neurotrauma 1996;12:527–546.

36. Polin RS, Alves WM, Jane JA. Sports and head injuries. In Evans RW (ed): Neurology and Trauma. Philadelphia, WB Saunders, 1996, pp 168–185.

37. Practice Parameter. The management of concussion in sports (summary statement). Neurology 1997;48:581–585.

38. Putukian M, Echemendia, RJ. Managing successive minor head injuries: Which tests guide return to play? Phys Sportsmed 1996;24:25–38.

39. Rimel RW, Giordani B, Barth JT, et al. Disability caused by mild head injury. Neurosurgery 1981;9:221–228.

40. Ross RJ, Casson IR, Siegel O, et al. Boxing injuries: Neurologic, radiologic, and neuropsychologic evaluation. Clin Sports Med 1987;6:41–51.

41. Ruff RM, Couch JA, Tröster AI, et al. Selected cases of poor outcome following minor brain trauma. Comparing neuropsychological and positron emission tomography assessment. Brain Inj 1994;8:297–308.

42. Rutherford WH, Merrett JD, McDonald JR. Symptoms at one year following concussion from minor head injuries. Injury 1979;10:225–230.

43. Saunders RL, Harbaugh RE. The second impact in catastrophic contact-sports head trauma. JAMA 1984;252:538–539.

44. Stiller JW, Weinberger DR. Boxing and chronic brain damage. Psychiatr Clin North Am 1985;8:339–356.

45. Spear J. Are footballers at risk for developing dementia? Int J Geriatr Psychiatry 1995;10:1011–1014.

46. Tegner Y, Lorentzon R. Concussion among Swedish elite ice hockey players. Br J Sports Med 1996;30:251–255.

47. Torg JS, Beer LA, Begso J. Head trauma in football players with mononucleosis. Phys Sportsmed 1989;17:573–578.

48. Tysvaer AT, Storli OV, Bachen NI. Soccer injuries to the brain: A neurologic and electroencephalographic study of former players. Acta Neurol Scand 1989;80:151–156.

49. Varney NR, Varney RN: Brain injury without head injury. Some physics of automobile collisions with particular reference to brain injuries occurring without physical head trauma. Appl Neuropsychol 1995;2:47–62.

50. Wilberger JE. Minor head injuries in American football: Prevention of long term sequelae. Sports Med 1993;15:338–343.

51. Williams DH, Levin HS, Eisenberg HM. Mild head injury classification. Neurosurgery 1990;27:422–428.

11

Concussions in Ice Hockey: The National Hockey League Program

Mark R. Lovell and Charles J. Burke, III

Over the last several years, the evaluation of concussion in athletes has become an area of intense interest among sports medicine practitioners. Much of the focus has been directed to the study of professional football and hockey athletes. The most recent outgrowth of this interest has been the development of comprehensive concussion evaluation programs within both the National Football League (NFL) and the National Hockey League (NHL).[1] These programs are structured to identify athletes immediately after injury and to avoid exposure to further injury. The NFL and NHL programs have also been developed to answer a number of important research questions. This chapter will provide an overview of the concussion program that has been developed for the National Hockey League (NHL). The current NHL evaluation and management protocol will be reviewed with special reference to return to play issues.

BIOMECHANICS AND PATHOPHYSIOLOGY OF CONCUSSION IN THE HOCKEY ATHLETE

The basic pathophysiology of concussion has been detailed elsewhere in this text and will not be reviewed in this chapter. However, it is important to briefly review the unique aspects of ice hockey that may at times contribute to concussions on the ice. Today's professional hockey players are larger, faster, and better conditioned than in past generations. In fact, a perusal of current NHL rosters reveals that the majority of the athletes weigh over 200 pounds and many are over 6 feet in height. A modern NHL player may reach speeds of almost 30 miles per hour during a game situation. In addition, the continuous rotation of rested players into the game maintains a high level of play and excitement but also maintains this level of speed on the ice. All of these factors combine to create the potential for high-speed collisions on the ice.

Mechanisms of Injury

Most of the concussions sustained by professional hockey athletes are the result of a collision with another object while skating at a high rate of speed. Such a collision can result in both deceleration and rotational injuries during which brain axons are stretched or torn.[2] That type of injury does not require direct trauma to the head and is not necessarily prevented through the use of protective headgear. In addition, direct contact of the head with the glass, boards, stick, elbow, or ice may result in direct trauma to the skull as well as contusion of the brain in more severe cases. The helmet is important in protecting the athlete against this type of injury. Finally, periodic fights on the ice may also result in a concussion, although preliminary data gathered through the NHL have indicated that on-ice skirmishes account for a relatively small number of concussions.

THE NHL CONCUSSION PROGRAM

The NHL concussion program was initiated to minimize concussive injuries in NHL players and involves the cooperative efforts of the NHL team physicians, athletic trainers, and consulting neuropsychologists. One of the primary goals of the project is to gather systematic league-wide statistics regarding the incidence of concussion. To facilitate this process, a concussion evaluation form was developed that is completed by the team physician following a suspected concussion. This form contains the physician's initial assessment of the player as well as a description of the characteristics of the injury (e.g., mid-ice collision, collision with boards). This information is then transferred to a central league-wide database for later study.

A second important aspect of the program involves the retrospective review of videotape of selected concussions in an attempt to better understand the biomechanics of the concussive injuries within the NHL and to reduce injuries in the future. Finally, the NHL has instituted a league-wide neuropsychologic testing program to assist in the assessment of a player's neurocognitive status following a suspected concussion.

THE NHL NEUROPSYCHOLOGIC TESTING PROGRAM

Historical Roots

The NHL neuropsychologic testing program represents the largest study of head injury in athletes to date. The use of neuropsychologic assessment procedures in sports has a relatively short history and began with the study of college football athletes by Jeffrey Barth and his colleagues at the University of Virginia in the 1980s. In this study, over 2300 athletes underwent preseason neuropsychologic testing as well as postinjury testing following a suspected concussion. Barth and his coinvestigators found subtle and rapidly resolving impairments in cognitive functioning on tests sensitive to information processing speed compared to a control group.[3, 4]

As a result of the interest generated by the University of Virginia study and based on the need for more sensitive clinical diagnostic procedures in professional athletes, a neuropsychologic evaluation program was begun with the Pittsburgh Steelers football team in 1993. This program was instituted by Joseph Maroon, M.D., Mark Lovell, Ph.D., and John Norwig, A.T.C.,[1] and represented the first clinically oriented project structured to assist team medical personnel in making return to play decisions following a

suspected concussion. This approach involved the formal evaluation of each player prior to the beginning of the season to provide the basis for comparison, in the event of a concussion during the season. Testing was then repeated within 24 hours after a suspected concussion, and again prior to the return of the athlete to contact (approximately 5 days postinjury). This project was subsequently adopted by the National Football League and is now being used by 20 NFL teams.

STRUCTURE OF THE NHL CONCUSSION EVALUATION PROGRAM

Rink-Side Evaluation

The initial evaluation of the concussed hockey player begins on the ice or at rinkside, and the first assessment of the athlete's status is usually completed by the team physician or athletic trainer. It is important both to evaluate the player's cognitive status via formal mental status testing and to document the athlete's reported symptoms. To facilitate the identification of concussion immediately after suspected injury, a pocket-sized card has been developed that lists frequently observed signs and symptoms of concussion (Fig. 11–1). This card is not meant to provide a comprehensive evaluation of signs or symptoms of concussion, but is constructed to assist the team physician or athletic trainer in evaluation of the players under the often chaotic conditions that surround the injury of the athlete (e.g., noisy arena, limited time until resumption of play).

At a minimum, this initial postinjury evaluation should involve an assessment of the player's orientation to place, game, and details of the contest. The athlete's recall of events preceding the collision (retrograde amnesia) is an important marker of injury severity that should also be evaluated. The ability to learn and retain new information (anterograde amnesia) should also be tested via a brief sideline memory test. In English-speaking athletes, the player should be asked to memorize five words. However, given the large number of players within the NHL for whom English is a second language, we suggest that familiar, hockey-specific words be used with non-native English speakers. For example, words such as

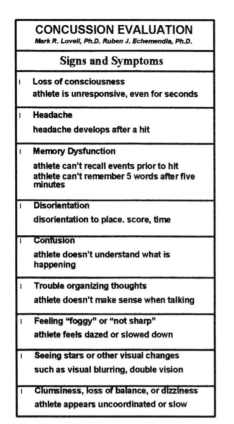

Figure 11–1. Rink-Side Concussion Evaluation.

"puck," "net," "goal," "stick," or "check" represent words with which most NHL players are familiar. Also, sequential pointing to body parts represents one method of evaluating memory without relying on language processes.[5] Regardless of whether sequence learning or word-list learning procedures are used, the athlete should be checked for recall of this list within approximately 5 minutes. Brief tests of attentional capacity such as recitation of digits in backward order or backward recitation of months of the year are also useful, but are not sufficient to evaluate concussion. Finally, the player should be observed for emerging postconcussive symptoms such as headache, nausea, dizziness, imbalance, or on-ice confusion.[6] The athlete should also be observed for the development of motor incoordination or any change in behavior.

Neuropsychologic Evaluation

The formal neuropsychologic evaluation of the athlete should take place within 24 to 48 hours of the suspected concussion, whenever possible. Although many athletes may appear to be symptom free, a neuropsychologic evaluation is recommended to evaluate more subtle aspects of cognitive functioning, such as information processing speed and memory.[7] If the athlete displays any cognitive deficits on testing or continues to exhibit postconcussive symptoms, return to play is contraindicated and a follow-up neuropsychologic evaluation is recommended within 5 to 7 days after injury. This interval represents a useful and practical time span and also appears to be consistent with animal brain metabolism studies, which have demonstrated metabolic changes in the brain which persist for days following injury.[8]

In the design of a league-wide neuropsychologic evaluation program, a number of factors had to be considered. While the time pressures in working with large groups of athletes are similar with all professional athletes, there are several factors that make the evaluation of the hockey athlete particularly challenging. First, the multiple languages spoken within the NHL make communication difficult, particularly during the somewhat chaotic game situations. While examination of each athlete in his native language may appear to be the most effective way of evaluating the athlete both at baseline and following a concussion, this is highly impractical and would require availability of multilingual neuropsychologists in all cities within a given league. For that reason, it is more practical to utilize test procedures that are not heavily language dependent. The assessment of players in their native tongue would also impede league-wide efforts to study performance on standardized tests because of limitations in translating languages directly. Therefore, neuropsychologic tests were selected that require relatively little familiarity with the English language.

In addition, the logistics of a typical professional hockey travel schedule, which often includes 2- to 3-week road trips, required a network approach through which injured players could be evaluated regardless of the city of their injury. If a player is injured while on a road trip, the athlete is evaluated by the athletic trainer under the supervision of the opposing team's physician. If neuropsychologic testing is indicated, the neuropsychologic consultant for the opposing team completes the evaluation and transmits the results of this evaluation to the neuropsychologic consultant from the player's team. The neuropsychologist then provides consultation to the athlete's team physician, who makes the return to play decision.

Importance of Baseline Testing

The importance of the baseline evaluation of the athlete, prior to exposure to injury, cannot be overemphasized. Individual players vary tremendously with regard to their life-long level of performance on tests of memory, attention/concentration, mental processing speed, and motor speed. These performance differences are often independent of their concussion history. For instance, some players perform poorly on the more demanding tests because of preinjury learning disabilities, attention deficit disorder, or other factors, such as test-taking anxiety. Additionally, language differences can also result in differences in performance on testing. Therefore, the only fair comparison of the athlete's test performance is with his own preinjury baseline. The use of baseline testing also allows for the evaluation of the player over time and will assist the NHL in tracking athletes throughout their careers.

Selection of a Neuropsychologic Test Battery for Ice Hockey

As noted previously in this chapter, the application of neuropsychologic assessment strategies to ice hockey provides specific challenges. As is the case with professional football, the need for brevity must be balanced against the need for sampling across multiple domains of neuropsychologic functioning. The test battery should be constructed to evaluate the athlete's functioning in the areas of attention, information processing speed, fluency, and memory. Although there are numerous tests that can provide information regarding the athlete's ability to function in these areas, procedures should also be selected that have multiple equivalent forms or that have been thoroughly researched with regard to the expected practice effects. The battery of tests adopted for the NHL study was constructed with these factors in mind. The NHL test battery was developed by the Neuropsychological Advisory Board, who serve as supervisors of the neuropsychologic testing component of the program. This group is composed of Drs. Mark Lovell and Ruben Echemendia, program codirectors; Drs. William Barr and Elizabeth Parker; and Dr. W. Gary Snow, NHL Players Association representative. The test battery can be administered in approximately 30 minutes and samples from the cognitive domains of memory, information processing speed, attentional processes, and visuomotor speed. The NHL test battery is presented in Table 11–1.

The Hopkins Verbal Learning Test[9] is a test of verbal memory, which involves the memorization of a 12-word list across three trials. This test involves a learning component (number of words learned over three trials) and a memory component (number of words recalled 20 minutes later). Ruff's Figure Fluency test[10] is a relatively new test that requires the athlete to rapidly draw a series of unique designs while under time pressure. Although the use of this test has yet to be formally evaluated with athletes, its nonverbal nature may be ideal for use with athletes for whom English is a second

Table 11–1. NHL Neuropsychological Test Battery

Test	Ability Evaluated
Orientation Questions	Retrograde and anterograde amnesia, orientation to place and time
Hopkins Verbal Learning Test (HVLT)* †	Word learning
Color Trail Making‡	Visual scanning, mental flexibility
Controlled Oral Word Association Test*§	Word fluency, word retrieval
Ruff Figural Fluency Test‖	Design fluency
Penn State Symbol Cancellation Test¶	Visual scanning, attention
Symbol Digit Modalities**	Visual scanning, immediate memory
Concussion Symptom Inventory	Postconcussive symptoms
Delayed recall from HVLT	Delayed recall for words

*Suggested for English-speaking athletes only.
†Brandt J. The Hopkins Verbal Learning Test: Development of a new memory test with six equivalent forms. Clin Neuropsychol 1991;5:125–142.
‡D'Elia L, Satz P. The Color Trail Making Test. Odessa, FL, Psychological Assessment Resources, 1989.
§Benton A, Hamsher K. Multilingual Aphasia Examination. Iowa City, IA, University of Iowa Press, 1978.
‖Ruff R. Ruff Figural Fluency Test. Odessa, FL, Psychological Assessment Resources, 1988.
¶Echemendia R. Penn State Symbol Cancellation Test (personal communication), 1999.
**Smith A. Symbol Digit Modalities Test Manual. Los Angeles, CA, Western Psychological Services, 1982.

language. The Color Trail Making[11] test was developed to provide a culturally neutral alternative to the widely used Trail Making Test[12] and requires the athlete to utilize visual scanning and sequencing skills while under time pressure. The Symbol Digit Modalities Test[13] measures mental processing speed and also has a memory component. The Penn State Cancellation Test[14] is a test that measures visual scanning and attentional processes and requires the athlete to cross out symbols that are imbedded within an array of other symbols. The Controlled Oral Word Association Test[15] is a test of verbal fluency, which is used only with English-speaking athletes.

In addition to the neuropsychologic tests listed above, the neuropsychologist should be careful to evaluate noncognitive symptoms of concussion. The Concussion Symptom Inventory scale has been found to be useful in this regard. This scale is presented in Figure 11–2. Finally, athletes should be checked for orientation to year, month, date of the month, and day of the week, and should also be questioned regarding their last memory prior to the hit (retrograde amnesia) and first memory following the hit (anterograde amnesia).

MAKING RETURN TO PLAY DECISIONS AFTER A SUSPECTED CONCUSSION

The decision to return a hockey player to the ice following a concussion should be made only after consideration of a number

of factors and a careful evaluation of the player's medical history, concussion symptoms, and performance on neuropsychologic testing. Although there is no magic formula for making return to play decisions, this section provides a general rationale for making these difficult decisions.

Neurobiologic Factors

Although the exact mechanisms that influence recovery from concussion are still unknown, preliminary studies of the recovery process have implicated a number of different factors. Current animal research has suggested that a sequence of neurophysiologic events may leave the brain in a state of vulnerability for days after trauma to the brain.[8] This area of research must be viewed as being preliminary at the current time and has yet to be adequately demonstrated in humans. However, the preliminary research has been sufficient to suggest caution when returning an athlete to the ice following a suspected concussion.

Player Concussion History

The team physician or athletic trainer should gather a complete concussion history of all athletes under his care. Current research, although somewhat scant, has suggested that multiple concussions may result in permanent brain injury and resulting disability.[16, 17] Although there is currently no absolute cutoff point at which a player

Patient/Athlete:_____   Team: _____

SYMPTOM	RATING			BASELINE Date:	TESTING 2 Date:	TESTING 3 Date:
	None	Mod.	Severe			
Headache	0 1 2 3 4 5 6					
Nausea	0 1 2 3 4 5 6					
Vomiting	0 1 2 3 4 5 6					
Balance problems	0 1 2 3 4 5 6					
Dizziness	0 1 2 3 4 5 6					
Fatigue	0 1 2 3 4 5 6					
Trouble falling asleep	0 1 2 3 4 5 6					
Sleeping more than usual	0 1 2 3 4 5 6					
Balance Problems	0 1 2 3 4 5 6					
Drowsiness	0 1 2 3 4 5 6					
Sensitivity to light	0 1 2 3 4 5 6					
Sensitivity to noise	0 1 2 3 4 5 6					
Irritability	0 1 2 3 4 5 6					
Sadness	0 1 2 3 4 5 6					
Nervousness	0 1 2 3 4 5 6					
More emotional than usual	0 1 2 3 4 5 6					
Numbness or tingling	0 1 2 3 4 5 6					
Feeling slowed down	0 1 2 3 4 5 6					
Feeling like "in a fog"	0 1 2 3 4 5 6					
Difficulty concentrating	0 1 2 3 4 5 6					
Difficulty remembering	0 1 2 3 4 5 6					
Other	0 1 2 3 4 5 6					
TOTAL SCORE						

Figure 11–2. NHL Concussion Symptoms Inventory. Lovell, M.R., and Echemendia, R., 1997.

should no longer compete, our experience with professional athletes has suggested that athletes who sustain multiple concussions within the same season are at increased risk for permanent disability. Therefore, the player's concussion history should be taken into consideration when return to play decisions are being made, and athletes who have suffered multiple concussions should be evaluated particularly carefully.

Initial Rink-Side Cognitive Screening

The athlete should be evaluated utilizing mental status evaluation or cognitive screening such as the rink-side cognitive screening evaluation described previously. This type of brief testing ideally should be incorporated into the player's preseason baseline assessment to ensure that the athlete can pass the screening items prior to injury. Specifically, the player should be evaluated for amnesia for events occurring before the injury (retrograde amnesia) and after the injury (anterograde amnesia). Additionally, the athlete should be evaluated for disruption of orientation and attentional processes. In general, the items that comprise the rink-side screening evaluation are sufficiently simple that athletes should be expected to complete all items successfully. If the player fails this evaluation, he should be observed, and formal neuropsychologic testing should be recommended.

Evaluation of Postconcussion Symptoms

Under no circumstances should a player be returned to competition while he is still symptomatic following a concussion. At the NHL level, the player's postinjury symptoms are measured initially at rink-side via the concussion card and by the concussion symptom inventory at the time of the neuropsychologic evaluation. The athlete's report of symptoms should be evaluated both at rest and following exertional activities, such as riding a stationary bicycle. If the player remains asymptomatic during this type of activity, we recommend re-evaluation of the player's symptoms during and following noncontact skating.

Neuropsychologic Test Results

Neuropsychologic testing has proven to be highly sensitive to even subtle variations in neurocognitive function in athletes and represents the most sensitive way of documenting changes in cognitive processes following concussion. However, at the current time, exact standards for determining readiness to play have yet to be derived, and each athlete's performance should be evaluated individually. Our initial experience with professional athletes has indicated that test performance following a concussion is variable, depending on the nature of the injury (i.e., blow to the head compared with deceleration injury), severity of injury, and the player's concussion history. We suggest that any decline in test performance following a concussion should be viewed as being significant. Although this strategy may eventually prove to be somewhat conservative, the adverse consequences of returning an athlete to the ice prematurely following a concussion argue for caution in medical decision making.

IMPORTANT RESEARCH QUESTIONS

As mentioned previously, in addition to providing important clinical data to the team physician, the NHL program has been structured to help answer a number of important questions regarding sports-related concussion. First, this project will allow the NHL to track the rate of concussion from season to season, team to team, and conference to conference, and will promote science-based decision making. One of the primary goals of this project is to help answer basic return to play questions such as: (1) How long should an athlete wait to return to maximize safety or prevent further injury? (2) How many concussions during any given season should result in termination of play for that season? (3) What specific criteria should be utilized in making return to play decisions? For instance, is loss of consciousness an important factor in determining recovery, or are other factors, such as duration of amnesia or concussion symptoms, relatively more important?

Second, this project should help to clarify issues regarding the different proposed grading systems for concussion, such as whether or not the current systems are sufficient, or whether there is a need for modification, based on more current scientific data.

Third, the NHL concussion project will promote a better understanding of the role of neuropsychologic testing in the assessment of athletes. The project will specifically answer questions such as: (1) Which neuropsychologic tests are sufficiently reliable and valid to allow their continued and more widespread use in organized athletics? (2) What exact neuropsychologic cutoff scores should be used in making return to play decisions? (3) To what extent do players' self-reported symptoms correlate with objective neuropsychologic test results?

SUMMARY

This chapter has provided a summary of the NHL concussion program and has focused on important issues regarding the evaluation and management of the concussed hockey player. Given the preliminary nature of this project, a clinical rather than a research perspective has been presented, and issues important to clinical decision making have been discussed. It is hoped that the NHL concussion program will result in a decrease in sports-related concussions and to a better understanding of sports-related concussion. It is also hoped that this project and others like it will promote better evaluation and management strategies for amateur athletes.

References

1. Lovell MR. Evaluation of the Professional Athlete. *In* Bailes JE, Lovell MR, Maroon JC (eds): Sports-Related Concussion. St. Louis, Quality Medical Publishers, 1998, pp 200–214.

2. Povlishock JT, Coburn TH. Morphopathological Change Associated With Mild Head Injury. *In* Levin HS, Eisenberg HM, Benton AL (eds): Mild Head Injury. New York, Oxford University Press, 1989, pp 37–53.
3. Barth J, Alves W, Ryan T, et al. Mild Head Injury in Sports: Neuropsychological Sequelae and Recovery of Function. *In* Levin HS, Eisenberg HM, Benton AL (eds): Mild Head Injury. New York, Oxford University Press, 1989, pp 257–276.
4. Macciocchi S, Barth J, Alves W, et al. Neuropsychological functioning and recovery after mild head injury in collegiate athletes. Neurosurgery 1997;39:510–514.
5. Echemendia R. Personal Communication, 1999.
6. Kelly JP, Nichols JS, Filley CM, et al. Concussion in sports: Guidelines for the prevention of catastrophic outcome. JAMA 1991;266:2867–2869.
7. Lovell MR, Collins MW. Neuropsychological assessment of the college football player. J Head Trauma Rehabil 1998;13:9–26.
8. Hovda DA, Prins M, Becker DP, et al. Neurobiology of Concussion. *In* Bailes J, Lovell MR, Maroon JC (eds): Sports-Related Concussion. St. Louis, Quality Medical Publishers, 1998, pp 12–51.
9. Brandt J. The Hopkins Verbal Learning Test: Development of a new memory test with six equivalent forms. Clin Neuropsychol 1991;5:125–142.
10. Ruff R. Ruff Figural Fluency Test. Odessa, FL, Psychological Assessment Resources, 1988.
11. D'Elia L, Satz P. The Color Trail Making Test. Odessa, FL, Psychological Assessment Resources, 1989.
12. Reitan R. Validity of the Trail Making Test as an indicator of organic brain damage. Percept Mot Skills 1958;8:271–276.
13. Smith A. Symbol Digit Modalities Test Manual. Los Angeles, CA, Western Psychological Services, 1982.
14. Echemendia R. Penn State Symbol Cancellation Test (personal communication), 1999.
15. Benton A, Hamsher K. Multilingual Aphasia Examination. Iowa City, IA, University of Iowa Press, 1978.
16. Gronwall D, Wrightson P. Cumulative effects of concussion. Lancet 1975;2:995–997.
17. Collins MW, Grindel SH, Lovell MR, et al. Relationship between concussion and neuropsychological performance in college football players. JAMA 1999;282:964–970.

12

Return to Play Guidelines After Concussion

Robert C. Cantu

IMMEDIATE TREATMENT ON THE FIELD

The major purpose of on-the-field evaluation of the injured athlete is to rule out a life threatening injury, especially a head injury, and a cervical spine fracture or spinal cord injury. Decisions must then be made as to the most appropriate and safest method of transporting the injured athlete off the field, and whether this transport is to the sidelines or directly to a facility with definitive neurosurgical capabilities.

After the athlete with a cerebral concussion has been reached, the initial evaluation should include the ABCs of first aid (airway, breathing, circulation). Is the airway obstructed? Is the athlete breathing? Does the athlete have a pulse? This evaluation must take place before a neurologic examination is undertaken. Only after the treating physician has determined that the airway is adequate and that circulation is being maintained should attention be directed to the neurologic assessment. If the athlete complains of neck pain or is unconscious, a cervical spine fracture must be assumed, the cervical spine must be immobilized, and the athlete must be transported as if a cervical spine fracture is present. Similarly, if the athlete is found to be without a pulse and is unconsciousness, the head and neck must be immobilized while cardiopulmonary resuscitation is initiated. Once the airway, breathing, and circulation have been determined to be unimpaired and the athlete noted to be conscious, a brief neurologic examination should be carried out on the field, including especially a brief mental exam with orientation to time, person, place, and situation. It is preferable that a Glasgow Coma Scale score (see Table 12–1)

be obtained quickly, and that eye contact with the individual and the briskness of responses to commands be documented. If the athlete is alert, the brief neurologic exam normal, and the athlete without neck symptoms, he may then be allowed to sit, and then to stand and walk off the field. If there are cervical symptoms, despite a normal neurologic exam, the neck should be immobilized and the athlete transported to a facility where radiographic and neuroradiologic capabilities are present.

Once the athlete has been transported or walks on his own off the playing field, a more detailed neurologic examination should be carried out on the sidelines, with particular recording of a more detailed mental examination that includes repeating the months of the year backward, repeating serial digits backward, or other mini-neuropsychologic mental status studies as

Table 12–1. Glasgow Coma Scale

Verbal	
None	1
Incomprehensible sounds	2
Inappropriate words	3
Confused	4
Oriented	5
Eye Opening	
None	1
To pain	2
To speech	3
Spontaneously	4
Motor	
None	1
Abnormal extension	2
Abnormal flexion	3
Withdraws	4
Localizes	5
Obeys	6
Normal	15

Table 12–2. Galveston Orientation and Amnesia Test (GOAT)[6]

Instructions: Error points (in parentheses) are scored for *incorrect* answers and are entered in the right column. Enter the total error points accrued for the different items in the lower right corner. The GOAT score equals 100 minus the error points. A score that is 85 or less should be considered to be a priority for special consideration and follow-up. Recovery of orientation can be plotted daily using the GOAT scores.

	Error Points
1. What is your name? (5) Where were you born? (4) Where do you live? (4)	_____
2. Where are you now? Participation area (5) City? (5)	_____
3. What is the *first* event you can remember *after* injury? (5)	
_____ _____	
Can you describe (type of play, teammates, etc.) the first event following injury? (5)	
	_____
4. What is the *last* event you can remember *before* the injury? (5)	
_____ _____	
Can you describe (type of play, teammates, etc.) the last event prior to the injury? (5)	_____
5. What time is it? (1 point for each half hour up to 5 points)	_____
6. What day of the week is it? (1 point for each day up to 5 points)	_____
7. What day of the month is it? (1 point for each day up to 5 points)	_____
8. What month is it? (5 points for each month up to 15 points)	_____
9. What year is it? (10 points for each year up to 30 points)	_____
If the patient is hospitalized, add the following question:	
10. On what date were you admitted to this hospital? (5) How did you get here? (5)	_____

From Levin HD, Williams H, Eisenberg W, et al. Serial MRI and neurobehavioral findings after mild to moderate closed head injury. J Neurosurg Psychiatry 1992;55:255–262.

suggested in Tables 12–2 and 12–3.[5, 6] The sideline neurologic exam should also include a more detailed evaluation of cranial nerve function and motor strength, coordination, and sensation.

Balance should be tested with Romberg's test and tandem gait. Symptoms of concussion, including lightheadedness, vertigo, headaches, tinnitus, blurred vision, difficulty concentrating, a feeling of lethargy, fatigue, or vagueness, should be determined.

If the athlete becomes asymptomatic with a normal neurologic evaluation at rest, exertional tests, having the individual do sprints, repetitive sit-ups, or push-ups, should be carried out to determine whether exertional tests provoke postconcussion or other neurologic symptoms.

Just as there are no lack of grading systems for concussion, similarly there are a number of guidelines for return to play after an initial concussion, as outlined in Tables 12–4, 12–5, and 12–6. Whereas there are minor differences in the duration of withholding an athlete from athletic competition according to the different guidelines, all the guidelines agree that no athlete who is still symptomatic with postconcussion symp-

toms should be allowed to return to competition.

Tables 12–7 and 12–8 provide guidelines for return to competition after a cerebral concussion, whether a Grade 1, Grade 2, or Grade 3, and whether a second or third concussion sustained in a given season. I believe it is important to realize, as I have indicated and shown (e.g., Table 12–8), that multiple guidelines for return to play exist.[1, 3, 4, 7] While none are in precise agreement as to the timing of return to play after various degrees and numbers of concussions received in a given season, and thus all are truly only guidelines, all do agree on one most salient point, that is, that no athlete who is still symptomatic from a previous injury should be allowed to risk a second head injury, either by practice or by participation. Therefore, while grading and return dates may vary slightly, all the guidelines will prevent the dreaded second impact syndrome.

In December 1997, the American Orthopedics Society for Sports Medicine hosted representatives from the American Academy of Neurology, American Academy of Pediatrics, American Academy of Orthopedic

Table 12–3. SAC: Standardized Assessment of Concussion[6]

NAME: _____

AGE: _____ SEX: _____ EXAMINER: _____

Nature of Injury: _____

Date of Exam: _____ Time: _____ No. ____

---

1) ORIENTATION:

Month: _____	0	1
Date: _____	0	1
Day of Week: _____	0	1
Year: _____	0	1
Time (within 1 hour): _____	0	1

Orientation Total Score _____ /5

---

2) IMMEDIATE MEMORY: (all 3 trials are completed regardless of score on trials 1 & 2; score equals sum across all 3 trials)

LIST	TRIAL 1		TRIAL 2		TRIAL 3	
Elbow	0	1	0	1	0	1
Apple	0	1	0	1	0	1
Carpet	0	1	0	1	0	1
Saddle	0	1	0	1	0	1
Bubble	0	1	0	1	0	1
Total						

Immediate Memory Score _____ / 15

---

3) CONCENTRATION:
Digits Backward: (If correct, go to next string length. If incorrect, read trial 2. Stop after incorrect on both trials.)

4-9-3	6-2-9	0	1
3-8-1-4	3-2-7-9	0	1
6-2-9-7-1	1-5-2-8-6	0	1
7-1-8-4-6-2	5-3-9-1-4-8	0	1

MONTHS IN REVERSE ORDER: (entire reverse sequence correct for 1 point)
DEC-NOV-OCT-SEP-AUG-JUL
JUN-MAY-APR-MAR-FEB-JAN   0 1

Concentration Total Score _____ / 5

EXERTIONAL MANEUVERS (When appropriate):

5 jumping jacks	5 push-ups
5 sit-ups	5 knee-bends

4) DELAYED RECALL

Elbow	0	1
Apple	0	1
Carpet	0	1
Saddle	0	1
Bubble	0	1

Delayed Recall Score _____ / 5

SUMMARY OF TOTAL SCORES:

Orientation	_____ /	5
Immediate Memory	_____ /	15
Concentration	_____ /	5
Delayed Recall	_____ /	5
OVERALL TOTAL SCORE	_____ /	30

From McCrea M, Kelly JP, Kluge J, et al. Standard assessment of concussion in football players. Neurology 1997;48:586–588.

Table 12–4. Cantu Guidelines for Return to Play After a First Concussion[1]

Grade	Guidelines for Return to Play After a First Concussion
1	May return to play if asymptomatic for one week.
2	May return to play if asymptomatic for one week.
3	Should not be allowed to play for at least one month. May then return to play if asymptomatic for one week.

From Cantu RC. Guidelines for return to contact sports after a cerebral concussion. Phys Sportsmed 1986;14:76–79. Used with permission of McGraw-Hill, Inc.

Table 12–5. Colorado Medical Society Guidelines for Return to Play After a First Concussion[4, 7]

Grade	Guidelines for Return to Play After a First Concussion
1	May return to play if asymptomatic at rest and exertion after at least 20 minutes observation.
2	May return to play if asymptomatic for 1 week.
3	Should not be allowed to play for at least 1 month. May then return to play if asymptomatic for 2 weeks.

From Kelly JP, Nichols JS, Filley CM, et al. Concussion in sports. Guidelines for the prevention of catastrophic outcome. JAMA 1991;266:2867–2869; Report of the Sports Medicine Committee. Guidelines for the management of concussion in sports. Colorado Medical Society, 1990 (revised May 1991). Class III.

Table 12–6. Jordan Guidelines for Return to Play After a First Concussion[3]

Grade	Guidelines for Return to Play After a First Concussion
1	May return to play if asymptomatic at rest and exertion.
2	May return to play if asymptomatic for 1 week.
3	Should not be allowed to play for at least 1 month. May return to play if asymptomatic for 1 week.
4	Should not be allowed to play for at least 1 month. May then return to play if asymptomatic for 2 weeks.

From Jordan BJ, Tsairis PT, Warren RF (eds). Head Injury in Sports. *In* Sports Neurology. Aspen Publishers, 1989, p 227.

Table 12–7. Cantu Guidelines for Return to Play After a Second or Third Concussion[1]

Grade	Second Concussion	Third Concussion
1	Return to play in 2 weeks if asymptomatic at the time for 1 week.	Terminate season; may return to play next season if asymptomatic.
2	Minimum of 1 month; may return to play then if asymptomatic for 1 week; consider terminating season.	Terminate season; may return to play next season if asymptomatic.
3	Terminate season; may return to play next season if asymptomatic.	

From Cantu RC. Guidelines for return to contact sports after a cerebral concussion. Phys Sportsmed 1986;14:76–79. Used with permission of McGraw-Hill, Inc.

Table 12–8. Colorado Guidelines for Return to Play After a Second or Third Concussion[4, 7]

Grade	Second Concussion	Third Concussion
1	Terminate contest or practice; may return to play if without symptoms for at least 1 week.	Terminate season; may return to play in 3 months if without symptoms.
2	Consider terminating season; may return to play in 1 month if without symptoms.	Terminate season; may return to play next season if without symptoms.
3	Terminate season; may return to play next season if without symptoms.	Terminate season; strongly discourage return to contact or collision sports.

From Kelly JP, Nichols JS, Filley CM, et al. Concussion in sports: Guidelines for the prevention of catastrophic outcomes. JAMA 1991;266:2867–2869; Report of the Sports Medicine Committee. Guidelines for the management of concussion in sports. Colorado Medical Society, 1990 (revised May 1991). Class III.

Surgeons, American Association of Neurological Surgeons, American College of Emergency Physicians, American Medical Society for Sports Medicine, Congress of Neurological Surgeons, American College of Sports Medicine, American Osteopathic Academy of Sports Medicine, National Athletic Trainers Association, National Collegiate Athletic Association, National Football League, National Hockey League, and other interested sports medicine specialists to a meeting entitled A Concussion in Sports Workshop. While that group was not able to settle the issue of a universal classification scheme for concussion, it did define concussion as "a brain injury produced by direct or indirect head trauma and manifesting one or more of the following signs or symptoms." The signs and symptoms that fell into the acute group included: posttraumatic amnesia; alteration of cognitive function, "memory/concentration"; headache; nausea; vomiting; photophobia; and balance disturbance, "dizziness/vertigo." Delayed signs and symptoms included any of the acute signs and symptoms that persisted plus sleep disturbance, fatigue, depression, and feelings of being slowed down or in a fog.

The classification group essentially divided concussion victims into two groups, those who could return to play the same day and those who could return to play after being asymptomatic for seven days at rest and exertion. The group whom it was felt safe to return to the contest the same day had the following criteria: (1) signs and symptoms had cleared within 15 minutes or less at rest and exertion; (2) normal neurologic evaluation; and (3) no documented loss of consciousness.

The group judged safe to return to competition only after being asymptomatic for 7 days both at rest and exertion included those in whom (1) signs and symptoms had not cleared by 15 minutes at rest and exertion, (2) there was documented loss of consciousness, and (3) at the time of return not only had the individual been asymptomatic for 7 days at rest and exertion, but also the neurologic evaluation was normal.

POSTCONCUSSION SYMPTOMS

A second, late effect of concussion is the postconcussion syndrome. This syndrome—consisting of headache (especially with exertion), dizziness, fatigue, irritability, and especially impaired memory and concentration—has been reported in football players, but its true incidence is not known. In my experience it is uncommon. The persistence of these symptoms reflects altered neurotransmitter function and usually correlates with the duration of posttraumatic amnesia.[2] When these symptoms persist, the athlete should be evaluated with a computed tomography (CT) scan and neuropsychiatric tests. Return to competition should be deferred until all symptoms have abated and the diagnostic studies are normal.

A FINAL COMMENT ON CONCUSSION

Following a concussion, a thorough review of the circumstances resulting in the concussion should occur. In my long experience as a team physician, those athletes subjected to repeated concussions were often using their heads unwisely, illegally, or both. If available, videotapes of the incident should be reviewed by the team physician, trainer, coach, and player to see whether this was a factor. Equipment should also be checked to be certain that it fits precisely, that the athlete is wearing it properly, and that it is being maintained, especially the air pressure in air helmets. Finally, neck strength and development should be assessed.

Furthermore, I am very well aware that lawyers read medical journals, and I want to make it bluntly clear that all of these guidelines listed for return to competition in contact sports after a concussion are just that, namely guidelines. The final decision on return to play is a clinical judgment in every case, and deviations based on the clinical judgment of the treating physician may be entirely appropriate. However, there is agreement that it is not appropriate for any athlete still symptomatic from a previous concussion to be allowed to return to play while symptomatic, and any athlete who is still symptomatic will require further medical evaluation to determine that he or she has become asymptomatic before being allowed to return.

References

1. Cantu RC. Guidelines for return to contact sports

after a cerebral concussion. Phys Sportsmed 1986;14:76–79.

2. Guthkelch AN. Post-traumatic amnesia, post-concussional symptoms and accident neurosis. Eur Neurol 1980;19:91.

3. Jordan BJ, Tsairis PT, Warren RF (eds). Head Injury in Sports. *In* Sports Neurology. Aspen Publishers, 1989, p 227.

4. Kelly JP, Nichols JS, Filley CM, et al. Concussion in sports: Guidelines for the prevention of catastrophic outcome. JAMA 1991;266:2867–2869.

5. Levin HD, Williams H, Eisenberg W, et al. Serial MRI and neurobehavioral findings after mild to moderate closed head injury. J Neurol Neurosurg Psychiatry 1992;55:255–262.

6. McCrea M, Kelly JP, Kluge J, et al. Standard assessment of concussion in football players. Neurology 1997;48:586–588.

7. Report of the Sports Medicine Committee. Guidelines for the management of concussion in sports. Colorado Medical Society, 1990 (revised May 1991). Class III.

LIFE THREATENING
HEAD INJURIES

CHAPTER

13

Intracranial Hematoma

Robert C. Cantu

HISTORICAL PERSPECTIVE

If we define a direct fatality as one occurring directly from participation in the skills of sports, as opposed to an indirect fatality, which is one caused by systemic failure as a result of exertion while participating in a sport, head injury, and intracranial hematoma in particular, is the most frequent direct cause of death in sports.[16, 17] Furthermore, injury to the head takes on a singular importance when we realize that the brain is neither capable of regeneration nor, unlike many other body parts and organs, of transplantation. Every effort must be made to protect the athlete's head, as injury can lead to dementia, epilepsy, paralysis, and death.

Starting with President Theodore Roosevelt's threat to ban American football in 1904, injuries from this sport have received more media attention and reports in the medical literature than any other organized sport because none has contributed more fatalities.[11] Starting with the 19 athletes killed or paralyzed from American football injuries in 1904, which led to the formation of the National Collegiate Athletic Association (NCAA)[1] as a governing body to establish rules for safer athletic competition, fatalities in American football peaked in 1964 at 30.[20] Between the years 1931 and 1986, at least 819 deaths were directly attributed to American football, most from head injury, followed in frequency by cervical spinal cord injury.[17] Fatalities in American football from 1973 to 1983 exceeded the deaths in all other competitive sports combined.[11]

Yet, per 100,000 participants, American football is not as likely to result in a fatal head injury as is horseback riding,[2, 3] sky diving,[12, 18] or automobile or motorcycle racing. It has about the same risk of a fatal head injury as gymnastics and ice hockey.[7, 9]

Other sports historically shown to have a high rate of head injury include boxing,[10, 13, 22] the martial arts,[15] and rugby football,[14, 19] though a fatal head injury in rugby is rare.[8, 18]

Those sports most likely to result in head and cervical spine injury are listed in Table 13-1.

Over the last 20 years there has been a dramatic decrease in the most serious head injuries—especially the incidence of subdural hematoma—owing to multiple factors, including rule changes (such as outlawing "spear tackling" and "butt blocking" in American football), improved equipment standards, better conditioning of the neck, and improved on-field medical care. The reduction in frequency of the most serious neck injury, quadriplegia, has been less impressive, likely because at present there is no equipment capable of preventing that injury.[4-6]

MECHANISM OF INJURY

Three distinct types of stress can be generated by an acceleration force to the head. The first is compressive; the second is tensile, the opposite of compressive and some-

Table 13-1. Sports Most Hazardous for the Head and Spine

1. Auto Racing	12. Martial Arts
2. Boxing	13. Motorcycling
3. Cheerleading	14. Parachute
4. Cycling	15. Rugby
5. Diving	16. Skating/Rollerblading
6. Equestrian Sports	17. Skiing
7. Football	18. Skydiving
8. Gymnastics	19. Soccer (Goalie)
9. Hang-gliding	20. Track (Pole Vaulting)
10. Ice Hockey	21. Trampolining
11. Lacrosse	22. Wrestling

times called negative pressure; and the third is shearing, a force applied parallel to a surface. Uniform compressive and tensile forces are relatively well tolerated by neural tissue, but shearing forces are extremely poorly tolerated.

The cerebrospinal fluid (CSF) that surrounds the brain acts as a protective shock absorber, converting focally applied external stress to compressive stress, because the fluid follows the contours of the sulci and gyri of the brain and distributes the force in a uniform fashion. The CSF, however, does not completely prevent shearing forces from being transmitted to the brain, especially when rotational forces are being applied to the head. These shearing forces are maximal where rotational gliding is hindered within the brain, such as at the dura matter–brain attachments, the rough, irregular surface contacts between the brain and the skull especially prominent in the floor of the frontal and middle fossas.

In understanding how acceleration forces are applied to the brain, it is important to keep in mind Newton's law: force = mass × acceleration; or, stated another way, force divided by mass equals acceleration. Therefore, an athlete's head can sustain far greater forces without injury if the neck muscles are tensed, as when the athlete sees the collision coming. In this state, the mass of the head is essentially the mass of the body. In a relaxed state, however, the mass of the head is essentially only its own weight, and therefore the same degree of force can impart far greater acceleration.

INJURY ASSESSMENT TECHNIQUES

In assessing a brain injury, if the athlete is unconscious, one must assume that there has been a neck fracture, and the neck must be immobilized. In assessment of an athlete with a head injury who is conscious, the level of consciousness or alertness is the most sensitive criterion both for establishing the nature of the head injury and for subsequent follow-up. Orientation to person, place, and time should be ascertained. The presence or absence of posttraumatic amnesia, and the ability to retain new information, such as the ability to repeat the names of four objects 2 minutes after having been given them, or the ability to repeat one's

assignments with certain plays of the contest, should be determined. It is also important to ascertain the presence, absence, and severity of neurologic symptoms such as headache, lightheadedness, difficulty with balance, coordination, and sensory or motor function. Whereas a complete but brief neurologic examination involving cranial nerve, motor, sensory, and reflex testing is appropriate, it is the mental examination and especially the level of consciousness that should be stressed.

Glasgow Coma Scale

When time permits, the use of the Glasgow Coma Scale (Table 13–2) can be very helpful not only in predicting the chances for recovery but also in assessing whether the injured athlete is improving or deteriorating from a given head injury. An initial score of greater than 11 is associated with more than a 90% chance of essentially complete recovery, whereas an initial score under 5 is associated with more than an 80% chance of death or survival in a vegetative state.

DIFFERENTIAL DIAGNOSIS

The differential diagnosis with a head injury includes a cerebral concussion, the second impact syndrome or malignant brain

Table 13–2. Glasgow Coma Scale = E + M + V

Eye Opening	(E)
Spontaneous	(4)
To Speech	(3)
To Pain	(2)
No Response	(1)
Motor Response	**(M)**
Obeys Commands	(6)
Localized Pain	(5)
Withdraws from Pain	(4)
Decorticate Posturing	(3)
Decerebrate Posturing	(2)
No Response	(1)
Verbal Response	**(V)**
Oriented	(5)
Confused Conversation	(4)
Inappropriate Words	(3)
Incomprehensible Words	(2)
No Response	(1)

edema syndrome, intracranial hemorrhage, and postconcussion syndrome.

Intracranial Hemorrhage

The leading cause of death from athletic head injury is intracranial hemorrhage. There are four types of intracranial bleeding to which the examining trainer or physician must be alert in every instance of head injury, epidural, subdural, and intracerebral hematoma, and subarachnoid hemorrhage. Because all four types of intracranial hemorrhage may be fatal, rapid and accurate initial assessment, as well as appropriate follow-up, is mandatory after an athletic head injury.

Epidural Hematoma

An epidural or extradural hematoma is usually the most rapidly progressing intracranial hematoma. It is frequently associated with a fracture of the temporal bone and results from a tear in one of the arteries supplying the covering (dura) of the brain (Fig. 13–1). The hematoma accumulates inside the skull but outside the covering of the brain (Fig. 13–2). Arising from a torn artery, it may progress quite rapidly and

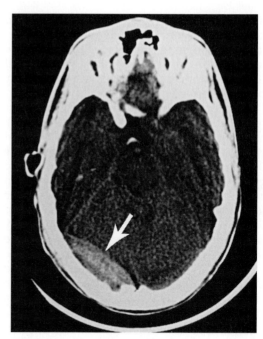

Figure 13–2. CT scan of epidural hematoma *(arrow)*. Note the lens shape of the clot.

reach a lethal size in 30 to 60 minutes. Occasionally the athlete may have a lucid interval, that is, initially the athlete may regain consciousness after the head trauma and before starting to experience increasing headache and progressive deterioration in the level of consciousness as the clot accumulates and the intracranial pressure increases. This lesion, if present, will almost always declare itself within an hour or two from the time of injury. Usually the brain substance is free from direct injury; thus, if the clot is promptly removed surgically, full recovery is to be expected. Because this lesion is rapidly and universally fatal if missed, all athletes receiving a head injury must be closely and frequently observed during the ensuing several hours, preferably the next 24 hours. This observation should be done at a facility where full neurosurgical services are immediately available.

The following case illustrates a typical epidural hematoma.

CASE 1. E.J.

E.J. was a pitcher on his baseball team and was running the bases between third base and home. In the process of sprinting home, his batting helmet, which did not have a chin strap, flew off his head. The throw to the catcher struck him in the area of the right temple, and he collapsed

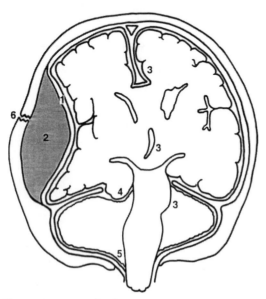

Figure 13–1. Epidural Hematoma. Key: 1. Dura; 2. Hematoma; 3. Midline shift; 4. Herniation of temporal lobe; 5. Herniation of cerebellar tonsil; 6. Skull fracture.

near home plate. He was unconscious about 30 seconds. Over the next minute, E.J. regained consciousness and was alert and oriented and only complained of pain in the area of his right temple, where he had been struck by the ball. He walked from home plate into the dugout. He was removed from the game and was sitting on the bench in the dugout when, about 15 minutes later, he reported that his headache was dramatically increasing in the area of his right temple, and he was feeling nauseated. Shortly thereafter he vomited and became stuporous and was rushed to the local hospital. Within 45 minutes of the incident, while a radiograph was being taken at the hospital, his right pupil began to dilate and within several minutes became fixed and dilated, as he became comatose with decerebrate posturing of his left limbs. Skull radiographs revealed a linear fracture in the right temporal area. I was summoned and saw this patient in the radiology department. In view of his rapid neurologic deterioration and the observed skull fracture, intravenous Decadron Phosphate (dexamethasone sodium phosphate), 12 mg, and 500 mL 20% mannitol were given, a Foley catheter was inserted, and he was taken directly to the operating room; computed tomography was forgone in the urgency of getting him into surgery. In the operating room, a left temporal craniectomy revealed a sizable epidural hematoma, which was evacuated in its entirety. Within several hours of surgery the patient had regained consciousness, and by the next day he was alert and oriented. Several weeks later a cranioplasty was carried out.

When the patient returned to school, he initially had some difficulty with concentration and was easily fatigued, but by the end of the school year, 6 weeks later, he was without any neurologic signs or symptoms of his head injury. Three months later, the patient was cleared to resume playing baseball, but his batting helmet was fitted with a special chin strap so that it could not come off his head.

Subdural Hematoma

A subdural hematoma, the second type of intracranial hemorrhage, occurs between the brain surface and the dura. Acute subdural hematoma is the leading cause of death in athletes.[21] It is located under the dura and directly on the brain. (See Fig. 13–3, a drawing, Fig. 13–4, a computed tomographic [CT] scan, and Fig. 13–5, a magnetic resonance image [MRI] of a subdural hematoma.) It often results from a torn vein running from the surface of the brain to the dura. It may also result from a torn venous sinus or even

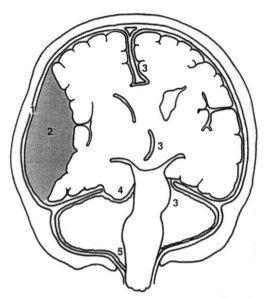

Figure 13–3. Subdural Hematoma. Key: 1. Dura; 2. Hematoma; 3. Midline shift; 4. Herniation of temporal lobe; 5. Herniation of cerebellar tonsil.

a small artery on the surface of the brain. With this injury, there is often associated injury to the brain tissue. If a subdural hematoma necessitates surgery in the first 24 hours, the mortality is high, not because of the clot itself but because of the associated brain damage. With a subdural hematoma

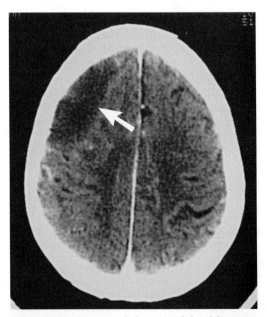

Figure 13–4. CT scan of chronic subdural hematoma *(arrow).* If this were an acute subdural, the hematoma would be white and not dark.

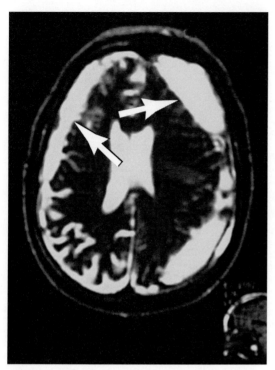

Figure 13–5. MRI of bilateral chronic subdural hematoma *(arrows).*

that progresses rapidly, the athlete usually does not regain consciousness, and immediate neurosurgical evaluation is obviously required. Occasionally, the brain itself will not be injured, and a subdural hematoma may develop slowly over a period of days to weeks. This chronic subdural hematoma, although often associated with headache, may initially cause a variety of very mild, almost imperceptible mental, motor, or sensory signs and symptoms. Since its recognition and removal will lead to full recovery, it must always be suspected in an athlete who has previously sustained a head injury and who, days or weeks later, is mildly symptomatic. A CT scan of the head will definitively show such a lesion.

The following cases are examples of subdural hematomas.

CASE 1. J.A.

On the third day of preseason camp, J.A., a 17-year-old senior defensive back/receiver, participated fully in the morning practice, culminating in five 80-yard wind sprints, without incident until near the end of practice, when he reported a headache and lightheadedness. About 10 min-

utes later, in the locker room, he sustained a grand mal tonic-clonic seizure with snorting respirations, fixed dilated pupils, and decorticate posturing for over 1 minute. His head and neck were immobilized, and at the conclusion of the seizure he became semilucid and vomited clear fluid.

By the time Emergency Medical Services arrived, about 5 minutes later, J.A. was more aware of his surroundings and was able to answer questions in relation to his head and neck evaluation. All vital signs were rechecked and oxygen was administered. Neurologic examination revealed no lateralizing deficits. J.A. could not recall having received a significant blow to the head.

He was taken to the local hospital emergency room, where the initial CT scan showed an acute subdural hematoma. Neurologic evaluation was completely intact, and the patient's Glasgow Coma Scale score was 15 on admission. He did have midline cervical spine tenderness and headache, but the spine series was completely normal. A second CT scan of his head confirmed an acute right frontal subdural hematoma. The patient was started on 1 g IV Dilantin (phenytoin sodium), and followed up with 100 mg three times a day. Following evacuation of the subdural hematoma, the patient remained neurologically intact and made a complete recovery.

Four months later, neurologically intact and off Dilantin, he was allowed to participate in basketball.

CASE 2. N.M.

N.M. is a 17-year-old soccer player who does not recall an incident of head trauma, but does recall that after doing wind sprints while conditioning for soccer, he had the worst headache of his life. It caused him to stop participating. The next day he awoke with a dull headache, which persisted. Two days later he experienced photophobia and a worsening of the headache that caused him to go to the hospital.

Examination at the hospital was notable for neck stiffness and a slight drift of his right arm. His neurologic examination was otherwise normal. Because of the nuchal rigidity, a spinal tap was performed that revealed xanthochromic fluid with 4480 RBC, 40 WBC, and normal glucose and protein. CT scan showed a small (8 mm), left temporal subdural hematoma with mild mass effect. MRI confirmed the same lesion. Bilateral carotid and vertebral arteriograms were normal. The patient was hospitalized 8 days, during which time his headache and meningismus and right arm drift abated. Two CT scans during the next week were unchanged.

A CT scan repeated 1 month later showed partial resolution of the subdural hematoma, and one done 2 months later was entirely normal. At that time all postconcussion symptoms of mild headache, mild fatigue, and some difficulty with learning new material had cleared.

Intracerebral Hematoma

An intracerebral hematoma is the third type of intracranial hemorrhage seen after head trauma. In this instance, the bleeding is into the brain substance itself, usually from a torn artery. (See Fig. 13–6, a drawing, and Fig. 13–7, a CT scan of an intracerebral hematoma.) It may also result from the rupture of a congenital vascular lesion, such as an aneurysm or arteriovenous malformation. Intracerebral hematomas are not usually associated with a lucid interval and may be rapidly progressive. Death occasionally occurs before the injured athlete can be moved to a hospital.

Because of the intense reaction such a tragic event precipitates among fellow athletes, family, students, and even the community at large, and because of the inevitable rumors that follow, it is imperative to obtain a complete autopsy in such an event to clarify the causative factors fully. Often the autopsy will reveal a congenital lesion that may indicate that the cause of death was other than presumed and was ultimately unavoidable. Only by such full, factual eluci-

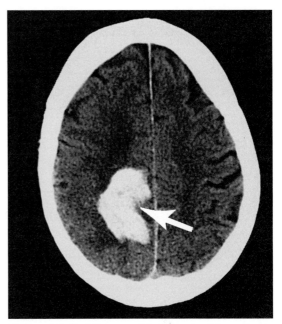

Figure 13–7. CT scan of intracerebral hematoma *(arrow).*

dation will inappropriate feelings of guilt in fellow athletes, friends, and family be assuaged.

Subarachnoid Hemorrhage

A fourth type of intracranial hemorrhage is subarachnoid, confined to the surface of the brain (Fig. 13–8). Following head trauma, such bleeding is the result of disruption of the tiny surface brain vessels and is analogous to a bruise. As with the intracerebral hematoma, there is often brain swelling, and such a hemorrhage can also result from a ruptured cerebral aneurysm or arteriovenous malformation. Because bleeding is superficial, surgery is not usually required unless a congenital vascular anomaly is present.

MANAGEMENT GUIDELINES

Immediate Treatment

The initial evaluation of intracranial hemorrhage, whether an epidural, subdural, intracerebral, or subarachnoid, is the same as for a Grade 3 concussion. The neck must be immobilized and assumed to be fractured.

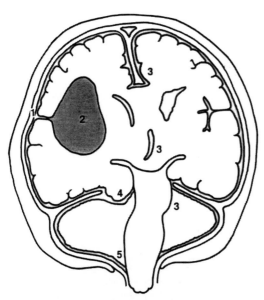

Figure 13–6. Intracerebral Hematoma. Key: 1. Dura; 2. Hematoma; 3. Midline shift; 4. Herniation of temporal lobe; 5. Herniation of cerebellar tonsil.

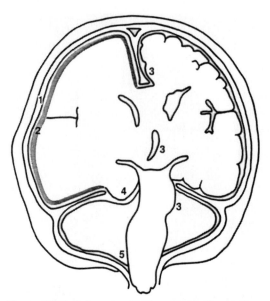

Figure 13–8. Subarachnoid Hemorrhage. Key: 1. Dura; 2. Hemorrhage; 3. Midline shift; 4. Herniation of temporal lobe; 5. Herniation of cerebellar tonsil.

The ABCs of first aid must be followed. Before a neurologic examination is undertaken, the treating physician must determine if the airway is adequate and that circulation is being maintained. Thereafter attention may be directed to the neurologic examination. Following the initial neurologic assessment, prompt transport with the head and neck immobilized to a hospital with neuroradiologic and neurosurgical capability should occur. There, definitive diagnosis is established with a head CT scan or MRI, and a decision is made regarding the need for surgical evacuation. While significant intracranial blood accumulations, whether subdural, epidural, or intracerebral, may require prompt surgical evacuation, the surgical treatment of each of these conditions is beyond the scope of this chapter.

OTHER CONDITIONS FOLLOWING SEVERE ATHLETIC HEAD INJURY

Diffuse Axonal Injury

This condition results when severe shearing forces are imparted to the brain, and axonal connections are literally severed in the absence of intracranial hematoma. The patient is usually deeply comatose, with a low Glasgow Coma Scale score and a negative head CT scan. Immediate neurologic evaluation for treatment of increased intracranial pressure is indicated.

Posttraumatic Seizure

If a seizure occurs in an athlete with a head injury, it is important to log-roll the patient onto his side. By this maneuver, any blood or saliva will roll out of the mouth or nose, and the tongue cannot fall back, obstructing the airway. If a padded tongue depressor or oral airway is available, it can be inserted between the teeth. Under no circumstances should fingers be inserted into the mouth of an athlete who is having a seizure, as a traumatic amputation can easily result from such an unwise maneuver. Usually such a traumatic seizure will last only for a minute or two. The athlete will then relax, and transportation to the nearest medical facility can be effected.

CONCLUSION

Intracranial hemorrhage is the leading cause of head injury death in sports, making rapid initial assessment and appropriate follow-up mandatory after a head injury. Although direct compressive forces may injure the brain, neural tissue is particularly susceptible to injury from shearing stresses, which are most likely to occur when rotational forces are applied to the head.

Although fatalities and catastrophic head injury will never be totally eliminated from athletics, their occurrence, especially in American football, is now low compared with previous decades. This reduction in incidence and severity of athletic head injury has been the result of changes and improvements instituted following constant study and research.

References

1. Albright JP, McCauley E, Mortin RK. Head and neck injuries in college football: An eight year analysis. Am J Sports Med 1985;13:147–152.
2. Barber HM. Horse-play: Survey of accidents with horses. BMJ 1973;iii:532.
3. Barclay WR. Equestrian sports. JAMA 1978;39: 1892.
4. Cantu RC. Minor Head Injuries in Sports. *In* Dy-

ment PG (ed): Adolescent Medicine: State of the Art Reviews. Philadelphia, Hanley & Belfus, 1991, pp 141–154.

5. Cantu RC. Second impact syndrome: Immediate management. Phys Sportsmed 1992;20:55–66.
6. Cantu RC. Second impact syndrome a risk in any contact sport. Phys Sportsmed 1995;23:27–34.
7. Fekete JF. Severe brain injury and death following rigid hockey accidents. The effectiveness of the "safety helmets" of amateur hockey players. CMAJ 1968;99:1234.
8. Gibbs N. Common rugby league injuries. Recommendation for treatment and preventative measures. Sports Med 1994;18:438–450.
9. Goldberg MJ. Gymnastic injuries. Orthop Clin North Am 1980;11:717.
10. Hillman H. Boxing. Resuscitation 1980;8:211.
11. Kraus JF, Conroy C. Mortality and morbidity from injuries in sports and recreation. Annu Rev Public Health 1984;5:163.
12. Krel FW. Parachuting for sport—Study of 100 deaths. JAMA 1965;194:264.
13. Lundberg GD. Boxing should be banned in civilized countries. JAMA 1983;249:250.
14. McCrory GF, Piggot J, Macafee AL, et al. Injuries of the cervical spine in schoolboy rugby football. J Bone Joint Surg Br 1984;66:500.
15. McLatchie GR, Davies JE, Caulley JH. Injuries in karate: A case for medical control. J Trauma 1980;2:956.
16. Mueller FO, Blyth CS. Survey of catastrophic football injuries: 1977–1983. Phys Sportsmed 1985;13:75.
17. Mueller FO, Schindler RD. Annual survey of football injury research, 1931–1986. Chapel Hill, NC, American Football.
18. Petras AF, Hoffman EP. Roentgenographic skeletal injury patterns in parachute jumping. Am J Sports Med 1983;11:325.
19. Ryan JM, McQuillen R. A survey of rugby injuries attending an accident and emergency department. Ir Med J 1992;82:72–73.
20. Schneider RC. Football head and neck injury. Surg Neurol 1987;27:505–508.
21. Coaches Association, NCAA, and National Federation of State High School Associations, 1987.
22. Van Allen MW. The deadly, degrading sport. JAMA 1983;249:250.

14

Malignant Brain Edema and Second Impact Syndrome

Robert C. Cantu

If we define a direct fatality as one occurring directly from participation in the skills of a sport as opposed to an indirect fatality, which is one caused by systemic failure as a result of exertion while participating in a sport, head injury is the most frequent direct cause of death in sport.[16] Furthermore, injury to the head takes on a singular importance when we realize the brain is neither capable of regeneration nor, unlike many other body parts and organs, of transplantation. Every effort must be made to protect the athlete's head, as injury can lead to dementia, epilepsy, paralysis, and death.

Over the last 20 years there has been a dramatic decrease in the most serious head injuries—especially the incidence of subdural hematoma—due to multiple factors including rule changes, such as outlawing "spear tackling" and "butt blocking" in American football, higher equipment standards, better conditioning of the neck, and improved on-field medical care.

During this same period, and especially since the early 1990s, there has been a dramatic increase in the literature citations of the second impact syndrome (SIS), with 17 of 24 citations coming between 1992 and 1998. We have no reason, however, to assume the incidence of SIS has increased as the number of cases seen annually in football has remained at one or two. Rather, we believe this condition is better recognized and reported by sports medicine professionals today.

Recognition of a head injury is easy if the athlete has lost consciousness. It is much more difficult to recognize the far more fre-

quent head injuries in which there is no loss of consciousness but rather only a transient loss of alertness. More than 90% of all cerebral concussions fall into this most mild category, where there has not been a loss of consciousness but rather only a brief period of posttraumatic amnesia or loss of mental alertness.[3, 4] Because the dreaded SIS can occur after a Grade 1 concussion, just as it can after more serious head injuries, it becomes very important to recognize all grades of concussion.[3, 6]

WHAT IS THE SECOND IMPACT SYNDROME?

What Saunders and Harbaugh[18] called "the second-impact syndrome of catastrophic head injury" in 1984 was described by Schneider in 1973.[19] The syndrome occurs when an athlete who sustains a head injury—often a concussion or worse injury, such as a cerebral contusion—sustains a second head injury before symptoms associated with the first have cleared.[5, 6, 14]

Typically, the athlete suffers postconcussion symptoms after the first head injury. These may include headache, labyrinthine dysfunction, visual, motor, or sensory changes or mental difficulty, especially the thought and memory process. Before these symptoms resolve, which may take days or weeks, the athlete returns to competition and receives a second blow to the head.

The second blow may be remarkably minor, perhaps only involving a blow to the chest that jerks the athlete's head and indirectly imparts accelerative forces to the brain. Affected athletes may appear stunned but usually do not lose consciousness and often complete the play. They usually re-

Reprinted with additional material from *Clinics in Sports Medicine*, Volume 17, Number 1 (January 1998).

main on their feet for 15 seconds to 1 minute or so but seem dazed, like someone suffering from a Grade 1 concussion without the loss of consciousness. Often, affected athletes remain on the playing field or walk off under their own power.

What happens in the next 15 seconds to several minutes sets this syndrome apart from a concussion or even a subdural hematoma. Usually within seconds to minutes of the second impact, the athlete—conscious yet stunned—quite precipitously collapses to the ground, semicomatose with rapidly dilating pupils, loss of eye movement, and evidence of respiratory failure.

The following five case histories taken from boxing illustrate the SIS.

CASE 1

A 17-year-old Golden Gloves boxer fought a difficult semifinal bout in a regional tournament. During the 2-day rest period before the final bout, he complained of a severe headache; his mother stated he had literally "eaten" two bottles of aspirin. On the morning of the final bout, he was in an automobile accident and struck his head forcefully. He felt nauseated on the way to the finals bout that evening, and his coach twice tried to pull the car over to the side of the road so the boxer could vomit. During the precompetition examination, the physician asked if there were any problems: The boy and his coach answered "none." After an uneventful first round and minor head blows during the second round, the boxer collapsed in the ring. Shortly thereafter he became decerebrate with fixed, dilated pupils.

He was intubated and taken to the hospital where, after he received intravenous mannitol and dexamethasone, his condition remained unchanged. Emergency computed tomographic (CT) scan showed massive brain swelling and a small left frontal subdural hematoma. After conferring with his parents, surgeons performed an emergency craniotomy. After removing the subdural hematoma, surgeons observed massive brain herniation out of the craniotomy defect and performed a decompressive craniectomy. Despite intensive treatment, the boxer's condition did not improve. Two postcraniotomy electroencephalograms were flat, and the patient died of cardiac arrest 1 week after surgery.

CASE 2

A 19-year-old boxer with the U.S. Marine Corps won the first bout of a camp tournament. He was knocked down in the bout and the next day complained of a headache. The following day he was allowed to box after a limited precompetition examination in which he reported a "slight headache." In the second round, he collapsed after receiving minor blows, experienced a seizure, and became decerebrate with fixed, dilated pupils.

At the hospital, an emergency CT scan revealed a small right subdural hematoma and massive brain swelling. The clot was removed surgically, and the swollen brain was observed to herniate from the skull opening. Despite hyperventilation, decompressive craniectomy, and intravenous mannitol, the postsurgical intracranial pressure was impossible to control, and the patient died 6 days later.

CASE 3

A 17-year-old amateur boxer fought poorly in his first bout in an international tournament. He received several standing 8-counts after being stunned by head blows. Afterward, he was obsessed with boxing again and (in retrospect) exhibited inappropriate obsessive behavior. Six hours later after another boxer's bout was canceled, he boxed again, encouraged by his coach. He again performed poorly, taking several severe hits that included two standing 8-counts, and the referee stopped the bout in the second round. A few minutes later, while the referee was announcing the winner and holding the contestants' hands, the injured boxer collapsed in the center of the ring. He immediately lapsed into a coma with fixed, dilated pupils.

Despite medical treatment that included decompression craniotomy, he died the next day. The autopsy showed severe cerebral edema with bilateral uncal herniation.

CASE 4

A 21-year-old college student prepared for a weekend fraternity smoker—an unofficial boxing match between two inexperienced boxers in which few rules were followed. He trained with an experienced boxer who inflicted head blows and other hits that were of considerable force. Afterward, the college student developed a headache and saw a physician at the student health center. He downplayed the severity of the pain and failed to keep a follow-up appointment. Two days later he sparred again in a training session without coaching or corner supervision. After 2 minutes of a light workout, he collapsed in the ring, lapsed into a coma with fixed, dilated pupils, became apneic, and died before medical attention could be obtained.

CASE 5

A 24-year-old novice boxer fought an extremely hard bout with a ranked boxer and received many forceful blows. During three rounds, he received four standing 8-counts—the fourth terminated the fight. He left the ring unassisted and returned to the dressing room. Within minutes he collapsed into a deep coma. He was taken to the hospital, but despite intensive medical treatment with a ventilator, mannitol, and corticosteroids, he died shortly thereafter. Autopsy revealed massively increased intracranial pressure from edema and vascular congestion and herniation that caused midbrain necrosis. No subdural hematoma was present.

What do these cases have in common? First, five patients had had a concussion with residual cerebral symptoms. In case 5, the patient sustained multiple Grade 1 concussive blows in the same bout. Second, all apparently lapsed into a coma with brain stem collapse from brain herniation secondary to massively increased intracranial pressure. The fatal lesion confirmed at surgery or autopsy was massive edema. Though subdural hematomas were present in two of the cases, they were small and of no clinical consequence. These extraordinary brain changes occurred with what appeared to be relatively minor head trauma and were refractory to medical treatment. In short, the findings of the six case studies are consistent with SIS.

CASE 6

A 16-year-old high school football player was riding his horse the day after a Friday night football game. He was thrown from his horse and struck his head upon landing and was unconscious for an undetermined length of time, perhaps as long as 30 minutes. When he regained consciousness, he was aware that he had a very severe headache but had no other neurologic signs or symptoms. The next day, Sunday, the headache remained intense, and he was nauseated and did not have any appetite. He did not go to school on Monday because of the intensity of his headache and its associated nausea and lack of appetite. No medical attention was sought. On Tuesday and Wednesday he went to school but did not participate in football practice because of his headache. He did not, however, tell his coach or any of his teammates of the reason why he was not coming to football practice. On Thursday, though he still had a headache, it was somewhat less and he did go to

football practice. Friday, his headache persisted, but, again, he did not tell his coaches or fellow players. His family was aware of his complaints of headache and lack of appetite, but no medical attention was sought. Friday evening he participated in the football game, and after a solid hit he was noted to appear stunned. He got up after making the tackle, but before he could walk off the field, he collapsed and within a matter of several minutes was noted to have decerebrate posturing and lapsed into coma. Resuscitative efforts at the scene by EMTs were carried out, and he was life-flighted to a nearby hospital, where a CT scan showed marked vascular congestion, and markedly elevated intracranial pressures were documented by an epidural pressure sensing device. With hyperventilation and osmotic diuretics (mannitol), the patient survived but remains at a vegetative level.

Comment

This case is cited because it points out that the first episode of head trauma need not necessarily have happened on the athletic field. The brain does not know whether it has been injured from football or from a fall. This also points out the importance of both the athlete's and the family's knowing what all coaches and medical personnel should know about the second impact syndrome, namely that any athlete still symptomatic from a prior head injury, no matter where or how it was incurred, should not be allowed to participate in contact or collision activities.

I believe it would be desirable if all football helmets carried a warning label similar to the following:

WARNING

Playing football may result in CONCUSSION which no helmet can prevent. Symptoms include: confusion, dizziness, headache, loss of consciousness or memory, or nausea. If you have these symptoms, immediately stop playing and report them to your coach, trainer, and parents.

Do not return to a game or practice until all symptoms are gone and you receive medical clearance. Ignoring this warning may lead to another and more serious or fatal brain injury.

Pathophysiology of Second Impact Syndrome

The pathophysiology of SIS is thought to involve a loss of autoregulation of the brain's blood supply. This loss of autoregulation leads to vascular engorgement within the cranium, which, in turn, markedly increases intracranial pressure and leads to herniation either of the medial surface (uncus) of the temporal lobe or lobes below the tentorium of the cerebellar tonsils through the foramen magnum (Fig. 14–1). Animal research has shown that vascular engorgement of the brain after a mild head injury is difficult, if not impossible, to control.[11, 15] The usual time from second impact to brain stem failure is rapid, taking 2 to 5 minutes. Once brain herniation and brain stem compromise occur, ocular involvement and respiratory failure precipitously ensue. Demise occurs far more rapidly than usually seen with an epidural hematoma. MR imaging and CT scan are the neuroimaging studies most likely to demonstrate the SIS. Although MR imaging is the more sensitive to traumatic brain injuries, especially true edema,[8, 9] the CT scan is usually adequate to show bleeding or midline shifts of the brain requiring neurosurgical intervention. This is important because CT scanning is cheaper, more widely available, and more quickly performed than MR imaging.

Incidence

Although the precise incidence per 100,000 participants is not known because the precise population at risk is unknown, the SIS is more common than previous reports have suggested. Between 1980 and 1993, the National Center for Catastrophic Sports Injury Research in Chapel Hill, N.C., identified 35 probable cases among American football players alone. Necropsy or surgery and MR imaging findings confirmed 17 of these cases. An additional 18 cases, though not conclusively documented with necropsy findings, most probably are cases of second impact syndrome. Careful scrutiny excluded this diagnosis in 22 of 57 cases originally suspected.[5]

SIS is not confined to American football players. Head injury reports of athletes in other sports almost certainly represent the syndrome, but do not label it as such. Fekete,[7] for example, described a 16-year-old high school hockey player who fell during a game, striking the back of his head on the ice. The boy lost consciousness and afterward complained of unsteadiness and headaches. While playing in the next game 4 days later, he was checked forcibly and again fell, striking his left temple on the ice. His pupils rapidly became fixed and dilated, and he died within 2 hours while in transit to a neurosurgical facility. Necropsy revealed contusions of several days' duration, an edematous brain with a thin layer of subdural and subarachnoid hemorrhage, and bilateral herniation of the cerebellar tonsils into the foramen magnum. Though Fekete did not use the label "second impact syndrome," the clinical course and necropsy findings in this case are consistent with the SIS.

Other cases include an 18-year-old male downhill skier described by McQuillen and associates,[14] who remains in a persistent vegetative state, and a 17-year-old football player described by Kelly and coworkers,[10] who died. Such cases indicate that the brain is vulnerable to accelerative forces in a variety of contact and collision sports. Therefore, physicians who cover athletic events, especially those in which head trauma is likely, must understand the SIS and be prepared to initiate emergency treatment.

Prevention of Second Impact Syndrome

For a catastrophic condition that has a mortality rate approaching 50% and a morbidity rate nearly 100%, prevention takes on the utmost importance. An athlete who is symptomatic from a head injury *must not* participate in contact or collision sports until all cerebral symptoms have subsided, and preferably not for at least 1 week after. Whether it takes days, weeks, or months to reach the asymptomatic state, the athlete must never be allowed to practice or compete while still suffering postconcussion symptoms.

Coaches, players, and parents as well as the physician and medical team must understand this. Files of the National Center for

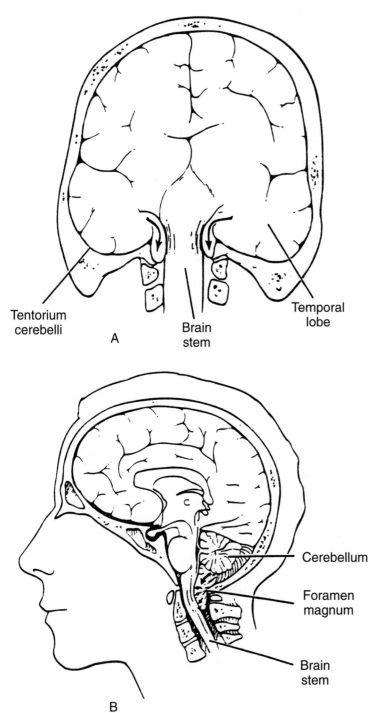

Tentorium
cerebelli

A

Brain
stem

Temporal
lobe

Cerebellum

Foramen
magnum

Brain
stem

B

Figure 14–1. In second impact syndrome, vascular engorgement within the cranium increases intracranial pressure, leading to herniation of the uncus of the temporal lobe *(arrows)* below the tentorium in this frontal section *(A)*, or to herniation of the cerebellar tonsils *(arrows)* through the foramen magnum in this midsagittal section *(B)*. These changes compromise the brain stem, and coma and respiratory failure rapidly develop. The shaded areas of the brain stem represent the areas of compression.

Catastrophic Sport Injury Research include cases of young athletes who did not report their cerebral symptoms. Fearing they would not be allowed to compete and not knowing they were jeopardizing their lives, they played with postconcussion symptoms and tragically developed SIS.

MALIGNANT BRAIN EDEMA SYNDROME

This condition is found in athletes in the pediatric age range and consists of rapid neurologic deterioration from an alert conscious state to coma and sometimes death, minutes to several hours after head trauma.[17, 20] Although this sequence in adults almost always is caused by an intracranial clot, in children pathology studies show diffuse brain swelling with little or no brain injury.[20] Rather than true cerebral edema, Langfitt and colleagues[12, 13] have shown that the diffuse cerebral swelling is the result of a true hyperemia or vascular engorgement. Prompt recognition is extremely important because there is little initial brain injury, and the serious or fatal neurologic outcome is secondary to raised intracranial pressure with herniation. Prompt treatment with intubation, hyperventilation, and osmotic agents has helped to reduce the mortality.[1, 2]

CONCLUSION

As can be seen from the preceding description, the malignant brain edema syndrome occurs in the pediatric age group after a first head injury and thus, unlike the SIS, is not preventable. Prompt recognition and treatment is thus vital. On the other hand, the SIS is preventable. Because the consequences of this syndrome are so catastrophic and because SIS is more common than previously thought and is not confined to football players, physicians covering all collision or contact sports must be aware of the syndrome, its prevention, and its immediate treatment. In addition, educating athletes and their parents about this condition and its prevention cannot be overemphasized.

References

1. Bowers SA, Marchall LF. Outcome in 200 consecutive cases of severe head injury treated in San Diego County: A prospective analysis. Neurosurgery 1980;6:237.
2. Bruce DA, Alavi A, Bilaniuk L, et al. Diffuse cerebral swelling following head injuries in children: The syndrome of "malignant brain edema." J Neurosurg 1981;54:170–178.
3. Cantu RC. Guidelines for return to contact sports after a cerebral concussion. Phys Sportsmed 1986;14:10.
4. Cantu RC. Minor head injuries in sports. In Dyment PG (ed): Adolescent Medicine: State of the Art Reviews. Philadelphia, Hanley & Belfus, 1991.
5. Cantu RC. Second impact syndrome: Immediate management. Phys Sportsmed 1992;20:55.
6. Cantu RC, Voy R. Second impact syndrome a risk in any contact sport. Phys Sportsmed 1995;23:27.
7. Fekete JF. Severe brain injury and death following rigid hockey accidents: The effectiveness of the "safety helmets" of amateur hockey players. CMAJ 1968;99:1234.
8. Gentry LR, Godersky JC, Thompson B, et al. Prospective comparative study of intermediate field MR and CT in the evaluation of closed head trauma. AJNR Am J Neuroradiol 1988;150:673.
9. Jenkins A, Teasdale G, Hadley DM, et al. Brain lesions detected by magnetic resonance imaging in mild and severe head injuries. Lancet 1986;iii:445.
10. Kelly JP, Nichols JS, Filley CM, et al. Concussion in sports: Guidelines for the prevention of catastrophic outcome. JAMA 1991;226:2867.
11. Langfitt TW, Weinstein JD, Kassell NF. Cerebral vasomotor paralysis produced by intracranial hypertension. Neurology 1965;15:622.
12. Langfitt TW, Kassell NF. Cerebral vasodilations produced by brainstem stimulation: Neurogenic control vs autoregulation. Am J Physiol 1978;215:90.
13. Langfitt TW, Tannenbaum HM, Kassell NF. The etiology of acute brain swelling following experimental head injury. J Neurosurg 1966;24:47.
14. McQuillen JB, McQuillen EN, Morrow P. Trauma, sports, and malignant cerebral edema. Am J Forensic Med Pathol 1988;9:12.
15. Moody RA, Ruamsuke S, Mullen SF. An evaluation of decompression in experimental head injury. J Neurosurg 1968;29:586.
16. Mueller FO, Blyth CS. Survey of catastrophic football injuries: 1977–1983. Phys Sportsmed 1985;13:75.
17. Pickles W. Acute general edema of the brain in children with head injuries. N Engl J Med 1950;242:607.
18. Saunders RL, Harbaugh RE. Second impact in catastrophic contact-sports head trauma. JAMA 1984;252:538.
19. Schneider RC. Head and neck injuries in football. Baltimore, Williams & Wilkins, 1973.
20. Schnitker MT. A syndrome of cerebral concussion in children. J Pediatr 1949;35:557.

CHAPTER

15

Return to Competition After Life Threatening Head Injury

Robert C. Cantu

Life threatening head injuries include the four types of intracranial bleeding; (epidural, subdural, and intracerebral hematoma, and subarachnoid hemorrhage), as well as the second impact syndrome, malignant brain edema syndrome, and diffuse axonal injury. Each of these areas will be discussed separately in this chapter. It must be made clear, however, that there are no guidelines for return to play after these life threatening injuries that are based on statistically significant data. This is because so few individuals have returned, either because they fail to achieve full neurologic recovery, or because those who do recover have little interest in returning after such injuries. Therefore, the accumulated scientific data is fairly minuscule. This chapter, therefore, is largely based on the author's 35 years' experience in neurosurgery, and on his experience in research on catastrophic head and spine injuries with the National Center for Catastrophic Sports Injury Research at Chapel Hill, North Carolina, as well as personal experience gained with colleagues at many sports medicine meetings through the last three decades.

Table 15–1 lists neurologic conditions that contraindicate return to contact sports after a head injury. These conditions include persistent postconcussion symptoms, symptomatic neurologic abnormalities about the foramen magnum, spontaneous subarachnoid hemorrhage, hydrocephalus, and permanent neurologic deficit from a brain injury. Theoretically, the door is left open for an athlete who makes a complete neurologic recovery following any of the life threatening head injuries to return to contact sports at a later time (usually at least 1 year post injury). However, extensive deliberations should occur before affirming such a deci-

sion, and documented informed consent from the patient and the patient's family is advised.

EPIDURAL HEMATOMA

An epidural hematoma occurs outside the dura, the covering of the brain, and therefore is not usually associated with a direct brain injury or disruption of the subarachnoid space. Neurologic symptoms usually occur because of pressure on the brain, but not direct contusion or disruption of brain tissue itself. Similarly, surgery for an epidural hematoma, which will usually involve a skull flap, is outside the surface of the dura, and usually the dura need not be violated by the surgery. Therefore, an athlete with an epidural hematoma who makes a complete neurologic recovery may be considered for return to a contact or collision sport after the skull plate has gone on to complete bony fusion. Such an athlete would not be expected to be at risk for greater neurologic injury than if the epidural hematoma had not occurred in the first place. In every instance return to competition will be an individual decision entered into by athletes and

---

Table 15–1. Conditions That Contraindicate Competition in Contact Sports

1. Persistent postconcussion symptoms
2. Permanent central neurologic sequelae from head injury (e.g., organic dementia, hemiplegia, homonymous hemianopsia)
3. Hydrocephalus
4. Spontaneous subarachnoid hemorrhage from any cause
5. Symptomatic neurologic or pain-producing abnormalities about the foramen magnum

their families, but there is no absolute contraindication for return to play following complete recovery from such an injury. Return will usually be deferred for 6 months to 1 year from the date of the initial injury.

SUBDURAL HEMATOMA

Death still occurs with an acute subdural hematoma in about a third of cases owing to the associated disruption of brain tissue incurred at the time of the head injury. In many cases, with subdural hematoma there is not only bleeding underneath the dura, but also very significant contusion, laceration, or disruption of brain tissue as well. Therefore, with the acute subdural hematoma, in a significant percentage of cases, there are residual neurologic deficits that would preclude the athlete from returning to a contact or collision sport.

Usually with a chronic subdural hematoma, there is no associated disruption of brain tissue, as is the norm for the acute subdural, but rather symptoms are caused by the pressure of the fluid on the brain itself. Chronic subdurals that do not resolve on their own can usually be evacuated surgically by means of a burr hole, as the hematoma is liquid in content and can be drained through a small opening in the skull. Thus, with the chronic subdural hematoma, complete neurologic recovery is common, and intervention, when necessary, is minor. In most cases, it will be safe to consider return to contact or collision sports.

With acute subdural hematomas that are small and produce minimal neurologic deficit, that do not require surgery, and in which all neurologic symptoms disappear, the athlete can be considered for return to a contact or collision sport when subsequent imaging studies, whether computed tomographic (CT) scan or magnetic resonance imaging (MRI), definitely establish that the hematoma has been completely absorbed and that there are no other intracranial sequelae such as hydrocephalus or an area of significant brain atrophy. After the athlete has made a complete neurologic recovery, and after complete absorption of the acute subdural has been documented, consideration of return to a contact or collision sport may occur, usually 6 months to a year after the initial incurrence of the acute subdural.

When the acute subdural hematoma requires surgical removal, which always involves a bone flap, return to play is more problematic, even for those who achieve complete neurologic recovery. The concern in individuals who have sustained acute subdurals that require surgery is that the surgery itself necessitates violation of the subarachnoid space, and that the brain dynamics, in terms of the ability of the brain to glide within the cranium, may be altered by scarring in the area of the craniotomy. Thus many experts believe that those individuals who have made a complete neurologic recovery following an acute subdural hematoma that required a craniotomy for evacuation should not be allowed to participate in sports in which repetitive acceleration forces to the brain would be expected. The concern is the possibility that the brain has become attached to the dura in the area of the surgery, and that this attachment will alter the protective absorbing capacity of the cerebrospinal fluid (CSF) in this area. Thus sports with expected repetitive acceleration forces, such as football, boxing, and so forth, would be contraindicated. Anyone trying to advise athletes or their families following surgically treated acute subdurals that required craniotomy should deliberate carefully, yet it must be made clear that no body of athletes that has been followed, following an acute subdural, is large enough to allow statistical documentation for this recommendation. In those situations following the acute subdural hematoma with surgical evacuation in which return to a collision sport is contraindicated, return to a noncollision sport would not be contraindicated if the neurologic recovery is complete. Again, extensive deliberations and informed discussions with the athlete and his or her family are urged in all instances.

SUBARACHNOID HEMORRHAGE

Subarachnoid hemorrhage secondary to a ruptured aneurysm or arteriovenous (AV) malformation that requires surgical correction poses a contraindication for returning to contact or collision sports. The ruptured aneurysm or other vascular malformation itself would certainly cause disruption of brain tissue in the area of the malformation, and in and of itself, extensive bleeding in the pia arachnoid of the brain; adhesion of the pia arachnoid of the brain to the dura, with loss of the normal cushioning effect of the CSF, would be anticipated. Ultimately such adhesion would be greatly augmented by the craniotomy that would be required to repair the vascular abnormalities. Therefore, following subarachnoid hemorrhage caused by a ruptured aneurysm or AV malformation, return to contact or collision sports is contraindicated, but if neurologic recovery is complete, return to a noncontact or non-collision sport is acceptable.

As discussed previously, spontaneous subarachnoid hemorrhage, which could be from a recognized aneurysm or AV malformation, but sometimes is from a smaller, cryptic, vascular malformation that is never identified by arteriography, still poses a contraindication for returning to a contact or collision sport, even if the athlete makes a complete neurologic recovery.

Traumatic subarachnoid hemorrhage associated with a contusion of the brain, usually along the undersurfaces of the frontal lobe or tips of the temporal lobe, does not pose a contraindication to return to collision sports in those athletes who make a complete neurologic recovery and who subsequently show complete resolution of the subarachnoid bleeding on neuroradiologic imaging studies (CT scan but preferably MRI) and no associated brain injury or secondary conditions such as hydrocephalus.

INTRACEREBRAL HEMATOMA

Traumatic intracerebral hematomas are usually accompanied by significant additional brain injury caused by disruption of brain tissue at the time of the bleed. Therefore complete neurologic recovery is unusual with significant intracerebral hematomas. In those intracerebral hematomas that require surgical evacuation, the same situation occurs as in subarachnoid hemorrhage, in which the subdural space is traumatized, thus setting up an adhesion of the pia arachnoid of the brain to the dura, with loss of the normal cushioning effect of the CSF. Therefore, even with complete neurologic recovery, if craniotomy was required to evacuate the intracerebral hematoma, return to a contact or a collision sport is felt to be contraindicated. On the other hand, if the intracerebral hematoma is small and spontaneously resorbs, and no underlying vascular

anomaly is documented, either by angiography or by MRI, and the athlete makes a complete neurologic recovery, return to contact or collision sport at a distant time may be considered on an individual basis after informed deliberations with the athlete and the family.

DIFFUSE AXONAL INJURY

Diffuse axonal injury results when severe shearing forces are imparted to the brain, and axonal connections are literally severed, in the absence of intracranial hematoma. The patient is usually deeply comatose with a low Glasgow Coma Scale and a negative head CT scan. Immediate neurologic assessment and transport for treatment of increased intracranial pressure are indicated. The diagnosis of this condition is usually established by the neurologic severity of injury and with a negative, for intracranial hematoma, head CT scan or more definitively with MRI scan. Following significant diffuse axonal injury, complete neurologic recovery is uncommon, and therefore return to a contact or collision sport is usually not a consideration.

MALIGNANT BRAIN EDEMA SYNDROME AND SECOND IMPACT SYNDROME

With each of these conditions, a complete neurologic recovery is usually not to be anticipated, and a very high mortality rate is the norm, as previously discussed in Chapter 14. Thus, return to a contact or collision sport following either of these conditions is usually not a consideration. However, consideration for return to a contact or collision sport could occur with the athlete who has an extremely mild second impact syndrome, who does make a complete neurologic recovery, and who did not require any intracranial surgery. On an individual basis following deliberation and informed discussion with the athlete and his or her family, return to a noncontact sport in such an instance would not be contraindicated.

SUMMARY

Conditions that contraindicate return to competition in contact or collision sports include persistent postconcussion symptoms, permanent neurologic sequels from head injury, hydrocephalus, spontaneous subarachnoid hemorrhage, and symptomatic neurologic pain-producing abnormalities about the foramen magnum.

From a practical standpoint, almost no athlete will recover without some residual neurologic damage following a diffuse axonal injury, or malignant brain edema, or second impact syndrome condition. Thus, in these conditions, return to a contact sport is essentially precluded.

After any of the intracranial hematomas except the subdural or the intracerebral, where surgery is required and the subdural space is traumatized, thus setting the stage for adhesion of the pia arachnoid of the brain to the dura and the consequent loss of the normal cushioning effect of the cerebrospinal fluid, return to a collision sport may be considered if complete neurologic recovery is experienced. In both situations in which craniotomy has occurred, whether it be for the subdural or for the intracranial hematoma, return to a collision sport is contraindicated, but return to a noncollision sport is usually believed to be safe. Again, extreme deliberateness and informed discussions with the athlete and his or her family are urged in every instance.

Bibliography

1. Cantu RC. Second impact syndrome: Immediate management. Phys Sportsmed 1992;20:55–66.
2. Cantu RC, Voy RO. Second impact syndrome: A risk in any contact sport. Phys Sportsmed 1995;23:27–34.
3. Cantu RC. Head injuries in sport. Br J Sports Med 1996;30:289–296.
4. Cantu RC. Head Injuries. *In* Safran M (ed): Spiral Manual of Sports Medicine. New York, Lippincott–Raven, 1998, pp 275–279.
5. Cantu RC. Second Impact Syndrome. *In* Cantu RC (ed): Clinics in Sports Medicine: Neurologic Athletic Head and Neck Injuries. Philadelphia, WB Saunders 1998, pp 37–45.
6. Cantu RC. Return to Play Guidelines After a Head Injury. *In* Cantu RC (ed): Clinics in Sports Medicine: Neurologic Head and Neck Injuries. Philadelphia, WB Saunders, 1998, pp 45–61.
7. Kelly JP, Nichols JS, Filley CM, et al. Concussion in sports: Guidelines for the prevention of catastrophic outcome. JAMA 1991;226:2867–2869.
8. Kelly JP, Rosenberg J. Practice parameter: The management of concussion in sport: Report of the Quality Standards Subcommittee. Neurology 1997; 48:581–585.
9. McQuillen JB, McQuillen EN, Morrow P. Trauma, sports, and malignant cerebral edema. Am J Forensic Med Pathol 1988;9:12–15.
10. Saunders RL, Harbaugh RE. The second impact in catastrophic contact sports head trauma. JAMA 1984;252:538–539.

PART

V

SPINE INJURIES

16

Athletic Cervical Spinal Cord and Spine Injuries

Jack E. Wilberger, Jr.

Many sports hold the potential for serious permanent spine and spinal cord injury. Fortunately, the incidence of catastrophic spine and spinal cord injuries has dramatically decreased since the mid-1980s. This decline is in part attributable to the development of sports-related spine injury registries, the elucidation of the pathomechanics of these injuries, the implementation of appropriate preventative measures, and the medical and surgical advances in the treatment of spine and spinal cord injuries. This chapter focuses on sports-related cervical spinal cord and spine injuries ranging from the mild "stinger" syndrome to complete quadriplegia. Epidemiology, etiology, and treatment of these injuries are reviewed, concluding with recommendations on return to competition.

EPIDEMIOLOGY

The list of athletic pursuits with potential for catastrophic injury is extensive. Sports bearing the highest risk of spinal cord injury include auto racing, motorcycle racing, diving, hang-gliding, football, and gymnastics. Sports considered high risk include horseback riding, ice hockey, mountain climbing, parachuting, ski jumping, sky gliding, snowmobiling, trampolining, and wrestling.

Fortunately, a relatively small number of all spine or spinal cord injury is sports-related. Of the 10,000 to 12,000 people in the United States who suffer a spinal cord injury every year, less than 10% to 15% of those injuries are related to recreational or organized sports.

While the occurrence of a spinal cord injury in the context of organized sports is generally high-profile and results in consid-

erable publicity, the vast majority of sports-related spinal cord injury occurs in recreational sports. For example, diving-related injuries account for two thirds of all sports-related spinal cord injuries, both in the United States and around the world. Recreational diving accounts for the majority of these cases, and it is rarely, if ever, seen in competitive diving.[1, 11, 19] Nevertheless, the majority of information available concerning sports-related spine and spinal cord injury has been collected from occurrences in organized sports.

In 1977, the National Collegiate Athletic Association (NCAA) initiated funding for a national survey of catastrophic football injuries, which was conducted at the University of North Carolina, Chapel Hill. In 1982, research was expanded to include all sports for both men and women, and a National Center for Catastrophic Sports Injury Research was established.

Of the school sports, football is associated with the greatest number of catastrophic injuries, but the incidence for injury per 100,000 participants is higher in a number of other sports (Table 16–1). Paralyzing injuries in football have been dramatically reduced when recent data are compared with data from the late 1960s and early 1970s. From 1971 to 1975, there were 259 cervical spine injuries (4.1 per 100,000 players) and 99 cases of permanent quadriplegia (1.58 per 100,000 players).[8] A careful evaluation of the data collected during that time led to the conclusion that one of the main contributing factors was inadequate head protection, and the problem was corrected with helmet redesign. As a result, the head became a primary contact point in blocking and tackling. Identifying this resultant problem provided the primary impetus for the 1976 NCAA

Table 16-1. Incidence of Sports-Related Neurologic Injury

Sport	Incidence/100,000 Participants*		
	Fatalities	Permanent Neurodeficits	Neurodeficits with Recovery
Football	0.25	0.75	0.81
Ice Hockey	0.43	1.73	0.86
Wrestling	0.08	0.66	0.37
Baseball	0.07	0.17	0.15
Gymnastics	1.75	1.75	0.00
Track	0.17	0.13	0.13

*Includes head and spinal cord injury.

football rule changes, which were intended to abolish the use of the head as an offensive weapon. After 1978, the incidence of spine injuries (1.3 per 100,000) and quadriplegia (0.4 per 100,000) declined dramatically and have remained relatively stable.[3] There were 26 serious spine injuries reported in football in 1996; 10 in high school, 14 in college, and 2 in professional football.[23]

In the mid-1970s, a perceived significant increased risk in hockey-related spine injuries led to the formation of the Canadian Committee on the Prevention of Spine and Head Injuries Due to Hockey.[6] Tator and Edmonds reported that from 1948 to 1973, there were no spinal cord injuries among hockey players, whereas from 1977 through 1981, hockey became the second most common cause of spinal cord injuries resulting from sports or recreational activities. From 1977 through 1983, the committee documented 42 spine injuries with 28 cases of spinal cord injury.[18] Careful analysis indicated that most resulted from a vertex blow to the head as a result of pushing or checking into uncushioned boards. As a result, in 1983, the committee issued guidelines aimed at decreasing the incidence of spine injuries in hockey: better enforcement of the rules against boarding and cross-checking; institution of rules against pushing or checking from behind; development of neck muscle conditioning programs; better player education regarding neck injuries; and helmet redesign to improve shape and shock absorbency. Primarily as a result of these efforts, spine injuries have decreased by more than 50% in hockey since the mid-1980s.

Almost all cases of serious spine injury in football and hockey involve the cervical spine. In a recent review of 34 spinal cord injuries, the most common level involved was C6. Only 4 of these 34 made a complete recovery.

Although less popular in the United States than in other countries, rugby is another organized sport that carries a certain risk of spinal injury. The "collapsing scrum" and "crashing of the scrum" are particularly dangerous aspects of the game in which the player may have his head pushed into the ground, often with the tremendous weight of many players driving him. More than 50% of the 30 reported catastrophic spinal injuries from rugby since 1976 have occurred in this manner.[4]

Neck injuries in wrestling are also common, but few are catastrophic. Wrestlers are usually in superior physical condition and have strong cervical muscle support.

ETIOLOGY

The pathomechanics of spine injuries in athletes appears to be similar regardless of the sport involved. Until the mid-1970s, hyperflexion of the cervical spine was thought to be the primary mechanism of spine injuries in athletes. However, careful analysis of these injuries by Torg and co-workers clearly established axial loading as the most common important biomechanical factor. Under normal circumstances, forces transmitted to the cervical spine are primarily dissipated by the cervical muscles, which allow for lateral bending, flexion, and extension. This force dissipation is most effective with the neck in an anatomic position—slightly extended because of normal cervical lordosis. However, when the neck is slightly flexed (approximately 30 degrees) and the normal lordosis is eliminated, the cervical spine becomes a single straight segmented column; thus any forces are transmitted directly to the bones, ligaments, and disks rather than to the muscles. When an athlete's head strikes another player, the ground, or the bottom of a pool, the cervical spine is compressed between the decelerated head and the force of the trunk. When sufficient force is applied, the bones, ligaments, or disks fail, resulting in various injuries.

The validity of this theory of biomechanics of athletic spine injuries has been underscored by many authors. For example, Scher studied spine injuries in rugby and stated: "When the neck is slightly flexed, the spine is straight. If significant force is applied to the vertex, the force is transmitted down the long axis of the spine. When the force exceeds the energy absorbing capacity of the structures involved, cervical spine flexion and dislocation will result."[17] Similarly, the most common mechanism of 28 severe hockey-related spinal injuries studied by Tator and Edmonds occurred from vertex impacts with the neck slightly flexed. The importance of these pathomechanics is also well established in diving injury.

When this mechanism is understood, it becomes clear that athletes occasionally use techniques and maneuvers that may place their cervical spines at risk of injury. Thus, more effective training, conditioning, and preventive measures can be instituted to further decrease the incidence of the more serious injuries.

PATHOPHYSIOLOGY OF SPINAL CORD INJURY

The pathophysiology of spinal cord injury related to athletic endeavors is no different from that related to any other cause (Fig. 16–1). The pathophysiology may be divided into two distinct phases, primary and secondary injury. Primary injury refers to the structural damage occurring instantly after the traumatic event. However, there may be further primary injury if an injured spine is not adequately immobilized. Secondary injury refers to a pathophysiologic cascade initiated shortly after injury, including such insults as ischemia, hypoxia, edema, and various harmful biochemical events. Since it is extremely rare for the primary injury to cause transection of the spinal cord, and it has been shown that less than 10% of the cross-sectional area of the spinal cord will support locomotion, it is very important to focus clinical attention on the secondary injury process.

Ischemia is a very prominent feature of post–spinal cord injury events. Within 2 hours of injury, there is a significant reduction in spinal cord blood flow. This ischemia may be confounded by loss of the normal autoregulatory response of the spinal cord vasculature. When autoregulation is lost, blood flow becomes dependent on systemic pressure. Thus, in the multitraumatized pa-

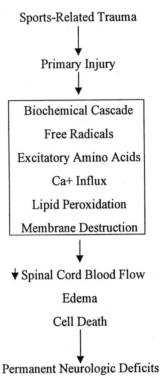

Figure 16–1. Pathophysiologic process of spinal cord injury following sports-related trauma.

tient or in the patient with vasogenic spinal shock complicating the spinal cord injury, severe systemic hypotension may exacerbate the spinal cord ischemia.

Edema formation is another feature of the secondary injury process. Edema develops first at the injury site and subsequently spreads into adjacent, and sometimes distant, segments of the cord. The relationship between this edema and worsening of neurologic function is not well understood.

Many biochemical mechanisms have been implicated in the evolution of the pathologic changes and physiologic derangements occurring after a spinal cord injury. Electrolyte disturbances have been well documented— increased intracellular calcium, increased extracellular potassium, increased sodium permeability. Other events, such as excitatory neurotransmitter accumulation, arachidonic acid release, endogenous opiate activation, and prostaglandin production, have all been implicated as damaging elements of the postinjury cascade. Another event, free radical production and lipid peroxidation, is believed to play a central role in this process. Ultimately, however, all of these events conspire to result in ischemia, edema formation, membrane destruction, cell death, and, eventually, permanent neurologic deficits.

IMMEDIATE CARE

All unconscious athletes and all injured athletes who complain of numbness, weakness, paralysis, or neck pain should be handled as if they have a cervical fracture and, thus, potentially an unstable spine. Moving and transporting the athlete off the field should be done with sufficient personnel so that the athlete's spinal column will not undergo motion. In particular, the caregiver should prevent flexion and extension movements that are likely to compromise the size of the cervical spinal canal. One designated person should be responsible only for immobilizing the cervical spine by cradling the shoulders and neck in his or her forearms while applying a mild traction force in the axial direction. This person should have no other role in transferring or supporting the weight of the body, and sufficient numbers of other personnel should be available or recruited so that the athlete can be easily moved without distracting the person at the head from maintaining proper cervical alignment. If necessary, the athlete's helmet can be safely removed by cutting the chin strap and pulling outward around the ear pads. This allows the helmet to be removed without movement of the neck. This maneuver is usually best accomplished once the athlete has been removed from the playing field. It is important to note that removal of a football helmet from a player wearing shoulder pads instantly forces the neck into hyperextension, and this must be avoided.

Injury Patterns and Classifications

A number of different classification schemes have been developed for athletic-related spinal cord and spine injury. Presentation of these injuries may vary from minor neck pain with associated significant underlying spinal and spinal cord abnormalities (i.e., cervical stenosis, Arnold-Chiari malformation) to unilateral upper extremity symptoms related to cervical root compression (stingers) to quadriplegia.

A general classification scheme that has proven useful in defining the severity of the injury, establishing treatment principles, and assisting in the determination as to safety for return to competition is as follows: serious spine injury with associated spinal cord injury, serious spine injury without associated spinal cord injury, minor spine injury, transient neurologic deficits with or without associated spine injury, and minimally symptomatic or asymptomatic underlying preexisting spine and/or spinal cord anomalies.

Spinal Cord Injury

Management of a spinal cord injury in an athlete generally raises few questions. If the athlete is fully conscious, cervical fracture with associated cervical cord injury usually is accompanied by rigid cervical muscle spasm and pain, which immediately alerts the athlete and the physicians to the presence of such an injury. It is the unconscious athlete with lax cervical musculature, who is unable to say that his neck hurts, who is most susceptible to cord injury if the possibility of an unstable cervical spine fracture is not considered. With an unconscious or obviously neck-injured athlete, it is important that no neck manipulation occur on the field.

The conscious athlete should be carefully questioned about the presence of any neck pain, weakness, numbness, or burning paresthesias. The burning hand syndrome has been classically described in association with athletic spinal cord injury. First elucidated by Maroon in 1977 and refined by Wilberger in 1986, the syndrome is now recognized as a variant of the central cord syndrome.[13, 25] The characteristic complaint is of burning paresthesias and dysesthesias in both arms or hands and occasionally in the legs; weakness does not necessarily occur. Burning hand syndrome has been associated with a bony or ligamentous spine abnormality in approximately 50% of affected individuals. Thus, any athlete with this syndrome should be treated as having a significant spinal cord injury until proven otherwise.

No athlete who has suffered a clear spinal cord injury with associated resulting neurologic deficits should be allowed to return to any type of sports activity that would increase the risk of further problems.

SERIOUS SPINE INJURY WITHOUT ASSOCIATED SPINAL CORD INJURY

For athletes who have suffered an unstable fracture or fracture-dislocation of the cervical spine and who have undergone spinal fusion, a return to any sport involving risk of further spine injury raises strong concerns. Even in the presence of an apparently stable spine as seen on flexion and extension radiographs, continued participation may not be advisable. There are no experimental or clinical data to help physicians predict the stability of healed spinal fractures or fusions when they are placed under extreme degrees of mechanical stress, as is frequently seen in athletic endeavors. There is increased mechanical stress above and below fused spinal segments, and repetitive microtrauma to a "stiff" spine exacerbates this stress. Torg and coworkers estimated that the forces involved in a football tackle may approach 18 g. Some attempt has been made to assess spinal strength following spinal injury with a Cybex dynamometer. The Cybex has been particularly useful in assessing muscle strength, power, and endurance, but its applicability to the spine has yet to be determined. In fact, there is no evidence that the injured cervical spine is made stronger than the normal, uninjured spine by fusion. Thus, in the absence of any objective ability to measure the degree of dynamic stress stability of the spine, any healed fracture (with the exception of minor spinal fractures), and any injury that has required internal stabilization, is highly suspect in its ability to withstand further challenges from contact sports.

This raises the question of what competitive sports, if any, a spine-injured athlete could safely resume without significant risk to neurologic or spinal integrity. Once again, there is little information to guide us. It has been reported that spine surgeons do not believe that fusion of the cervical spine is a contraindication to participation in contact sports unless the fusion is at C1 or C2. However, laminectomy, disk surgery, and spinal instrumentation have been considered contraindications to continued participation. A number of college and professional athletes have had disk surgery or fusions for various nontraumatic reasons (cervical disk disease, spondylolisthesis) and continued to participate without difficulty or apparent in-

Table 16–2. Sports Classification

Contact/Collision	Limited Contact/Impact
Football	Baseball
Boxing	Basketball
Soccer	Diving
Ice Hockey	Gymnastics
Wrestling	Skiing
Strenuous/Noncontact	**Nonstrenuous/Noncontact**
Aerobics	
Running	Badminton
Swimming	Cycling
Tennis	Archery
Track	Golf

creased risk of injury. The American Academy of Pediatrics has classified sports according to degree of contact, impact, and exertion involved in order to help physicians determine the appropriateness of allowing children with serious spine trauma to participate in these endeavors (Table 16–2). Given the lack of any more objective data, these guidelines may be reasonable for adult athletes as well.

MINOR SPINE INJURY

As noted previously, there are no definitive data that fully assess spinal stress tolerance after injury. Thus, isolated wedge fractures and chip fractures of the vertebral body in the absence of subluxation, laminar fracture, and spinous process fracture would seem to pose no long-term problem once adequate healing has occurred. However, there may be an exception to this general rule if the angular deformity of the end plate of the vertebral body fracture is greater than 11 degrees, compared with the adjoining normal vertebrae. White and coworkers suggested that such a degree of deformity may predispose to chronic instability. When such an injury occurs, the athlete should discontinue all contact and competitive sports for at least 6 months. If the athlete is asymptomatic and if dynamic films show fracture healing without evidence of instability, return to competition is unlikely to be associated with a significant risk of further injury.[24]

Most cervical injuries will involve a ligament sprain, muscle strain, or contusion. With such injuries, there is no neurologic or osseous injury, and return to competition can occur when the athlete is free of neck pain with and without axial compression, range of motion is full, and the strength of the neck is normal. Cervical radiographs should show no subluxation or abnormal curvatures. It is preferable that athletes not return to competition until they are asymptomatic and can perform at the level of their pre-injury profile.

It is well known that ligament damage may accompany a cervical spine injury and can occur in the absence of bony injury. Generally, this is minor and self-limited, but on occasion, it may result in progressive instability, cervical spine deformity, and spinal cord injury. There are guidelines to assist in determining ligament stability. Under normal circumstances, conditions permit very little motion between the cervical vertebrae. In cadaver studies with all ligaments intact, horizontal movement of one vertebral body on the next does not exceed 3.5 mm, and the angular displacement of one vertebral body on the next is always 11 degrees or less. Only when most of the restraining ligaments are injured or destroyed do motions in excess of these occur. In the clinical setting, measurements of the horizontal or angular displacement can be made on neutral or flexion/extension radiographs.

Incipient, severe ligamentous injury in the acutely injured athlete may not be recognized because a normal degree of spinal ligamentous laxity in younger patients is generally accepted, and cervical muscle spasm, which may compensate for ligamentous instability, may be present. For these reasons, when any subluxation is seen after a sports-related injury, the patient should wear a hard cervical collar, and flexion/extension films of the cervical spine should be repeated 2 to 4 weeks after injury. If the films show no evidence of progression or if there is a return to normal, it is unlikely that any significant injury has occurred, and the athlete can most likely return safely to his or her competitive sport.

TRANSIENT NEUROLOGIC DEFICITS

Transient neurologic symptoms are relatively common in athletes and need not be associated with significant underlying spine or spinal cord injury.

"Stingers" or "burners" are colloquial terms used by athletes and trainers to describe a set of symptoms that involve pain, burning, or tingling down an arm, occasion-ally accompanied by localized weakness. The symptoms typically resolve within seconds or minutes, rarely persisting for days. It has been estimated that a stinger will occur at least once during the career of over 50% of athletes.

There are two typical mechanisms by which stingers may occur, traction on the brachial plexus, or nerve root impingement within the cervical neural foramen. The majority of high school–level injuries are of the brachial plexus type, whereas most at the college level and virtually all in the professional ranks result from a pinch phenomenon within the neural foramen.

With either type of stinger, the athlete experiences a shocklike sensation of pain and numbness radiating into the arm and hand. The symptoms typically are purely sensory in nature and most commonly involve the C5 and C6 dermatomes. On occasion, weakness may also be present. The most common muscles involved include the deltoid, biceps, supraspinatus, and infraspinatus. Stingers are almost always unilateral and never involve the lower extremities. Thus, if symptoms are bilateral or involve the leg, the burning hand syndrome or some other type of transient neurologic phenomenon, with all of their implications, must be considered.

Other types of symptoms that strongly implicate the spinal cord as the source include quadriplegia, quadriparesis, hemiplegia, paraplegia, and bilateral sensory loss. A 1984 survey of over 500 NCAA football players found that the incidence of transitory paresis and paresthesias was 1.3 per 10,000 participants, and the incidence of numbness and tingling was 6.0 per 10,000 participants.

Torg and colleagues in 1986 reported on 32 athletes with what he termed neurapraxia of the cervical cord with associated transient quadriplegia. In all instances, minor abnormalities were found on cervical spine films. The quadriplegia lasted from 1 minute to 48 hours, and in all cases resolved completely. A magnetic resonance image (MRI) was obtained in only one patient, and no intrinsic cord abnormalities were identified.[21]

To determine the relative risk of future neurologic consequences to athletes, Ladd and Scranton conducted a retrospective analysis on 117 quadriplegic athletes studied in the National Football Head and Neck Registry. None of the athletes reported any episodes of transient motor weakness prior to their permanent cord injury.[12] Only one reported prior transient sensory symptoms.

In the data from the National Center for Catastrophic Sports Injury Research between the years 1989 and 1991, there were 22 cases of quadriplegia and 3 cases of transient quadriplegia. Once again, none of these individuals with transitory symptoms went on to significant injury.

It has been subsequently shown by Torg and coworkers that athletes who suffer one episode of transitory neurologic dysfunction are more likely to suffer additional episodes even if no underlying etiology can be demonstrated.[22]

When faced with an athlete who has suffered a transient neurologic deficit, the physician must do a thorough workup to rule out bony or ligamentous injury to the spine. Plain cervical spine films with flexion and extension views are essential. A computed tomographic (CT) scan or polytomography may be necessary to evaluate subtle bony injury. If no bony or ligamentous abnormalities are identified in a patient with transient neurologic deficit, the physician must rule out ongoing extrinsic cord or nerve root compression or intrinsic cord abnormalities. This is most readily accomplished by MRI. Somatosensory evoked potentials may also prove useful in documenting physiologic cord dysfunction. Special concerns should be raised if any intrinsic abnormalities are seen on MRI or documented by somatosensory evoked potentials, as this provides direct evidence of an overt, though mild, spinal cord injury and should preclude a return to sports. If no evidence of spinal cord injury is found, and no bony or ligamentous problems are identified, return to competition is probably safe. A second episode of transient neurologic deficit should initiate another complete workup. If all studies remain normal, a return to competition need not be precluded; however, concerns should be raised about the recurrent nature of the problem and consideration given to limiting further athletic activity.

ASYMPTOMATIC OR MINIMALLY SYMPTOMATIC SPINE ANOMALIES IN THE ATHLETE

Spear Tackler's Spine

Recently, the entity of "spear tackler's spine" has been defined based on informa-

tion from the National Football Head and Neck Injury Registry. This entity refers to a combination of cervical spine abnormalities including developmental narrowing, reversal of the normal cervical lordosis or the presence of kyphosis, and minor vertebral body abnormalities (i.e., wedge compressions); all in the setting of an individual who employs spear tackling techniques. Recently, two cases with pre-injury radiographs as well as video documentation of the mechanism of injury resulted in cervical fracture-dislocations with associated quadriplegia. Whether the straightened, segmented column alignment of the spine, or the head-first axial loading type of tackling technique, or a combination of the two, predisposes those with spear tackler's spine to catastrophic injury is not clear. However, at present, this combination of factors is generally believed to constitute an absolute contraindication to further participation in contact sports.[22]

Spine Anomalies

Hensinger has stated, "Patients with congenital anomalies of the odontoid are leading a precarious existence. The concern is that a trivial insult superimposed on an already weakened or compromised bony structure may be catastrophic."[22] In 1989, an 18-year-old high school football player became quadriplegic after making a head-first tackle. Radiographs taken subsequent to the injury revealed the presence of an os odontoideum. Thus, the presence of odontoid agenesis, odontoid hyperplasia, or os odontoideum all appear to be absolute contraindications to participation in contact sports.

Kipple-Feil anomaly is the eponym applied to congenital fusion of two or more cervical vertebrae. Pizzutillo has pointed out that "children with congenital fusion of the cervical spine rarely develop neurologic problems or signs of instability." However, he goes on to state that "the literature reveals more than 90 cases of neurologic problems . . . that developed as a consequence of occipital cervical anomalies, late instability, disc disease, or degenerative joint disease."[20] These reports included cervical radiculopathy, spasticity, pain, quadriplegia, and sudden death. Also, "more than two-thirds of the neurologically involved patients had single-level fusion of the upper area whereas many cervical patients with extensive fusions of five to seven levels, had no associated neurologic loss."[22] It is thus believed that extensive fusion anomalies of the cervical spine with associated limited motion or associated occipital cervical anomalies constitute a clear contraindication to participation in contact sports. However, a single-level fusion without other associated anomalies or evidence of instability should present no increased risk to the athlete participating in contact sports.

Cervical Stenosis

Cervical spinal canal stenosis in the athlete may be a developmental or congenital condition or may be caused by acquired degenerative changes of the spine. In addition, recently, a report of neurologic disability in an athlete with an Arnold-Chiari I malformation and associated spinal stenosis has created additional concerns. It is well known that long-term sports participation predisposes the athlete to degenerative changes. When the minimum anteroposterior diameter of the cervical spine in the general population is compared with that of patients with cervical spondylitic myelopathy, it is clear that a substantial number of individuals have a constitutionally narrow spinal canal. The primary question, however, is whether a narrow canal alone predisposes to the development of myelopathy. In sports, most attention is focused on developmental spinal stenosis as a result of dramatic cases of spinal cord injury associated with a congenitally small spinal canal in several football players.[7] In spite of this, however, there is little information concerning the risk of an asymptomatic narrow canal in an athlete.[9]

There has been considerable debate over what constitutes spinal stenosis. The literature on this subject is so confused by a multiplicity of definitions as to make it impossible to compare articles by different authors, as the same structural entity is not uniformly being compared. For many years, the height of the spinal canal as measured from the midpoint of the vertebral body up to the spinolaminar line was used by radiologists to determine the presence of spinal stenosis. The general consensus was that between C3 and C7, canal heights were normal when

this measurement corrected for magnification error was 15 mm or more, and spinal stenosis was present when the measurement was 12 to 13 mm or less. To eliminate the need for correcting for radiographic magnification error, Torg and colleagues, in 1985, and Pavlov and coworkers, in 1987, put forward a new "ratio" method for radiographically assessing cervical spinal stenosis.[16, 20] This ratio method measured the height of the spinal canal from the midpoint of the posterior surface of the vertebral body up to the spinolaminar line and the height of the corresponding midvertebral body. These authors concluded that a "significant spinal stenosis" was present when the canal/vertebral body ratio was 0.8 or less. Based on their experience, the authors also concluded that "our data clearly indicate that athletes who have developmental spinal stenosis are not predisposed to more severe injuries with associated permanent neurological sequelae."

More recently, the ratio method as a means of defining cervical spinal stenosis has been called into question. In 1990, the Kerlan Jobe Clinic published data indicating that 33% of professional football players studied had spinal stenosis by the ratio method.[15] Herzog and colleagues, also found abnormal ratios below 0.8 in 49% of the professional football players they studied in the 1989 San Francisco 49ers training camp.[10] They concluded that this ratio was highly unreliable in determining spinal stenosis, with a positive predictive value of only 12%. Thus, spinal stenosis cannot be defined by bony measurements alone.

"Functional" spinal stenosis, defined as loss of the cerebrospinal fluid around the spinal cord or, in more extreme cases, deformation of the spinal cord whether documented by contrast CT, myelography, or MRI is a more accurate measure of stenosis. The term "functional" is taken from the radiographic term "functional reserve," as applied to the protective cushion of cerebrospinal fluid around the spinal cord in a nonstenotic canal. In a 1993 study where MRI was used to document the presence or absence of spinal stenosis in 11 athletes rendered quadriplegic, 6 had functional stenosis.[2]

Numerous reports suggest that spinal stenosis predisposes to spinal cord injury. Matsuura and coworkers compared 42 patients with spinal cord injuries with 100 normal controls and found that "the sagittal diameters of the spinal canals of the control group were significantly larger than those of the spinal cord injured group."[14] Ladd and Scranton further concluded that "patients who have stenosis of the cervical spine should be advised to discontinue participation in contact sports."[12] Eismont and co-workers found that the greater the degree of spinal stenosis, the higher the risk of permanent neurologic injury in patients who had suffered spinal cord injury.[5]

Anyone with developmental or spondylitic narrowing of the spinal canal is especially at risk for neurologic injury during hyperextension. Generally, an anteroposterior diameter of less than 15.5 mm in a cross-sectional area of less than 55 mm² puts an individual at high risk. When the neck is hyperextended, the sagittal diameter of the spinal canal is further compromised by as much as 30% by infolding of the intralamellar ligaments. Thus, it is understood how hyperextension is the mechanism most likely to further compromise an already narrow spinal canal and lead to neurologic symptoms. However, as previously noted, axial loading combined with flexion rather than hyperextension is the most important factor in sports-related spinal cord injury. Thus, the athlete might be at less risk than expected.

Whether cervical stenosis in an athlete increases the risk of spinal cord injury has yet to be adequately resolved. There are, however, sufficient data to draw some conclusions. The evidence at this point does suggest an increased neurologic risk to an athlete with functional cervical stenosis.

Nevertheless, there are still no good guidelines to help the physician manage an athlete with a narrow, asymptomatic cervical spinal canal. When such an abnormality is encountered, management must be individualized according to the patient's symptoms, the degree of canal stenosis, and the perceived risk of permanent neurologic injury.

References

1. Albrand WO, Corkill G. Broken necks from diving accidents: A summer epidemic in young men. Am J Sports Med 1976;4:107–110.
2. Cantu RC. Functional cervical spinal stenosis: A contraindication to participation in contact sports. Med Sci Sports Exerc 1993;25:316–317.
3. Cantu RC, Mueller FO. Catastrophic spine injuries in football. J Spinal Disord 1990;3:227–231.
4. Duda M. Reducing catastrophic injuries in Rugby. Phys Sportsmed 1988;16:29.
5. Eismont FJ, Clifford S, Goldberg M, et al. Cervical sagittal spinal canal size and spinal injury. Spine 1984;9:663–666.
6. Feriencik K. Trends in ice hockey injuries, 1965–1977. Phys Sportsmed 1979;7:81–84.
7. Firooznia H, Ahn J, Rafii M, et al. Sudden quadriplegia after a minor trauma: The role of preexisting spinal stenosis. Surg Neurol 1985;23:165–168.
8. Funk FJ, Wells RE. Injuries of the cervical spine in football. Clin Orthop 1975;109:50–58.
9. Grant TT, Puffer J. Cervical stenosis: A development anomaly with quadriparesis during football. Am J Sports Med 1976;4:219–221.
10. Herzog RJ, Weins JJ, Dillingham MF, Sontag MJ. Normal cervical spine morphometry and cervical spinal stenosis in asymptomatic professional football players. Spine 1991;16:178–186.
11. Kewalramani LS, Taylor RG. Injuries to the cervical spine from diving accidents. J Trauma 1975; 15:130–142.
12. Ladd AL, Scranton PE. Congenital cervical stenosis presenting as transient quadriplegia in athletes. J Bone Joint Surg 1986;68:1371–1374.
13. Maroon JC. Burning hands and football spinal cord injury. JAMA 1977;238:2049–2051.
14. Matsuura P, Waters RL, Adkins RH, et al. Comparison of computerized tomography parameters of the cervical spine in normal control subjects and spinal cord injured patients. J Bone Joint Surg 1989;71:183–188.
15. Odor JM, Watkins RG, Dillin WH, et al. Incidence of cervical spinal stenosis in professional and rookie football players. Am J Sports Med 1990;18:507–509.
16. Pavlov H, Torg JS, Robie B, Jahre C. Cervical spinal stenosis determination with vertebral body ratio method. Radiology 1987;164:771–775.
17. Scher AT. Vertex impact and cervical dislocation in rugby players. S Afr Med J 1981;59:227–228.
18. Tator CH, Edmonds VE. National survey of spinal injuries in hockey players. CMAJ 1984;130:875–880.
19. Tator CH, Edmonds VE, New ML. Diving: A frequent and preventable cause of spinal cord injury. CMAJ 1981;124:1323–1324.
20. Torg JS. Epidemiology, pathomechanics, and prevention of athletic injuries to the cervical spine. Med Sci Sports Exerc 1985;17:295–303.
21. Torg JS, Pavlov H, Genuano SE, et al. Neurapraxia of the cervical spinal cord with transient quadriplegia. J Bone Joint Surg 1986;68a:1354–1370.
22. Torg JS, Sennett H, Pavlov H, et al. Spear tackler's spine: An entity precluding participation in tackle football and collision activities that expose the cervical spine to axial energy inputs. Am J Sports Med 1993;21:640–649.
23. Torg JS, Vegso JJ, Sennett H, et al. The National Football Head and Neck Injury Registry: 14-year report of cervical quadriplegia, 1971–1984. JAMA 1985;254:3439–3443.
24. White AA, Johnson RM, Panjabi MM, et al. Biomechanical analysis of clinical stability in the cervical spine. Clin Orthop 1975;109:85–96.
25. Wilberger JE, Abla A, Maroon JC. Burning hand syndrome revisited. Neurosurgery 1986;19:1038–1040.

CHAPTER

17

Guidelines for Return to Contact or Collision Sport After a Cervical Spine Injury

Robert C. Cantu, Julian E. Bailes, and Jack E. Wilberger, Jr.

SPRAIN/STRAIN— LIGAMENTOUS INJURY

Most cervical injuries will involve a ligament sprain, muscle strain, or contusion. With such injuries, there is no neurologic or osseous injury, and the athlete can return to competition when he or she is free of neck pain with or without axial compression, range of motion is full, and the strength of the neck is normal. Cervical radiographs should show no subluxation or abnormal curvatures. It is preferable that athletes not return to competition until they are asymptomatic and can perform at the level of their pre-injury abilities.

It is well known that ligament damage may accompany a cervical spine injury and can occur in the absence of bony injury. Generally, this is minor and self-limited but, on occasion, it may result in progressive instability, cervical spine deformity, and spinal cord injury. There are guidelines to assist in determining ligament stability. Under normal circumstances, conditions permit very little motion between the cervical vertebrae. In cadaver studies with all ligaments intact, horizontal movement of one vertebral body on the next does not exceed 3.5 mm, and the angular displacement of one vertebral body on the next is always 11 degrees or less. Only when most of the restraining ligaments are injured or destroyed do motions in excess of this occur. In the clinical setting, measurements of the horizontal or

Adapted from Cantu RC (ed): Neurologic Athletic Head and Neck Injuries, *Clinics in Sports Medicine,* Philadelphia, WB Saunders, 1998.

angular displacements can be made on neutral or flexion/extension radiographs. It is important, however, to remember that the younger the athlete, the more likely there is to be ligamentous laxity, and the above criteria may not always be applicable.[20]

Incipient, severe ligamentous injury in the acutely injured athlete may not be recognized because a normal degree of spinal ligamentous laxity in younger patients is generally accepted, and cervical muscle spasms, which may compensate for ligamentous instability, may be present. For these reasons, when any subluxation is seen after a sports-related injury, the patient should wear a hard cervical collar, and flexion/extension films of the cervical spine should be repeated 2 to 4 weeks after injury. If the films show no evidence of progression, or if there is a return to normal, it is unlikely that any significant injury has occurred, and the athlete can most likely return safely to his or her competitive sport.

SPEAR TACKLER'S SPINE

The entity of spear tackler's spine was originally described in 1993 after careful evaluation of data from the National Football Head and Neck Injury Registry.[20] Permanent neurologic injury occurred in four athletes who were identified as having the following characteristic combination of abnormalities on plain cervical spine films: (1) developmental narrowing of the cervical spinal canal; (2) straightening or reversal of the normal cervical lordotic curve; and (3) pre-existing minor posttraumatic radiographic evidence of bony or ligamentous injury. In addition to these radiographic criteria, all of these players were documented as having used spear-tackling techniques.

The existence of a spear tackler's spine, in some authors' opinions, absolutely prohibits the return to contact or collision sports, even if the abnormality is an incidental finding because of minor complaints or symptoms. Other experts believe that although concerns should be raised, if the normal cervical lordosis is restored by treatment, and the athlete refrains from any further spear-tackling techniques, then there is not a high degree of risk for injury from allowing return to athletic activity.

CERVICAL SPINE FRACTURE

Some bony injuries, such as spinous process fractures or unilateral laminar fractures, may require no treatment or only immobilization in a cervical collar. Others, such as the bilateral pars interarticularis fracture of C2 ("hangman's fracture") often may be treated with a cervical collar or, in some cases, halo vest immobilization. Unstable injuries should initially be reduced and temporarily stabilized with cervical traction using Gardner-Wells tongs or a halo ring device. Contrast-enhanced computed tomographic (CT) scan or magnetic resonance (MR) imaging of the cervical spine often should be obtained before fracture reduction to rule out the presence of retropulsed intervertebral disk material. Unrecognized retropulsed disk material has been implicated in the sudden neurologic deterioration of patients undergoing reduction of their cervical fractures.[5] Surgical treatment may subsequently be required for severe comminuted vertebral body fractures, unstable posterior element fractures, type 2 odontoid fractures, incomplete spinal cord injuries with canal or cord compromise, and in those patients with progression of their neurologic deficit to higher levels of spinal cord function.[10, 13]

Any athlete with a permanent neurologic injury should be prohibited from further competition. Those without cord injury, however, who have stable fractures as evidenced by flexion/extension radiographs, should be allowed to return to their normal daily activities. Athletes with burning hands syndrome or brachial plexus injuries may be considered healed and safe for return to play when their neurologic examinations return to normal, and they are symptom free.[11] Those whose fractures require halo vest or surgical stabilization are considered to have insufficient spinal strength to safely return to contact sports unless biomechanics are shown to be normal. Even after the fracture has healed, the altered biomechanics in surrounding spinal segments and loss of normal motion may produce high risk of future sports-related injury.[2]

Generally, stable fractures that have healed completely will allow the player to return by the next season. If there is a one-level anterior or posterior fusion for a fracture, athletes are usually allowed to go back when the neck pain is gone, the range of motion is complete, muscle strength of the neck is normal, and the fusion is solid. For any athlete with a fractured neck, proper warnings against contact or collision sports are advisable until it is certain that the patient is completely healed.

Managing athletes with traumatic spine or spinal cord injury presents unique challenges for the spinal surgeon. Even in the presence of an apparently stable spine, as seen on flexion/extension radiographs, and a normal-sized spinal canal, continued participation may not be advisable. Currently, there are no experimental or clinical data to help physicians predict the stability of healed spinal fractures or fusions when they are placed under extreme degrees of mechanical stress. There is increased mechanical stress above and below fused spinal segments, and repetitive microtrauma to a stiff spine exacerbates the stress. Torg and co-workers estimated that the forces involved in a football tackle may approach 18 g. Some attempt has been made to assess spinal strength following spinal injury with a Cybex dynamometer. The Cybex has been particularly useful in assessing muscle strength, power, and endurance, but its applicability to the spine is yet to be determined. In fact, there is no conclusive evidence that the injured cervical spine is made stronger than normal by fusion. Thus, in the absence of any objective ability to measure the degree of dynamic stress stability of the spine, any healed fracture (with the exception of chip, minor wedge/compression, isolated laminar, or spinous process fractures) or any injury that has required internal stabilization is suspect in its ability to withstand further challenges from contact or collision sports.

Where there are multilevel fusions or a fusion involving C1–C2 or C2–C3, return to contact or collision sports is contraindicated, but the athlete could participate in a noncontact sport at low risk of neck injury, such as tennis or golf.

RETURN TO PLAY CRITERIA AFTER A BURNER

Roughly, half of so-called burners or stingers in football at the high school level involve a brachial plexus stretch injury. Most burners at the college and professional level involve a cervical nerve root "pinch" phenomenon within the neural foramen. Because the dorsal root ganglion occupies most of the space within the foramen and lies underneath the subluxing facet, it often takes the brunt of the injury, and symptoms may be purely sensory in a dermatomal distribution. This is especially true if the athlete has had similar symptoms before. If there are any residual symptoms, neck pain, incomplete range of motion, or suspicion of a neck injury, return to play should be deferred.

RETURN TO PLAY CRITERIA AFTER TRANSIENT QUADRIPLEGIA

What factors predispose athletes to quadriplegia and when should athletes be withheld from future participation in contact or collision sports after an episode of transient quadriplegia? What are the appropriate circumstances to allow return after transient quadriplegia and what are relative and absolute contraindications for return? In presenting and discussing three case histories seen in the first author's practice, these questions are answered.

Case Histories

CASE 1

Case 1 involved a 27-year-old National Football League linebacker who experienced transient up-per and lower extremity paralysis and numbness after tackling a 225-lb (102-kg) opponent. The patient made contact sufficient to dent the forehead portion of his helmet and appeared to sustain an axial load injury with some hyperextension. Paralysis lasted 4 minutes; then, over the next 10 to 20 minutes, motor and sensory function returned beginning in the lower extremities. On arrival at the hospital, the patient was complaining of a burning sensation across his neck and shoulders. He denied any loss of consciousness, and there was no loss of bowel or bladder function.

On physical examination, higher cortical functions were intact. Motor examination results were 5/5 throughout, and reflexes were 2+ and symmetric, except for the ankles, which were 1+ and symmetric. Plantar response was downgoing bilaterally. Sensory examination results were positive to light touch and pinprick. The cerebellum was intact on examination.

Plain films of the cervical spine showed no evidence of fracture, dislocation, subluxation, or degenerative disk disease. The canal height measured within normal limits: 15 mm at C3 and C4, and 20 mm at C6. Torg ratios were C3 = 15/24 = 0.63, C4 = 15/22 = 0.68, C5 = 17/20 = 0.85, C6 = 20/22 = 0.91. MR imaging showed no evidence of fracture, canal compromise, or contusion. Flexion and extension views of the spine showed no instability. Cervical CT and MR imaging showed a functional reserve of cerebrospinal fluid (CSF) around the cord.

CASE 2

Case 2 involved a 23-year-old hockey player, drafted into the National Hockey League, who was injured while filming a team advertisement. Bending at the waist with his neck flexed, he unexpectedly collided with another player. The top of the patient's helmet struck the other player's abdomen. The patient's neck was relaxed because he was not expecting impact. Each player had taken one stride before the impact. The patient had immediate neck pain and felt something was wrong with his arms and legs. He fell to his side and rolled over on the ice onto his back. After 1 minute, he was aware that he could move his fingers in his gloves and his toes in his skates. A pins-and-needles sensation extended into both hands and to a lesser extent, his torso and legs. He was aware of a rigid painful neck within minutes. When he moved his head, a shocklike sensation traveled down his spine to his buttocks. It was about 4 or 5 minutes before he could rise from the ice. Neurologic symptoms persisted at highest intensity for approximately 5 minutes, then gradually subsided, first in his legs and then his arms. It was 2 weeks before all paresthesias disappeared. Other than a brief concussion in 1984, when his helmeted head struck the boards, he denied any significant prior injury.

Two weeks after injury, the patient had normal range of neck motion. No radiating symptoms could be elicited by compression of his spinous processes or by mild axial loading (negative Spurling's maneuver). No neurologic deficit was detected. Strength and tone were normal throughout. Plantar responses were downgoing. No clonus or abnormal reflexes were present. Upper extremity reflexes were 1+ and lower extremity reflexes were 2+. Gait proved normal, and no sensory loss for pinprick, vibration, or position sense was found.

Plain films showed no evidence of degenerative disk disease, subluxation, or fracture. The height of the canal at all levels exceeded 15 mm. Torg ratios measured C3 = 17/24 = −0.71; C4 = 15/23 = 0.65; C5 = 15/26 = 0.68; C6 = 16/23 = 0.70. MR imaging revealed mild disk bulging at C3–C4 but did not show spinal cord encroachment, and did show a functional reserve of CSF around the cord at all levels. Myelogram and CT showed a slight disk bulging at C3–C4 but also CSF around the spinal cord at all levels, including C3–4.

CASE 3

The athlete in case 3 first injured his neck as a high school football player in 1987. On making what he remembers to be a head-up tackle, he fell to his side and was unable to get up or roll onto his back. Sensation and motor movement were absent from the neck down. Gradually, motor function and sensation returned, first in his feet and then his hands. He could not move his head because of cervical spasm, and any attempts to do so produced jabs of pain running from his neck to his head. After several minutes, he was able to stand and walk off the field unassisted, although his legs felt very weak. His neck was rigid on the sidelines and he did not return to play. No radiographs were taken at that time, and no medical attention was sought. The patient played the following week with a neck collar. He reported that his neck was rigid, and thus he performed poorly. He did not play for the next 2 weeks because of continued rigidity and severe neck pain. Three weeks after the injury, because of persistent neck pain and stiffness, he sought medical attention at a sports medicine facility. There, cervical spine radiographs were taken. Although canal heights and Torg ratios were not measured, subsequent review of those films revealed canal heights of 12 mm, consistent with spinal stenosis, and abnormal Torg ratios at C4 = 12/25 = 0.48, and C5 = 12/24 = 0.50. After 2 weeks, the patient returned to competition, his neck pain and stiffness relieved. He played his senior season without further cervical symptoms.

The following fall, as a college freshman on full athletic scholarship, the patient squatted to make a tackle, hitting face to face and chest to chest. With head tilted up, his facemask made first contact. He fell backward on the ground, unable to move and without sensation from the neck down. Over the next few minutes, movement began to return to his right side and patchy sensation to his left side. He was transported to the hospital, where physical examination showed cranial nerves to be intact. There was a Brown-Séquard syndrome with right-sided hemisensory loss and a nearly flaccid left side. Muscle strength was 4/5 on the right, except the intrinsic muscles of the hand, which were 3/5. Biceps reflex was 1+ and symmetric, triceps reflex was 2+ on the right and absent on the left, knee jerk reflex was 2+ on the right and absent on the left, ankle jerk reflex was 2+ on the right and 1+ on the left. There were three beats of clonus in both ankles.

Radiographs, CT scans, and MR images were taken. The films revealed cervical stenosis and posterior disk herniation at C3–C4 with displacement of cord and thecal sac to the right. Torg ratios measured C2 = 20/23 = 0.87; C3 = 13/23 = 0.52; C5 = 12/24 = 0.50. C6 and C7 could not be read. Edema was found within the spinal cord from C2 to C5. Surgery was performed without complications, but the patient remained paralyzed immediately afterward. A second exploration did not find bleeding. The patient went to rehabilitation and remained in a wheelchair for 8 months before walking. Presently, he has recovered to a spastic quadriparetic state.

DISCUSSION

All three athletes in these cases suffered a bout of transient quadriplegia. Although such an event may occur after hyperextension or hyperflexion, it most frequently occurs with an axial load injury to the cervical spine, as described by Torg and associates.[18] In all cases, the symptoms were consistent with variations of the central spinal cord syndrome as described by Schneider and coworkers.[17]

Cervical spinal stenosis is known to increase the risk of permanent neurologic injury.[1, 12–15] Firooznia and associates[7] presented three case reports of patients who became quadriplegic after only "minor trauma." In all three patients, radiologic studies revealed "marked stenosis of the spinal canal." Some debate exists, however, over the definition of spinal stenosis. In the past, anteroposterior (AP) diameter of the spinal canal, measured from the posterior aspect of the vertebral body to the most anterior point on the spinolaminar line, determined the presence of stenosis. General consensus has been that between C3 and C7, canal heights are normal above 15 mm and spinal stenosis is present below 13 mm.[21] Resnick says CT scan and myelography are the "most sensitive diagnostic modalities" in determining spinal stenosis.[16] He points out that roentgenography fails to appraise the width of the cord and is not useful when stenosis results from ligamentous hypertrophy or discal protrusion. Ladd and Scranton[9] state that the AP diameter of the spinal canal is "unimportant" if there is total impedance of the contrast medium. They argue that metrizamide-enhanced myelogram is needed for the injured athlete because CT scan alone fails to reveal neural compression adequately. Thus, spinal stenosis cannot be defined by bony measurements alone. "Functional" spinal stenosis, defined as loss of the CSF around the cord or, in more extreme cases (i.e., Case 3), deformation of the spinal cord, whether documented by CT scan, MR imaging, or myelography, is a more accurate measure of stenosis.[4] The term *functional* is taken from the radiologic term *functional reserve* as applied to the protective cushion of CSF around the spinal cord in a nonstenotic canal.[8] In the data from the National Center for Catastrophic Sports Injury Research, cases of quadriplegia without spine fracture have been seen only when functional spinal stenosis is present.[4] Also, complete recovery of neurologic function after initial neurologic deficit from spine fracture or dislocation has been seen only in the absence of functional spinal stenosis.[4]

Of the three athletes presented, only the patient in Case 3 was documented as having cervical spinal stenosis as determined by AP diameter alone (12 mm at C4 and C5). In both Cases 1 and 2, the narrowest AP diameter measured 15 mm. In Case 1, CT scan and MR imaging showed no abnormalities and did show a functional reserve of CSF around all levels of the cord. In Case 2, CT scan, MR imaging, and myelogram all showed slight disk bulging at C3–C4, but again showed a reserve of CSF around the cord at all levels. After the second injury, in Case 3, the patient was shown to suffer functional cervical spinal stenosis. CT scan and MR imaging also showed spinal cord edema and displacement of the cord secondary to disk herniation.

Torg ratios were abnormal for all three athletes, with minimum ratios of 0.63 for Case 1, 0.65 for Case 2, and 0.40 for Case 3. This ratio (canal height/vertebral body AP diameter) of less than 0.80 has been defined as spinal stenosis.[3] For Cases 1 and 2, this ratio is misleading because the large vertebral body, not a narrow canal, produced ratios less than 0.80. This is consistent with other reports that an abnormal Torg ratio is a poor predictor of true functional stenosis.[8] Although the ratio leads to many false-positive results (positive predictive value at 12%),[8] it rarely is normal when true stenosis documented by MR imaging is present (sensitivity = 92%).[8] Thus, an abnormal ratio in an athlete with spinal cord symptoms means that evaluation with MR imaging, myelogram, or contrast-positive CT scan should be done.

Given an athlete who has suffered transient quadriplegia, what criteria should be followed for his or her return to contact sports? Case 1 is an example of an athlete who has never had these symptoms. This athlete had complete neurologic recovery and full range of cervical spine movement. AP diameter was normal at all levels; CT scan and MR imaging showed no evidence of functional stenosis. Thus, there were no neurologic, mechanic, symptomatic, or structural (functional spinal stenosis) contraindications for return to competition. Understanding that he may be at a slightly greater risk for a second event, the athlete returned to competition and has had no further symptoms.

Case 2 involved an athlete who has two relative contraindications for returning to play, namely, mild disk bulging at C3–C4, and the fact that the impact that produced the transient quadriplegia seemed relatively minor (head-to-abdomen contact from one step apart). Because myelogram and CT scan did not show functional stenosis and his cervical strength and range of motion returned to normal, there was not an absolute contraindication to return to play. After consideration of the relative contraindications, this athlete chose not to return to professional hockey.

Case 3 is an example of an athlete with an absolute contraindication for return. In addition to a stenotic canal according to AP diameter (12 mm), he had functional stenosis on CT scan and MR imaging, with cord displacement, edema, and lack of reserve of CSF around the cord at all levels secondary to disk herniation. Because studies were not performed after his initial injury, it is not known whether he had a cord displacement at that time, but the stenosis was present. This should have been evaluated by MR imaging, myelogram, or CT scan and the presence of functional stenosis should have terminated his football career after the initial episode of transient quadriplegia. If he had not had severe spinal stenosis, it is probable his subsequent disk herniation would have produced radicular symptoms alone instead of severe spinal cord injury.

Given an athlete with cervical spinal stenosis, what is the mechanism of injury causing transient or permanent neurologic deficit? Eismont and coworkers[6] state that such athletes are "remarkably susceptible to hyperextension injuries known to produce maximal narrowing (up to 2 mm) of the ventrodorsal diameter of the spinal canal." Torg and others[19] note that hyperextension causes "an inward indentation of the ligamentum flavum," which can compress the cord. Penning[16] described a "bony pincers" mechanism in hyperextension in which the cord is compressed between the vertebral body and the closest portion of the spinolaminar line of the inferior vertebra. The athlete in Case 3 appeared to suffer a hyperextension injury making contact with the facemask, and it was spinal stenosis that predisposed him to neurologic injury. For the athletes in Cases 1 and 2, although the force of the blow was not great, the contact was not expected, and therefore their neck muscles were relaxed, causing greater forces to be transmitted directly to the spine instead of being dissipated in the muscles.

These athletes present a spectrum of when to allow return to competition in contact or collision sports after an episode of transient quadriplegia. It is important to realize that normal canal size on lateral radiograph does not preclude the possibility of functional spinal stenosis—an absolute contraindication for return. For this diagnosis, myelogram, CT scan, or MR imaging is needed.

CONCLUSION

Return to play decisions after traumatic spine or spinal cord injury are not always clear cut and often require individualization. This chapter has attempted to provide a framework for these decisions. The classification scheme previously described by Cantu in Chapter 15 is useful in decision-making regarding the return to play status of these athletes. Type 1 athletic injuries are those with permanent neurologic injury and preclude the player from further participation in contact sports. Type 2 injuries consist of transient neurologic disturbances with normal radiographic studies. If the complete workup reveals no injury, these players may return to competition once they are symptom free. Type 3 injuries are heterogeneous, including all players with radiographic abnormalities. Those athletes with significant bony or ligamentous spinal instability, or spinal cord contusion, are advised not to return to contact sports. Other radiographic abnormalities, such as spear tackler's spine, posterior ligamentous injury, congenital fusion or stenosis, herniated disks, or degenerative spondylitic disease, require consideration on an individual basis.

References

1. Alexander MM, Davis CH, Field CH. Hyperextension injuries of the cervical spine. Arch Neurol Psychiatry 1958;79:146–150.
2. Bailes JE, Hadley MN, Quigley MR, et al. Management of athletic injuries of the cervical spine and spinal cord. Neurosurgery 1991;29:4.
3. Boijsen E. The cervical spinal canal in intraspinal expansive processes. Acta Radiol 1954;42:101–115.
4. Cantu RC. Functional cervical spinal stenosis: A contraindication to participation in contact sports. Med Sci Sports Exerc 1993;25:1082–1083.
5. Chestnut RM. Emergency management of spinal cord injury. In Narayan RK, Wilberger JE Jr, Povlishock JT (eds): Neurotrauma. New York, McGraw-Hill, 1996, p 1121.
6. Eismont FJ, Clifford S, Goldberg M, et al. Cervical sagittal spinal canal size in spinal injury. Spine 1984;9:663–666.
7. Firooznia H, Ahn J, Rafii M, et al. Sudden quadriplegia after a minor trauma: The role of pre-existing spinal stenosis. Surg Neurol 1985;23:165–168.
8. Herzog RJ, Weins JJ, Dillingham MF, et al. Normal cervical spine morphometry and cervical spinal stenosis in asymptomatic professional football players. Spine 1991;16:178–186.
9. Ladd AL, Scranton PE. Congenital cervical stenosis presenting as transient quadriplegia in athletes. J Bone Joint Surg 1986;68:1371–1374.
10. Maroon JC, Bailes JE. Athletes with cervical spine injury. Spine 1996;21:19.
11. Maroon JC. "Burning hands" in football spinal cord injuries. JAMA 1977;238:2031–2049.
12. Matsuura P, Waters RL, Adkins RH, et al. Compari-

son of computerized tomography parameters of the cervical spine in normal control subjects and spinal cord-injured patients. J Bone Joint Surg 1989;71:183–188.

13. Mayfield FH. Neurosurgical aspects of cervical trauma. *In* Clinical Neurosurgery, vol. 2. Baltimore, Williams & Wilkins, 1955.

14. Nugent GR. Clinicopathologic correlations in cervical spondylosis. Neurology 1959;9:273–281.

15. Penning L. Some aspects of plain radiography of the cervical spine in chronic myelopathy. Neurology 1962;12:513–519.

16. Resnick D. Degenerative Disease of the Spine. *In* Diagnosis of Bone and Joint Disorders. Philadelphia, WB Saunders, 1981, pp 1408–1415.

17. Schneider RS, Reifel E, Crisler H, et al. Serious and fatal football injuries involving the head and spinal cord. JAMA 1961;177:362–367.

18. Torg JS, Pavlov H, Genuano SE, et al. Neuropraxia of the cervical spinal cord with transient quadriplegia. J Bone Joint Surg 1986;68A:1354–1378.

19. Torg JS, Sennett B, Pavlov H, et al. Spear Tackler's Spine: An entity precluding participation in tackle football and collision activities that expose the cervical spine to axial injury inputs. Am J Sports Med 1993;21:640–649.

20. White AA, Johnson RM, Pangabi MM, et al. Biomechanical analysis of clinical stability in the cervical spine. Clin Orthop 1975;109:85–89.

21. Wolfe BS, Khilnani M, Malis L. The sagittal diameter of the bony cervical spinal canal and its significance in cervical spondylosis. J Mt Sinai Hosp 1956;23:283–292.

18

Cervical Spinal Stenosis: Diagnosis and Return to Play Issues

Robert C. Cantu

Just as is true of other neurologic conditions, such as concussions, the world medical literature on spinal stenosis is confused by a multiplicity of definitions. This confusion renders a comparison of different articles on the subject extremely difficult, if not impossible, because identical structural entities are not being compared, much as in the proverbial comparison of apples with oranges or even pears, not just with other apples.

The purpose of this chapter is to define cervical spinal stenosis in terms of 1990s imaging technology, the magnetic resonance (MR) image, and, based on the experience of the National Center for Catastrophic Sports Injury Research, to give clear indications for sports participation once this condition has produced symptoms.

In a 1956 study of 200 randomly selected asymptomatic subjects who underwent lateral cervical spine radiograph examinations at a fixed target distance of 72 inches, Wolfe and associates[20] established the normal values of the sagittal diameters of the cervical spine. Canal height, sagittal diameter, was defined as the anteroposterior diameter measured from the posterior aspect of the vertebral body to the most anterior point on the spinolaminar line (Fig. 18–1, a). Wolfe and colleagues found that the average anteroposterior diameter was 22 mm at C1, 20 mm at C2, and 17 mm at C3–C7. General consensus has been that between C3 and C7, canal heights are normal above 15 mm,[1, 2] and spinal stenosis is present below 13 mm.[8, 12]

In 1986, Torg and coworkers[19] and, in 1987, Pavlov and coworkers[16] described a new method to assess cervical spinal stenosis radiographically using a ratio method to eliminate the need to correct for radiographic magnification error. The height of the spinal canal as measured from the midpoint of the posterior surface of the vertebral body to the spinolaminar line is the numerator, and the denominator is the height of the corresponding midvertebral body (Fig. 18–1, b). A vertebral canal/vertebral body ratio under .80 was defined as "significant spinal stenosis." The authors also concluded that their "data clearly indicate that athletes who have developmental spinal stenosis are not predisposed to more severe injuries associated with permanent neurological sequelae."[19]

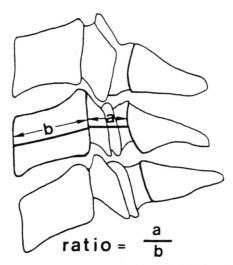

$$\text{ratio} = \frac{a}{b}$$

Figure 18–1. The spinal canal/vertebral body ratio is the distance from the midpoint of the posterior aspect of the vertebral body to the nearest point on the corresponding spinolaminar line (a) divided by the anteroposterior width of the vertebral body (b). Pavlov's ratio is a/b. From Torg JS, Pavlov H, Gennario SE, et al. Neurapraxia of the cervical spinal cord with transient quadriplegia. J Bone Joint Surg 1986; 68A:1354–1370, with permission.

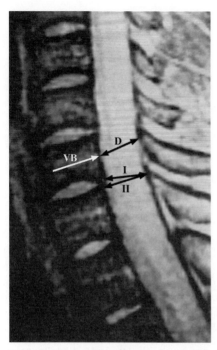

Figure 18–2. MR imaging showing functional spinal stenosis as the canal is so small that no CSF is around the spinal cord. From Clinics in Sports Medicine 1998;17:123, with permission.

Beginning about 1990, the ratio method as a means to define spinal stenosis has been shown to be of low predictive value. First, the Kerlan Jobe Orthopedic Clinic found the incidence of spinal stenosis using the Torg ratio to be 33% in 124 professional and 100 rookie football players.[15] Then Herzog and associates[10] found in 80 asymptomatic professional football players that 49% had abnormal ratios below .80 at one or more cervical levels. They also found the ratio to be highly unreliable in determining spinal stenosis, with a positive predictive value of only 12%. Herzog and colleagues[10] theorized that the Torg ratio had a high rate of false positives (88% of the time) because the large vertebral bodies of larger athletes skewed the ratio, and they were correct. The cervical spinal canal heights (numerator) of all the athletes they studied were within normal limits. The athletes with the abnormal Torg ratios had extremely large vertebral bodies (denominator), which brought the ratio below .80.

They thus concluded, "If an abnormal Torg ratio is detected, further evaluation is necessary before an athlete can be diagnosed as 'significantly spinal stenotic.'"[10] This is extremely important to understand because

commentary in any literature that used the ratio method to define stenosis is very suspect because true stenosis was likely not present in 88% of the cases.

Even in the small percentage of professional football players in Herzog and his colleagues' study[10] (with spinal stenosis defined as canal size by MR image two standard deviations below the mean), none had experienced spinal cord symptoms and none had "functional cervical spinal stenosis" defined as a cervical spinal canal so small as to obliterate the protective cushion of cerebrospinal fluid (CSF) (Fig. 18–2), or in more extreme cases, deformation of the spinal cord itself (Fig. 18–3).

HOW BEST TO DEFINE CERVICAL SPINAL STENOSIS

Resnick[18] stated that computed tomography (CT) and myelography are "the most sensitive diagnostic modalities" in determining spinal stenosis. He pointed out that spine radiographs fail to appraise the width of the cord and are not useful when stenosis results from ligamentous hypertrophy or discal protrusion. Ladd and Scran-

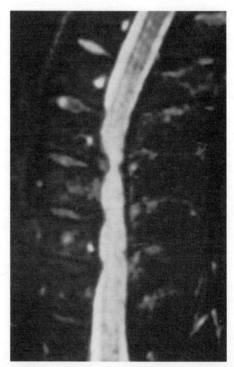

Figure 18–3. MR imaging showing deformation of the spinal cord by extreme functional spinal stenosis. From Clinics in Sports Medicine 1998;17:123, with permission.

ton[11] reported that the anteroposterior diameter of the spinal cord is "unimportant" if there is total impedance of the contrast medium. They argued that a metrizamide-enhanced myelogram is needed in the injured athlete because CT alone fails to adequately reveal dural compression. Thus, spinal stenosis cannot be defined by bone measurements alone. "Functional" spinal stenosis, defined as a loss of the CSF around the cord (see Fig. 18–2), or, in more extreme cases, as deformation of the spinal cord itself (see Fig. 18–3), whether documented by contrast-enhanced CT, magnetic resonance imaging (MRI), or myelography, is a more accurate measure of stenosis.[3, 4] The term *functional* is taken from the radiologic term *functional reserve* as applied to the protective cushion of CSF around the spinal cord in a nonstenotic canal.[10]

Does Functional Spinal Stenosis Increase the Risk of Neurologic Injury With Cervical Spine Trauma?

The author agrees that functional spinal stenosis is what neurosurgeons and team physicians should be concerned with, and, if present, especially if the athlete incurs spinal cord symptoms, no further participation in contact or collision sports should occur. Cervical spinal stenosis is known to increase the risk of permanent neurologic injury. Firooznia and associates[9] presented the case reports of three patients "with marked stenosis of the spinal canal" who became quadriplegic after only "minor trauma." These findings are consistent with those of Matsuura and coworkers,[12] who found in 42 spinal cord injuries compared with 100 controls that "the sagittal diameter of the spinal canals of the control group were significantly larger than those of the spinal cord injured group." Eismont and colleagues[7] concluded, "Our results provide evidence that the sagittal diameter of the spinal canal of some individuals may be inherently smaller than normal, and that this reduced size may be a predisposing risk factor for spinal cord injury." Others who have concluded that spinal stenosis predisposes to spinal cord injury include Wolfe and coworkers,[20] Penning,[17] Alexander and associates,[1] Mayfield,[13] Nugent,[14] and Ladd and Scranton,[11] who conclude, "Patients who have stenosis of the cervical spine should be advised to discontinue participation in contact sports."

In data from the National Center for Catastrophic Sports Injury Research, in research conducted from 1987 to 1998, no quadriplegic patients with cervical spine fracture-dislocation and functional spinal stenosis recovered completely, compared with nearly 20% of quadriplegic patients with fracture dislocation who had normal-sized spinal canals who went on to a complete neurologic recovery. During this same period, cases of quadriplegia that occurred without fracture dislocation were recorded, and in every instance, severe functional spinal stenosis was present. Thus, in the experience of the National Center for Catastrophic Sports Injury Research, a small cervical spinal canal predisposes the athlete to a worse neurologic outcome when spinal cord injury occurs.

What About the Workup?

When an athlete has symptoms referable to the spinal cord or nerve roots, radiographs to detect subluxation or fracture should be a part of the initial workup. Radiographic bone measurements are still a useful screening tool; an abnormal Torg ratio should suggest the need for further workup. Though the ratio overestimates the presence of spinal stenosis 88% of the time, if a patient has spinal stenosis, the ratio is almost always abnormal.

If an athlete exclusively has neck symptoms, such as pain or rigidity, that promptly resolve, cervical spine films are usually sufficient. If, however, the patient has symptoms such as transient quadriplegia, burning hands syndrome, or other bilateral motor or sensory symptoms that suggest spinal cord involvement, the physician should order an MR image after obtaining radiographs.

Contrast-positive CT and myelography are useful for defining the degree of spinal stenosis; however, both techniques are invasive and usually not needed, as the MRI in most cases is sufficient. In some difficult cases, contrast-positive CT, which is more sensitive than MRI for fractures and bony abnormalities, and myelography provide a better view of spinal cord compression than MRI.

RETURN TO PLAY ISSUES

When asked if he advocates MRI to screen all athletes who play contact sports for spinal stenosis, the author's answer is no. MRI of all players would not be cost-effective, and the data is insufficient to suggest that it would be appropriate to screen athletes in this manner.

When a player has spinal cord symptoms after an injury and is shown to have an abnormal Torg ratio, MRI can better define whether that player should or should not return to play. The author believes very strongly that those who have had spinal cord symptoms from sports-related injuries and are shown to have true functional spinal stenosis on MRI should not be allowed to return to contact sports.

Guidelines for Return to Contact Sports After Transient Quadriplegia

Based on three cases treated by the senior author,[5, 6] Cantu and Cantu proposed acceptable circumstances, as well as relative and absolute contraindications, for athletes to return to contact or collision sports after an episode of transient quadriplegia. Return after a first episode of transient quadriplegia is deemed acceptable if the athlete has complete resolution of symptoms, full range of motion, a normal curvature of the cervical spine, as well as no evidence of spinal stenosis on MRI, contrast-enhanced CT scan, or myelography. Relative contraindications, as seen in Case 2 (described hereafter), involve a mild intervertebral disk bulge that does not obliterate the reserve of CSF around the cord and transient quadriplegia caused by minimal contact. In Case 3 true spinal stenosis documented by MRI illustrates an absolute contraindication for return to contact or collision sports after an episode of transient quadriplegia, and what can happen if return is allowed. The authors recognize that these are guidelines that would be difficult to prove in a scientific fashion, and that, in any case, the legal and moral consequences would be too serious to allow a controlled trial.

CASE 1

This 27-year-old National Football League linebacker experienced transient upper- and lower-extremity paralysis and numbness after an axial load spear tackle of a 255-pound fullback. Paraly-

sis lasted for 4 minutes; during the next 10 to 20 minutes, complete motor and sensory function returned, beginning with the lower extremities. On his arrival at the hospital, his neurologic examination was normal. Cervical spine films showed no evidence of fracture, dislocation/subluxation, or degenerative disk disease. The canal height at all levels measured within normal limits (> 15 mm). There was no evidence of fracture, canal compromise, or contusion on MRI, and flexion and extension views of the spine showed no instability.

This case is an example of an athlete who has no contraindications for returning to his sport, except for the fact that one episode of transient quadriplegia may make him more likely to have a second than an athlete who has never had these symptoms. This athlete had a complete neurologic recovery and full range of cervical spine movement. The anteroposterior (AP) diameter of the canal was normal at all levels; CT scan and MRI showed no evidence of functional stenosis. Thus, there were no neurologic, mechanical, symptomatic, or structural (functional spinal stenosis) contraindications for returning to competition. Understanding that he may be at slightly greater risk for a second event, the athlete returned to competition and has had no further symptoms.

CASE 2

This 33-year-old National Hockey League player was rendered transiently quadriplegic while filming a team advertisement. Bending at the waist with his neck flexed, he unexpectedly collided with another player. The top of the patient's helmet struck the other player's abdomen. His neck was relaxed because he was not expecting impact. Each player had taken one stride prior to impact. The patient had immediate neck pain and felt that something was wrong with his arms and legs. He fell to his side and rolled over on the ice onto his back. After 1 minute, he was aware that he could move his fingers in his gloves and his toes in his skates. A pins-and-needles sensation extended into both hands and, to a lesser degree, his torso and legs. Within minutes he was aware of a rigid, painful neck; upon moving his head, a shocklike sensation traveled down his spine to his buttocks. It was about 4 or 5 minutes before he could rise from the ice. Neurologic symptoms persisted at highest intensity for approximately 5 minutes, then gradually subsided, first in his legs and then in his arms. It was 2 weeks before all paresthesias had disappeared; at that time, the patient had normal range of motion and a normal neurologic examination. Plain films showed no evidence of degenerative disk disease, subluxation, or fracture. Height of the spinal canal exceeded 15 mm at all levels. MR imaging revealed mild disk bulging at C3–4 but no spinal cord encroachment; it showed a functional reserve of CSF around the cord at all levels. Myelography and contrast-enhanced CT scan also showed slight disk bulging at C3–4, but CSF around the spinal cord at all levels, including C3–4.

This athlete has two relative contraindications for returning to play: (1) mild disc bulging at C3–-4, and (2) the fact that the impact that produced the transient quadriplegia seemed relatively minor (head to abdomen contact from one step apart). Since the myelogram and CT scan did not show functional stenosis, and his cervical films were normal, there was no absolute contraindication to return to play. After consideration of the relative contraindications, this athlete chose not to return to professional hockey.

CASE 3

This athlete first injured his neck making a head-up tackle as a high school football player. He fell to his side unable to rise or to roll onto his back. Sensation and motor movement were absent from the neck down. Gradually, motor function and sensation returned, first to his feet and then to his hands. After several minutes, he was able to stand and walk off the field unassisted, although his legs felt very weak. On the sidelines his neck was rigid and he did not return to play. No radiographs were obtained at that time, and no medical attention was sought. Three weeks after the injury, because of persistent neck pain and stiffness, he sought medical attention at a sports medicine facility, where cervical spine radiographs were taken. Subsequent review of these films revealed canal heights of 12 mm, consistent with spinal stenosis. Two weeks thereafter, the patient returned to competition, his neck pain and stiffness relieved. He played throughout his senior season without further cervical symptoms.

The following fall, as a college freshman on full athletic scholarship, he was rendered quadriplegic making a face-to-face and chest-to-chest tackle. Over the next few minutes, movement began to return to his right side and patch sensation to his left side. Neurologic examination at the hospital revealed a Brown-Séquard syndrome with right-sided hemisensory loss and a nearly flaccid left side. Radiographs, CT scans, and MRI images were obtained. The films revealed cervical stenosis and posterior disk herniation at C3–4, with displacement of the cord and thecal sac to the right. Edema was found within the spinal cord from C2 to C5. Surgery was performed without complications, but the patient remained paralyzed immediately afterward. At a second exploration no bleeding was found. The patient went to rehabilitation and remained in a wheelchair for 8 months before walking. He has ultimately recovered to a spastic quadriparetic state.

This case is an example of an athlete with an absolute contraindication for return to competition. In addition to a stenotic canal with an AP diameter of 12 mm, he had a functional stenosis on CT and MR images with cord displacement and edema secondary to disk herniation. Since studies were not performed following his initial injury, it is not known whether he had cord displacement at that time, but the stenosis was present. This should have been evaluated by MRI, myelography, or contrast-enhanced CT scan, and the presence of functional stenosis should have terminated his football career after the initial episode of transient quadriplegia. If he had not had severe spinal stenosis, it is probable that his subsequent disk herniation would have produced radicular symptoms alone instead of severe spinal cord injury.

These three athletes present a spectrum of whether to allow return to competition in contact or collision sports following an episode of transient quadriplegia. It is important to realize that a normal canal size on lateral radiographs does not preclude the possibility of functional spinal stenosis as an absolute contraindication for return to sport. For this diagnosis, a myelogram, contrast-enhanced CT scan, or MRI image is needed.

CONCLUSIONS REGARDING SPINAL STENOSIS

The following conclusions can be drawn:

1. In the 1990s, realizing the size of the spinal cord may vary as may the size of the spinal canal, the definition of spinal stenosis should *not* be made on bone measurements alone.

2. Functional spinal stenosis defined as a loss of CSF around the spinal cord or, in more extreme cases, deformation of the spinal cord, whether documented by MR imaging, positive contrast CT, or myelography, should be the 1990s standard to define significant spinal stenosis.

3. Experience with the National Center for Catastrophic Sports Injury Research, as well as literature review, leads to the conclusion that an athlete with significant spinal stenosis, as defined by a loss of functional reserve by MR imaging, is at increased risk of quadriplegia and should not participate in contact or collision sports.

4. The presence of spinal stenosis as defined by the ratio method is common in professional football players and has a very low predictive value for the actual presence of functional spinal stenosis.

5. Any conclusions or recommendations regarding spinal stenosis based on the ratio method must be held suspect, as functional or true spinal stenosis was likely not present.

References

1. Alexander MM, Davis CH. Field CC. Hyperextension injuries of the cervical spine. Arch Neurol Psychiatry 1958;79:146.
2. Boijsen E. The cervical spinal canal in intraspinal expansive processes. Acta Radiol 1954;42:101.
3. Cantu RC. Functional cervical spinal stenosis: a contraindication to participation in contact sports. Med Sci Sports Exer 1993;25:316–317.
4. Cantu RC. Cervical spinal stenosis: Challenging an established detection method. Phys Sportsmed 1993;21:57–63.
5. Cantu RV, Cantu RC. Guidelines for return to contact sports after transient quadriplegia. J Neurosurg 1994;80:592–594.
6. Cantu RC. Transient quadriplegia: To play or not to play. Sports Med Digest 1994;16:1–4.
7. Eismont FJ, Clifford S, Goldberg M, et al. Cervical sagittal spinal canal size in spinal injury. Spine 1984;9:663–666.
8. Epstein JA, Carras R, Hyman RA, et al. Cervical myelopathy caused by developmental stenosis of the cervical canal. J Neurosurg 1979;51:362–367.
9. Firooznia H, Ahn J, Raffi M, et al. Sudden quadriplegia after a minor trauma: The role of preexisting spinal stenosis. Surg Neurol 1985;23:165–168.
10. Herzog RJ, Weins JJ, Dillingham MF, et al. Normal cervical spine morphometry and cervical spinal stenosis in asymptomatic professional football players. Spine 1991;16:178–186.
11. Ladd AL, Scranton PE. Congenital cervical stenosis presenting as transient quadriplegia in athletes. J Bone Joint Surge 1986;68:1371–1374.
12. Matsurra P, Waters RL, Adkins RH, et al. Comparison of computerized tomography parameters of the cervical spine in normal control subjects and spinal cord-injured patients. J Bone Joint Surg 1989;71:183–188.
13. Mayfield FH: Neurosurgical Aspects of Cervical Trauma. *In* Clinical Neurosurgery, vol. 2. Baltimore, Williams & Wilkins, 1995.
14. Nugent GR. Clinicopathologic correlations in cervical spondylosis. Neurology 1959;9:273.
15. Odor JM, Watkins RG, Dillin WH, et al. Incidence of cervical spinal stenosis in professional and rookie football players. Am J Sports Med 1990;18:507–509.
16. Pavlov HJ, Torg S, Robie B, et al. Cervical spinal stenosis: Determination with vertebral body ratio method. Radiology 1987;164:771–775.
17. Penning L. Some aspects of plain radiography of the cervical spine in chronic myelopathy. Neurology 1962;12:513–519.
18. Resnick D. Diagnosis of Bone and Joint Disorders. Philadelphia, WB Saunders, 1981, pp 1408–1415.
19. Torg JS, Pavlov H, Genuano SE, et al. Neuropraxia of the cervical spinal cord with transient quadriplegia. J Bone Joint Surg 1986;68A:1354–1370.
20. Wolfe BS, Khilnani M, Malis L. The sagittal diameter of the bony cervical spinal canal and its significance in cervical spondylosis. J Mt Sinai Hosp 1956;23:283.

19

Thoracic and Lumbar Spine Injuries in Athletics

Arthur L. Day and Mark A. Giovanini

The increased number of adults and adolescents who regularly participate in a fitness (e.g., jogging) or highly competitive athletic program has led to a substantially increased incidence and awareness of athletics-related thoracic and lumbar spinal problems. Most of these injuries are caused by bruising, overstretching, or tearing of paraspinal soft tissues (e.g., muscles, ligaments). In such cases, proper training techniques and avoidance of aggravating activities may allow continued athletic participation while the pain resolves over several weeks. Other types of injury, however, pose a major obstacle to continued competition, and may require specific types of intervention to optimize recovery. The purpose of this chapter is to examine the unique clinical features of athletics-related thoracic and lumbar spinal problems, and to present the specifics of evaluation and treatment that separate athletes from the general population.

DIFFERENCES IN ATHLETES

An *athlete* is defined herein as an individual who participates at the highest levels of competition in a physically demanding sport. This definition could include adolescents (younger than 18 years old) as well as those who compete at collegiate, Olympic, "serious" amateur, or professional levels. In most instances, success will be determined by dedication to the sport and to intense and frequent training routines. This definition is not intended to insult the millions of people who participate in recreational athletics, many of whom excel and take their sport and training quite seriously. Recreational athletes, however, generally have other jobs and goals outside athletics, and could stop their athletic participation without loss of livelihood or future earning potential. The top-level athlete with a lumbar spine problem often has specific physical, motivational, and therapeutic goals different from the general population.[34]

Physical

Despite the complex movements necessitated by many sports, during which the thoracolumbar spine is subjected to a combination of extreme forces simultaneously, athletes appear to have a lower incidence of serious back injuries than expected, and a reduced severity of clinical complaints once the injury occurs.[16] These differences may be explained by several factors, including age, natural selection, training routines, and humoral factors.

Age

The age of participation is a substantial factor in both the type and frequency of lumbar region injuries.[46] The differential diagnosis in adolescents is distinctly different than in adults.[20] Micheli found that injuries to the posterior elements comprised 73 out of 100 injuries in adolescents, whereas discogenic causes were prominent in adults. The physical demands placed on the young, skeletally immature spine, and the growth spurt, which produces asynchronous development between bony and musculoligamentous elements, make the young athlete vulnerable to specific types of injuries, including spondylolysis, Scheuermann's disease, and hyperlordotic mechanical low back pain.[24, 26, 33, 46]

Selection Bias

To a large degree, most top-level athletes are preselected at an early age according to such natural talents as, for example, flexibility, strength, and coordination that allow them to excel and advance to higher levels. This enhanced "athleticism" may provide protection to that individual from a variety of injuries, as he or she has more body control and skill to avoid dangerous activities or positions.

Physical Conditioning and Training Techniques

Although somewhat difficult to quantify, training routines can strengthen the supplementary muscles and ligaments that support and protect the spine during extremes of movement and loading. Strong abdominal and paraspinous musculature, proper warm-up and stretching, and attention to precision techniques are qualities particularly well developed and emphasized by the top-level athlcte, and may serve to protect from lumbar region injury. It is unclear, however, whether such training can actually strengthen or thicken adjacent ligaments to decrease the propensity to disk rupture. The incidence of free-fragment disk rupture through the posterior longitudinal ligament is significantly less in an athletic population than in the general group, a characteristic that could easily be attributable to the differences in disk and ligamentous character associated with age rather than those induced by training.[7]

Conversely, poor physical conditioning predisposes to acute and overuse injuries in the thoracic and lumbar spine. The abdominal and paraspinal muscles provide support to the axial spine, and weakness or imbalance in these muscle groups puts abnormal constraints on tendons, ligaments, and bony elements, thus subjecting them to injury.[13] Improper training techniques that abnormally load the axial skeleton may also promote injury. These injuries are typically seen with weightlifting, either as a primary discipline or as a training regimen for another sport. Inflexibility of the hamstring muscles places the axial spine in a hyperlordotic posture, a position that may make the spine less resilient to axial loading and pre-disposes to injuries such as spondylolysis.[5, 6, 39, 43]

Humoral Factors

Top-level athletes often have alterations of pain perception or an enhanced ability to suppress discomfort associated with minor injuries. Athletes are often able to tolerate symptoms that would incapacitate "unathletic" people by entering an "analgesic" state, during which there is some evidence of increased liberation of beta-endorphins and other substances that have direct effects on pain appreciation and mood.

Motivation

Successful athletes invariably have an intense competitive spirit and desire to win. They are generally not interested in disability, but only in ways to enhance their own physical performances. Depending on their age, type of athletic activity, and capability level, fame, education, or monetary gain (present or potential) may also be significant motivating factors. Adolescents may derive substantial personal pleasure from their sport, and may gain further support and motivation from their peers or parents. High schoolers may view athletics as a way to further their education via a college scholarship. Collegiate athletes may aspire for lucrative professional career opportunities. The financial rewards to some sports professionals are staggering, and are obvious goals for many young athletes, worthy of great sacrifice and effort, potentially by both the individual athlete and his treating physicians.

Return to Activity

The athlete with a thoracolumbar-region injury is anxious to return to competition, and the treating physician must recognize the special goals of therapy.[4, 10, 18, 30, 38, 40, 41] First, the desired end product is a "perfect" result, which allows the athlete to have unrestricted flexibility, strength, and agility at former levels; a good outcome is not acceptable. Second, the cause of the injury is often expected to continue, especially in traumatic sports such as football, running, and weightlifting. The final decision regarding treatment and return to activity is a complicated one, especially in the top-level athlete. In our opinion, a neurologic specialist (ideally a neurosurgeon) should be consulted prior to the athlete's return to participation whenever there are neurologic deficits or risks of new or further neurologic deterioration.

TYPE OF SPORT AND LEVEL OF COMPETITION

Most thoracolumbar spine injuries are caused either by acute traumatic events or by repetitive overuse maneuvers. Acute injuries usually arise as a result of blunt trauma, and include soft tissue contusions, sprains, strains, and fractures, and are particularly common in contact sports such as football and rugby. Up to 30% of football players lose playing time from low back pain.[40] In a review of 506 collegiate level football players, 27% had complaints of low back pain, most commonly a soft tissue injury from a blow to the low back resulting in some form of a musculoligamentous injury.[42] Spondylolysis defects have been noted in up to one third of all linemen.[12] Weight lifters show a high incidence of premature degenerative disk disease.[36, 48] Eighty percent of male lifters demonstrate evidence of compression fractures, spondylolysis, or disk injuries by age 40, presumably from poor lifting techniques and excessive axial loading. Physical size differences and the duration of exposure to high-level training also contribute, with increasing frequency and extent of injury noted in collegiate and professional football players compared with younger groups.

In noncontact sports, most low back injuries are the result of repetitive microtrauma to the lumbar spine and surrounding structures. The extreme and repetitive torsional and flexion/extension motions associated with sports such as gymnastics, running, golf, and diving place unusual demands on certain regions of the lumbar spine not necessarily designed to support such activities. Gymnasts have a particularly high rate of spine injury, with the rate related to the level of competition and the type of event (i.e., floor exercises, balance beam, and parallel bar routines).[19, 20, 21] Gymnastics and diving have a very high incidence of spondylolysis compared with other sports and the general population.[5, 9, 10, 16, 32, 35, 39, 43, 48] Runners show a degree of premature disk degeneration and herniation from repetitive axial loading.

COMMON TYPES OF LUMBAR INJURIES

Isolated thoracic injury is quite uncommon in athletics, and is herein joined with lumbar region abnormalities. Lumbar spine injuries differ from those in the cervical or thoracic region, in that the spinal cord and cerebral vasculature are not at risk. The risks and extent of neurologic injury, therefore, are substantially milder, and are usually limited to a single nerve root. One or more spinal elements may be affected, including soft tissues (muscles, ligaments), intervertebral disk, bones, and neural elements. Lumbar spine injuries are herein separated into four categories: soft tissue injuries, fractures, disk injuries, and pars interarticularis defects. Each type of injury has its own individual mechanisms of development, signs and symptoms, radiographic features, treatment, and return to play decisions.

Soft Tissue Injuries

Most acute low back pain problems are caused by soft tissue injuries and will resolve with time and rest without subsequent restrictions.[16] Symptoms that persist beyond the acute stage may represent a more serious process needing more careful investigation. Soft tissue injuries include contusions, strains, and sprains.

Incidence, Clinical Features, and Differential Diagnosis

Contusions are usually the result of direct trauma, such as a knee or helmet striking the lumbar area during football. Physical findings include focal low back pain and tenderness, sometimes confirmed by later bruising over the painful area. Back spasm is often an early accompaniment and may last for several days. Extensive bruising may indicate deeper injuries to a transverse process, the kidneys, or ureter. No neurologic abnormalities are identified, as the nerve roots are well protected by the thick lumbar paraspinous musculature.

A sprain refers to damage to a ligament, while a strain indicates an injury to a muscle, tendon, or musculotendinous junction.[16] The clinical findings in the two conditions are quite similar, and differentiation may be quite difficult and probably unnecessary. Sprains and strains are primarily due to improper body mechanics, conditioning, or stretching, and their onset is most commonly associated with weightlifting, or improper warm-up, or stretching. Symptoms typically develop suddenly following overload of the musculotendinous units during sprints or heavy weightlifting exercises. A chronic form can also occur following repeated overload during endurance training or highly repetitive activities. Clinical findings include back and paraspinous pain without radiculopathy that is accentuated by bending, twisting, or weight bearing. The pain may be located on one or both sides of the midline, and may extend into one or both hips secondary to spasm of the lumbodorsal fascia extending into the tensor fascia lata. Neurologic findings are absent, and if present should prompt a search for an intraspinal cause.

Evaluation

Radiographic studies are generally normal, other than straightening of the lumbar spine from spasm or the secondary osseous abnormalities from chronic athletic endeavors (accelerated degenerative changes in the end plates, facet joints, pars interarticularis, or disk spaces).

Treatment and Return to Play

For contusions, symptoms will usually resolve within a few days. The injury may initially respond to ice and cold packs to reduce pain and swelling. Later, heat, massage, and restricted activity is advised until the discomfort is largely resolved, at which time the athlete may return to play without restrictions.[4, 18]

With sprains or strains, treatment depends on the severity of the injury, as the healing phase is variable, sometimes prolonged up to 6 to 8 weeks. Initial treatment includes relative immobilization and ice to the affected area, with avoidance of extreme ranges of motion. In severe cases, bracing may provide some comfort. After the initial discomfort has improved, a rehabilitation process consisting of stretching, flexing, and strengthening of the lumbar axial and abdominal muscles is begun, with return to competition permitted once the injury has resolved. The exercises should be maintained so as to reduce the chances of a repeat injury.

Fractures

Major fractures threatening the stability or neural elements of the lumbar spine are quite uncommon in most athletics-related activity, with the exception of sports such as auto racing, skiing, and so forth, where very high speeds are reached or immobile objects are met at inopportune intersections. Most lumbar fractures in athletes are minor, as the bones are quite large and well supported by ligamentous and muscular structures. Several types of fractures can be identified, including those to the transverse or spinous processes, facets, vertebral bodies, and end plates.

Incidence, Clinical Features, and Differential Diagnosis

Transverse process fractures are usually the result of a direct blow to the back, and are generally accompanied by a severe muscular contusion. Spinous process fractures are exceedingly rare in the lumbar spine, as the force necessary to generate these types of injuries is not experienced in most types of athletic activity. Lumbar facet injuries are found in athletes performing repeated forceful hyperextension motions, such as football linemen, gymnasts, wrestlers, and golfers.[16] Mild compression fractures are not uncommon, particularly in individuals who have been training for many years with heavy weightlifting. The anterior portion of the vertebral body lacks horizontal trabeculations, and exercises such as squats or military presses can generate significant flexion-compression forces that lead to repetitive end plate fractures, collapse of the disk space, and ultimately to compression fractures of the vertebral bodies.[44] End plate fractures are more common in young, skeletally immature athletes. When the end plate fails, the nucleus pulposis may herniate into the fracture, producing a Schmorl's nodule.

Another vertebral body injury is Scheuermann's disease, an entity traditionally found in the thoracic spine of adolescents.[2, 26, 45, 46] Typical Scheuermann's disease results in progressive thoracic kyphosis due to anterior wedging (greater than 5 degrees) of three or more consecutive vertebral bodies. The thoracic form occurs most commonly from T7 to T10. Atypical Scheuermann's disease affects the thoracolumbar junction, most commonly L1, and is more strongly associated with athletes, implicating training and repetitive trauma as potential causative factors. In the atypical form, one or more thoracolumbar segments may be affected. The etiology is unknown, and theories include congenital disorders of endochondral ossi-

fication and repetitive axial flexion forces. Clinically, the athlete may present with a kyphotic posture that may or may not be associated with back pain. If back pain is prominent, it usually begins during the growth spurt, becomes maximal at the end of bone maturity, and resolves when growth is completed. Neurologic deficits are rare, but may become manifest with severe degrees of kyphosis.

Acute fractures produce acute back pain very similar to that associated with contusions or sprains. Paraspinous muscle spasm is common and is usually bilateral, may extend into the buttocks, and may be restimulated by movement or palpation of the affected region. The clinical findings of facet fractures are more unilateral, and include paralumbar tenderness, pain exacerbated by hyperextension, and ipsilateral hip and buttock pain referred to the groin, hip, and posterior thigh. The neurologic examination is usually normal, although uncommonly a

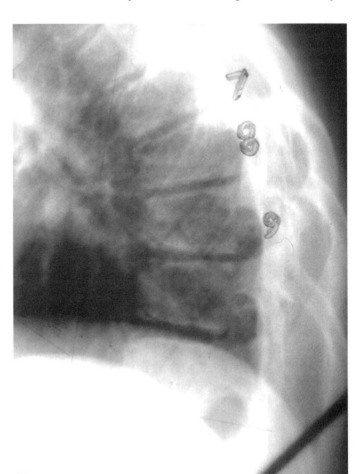

Figure 19–1. Scheuermann's disease. Thoracic spine radiograph (lateral view) showing lower thoracic kyphosis due to anterior wedging of multiple vertebral bodies. Note irregular upper and lower end plates and loss of disk height.

transverse process or facet fracture may contuse an adjacent exiting nerve root.

Evaluation

Diagnostic evaluation should include plain films and a computed tomographic (CT) scan, with the addition of a urinalysis and intravenous pyelogram (IVP) if a transverse process fracture is identified. A bone or single photon emission computed tomography (SPECT) scan may help to delineate acute from chronic osseous injuries.[1, 3] In Scheuermann's disease, radiographic findings include irregular upper and lower end plates, loss of disk space height, greater than 5 degrees of wedging in one or more vertebrae, and kyphosis of greater than 40 degrees (Fig. 19–1).

Treatment and Return to Play

With conservative care, most lumbar spine fractures have an excellent prognosis, with little or no residual back pain.[4, 18] Treatment is similar to that of severe sprains and strains. Movements and axial loading are restricted until the acute pain resolves, followed thereafter by progressively increasing activities and range of motion, until the athlete can return to former activity levels without significant pain. Radiographic follow-up is usually not necessary, as instability, unlike that of the cervical spine, is not likely to be progressive. A course of anti-inflammatory medications may reduce the general discomfort and inflammation during rehabilitation, and promote earlier return to play. Surgical intervention is rarely necessary unless other injuries are also present. For symptomatic Scheuermann's disease, treatment ranges from withdrawal from activity to bracing. Surgical correction of the kyphosis is rarely required, and generally is considered only in extreme cases for cosmetic reasons.

Pars Interarticularis Defects

The pars interarticularis represents the bone isthmus that separates the two facet joints of an individual vertebra. Microtrauma and shear forces placed on the posterior elements during repetitive hyperextension maneuvers can produce a fatigue failure or stress fracture of this area.[5, 6, 31, 32] Early in the clinical course, the region becomes stressed and may remodel, but the integrity of the pars is maintained. With time, however, the inflammatory condition converts to a frank dissolution of the pars (spondylolysis). Once the fracture is firmly established, spondylolisthesis, or slippage of the two adjacent vertebrae, may occur.

Incidence, Clinical Features, and Differential Diagnosis

Pars interarticularis defects are thought to occur only in humans, as a consequence of bipedal locomotion in an upright posture. Most evidence indicates that these are acquired defects, in that they are not identified at birth, and the radiographic manifestations do not appear for 5 to 7 years.[5] Once spondylolysis occurs, associated vertebral slippage (spondylolisthesis) may develop and progress until skeletal maturity, at which point it usually ceases. The period of most rapid slippage occurs between ages 9 to 15 years, and is rare after this time.[37]

The distribution of structural lesions of the spine in athletes younger than 18 years old is divided between pars defects (40%), end plate or growth plate fractures (40%), spondylolisthesis with instability (10%), and herniated disk (10%).[20] With age, the incidence of disk rupture goes progressively higher, while the incidence of pars defects lessens. The incidence of spondylolysis is approximately 6% in the normal population, but in certain athletic populations, the incidence reaches as high as 25% to 50% of participants.[19, 43] Athletes involved in repetitive hyperextension, such as weightlifters, interior linemen, or gymnasts, are particularly prone to this disorder.

Symptomatic pars defects characteristically cause back pain that occurs during performance or training maneuvers, particularly those that require hyperextension. The onset of symptoms may be acute, subacute, or chronic, and may be accompanied by progressive signs of decreased performance. Initially, the diagnosis is difficult to discern from a sprain, strain, or end plate fracture. Symptoms are usually unilateral, with pain in the paraspinous musculature near the midline that often extends into the ipsilateral hip or thigh. Symptoms can often be accentuated by standing the athlete on the affected leg, then leaning backwards toward the same side. This test, known as the one-legged hyperextension test, places the spine in a position that stresses the ipsilateral posterior elements.

Once the spondylolysis becomes established, spondylolisthesis may develop. The majority of adolescent athletes with Grade I spondylolisthesis are relatively asymptomatic.[16, 20, 25] Those with symptoms often complain of bilateral radicular pain. Hamstring spasm may also be noted as a postural reflex aimed at stabilizing the painfully displaced segment.

Evaluation

Early in the course, plain radiographs may be normal, but a bone or SPECT scan will show increased metabolic activity in the posterior elements in the region of the pars (Fig. 19–2).[1] At this stage, the defect is a stress fracture, and may heal with immobilization and rest. With time, however, the stress fracture will frequently progress to frank dissolution of the pars, at which time it will become evident on an oblique lumbar plain film or CT scan. When chronic, the bone or SPECT scans may no longer "light up" in the area of the fracture. A lateral plain film will then delineate the degree and progression of any subluxation related to the spondylolysis.

Treatment and Return to Play

For spondylolysis without spondylolisthesis, treatment is conservative.[4, 18, 34, 35] Initial treatment regimens should include rest and restricted activities, combined with anti-inflammatory drugs. If pain worsens or continues despite activity restriction, bracing should be considered, particularly in young individuals who have only stress fractures. Treatment should continue until symptoms resolve, ideally until the SPECT scan has returned to normal.

Treatment of spondylolisthesis is based upon the degree of slippage and the clinical symptoms. In asymptomatic patients with low-grade subluxation (less than 25%), the risk of increased displacement from intensive training is minimal, and continued activity is not contraindicated.[35] If symptoms develop, conservative measures are instituted and may include withdrawal from competition, restricted activities, and bracing. Athletes with subluxations greater than 50% are generally advised not to compete in sports with high potential for back injury. Surgery is rarely required, and only when

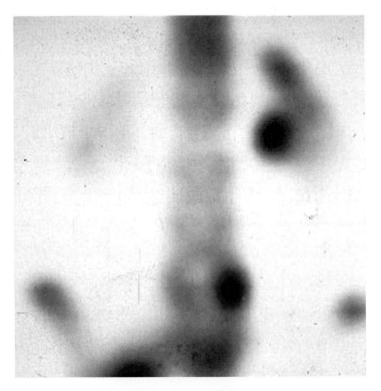

Figure 19–2. Stress fracture of pars interarticularis (spondylolysis). SPECT scan of a 21-year-old college sprinter with recent onset of lower back pain and paraspinous discomfort and tightness. Straight leg raise test and neurologic exam were normal. Symptoms were reproduced by hyperextension and rotation of lumbar spine. Note "hot spots" at L5 vertebra in the region of the pars interarticularis. Later plain spine films confirmed fractures bilaterally.

signs of progressive instability are obvious, and when conservative measures fail.

Disk and End Plate Injuries

Most young athletes do not experience clinically significant disk degeneration during their competitive years. The adolescent disk is substantially more viscous, malleable, and forgiving than the mature (and aging) specimen. In sports that are particularly stressful on the spine, such as gymnastics, wrestling, weightlifting, and football, however, radiographic evidence of disk injury is far more common and appears earlier than expected in similar age-matched general populations.[3, 17, 27, 46, 47] Intensive weight training and repetitive axial loading appear to significantly accelerate the degenerative process, and can lead to failure of even non-degenerated disks. Continued high-intensity training may cause repetitive injury to the disk and end plate, resulting in three types of problems, including disk rupture, spondylosis, and lumbar stenosis.

Incidence, Clinical Features, and Differential Diagnosis

Lumbar disk disease is very uncommon in young athletes and accounts for 10% or less of athletics-related chronic lumbar spine injuries before the age of 18 years.[15, 20, 21, 23, 24, 52] Younger athletes are quite susceptible to end plate fractures or transient syndromes where bony growth of the spine surpasses that of the adjacent ligaments and tendons (during the second or pubertal growth spurt). Such imbalances may cause

excessive tightness, postural alterations, or even spinal deformity. Athletics begun at young ages also place heavy stress on the developing disks, which may accelerate the degenerative process and lead to premature lumbar disc desiccation and collapse, osteoarthritis, and lumbar stenosis at ages considerably younger than that seen in the general population.[50]

By age 30, disk herniations and degeneration become more clinically relevant.[36, 47, 53] This age transition interval occurs in part because the disk becomes avascular by the mid-teens. Thereafter, the disk begins to lose its water content, and its viscoelastic and structural properties begin to degenerate, making it more susceptible to rupture. The differential diagnosis of back and leg pain of the athletes at risk, their predisposing activities, and the types of lumbar spine injury incurred are outlined in Table 19–1.

DISK HERNIATION

The onset of symptoms often begins during weight training or some sudden pivot, turn, or strain. In other situations, there is no preceding event, indicating that the final disk rupture followed the accumulation of multiple smaller injuries over an extended length of time. Older athletes tend to present with the classic findings of disk herniation, including back and unilateral leg/hip pain, with neurologic radicular findings on examination depending on the level of disk disruption.

Younger athletes usually present with subtle clinical findings, and complain of back pain and muscle spasm with little or no radicular components.[7, 8, 11, 14, 47, 51] Physi-

Table 19–1. Lumbar Region Athletic Injuries: Predisposing Activities

Athlete at Risk	Predisposing Activity	Type of Spinal Lesion
Football players	Poor technique Field trauma	Facet, transverse process fracture Vertebral compression fracture Disk degeneration, herniation End plate fracture, spondylosis Spondylolysis, spondylolisthesis
Weight lifters	Poor technique	Vertebral compression fracture Disk degeneration, herniation End plate fracture, spondylosis Spondylolysis, spondylolisthesis
Gymnasts, divers	Repetitive axial loading in hyperextension	Disk degeneration Intraosseous disk herniation Spondylolysis, spondylolisthesis
Runners, dancers	Repetitive axial compression	Disk degeneration, herniation

cal findings are minimal and may only consist of stiffness, mild scoliosis, or unilateral hamstring tightness. The straight leg raise test is often not strikingly positive. Motor deficits are difficult to elicit, given the great strength of these well-conditioned athletes. The reasons for the lack of distinctive clinical findings are unclear, but may reflect the younger age, increased flexibility, or increased pain threshold of the affected individuals. Pathologically, the younger athlete invariably has a protruded disk bulge contained within the annulus rather than a free-fragment herniation, which could lessen the amount of nerve root impingement.[7, 36]

SPONDYLOSIS

Spondylosis occurs as an end result of multilevel or repetitive disk or end plate injuries. Usually, individuals who develop this problem have been chronic heavy weight lifters or involved in activities with repetitive hyperextension or axial loading. Spondylosis often mimics an arthritic process, with many episodes of back discomfort but none particularly dramatic. The individual often "plays through" the pain, as it is not severe or associated with neurologic signs. Symptoms usually begin with an episode of lower back pain associated with unilateral or midline paraspinous pain and spasm that refers to one or both hips or thighs.

Evaluation

Plain films of the lumbar spine should include AP, lateral, and oblique views. The demonstration of one or more bony abnormalities is not uncommon, as their incidence, even in the presence of a clearly ruptured disk, is very high.[25] The diagnosis of spondylolysis must be considered, especially in young athletes, and bone or SPECT scans may be required in complex cases. Plain CT scanning is very helpful in further differentiating chronic bony conditions, and may also demonstrate a herniated lumbar disk. Bone windows can distinguish facet fractures not apparent on plain films that could compress a nerve root and closely mimic a ruptured disk clinically. MR scanning is very useful in defining disk herniation, with myelography and postmyelography CT scanning added in questionable cases (Fig. 19–3). Electromyography/nerve conduction velocity (EMG/NCV) testing can occasionally be helpful in confirming a suspected radiculopathy, but is superfluous in

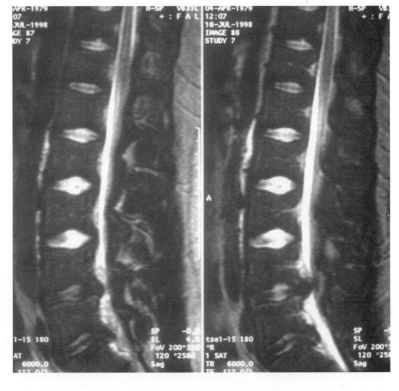

Figure 19–3. Herniated lumbar disk. An 18-year-old college football player (defensive back) with acute onset of unrelenting low back and radicular pain associated with weightlifting (squats). Examination revealed mildly positive straight leg raise test and mild unilateral weakness and numbness in L5 distribution. MRI scan (lateral view) reveals collapse and dessication of L4–L5 and L5–S1 disk spaces, associated with apparent disk herniations. Symptoms did not resolve with two months of complete activity restriction. Surgery (microdiskectomy) confirmed large disk herniation at both levels. The patient was able to resume his college career without restrictions.

most instances. We have not found the routine use of thermography or discography beneficial in clinical decision making in this population.

With spondylosis, plain radiographs demonstrate multiple asymmetrically collapsed disks or Schmorl's nodules, and an MRI scan shows accelerated degenerative changes and loss of water content of the disk spaces (Figs. 19–3 to 19–5). The affected disks appear to bulge, but do not substantially compromise the spinal canal and neural foramen.

Treatment and Return to Play

Initially, the primary mode of therapy should be conservative, as the acute episode

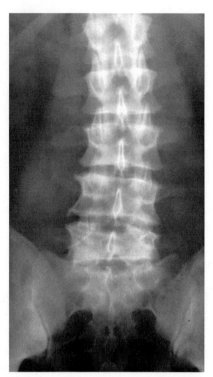

Figure 19–5. Accelerated lumbar spondylosis. Lumbar spine radiograph in a 35-year-old former college offensive lineman with many years of extensive heavy weight training. He had a prior history of intermittent lower back pain that resolved with rest and recent onset of increasingly frequent episodes, now associated with neurogenic claudication symptoms in both lower extremities. Note the multiple level disk collapse and compression of vertebral bodies.

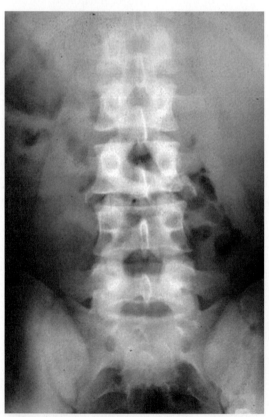

Figure 19–4. Focal spondylosis. Lumbar spine radiograph (AP view) of a 19-year-old college offensive lineman with repeated episodes of low back pain associated with weightlifting (squats), now associated with unilateral burning pain into the anterior thigh. Note large focal osteophyte at L3–L4 level, presumably representing old disk or end plate injury. Symptoms resolved with rest and elimination of squats and military presses from the patient's training regimen. He was able to complete his college career with no substantial recurrent problems other than occasional lumbar paraspinous "tightness."

will often resolve and allow the athlete to gradually return to full activity and participation in sport.[38, 40, 41] Since the risks of neurologic sequelae following such injuries are low, continued athletic participation, with appropriate alterations in training, can often be allowed. The goal of therapy should be to return the athlete to competition as soon as possible, while maintaining the highest regard for the athlete's safety.

DISK HERNIATION

Acute lumbar disk herniations presenting with severe back and radicular pain are treated with bed rest, analgesics, muscle relaxants, and nonsteroidal anti-inflammatory medications. Less dramatic presentations can be treated with restriction of exertional activity and heavy lifting in combination with mild analgesics and some time off from practice or competition. Once symptoms lessen, lumbar and abdominal stretching and strengthening exercises can begin, followed by gradual increases in weight training and other routine practice activities that do not place the spine in extremes of axial loading, flexion, and rotation. Continued emphasis on back strengthening and flexibility should become a routine part of the athlete's training from that time forward to reduce the chance of recurrence.

The chances of impairing the athlete's ability to compete successfully should be weighed against the time lost pursuing a likely unsuccessful conservative treatment regimen. The amateur athlete is usually urged to discontinue that particular sport indefinitely, and to try to find another type of competition that is less stressful physically. Surgery is generally reserved in this population for those conditions that remain symptomatic despite cessation of the offending activity. In the "top level" athlete, in whom years of training have been invested and potentially great financial or other rewards are active or anticipated, cessation of competition has much greater consequences, and cannot be so easily accepted. Indications for operative intervention are: (1) significant neurologic compromise (cauda equina syndrome, foot drop, or other major motor deficit); (2) severe, incapacitating back and radicular pain that does not respond to conservative therapy; and (3) chronically recurring symptoms that persist despite adequate conservative therapy.

Once a decision has been made to operate, the likelihood of the athlete returning to play is enhanced by selecting a procedure that will relieve the patient's symptoms with minimal disruption of bony, muscular, and ligamentous structures.[7, 28, 49] Since the early 1990s, surgical advances have greatly changed attitudes about the effects of intervention on an athlete's career.[30] In years past, surgery would only be considered as a last alternative, after many weeks, months, or even years of conservative therapy. With minimally invasive techniques, however, most athletes can return to their sport, often during the same season, with no significant loss of flexibility or strength.

The standard intervention is a microdiskectomy, during which the offending fragment is directly extracted.[7, 49] Using a small incision and a surgical microscope, the fragment can be removed rapidly and reliably, with minimal disruption of the lumbar paraspinous musculature. Variations

of this technique holding future promise include a microendoscopic or percutaneous diskectomy.[28, 29] Complete bilateral laminectomy and diskectomy should generally be discouraged except in large central disk herniations with cauda equina syndrome or a disk rupture in combination with significant spinal canal stenosis. Bilateral laminectomy typically requires a longer incision, more extensive muscle dissection, and may put the athlete at greater risk of postoperative instability or pain syndromes than a less disruptive procedure. Accompanying degenerative changes such as spondylosis or spondylolysis, if asymptomatic, should not be disturbed, as a more involved and prophylactic procedure, such as a lumbar fusion, stands a high likelihood of ending the career of most athletes.[7, 49]

Postoperative hospitalization is often not required, and the athlete feels better immediately, except for some incisional soreness. After several weeks of rest and restricted activity, a program is begun to reestablish flexibility and strength, after which the athlete is allowed to return to play.[4, 18] The exact timing of return should be based on a number of factors, but can be as early as 4 to 6 weeks after the initial surgical procedure. Future training would include maintenance of strong paraspinous muscular support and flexibility, so as to minimize the chance of recurrence.

SPONDYLOSIS

Initial treatment should include rest, restricted activities, physical therapy, and anti-inflammatory drugs during acute flare-ups. Usually spondylosis becomes a chronic disorder that is overcome by the determination of the athlete and his or her high endurance of discomfort. As there is no significant risk of neurologic injury, the athlete may return to play whenever symptoms resolve enough to allow comfortable participation.

Advanced cases may ultimately lead to the classic degenerative changes of lumbar stenosis: disk desiccation and collapse, osteophyte formation along the disk spaces, multiple level facet hypertrophy, and narrowing of the spinal canal. By that time, the athlete's career has invariably ended, so rehabilitation and return to play decisions are not issues. Surgery should be considered if symptoms suggestive of instability or of typical lumbar stenosis are refractory to conservative measures. An extensive procedure, combined with long-term postoperative activity restrictions, make return to the athletic field unlikely. Modern neurosurgery, however, now includes techniques that are minimally invasive, with little disruption of the lumbar paraspinous musculature following such procedures. Excellent results can be achieved with certain types of athletes, particularly golfers, in returning to play without major restrictions. Whether such procedures would stand up to the rigors of professional weightlifting or football, however, is unclear.

CONCLUSION

Lumbar spinal injuries in athletes are common. Many are related to training errors, while others are caused by the demands of a specific type of athletic activity. Management is often more complex than for nonathletes, as the athlete will invariably be returning to the exact type of activity that precipitated the injury. The primary treatment objective is protection and preservation of the nervous system for the remainder of the individual's life. Fortunately for most, this can now be accomplished, even if surgery is required, allowing the athlete to continue his or her career under most circumstances.

References

1. Bellah RD, Summerville DA, Treves ST, et al. Low-back pain in adolescent athletes: Detection of stress injury to the pars interarticularis with SPECT. Radiology 1991;180:509–512.
2. Blumenthal SL, Roach J, Herring JA. Lumbar Scheuermann's: A clinical series and classification. Spine 1986;12:929–932.
3. Cacayorin E, Hochhauser L, Petro GR. Lumbar and thoracic spine pain in the athlete: Radiographic evaluation. Clin Sports Med 1987;6:767–783.
4. Chilton MD, Nisenfeld FG. Nonoperative treatment of low back injury in athletes. Clin Sports Med 1993;12:547–555.
5. Ciullo JV, Jackson DW. Pars interarticularis stress reaction, spondylolysis, and spondylolisthesis in gymnasts. Clin Sports Med 1985;4:95–110.
6. Commandre FA, Taillan B, Gagnerie F, et al. Spondylolysis and spondylolisthesis in young athletes: 28 cases. J Sports Med Phys Fitness 1988;28:104–107.
7. Day AL, Friedman WA, Indelicato PA. Observations on the treatment of lumbar disc disease in college football players. Am J Sports Med 1987;15:72–75.
8. DeOrio JK, Bianco AJ. Lumbar disc excision in children and adolescents. J Bone Joint Surg Am 1982;64:991–996.
9. Deusinger RH. Biomechanical considerations for clinical application in athletes with low back pain. Clin Sports Med 1989;8:703–715.
10. Dreisinger TE, Nelson B. Management of back pain in athletes. Sports Med 1996;21:313–320.
11. Epstein JA, Epstein NE, Marc J, et al. Lumbar intervertebral disc herniation in teenage children. Spine 1984;9:427–432.
12. Ferguson RJ, McMaster JH, Stanitski CL. Low back pain in college football linemen. Am J Sports Med 1974;2:63.
13. Foster DN, Fulton MN. Back pain and the exercise prescription. Clin Sports Med 1991;10:197–209.
14. Ghabrial YAE, Tarrant MJ. Adolescent lumbar disc prolapse. Acta Orthop Scand 1989;60:174–176.
15. Goldstein J, Berger PE, Windler GE, Jackson DW. Spine injuries in gymnasts and swimmers. Am J Sports Med 1991;19:463–468.
16. Harvey J, Tanner S. Low back pain in young athletes: A practical approach. Sports Med 1991;12:394–406.
17. Hellstrom M, Jacobsson B, Sward L, Peterson L. Radiologic abnormalities of the thoracolumbar spine in athletes. Acta Radiol 1990;31:127–132.
18. Hopkins TJ, White AA. Rehabilitation of athletes following spine injury. Clin Sports Med 1993;12:603–619.
19. Jackson D, Forman W, Benson B. Patterns of injuries in college athletes: A retrospect of study of injuries sustained in intercollegiate athletics in two colleges in a two year period. Mt. Sinai J Med 1980;47:423–426.
20. Jackson DW, Wiltse LL, Cirincione RJ. Spondylolysis in the female gymnast. Clin Orthop. 1976;117:68–73.
21. Jackson D. Low back pain in young athletes. Evaluation of stress reaction and discogenic problems. Am J Sports Med 1979;7:364–366.
22. Keene JS, Albert MJ, Springer SL, et al. Back injuries in college athletes. J Spinal Disord 1989;2:190–195.
23. Keene JS: Low back pain in the athlete. From spondylogenic injury during recreation or competition. Postgrad Med 1983;74:209–217.
24. Klemp P, Learmonth ID. Hypermobility and injuries in a professional ballet company. Br J Sports Med 1984;18:143–148.
25. Kraus D, Shapiro D. The symptomatic lumbar spine in the athlete. Clin Sports Med 1989;8:59–69.
26. Lowe TG. Current concepts review: Scheuermann disease. J Bone Joint Surg Am 1990;72:940–945.
27. Maffuli N. Intensive training in young athletes. The orthopaedic surgeon's viewpoint. Sports Med 1990;9:229–243.
28. Maroon JC, Onik G, Day AL. Percutaneous automated discectomy in athletes. Phys Sports Med 1988;16:61–73.
29. Mayer HM, Brock M. Percutaneous endoscopic discectomy: Surgical technique and preliminary results compared to microsurgical discectomy. J Neurosurg 1993;78:216–225.
30. Mazur LJ, Yetman RJ, Risser WL. Weight-training injuries. Common injuries and preventative methods. Sports Med 1993;16:57–63.
31. Meeusen R, Borms J. Gymnastic injuries. Sports Med 1992;13:337–356.

32. Micheli LJ. Back injuries in gymnastics. Clin Sports Med 1985;4:85–93.
33. Micheli LJ. Back injuries in dancers. Clin Sports Med 1983;2:473–484.
34. Micheli LJ. Sports following spinal surgery in the young athlete. Clin Orthop 1989;198:152–157.
35. Micheli LJ, Wood R. Back pain in young athletes. Arch Pediatr Adolesc Med 1995;149:15–18.
36. Miller JA, Schmatz C, Schultz AB. Lumbar disc degeneration correlation with age, sex and spine level in 600 autopsy specimens. Spine 1988;13:173–178.
37. Muschik M, Hahnel H, Robinson PN, et al. Competitive sports and the progression of spondylolisthesis. J Pediatr Orthop 1996;16:364–369.
38. Ohnmeiss DD. Non-surgical treatment of sports-related spine injuries. In Hochschuler (ed): The Spine in Sports. Philadelphia, Hanley & Belfus, 1990, pp 241–260.
39. Rossi F, Dragoni S. Lumbar spondylolysis: Occurrence in competitive athletes. Updated achievements in a series of 390 cases. J Sports Med Phys Fitness 1990;30:450–452.
40. Saal JA. Rehabilitation of football players with lumbar spine injury. Phys Sports Med 1988;16:117–127.
41. Saal JA, Saal JS. Non-operative treatment of herniated lumbar intervertebral disc with radiculopathy: An outcome study. Spine 1989;14:431–437.
42. Semon RL, Spengler D. Significance of lumbar spondylolysis in college football players. Spine 1981;6:172–174.
43. Stinson JT. Spondylolysis and spondylolisthesis in the athlete. Clin Sports Med 1993;12:517–528.
44. Stinson JT. Spine problems in the athlete. Md Med J 1996;45:655–658.
45. Swärd L, Hellström M, Jacobsson B, Karlsson L. Vertebral ring apophysis injury in athletes. Is the etiology different in the thoracic and lumbar spine? Am J Sports Med 1993;21:841–845.
46. Swärd L. The thoracolumbar spine in young athletes. Current concepts on the effects of physical training. Sports Med 1992;13:357–364.
47. Swärd L, Hellström M, Jacobsson B, et al. Disc degeneration and associated abnormalities of the spine in elite gymnasts. A magnetic resonance imaging study. Spine 1991;16:437–443.
48. Tall RL, DeVault W. Spinal injury in sport: Epidemiologic considerations. Clin Sports Med 1993;12:441–448.
49. Wang JC, Shapiro MS, Hatch JD, et al. The outcome of lumbar discectomy in elite athletes. Spine 1999;24:570–573.
50. Watkins RG, Campbell DR. The older athlete after lumbar spine surgery. Clin Sports Med 1991;10:391–399.
51. Watkins RG, Dillin WH. Lumbar spine injury in the athlete. Clin Sports Med 1990;9:419–448.
52. Wroble R, Albright JP. Neck and low back injuries in wrestling. Clin Sports Med 1986;5:295–326.
53. Young JL, Press JM, Herring SA. The disc at risk in athletes: Perspectives on operative and non-operative care. Med Sci Sports Exerc 1997;29:S222–232.

20

Assessment and Rehabilitation of the Athlete With a Stinger

Stuart M. Weinstein and
Stanley A. Herring

Cervical and shoulder girdle nerve injuries do occur in athletics, accounting for approximately 5% of all peripheral nerve injuries.[8, 21] Whereas cervical radiculopathies typically are caused by acute overload of the cervical spine from contact or collision sports, shoulder girdle neuropathies more commonly develop from chronic repetitive exertion, such as in the throwing, or overhead, athlete. The nerves of the brachial plexus are particularly at risk owing to the extensive functional range of motion of the shoulder joint, tremendous forces across the shoulder complex, and tendency for muscular hypertrophy and inflexibility. The differential diagnosis of the dead-arm syndrome includes several sites of peripheral nerve injury, including cervical radiculopathy; thoracic outlet syndrome; suprascapular neuropathy; and axillary neuropathy.

These nerve injuries pose unique rehabilitation challenges to the sports medicine practitioner. First is the ability to diagnose the condition, especially if the primary presenting symptom is pain, not weakness or sensory disturbance. A knowledge of the sport and mechanism of injury, a high index of suspicion, and appropriate use of ancillary tests such as electrodiagnostics and imaging optimize the diagnostic process. Second, the extent of neurologic damage, when present, dictates when to initiate an aggressive strengthening program. Early progressive resistance exercises in the presence of axonal dysfunction could retard or reverse spontaneous neurologic recovery. Third, the functional postural dysfunctions that contributed to, and the maladaptations that resulted from, the development of the peripheral nerve injury must be identified and treated in order to prevent recurrences. Re-

habilitation of the upper quarter and the entire kinetic chain is often necessary to maximize performance. Finally, conservative treatment does not always equate with nonoperative rehabilitation. If surgical intervention is the appropriate treatment option (e.g., in the clinical setting of progressive weakness following nerve injury), early referral is key to minimizing permanent nerve dysfunction, secondary deconditioning, and time lost from competition.

This chapter will present a review of the athletically-induced peripheral nerve injury known as the "stinger," including a discussion of epidemiology, pathomechanics, assessment, rehabilitation, and return to play decisions. As will be demonstrated, the rehabilitation principles described for this particular injury can be applied to most cervical spine injuries.

EPIDEMIOLOGY

Disability or lost playing time can be substantial for athletes sustaining peripheral nerve injuries. The National Football League (NFL), via the National Football League Injury Surveillance System and Med Sports Systems (MSS, Iowa City, Iowa), has collected data for a spectrum of injuries, including nerve-related injuries, from 1980 through 1997, the most recent year for which data has been compiled. All NFL teams are required to submit injury data to the league from the start of summer training camp through the Super Bowl, based on a minimum reportable criterion of 2 days lost playing time from 1980 through 1994 and 1 day lost playing time beginning in 1995.

Many athletic organizations, including the

National Collegiate Athletic Association and the NFL, do not collect injury data for the specific diagnosis of stinger. When analyzing the NFL injury data for the 18-year period during which this information has been collected, it is evident that different diagnostic categories may have served as the catch basin for the stinger, including brachial plexus compression and stretch, cervical impingement (various levels), cervical disk bulge (various levels), cervical disk herniation (various levels), cervical disk rupture (various levels), cervical plexus compression and stretch, neck nerve contusion with motor and/or sensory loss, neck nerve disorder with motor and/or sensory loss, and neck neurotrauma. The more specific diagnostic categories probably parallel the availability of more advanced diagnostic tools, such as magnetic resonance imaging (MRI).

The vast majority of stingers are probably coded as brachial plexus compression or stretch injuries, and for purposes of this data review, this pathoanatomic diagnosis will be accepted. (Although this categorization is probably widely accepted as the one most closely representing the stinger, anatomic facts and pathomechanical principles, as described hereafter, contradict this classification, suggesting that stingers are primarily cervical nerve root injuries.) Using epidemiologic data from the player group classified as brachial plexus injured, it is apparent that substantial time loss does occur; yet, this probably underestimates the true incidence and disability. Table 20–1 demonstrates the four positions that incur the highest number of cases and total and mean lost playing days and missed games. These positions are linebacker, offensive lineman, defensive lineman, and defensive secondary. Among all the remaining diagnostic categories, cervical disk rupture showed the greatest number of cases, lost days, missed practices, and highest total games missed, as well as the highest mean games missed, higher even than brachial plexus injuries. The position breakdown is very similar to brachial plexus injuries. However, the specific neurologic injury, if any, associated with these cervical disk ruptures is not known, thus the difficulty in including these cases when determining disability statistics attributable solely to players with stingers.

Given that the occurrence of one subtype of the stinger is inversely proportional to the skill level and neck/shoulder area strength of the athlete (see below), one may conclude that the incidence of stingers in lower levels of competition (e.g., high school and college) is greater. However, no specific data exist to demonstrate this hypothesis.

PATHOMECHANICS

Stingers are also known as "burners," both terms descriptive of the upper limb sensory disturbance that the athlete experiences at the time of the injury. Stingers are peripheral nerve injuries, not spinal cord injuries, and are not directly related to the presence of central cervical spinal stenosis. However, burners are distinct from the burning hands syndrome,[13] which is a separate clinical entity, describing bilateral upper limb involvement, which is reflective of a cervical spinal cord injury.

Historically, both compressive and tensile (i.e., traction or stretch) overload have been implicated as the pathomechanics of the stinger, although precise localization of this injury—cervical spine versus brachial plexus—has been controversial. A variety of mechanisms have been described, including tensile injury to the upper trunk of the bra-

Table 20–1. Brachial Plexus Stretch and Compression Injuries in the National Football League, 1980–1997

Position	N (#cases)	Days Lost (Sum)	Days Lost (Mean)	Games Missed (Sum)	Games Missed (Mean)
Linebacker	98	1953	20	191	2
Offensive lineman	92	1974	21	173	2
Defensive lineman	73	1036	14	106	1
Secondary	39	938	24	93	2

Permission to use statistics authorized by the National Football League.

chial plexus,[1, 2, 5, 9, 10, 17, 26] tensile injury to the cervical nerve root–spinal nerve complex,[3, 5, 14, 19, 23] compressive injury to the cervical nerve root–spinal nerve complex,[16, 18, 23, 26] and compressive injury to the brachial plexus.[4, 12] The following neuroanatomic features of the cervical nerve root–spinal nerve complex provide compelling evidence that these peripheral nerves of the cervical spine are in fact at greater risk than the brachial plexus for injury.[20]

In general, neural tissue resistance to tensile load is proportional to the number of funiculi (i.e., one nerve bundle, the aggregate of which comprise the nerve trunk) and the amount of perineurial tissue, whereas the resistance to compressive load is proportional to the size of the nerve pathway (i.e., intervertebral neuroforamen) and the amount of epineurial tissue. In comparing the nerve root–spinal nerve complex to the brachial plexus, it is apparent that the former is more susceptible to both compressive and tensile load for the following reasons: The motor (i.e., anterior or ventral) and sensory (i.e., posterior or dorsal) nerve roots lack perineurial tissue, which develops as an extension of the dura around the spinal nerve; the spinal nerve exists as a single funiculus of a motor and sensory nerve root; the neuroforamen is narrowed with movement of the head and neck into the posterolateral quadrants; and epineurial tissue is lacking about the spinal nerve. Furthermore, the anterior nerve root is more vulnerable than the posterior nerve root to traction injury, as it lacks the dampening effect of the dorsal root ganglion; it has a thinner dural sheath; and it directly aligns with the spinal cord (Fig. 20–1). This may explain why motor impairment is more typical than sensory impairment in athletes who have residual neurologic deficits following a stinger. Weakness is the one consistent reported clinical finding in many of the studies previously cited.

Conversely, the brachial plexus resists tensile load owing to its plexiform nature, the presence of perineurial tissue, and multiple funiculi. It also resists compressive load owing to epineurial tissue, which is an extension of the loosely organized epidural sheath of the spinal nerve. Therefore, if the mechanism of the stinger is either traction or compression, it is most likely that the nerve root–spinal nerve complex is at

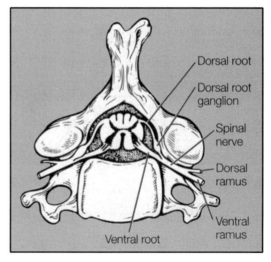

Figure 20–1. Cross-sectional representation of a typical cervical segment emphasizing the relationship of the ventral (motor) and dorsal (sensory) nerve roots to the spinal cord. The ventral nerve root is more vulnerable to traction injury because of its more linear orientation to the spinal cord, the lack of a dorsal root ganglion, and its thinner dural sheath (not depicted). From Vereschagin KS, Wiens JJ, Fanton GS, Dillingham MF. Burners: Don't overlook or underestimate them. Phys Sportsmed 1991;9:100, Figure 1. Permission granted by McGraw-Hill and Mary Albury-Noyes.

greater risk than the brachial plexus for sustaining injury.

ASSESSMENT

The clinical assessment of the stinger requires an understanding of the sport and of the skill level of the athlete. For example, a tensile overload mechanism of injury occurs when the head and shoulder of the symptomatic limb are forcefully moved in opposite directions, resulting in widening of the acromiomastoid distance (Fig. 20–2A). A compressive overload mechanism occurs when the head and neck are forced into the extreme of the ipsilateral posterolateral quadrant, narrowing the cervical intervertebral foramen and compressing the cervical nerve root–spinal nerve complex (Fig. 20–2B). In football, tackling and blocking are the most common activities that cause stingers, with the tacklers or blockers usually sustaining the injuries. In the tensile overload model, a relative lack of neck and shoulder girdle strength is probably as important as errors in tackling technique, which may explain the propensity of this particular mechanism to occur in the skele-

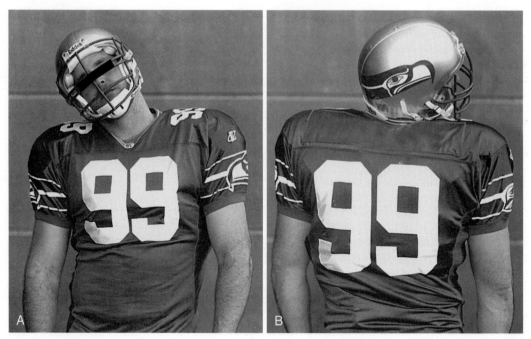

Figure 20–2. Pathomechanisms of the stinger. *A,* Traction injury: The head and neck are forcefully moved away from the symptomatic arm, widening the acromiomastoid distance. *B,* Compression injury: The head and neck are forcefully moved into the posterolateral quadrant toward the symptomatic arm, narrowing the intervertebral foramen.

tally immature athlete. With the compressive overload mechanism, breakdown in technique and the relatively greater force of the contact or collision are usually more important factors. Owing to the inherent mobility of the midcervical segments, the fifth, sixth, and seventh nerve root–spinal nerve complexes are most susceptible to injury.

The hallmark of the stinger is unilateral upper limb involvement following a traumatic event as described. The development of simultaneous bilateral cervical radiculopathy is very uncommon, and involvement of more than one limb should always prompt the consideration of a spinal cord injury. The athlete typically experiences lancinating, burning pain and dysesthesias, usually in a dermatomal pattern. If the player remains on the playing surface, the possibility of a spinal cord injury must be considered and ruled out before he is allowed to walk away from the site of injury. A detailed assessment on the sidelines should include determination of the mechanism of injury; distribution and duration of symptoms; evaluation of active cervical range of motion only within pain tolerance

to determine the presence of rigidity and for pain provocation (passive range of motion examination on the sidelines is contraindicated if the player is symptomatic, to avoid the development of complications from a potentially unstable spine); palpation for muscle spasm and localized bony tenderness; and a detailed neurologic examination emphasizing the motor deficits in the fifth, sixth, and seventh myotomes. Therefore, a "quick" neurologic assessment that measures only grip or finger strength as the basis for determining normal motor function is wholly inadequate, as these muscles are primarily supplied by the seventh and eighth cervical and first thoracic segments. At a minimum, testing of the rhomboid, spinatii, deltoid, biceps, triceps, and wrist flexors and extensors is mandatory (Table 20–2). Testing of the rhomboid is particularly useful in determining fifth cervical involvement, since it is the only shoulder girdle and upper extremity muscle that is innervated solely through a single nerve root. Identifying mild weakness in these athletes may require repetitive testing of any given muscle to fatigue, since a single manual muscle test may be unreliable given the relatively

Table 20–2. Innervation of Muscles Commonly Affected Following a Stinger

Muscle	Myotome	Peripheral
Rhomboid	C5	Dorsal scapular
Supraspinatus	C5, 6	Suprascapular
Infraspinatus	C5, 6	Suprascapular
Deltoid	C5, 6	Axillary
Biceps	C5, 6	Musculoskeletal
Wrist flexors	C6, 7	Median
Wrist extensors	C6, 7	Radial
Triceps	C7, 8	Radial

greater baseline level of strength of these athletes. The unaffected extremity should be used as a control.

For any given episode, the duration of the pain symptomatology following a stinger varies from seconds to hours, rarely persisting for days or longer. However, specific myotomal weakness without pain may continue for days or longer, demanding frequent, serial examination in the acute postinjury period; initially on the sidelines and subsequently in the health care provider's office or in the training room. If weakness persists for more than 2 weeks, or worsens over the first few postinjury days, ancillary testing is reasonable and appropriate to precisely determine the site of injury and the degree of axonopathy.[24]

Electrodiagnostics can be performed as early as 7 to 10 days following the onset of symptoms.[6] Electromyography (EMG) may be the most sensitive technique for evaluating axonal loss in the presence of continued clinical weakness. However, the milder the injury, the more difficult it may be to identify abnormalities. Typically, these injuries result in a relatively mild degree of axonal injury and a variable degree of neurapraxia (i.e., conduction block). The amount of membrane instability (i.e., positive sharp waves and fibrillation potentials) is proportional to axonal disruption. Motor unit recruitment abnormalities in the affected muscles will also develop after axonal injury, but may be the sole abnormal finding with a neurapraxic lesion. Although EMG should be able to differentiate a brachial plexus injury from cervical radiculopathy, particularly through examination of the paraspinal musculature, early reinnervation of the cervical paraspinals following nerve root trauma may preclude identifying these abnormalities. Thus, the timing of performing an electrodiagnostic study is critical; usually between 2 and 4 weeks is ideal. Electromyographic findings are also a determinant of return to play decisions (discussed later). To further assess muscle weakness following a stinger, nerve conduction techniques have also been used, such as stimulation over Erb's point, cervical nerve root stimulation, and long latency conduction (e.g., F waves), but the proximal location of these injuries presents technical challenges with these nerve conduction studies.

Imaging studies are valuable in the assessment of the stinger. Plain radiographs with dynamic flexion and extension views will provide information regarding neuroforaminal encroachment due to zygapophyseal (previously known as facet) or uncovertebral joint arthropathy; postural dysfunction, including loss of the cervical lordosis; and hypermobility (see hereafter). Advanced techniques such as MRI can more readily demonstrate neuroforaminal stenosis and disk abnormalities, including herniation and degenerative disk changes. A cervical MRI will almost always be obtained if an athlete experiences severe unrelenting pain, if the neurologic examination demonstrates profound weakness, or if there is a delayed recovery.

A 1997 study of athletes sustaining stingers demonstrated that 87% had MRI evidence for degenerative disk abnormalities, primarily at the C4–C5, C5–C6, and C6–C7 levels, whereas 93% had either disk abnormalities or foraminal narrowing.[11] Another group evaluated the relationship of the Torg ratio with the occurrence of stingers in collegiate football players, finding that the mean Torg ratio was significantly smaller for the athletes with stingers as compared with a control group.[15] They concluded that spinal stenosis increases the risk for having stingers with complicated clinical courses. Although the results of this study are intriguing, in that the use of plain radiographs was determined to be predictive of developing a specific event, two distinct problems arise. First, stingers are peripheral nerve injuries and are not directly related to the presence of central spinal stenosis, which is what the Torg ratio is purported to assess, unless one extrapolates this to include uncovertebral arthropathy, which may contribute to foraminal stenosis (Fig. 20–3). Second, the Torg ratio has been shown to have a very low positive predictive value for spinal

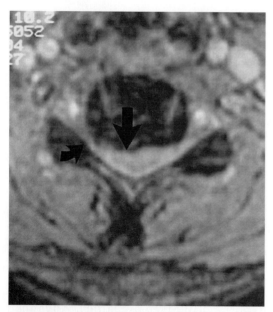

Figure 20–3. Cervical MRI in an athlete with a stinger. This T_2-weighted axial image through the cervical spine demonstrates degenerative processes contributing to both central (posterior vertebral body osteophyte [straight arrow]) and right-sided neuroforaminal stenosis (uncovertebral arthropathy [curved arrow]).

stenosis,[7] and further review of the article by Meyer and associates[15] revealed that there was not a significant difference between canal diameter on plain radiograph between the stinger group and the control group. Advanced imaging was not routinely performed in this study. Thus, one must conclude that the observation made by Meyer and associates[15] does not have a clear anatomic correlate.

REHABILITATION

Successful rehabilitation of any neuromuscular or musculoskeletal condition does not occur in a black box. Following an athletic injury, the decision to return an athlete to competition is highly dependent upon a well-designed treatment program. A conservative treatment plan, especially for a high-caliber or elite athlete, does not necessarily imply a wait-and-see approach; rather, the plan should be proactive and aggressive.

A comprehensive cervical spine rehabilitation program progresses over specific stages: protection of the injured structure, control of pain and inflammation, correction of flexibility and strength imbalances, cor-

rection of postural dysfunction, emphasis on sport-specific exercise, reversal of deconditioning effects, prevention of recurrent injury, and return to competition. Although this discussion will specifically relate to the stinger, the principles and practice of this rehabilitation plan can be applied to most cervical spinal injuries. For purposes of this chapter, emphasis is placed on postural correction and normalization of flexibility and strength imbalances.

Postinjury cervical radiographs frequently demonstrate either reduction or absence of the normal cervical lordosis. Whether this finding is a cause or effect of the injury (i.e., did the straightening of the lordosis predate the injury?), it is often followed by a prescription from the sports medicine practitioner to "correct" the lordosis prior to allowing the athlete to return to play. It is hypothesized that the absence of cervical lordosis contributes to a football-related spinal cord injury known as spear tackler's spine, and that persistent loss of the lordosis is one criterion that prevents an athlete from returning to competition.[22] Although the stinger is not a spinal cord injury, treatment of reduced or absent lordosis following a stinger is a key element in the rehabilitative process, since this represents a more generalized dysfunction characterized by the forward head postural attitude (Fig. 20–4A and B). This common abnormal posture, with a multifactorial cause that includes sedentary lifestyle; prolonged inactivity such as that following injury; strength and flexibility imbalances about the cervical and thoracic spine and shoulder girdle; and probably genetics, predisposes to the development of cervical nerve injury.

The following structural and myofascial abnormalities are typically found with the forward head posture: increase in the thoracic kyphosis; excessive scapular protraction and glenohumeral internal rotation; hyperflexion of the lower cervical and upper thoracic segments, with resultant hypomobility of the corresponding zygapophyseal joints; hyperextension of the upper cervical segments, with associated hypomobility of the zygapophyseal joints; relative segmental hypermobility (not necessarily gross instability) of the midcervical segments due to unloading of the zygapophyseal joints; and weakening of many muscle groups due to either shortening or lengthening with alteration of their normal length–tension rela-

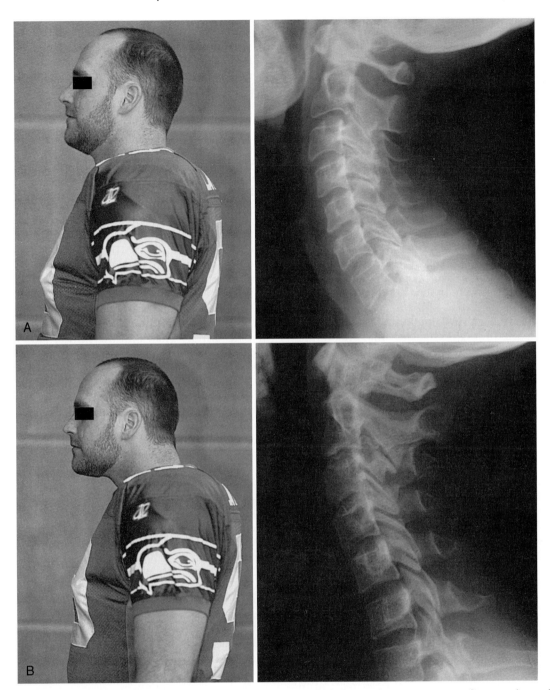

Figure 20–4. Clinical and radiographic demonstration of normal and abnormal posture. *A,* Normal posture (neutral head and neck position) with lateral cervical radiograph demonstrating relatively normal cervical lordosis. *B,* Forward head posture with lateral cervical radiograph demonstrating straightening or loss of the usual lordosis. It is important to recognize that the forward head posture does not result in an increase in cervical lordosis. Whereas cursory clinical examination may suggest cervical hyperlordosis, only the upper cervical segments are typically hyperextended.

tionship. Muscles that are shortened include the capital and cervical extensors, sternocleidomastoid, upper trapezius, levator scapula, pectoralis minor and major, anterior deltoid, subscapularis, serratus anterior, and the anterior scalene. Those lengthened include the capital and cervical flexors, middle and lower trapezius, rhomboids, thoracic extensors, and latissimus dorsi.

The midcervical hypermobility may promote early degenerative changes of these segments. Degenerative disk changes and uncovertebral joint arthropathy may contribute to fixed neuroforaminal narrowing. This would predispose an athlete who sustains either a dynamic compressive or tensile overload injury to the cervical spine, as discussed previously, to develop nerve root or spinal nerve pathology. As previously shown, a large proportion of athletes who experience a stinger have advanced imaging evidence for these degenerative changes.[11]

With this as a basis, the implementation of a rehabilitation program follows the principles outlined previously. Initially, pain control can be accomplished through a combination of relative rest, the use of a cervical collar to avoid cervical extension (therefore the smaller component is placed in front), maintenance of a chin tuck position, thermal and electrical modalities, and medication (including analgesics and anti-inflammatories). Traction may be used as an analgesic tool, with manual traction more easily tolerated because it places the athlete at ease, allows graded force application, and provides better control of neck position by maintaining slight cervical flexion to open the neuroforamina. In the presence of significant foraminal degenerative changes, manual or mechanical traction may be irritative if the spinal nerve is fixed owing to scarring or bony spurring. Although pain associated with the stinger tends to resolve relatively quickly, persistent or residual radicular pain that interferes with daily activities or with progression of the rehabilitation program may be managed by selective spinal injection, such as an epidural steroid injection, or selective nerve root sheath injection, performed with fluoroscopic guidance.[25] An advanced imaging study such as MRI would be required prior to instituting this treatment option to confirm the proper segmental level as well as to assess the pathoanatomy, which may alter the technical aspects of the injection.

Manual therapy techniques performed by qualified experts provide analgesic benefit as well as normalization of the previously mentioned segmental and myofascial dysfunctions in order to regain the cervical lordosis and normal spinal mechanics as much as possible. Mobilization and manipulation (the highest grade of mobilization) may improve zygapophyseal joint mobility and glide, but must be precisely directed to hypomobile segments only. Forceful manipulation in the presence of significant neuroforaminal compromise could potentially be aggravating or damaging. Myofascial stretching techniques such as myofascial release and massage should be used to lengthen the shortened and weakened musculature. Improved soft-tissue extensibility will also improve segmental motion at the hypomobile levels; however, release of the tight paraspinal musculature may uncover hypermobilities that had been splinted or protected in the midcervical spine. Thus, the next step in the rehabilitative process is the initiation of a postural stabilization exercise program.

Cervicothoracic stabilization training is sequenced through isometric, isotonic, and multiplanar strengthening techniques. Isometrics begin with a neutral position with the head supported in order to avoid cervical nerve irritation. Positions are varied relative to gravity (i.e., supine, prone, side-lying), and gradually the starting position of the head is progressed out of neutral. Isotonic exercise initially emphasizes concentric strengthening of the lengthened musculature. Head and neck positions that may compromise the cervical nerves, such as the extreme of the posterolateral quadrants and excessive flexion, are avoided. Positions are again varied against gravity. At this point, strengthening of the shoulder girdle (i.e., scapular stabilizer) and thoracic extensor musculature is begun and is eventually coupled to upper limb strengthening. Cocontraction of the axial musculature while simultaneously performing upper extremity strengthening maximally recruits these spinal stabilizers. Balanced strengthening of the anterior and posterior shoulder girdle musculature is critical in preventing the rounding of the shoulders. Because the shoulder girdle and proximal upper limb musculature are usually most involved following a stinger, caution must be used when initiating a strengthening program that includes these weak muscles if a significant axonal injury has occurred. The results of EMG testing are very helpful in determining how early and how aggressively these strengthening exercises can be initiated. The final phase of rehabilitation involves functional tasks to specifically match the complex movement patterns of the individual athlete's sport and position within that sport. Multiplanar patterned movements are emphasized, initially without and then with progressive resistance, to promote strength, balance, and endurance. Finally, training in sport- and position-specific skills (e.g., blocking and tackling) completes the rehabilitation process.

RETURN TO PLAY GUIDELINES

Return to play decisions should be based on clinical, electrodiagnostic, and imaging findings with additional consideration given to whether the injury is a first-time or recurrent problem (Table 20–3). In any case, there must be full recovery of strength in the affected muscle(s). Furthermore, the player must have completed a comprehensive rehabilitation program as described. Following this program, the athlete should exhibit balanced flexibility and strength through the cervicothoracic spine and shoulder girdle. However, complete correction of the cervi-

---

Table 20–3. Summary of Guidelines for Return to Competition Following a Stinger

Clinical

Asymptomatic
Full recovery of strength in affected muscles
Full pain-free cervical range of motion

Rehabilitation

Correction of postural faults, including soft tissue and joint imbalances
Completion of cervicothoracic stabilization program
Sports-specific retraining

Electrodiagnostics

No acute axonopathy in shoulder girdle or extremity muscles

Imaging

Absence of a substantial nerve root compressive lesion, including a disk herniation or foraminal stenosis

Timing of Return to Competition

Following 1st Stinger

If full clinical recovery within 15 minutes, return to same game.
If full clinical recovery within 48–72 hours, return in 1 week.

Following a Recurrent Stinger in Same Season

(Assumes higher likelihood of residual weakness)
Hold from practice and competition for the number of weeks that corresponds to the number of that stinger.
After 3 or more stingers, consider ending season, especially if associated with acute EMG findings and imaging evidence for a neurocompressive lesion.

---

cal lordosis may not be achievable and should not be considered an absolute contraindication to return to play following a stinger. For this reason, repeat cervical radiographs are not routinely obtained.

Electrodiagnostics plays a key role in determining return to play. Fibrillation potentials, either of at least a moderate degree or of a mild degree but with clinical weakness, justify withholding the athlete from competition. Mild or scattered positive waves should not serve as the sole criterion to prevent return to play because these may develop following local muscle trauma, but moderate positive waves in the face of weakness in the same muscles should raise concern. Sequential studies are mandatory if weakness persists. If repeat study in a player previously held from competition demonstrates no spontaneous potentials or only scattered positive waves, and motor unit recruitment reveals polyphasic potentials without significant increase in the firing rate, which is suggestive of reinnervation, then return to play should be allowed. Reestablishment of a normal EMG is not a criterion for return to play as long as the residual findings suggest reinnervation. No further studies are necessary unless reinjury occurs. Repeat EMG is then mandatory to observe for any new findings.

Although advanced imaging is not always necessary, an acute disk herniation should be ruled out prior to return to play if significant and persistent pain and weakness have occurred. Finally, equipment may be modified, including the attachment of collars to the shoulder pads to prevent excessive excursion of the head and neck into the posterolateral quadrants, to complete the criteria for return to play.

The timing of returning an athlete to competition following a stinger should also be based on the number of previous stingers, if any, that the athlete has experienced in that season. The basis for this reasoning is that prolonged and more significant motor impairments are more likely to occur with recurrent episodes. Following a first time stinger, if full clinical recovery happens within 15 minutes, return to that same game or competition is allowed. If full clinical recovery occurs within the first 48 to 72 hours, then return in 1 week is allowed; otherwise, the resumption of practice and play is delayed until further assessment is completed as described previously. For recurrent stingers in the same season, the guideline is to withhold an athlete from competition for at least the number of weeks that corresponds to the number of that stinger (e.g., 2 weeks for the second stinger). If an athlete sustains more than three stingers in a season, then consideration should be given to ending that season, particularly if there is persistent muscle weakness, persistent acute EMG abnormalities, and if advanced imaging reveals a cervical disk herniation or significant foraminal stenosis. These guidelines, however, do not necessarily apply to all possible scenarios. As with any other athletic injury, other medical and nonmedical factors may play a role in determining when an athlete can and should return to competition following a stinger.

References

1. Archambault JL. Brachial plexus stretch injury. J Am Coll Health 1983;31:256–260.
2. Clancy WG, Brand RL, Bergfled JA. Upper trunk brachial plexus injuries in contact sports. Am J Sports Med 1977;5:209–215.
3. Chrisman OD, Snook CA, Stanitis JM, et al. Lateral flexion neck injuries in athletic competition. JAMA 1965;192:613–615.
4. DiBennedetto M, Markey K. Electrodiagnostic localization of traumatic upper trunk brachial plexopathy. Arch Phys Med Rehabil 1984;65:15–17.
5. Funk FJ, Wells RE. Injuries of the cervical spine in football. Clin Orthop 1975;109:50–58.
6. Herring SA, Weinstein SM. Electrodiagnosis in sports medicine. Phys Med Rehabil: State of the Art Reviews. 1989;3:809–822.
7. Herzog RJ, Wiens JJ, Dillingham MF, et al. Normal cervical spine morphometry and cervical spinal stenosis in asymptomatic professional football players. Plain radiography, multiplanar computed tomography, and magnetic resonance imaging. Spine 1991;16:S178–S186.
8. Hirasawa Y, Sakakida K. Sports and peripheral nerve injury. Am J Sports Med 1983;11:420–426.
9. Hunter C. Injuries to the brachial plexus: Experience of a private sports medicine clinic. J Am Osteopath Assoc 1982;91:757–760.
10. Jackson DW, Lohr FT. Cervical spine injuries. Clin Sports Med 1986;5:373–386.
11. Levitz CL, Reilly PJ, Torg JS. The pathomechanics of chronic, recurrent cervical nerve root neurapraxia. The chronic burner syndrome. Am J Sports Med 1997;25:73–76.
12. Markey KL, DiBennedetto M, Curl WW. Upper trunk brachial plexopathy. The stinger syndrome. Am J Sports Med 1993;21:650–655.
13. Maroon JC. "Burning hands" in football spinal cord injuries. JAMA 1977;238:2049–2051.
14. Marshall TM. Nerve pinch injuries in football. J Ky Med Assoc 1970(Oct):648–649.
15. Meyer SA, Schulte KR, Callaghan JJ, et al. Cervical spinal stenosis and stingers in collegiate football players. Am J Sports Med 1994;22:158–166.
16. Poindexter DP, Johnson EW. Football shoulder and neck injury: A study of the "stinger." Arch Phys Med Rehabil 1984;65:601–602.
17. Robertson WC, Eichman PL, Clancy WG. Upper trunk brachial plexopathy in football players. JAMA 1979;241:1480–1482.
18. Rockett FX. Observations on the "burner." Traumatic cervical radiculopathy. Clin Orthop 1982;164:18–19.
19. Speer KP, Bassett FJ, III. The prolonged burner syndrome. Am J Sports Med 1990;18:591–594.
20. Sunderland S. The Brachial Plexus Normal Anatomy. In Nerves and Nerve Injuries, 2nd ed. New York, Churchill Livingstone, 1978, p 856.
21. Takazawa H, Sudo N. Statistical observation of nerve injuries in athletes. Brain Nerve Inj 1971;3:11–17.
22. Torg JS, Sennet B, Pavlov H, et al. Spear tackler's spine: An entity precluding participation in tackle football and collision activities that expose the cervical spine to axial energy inputs. Am J Sports Med 1993;21:640–649.
23. Watkins RG. Nerve injuries in football players. Clin Sports Med 1986;5:215–246.
24. Wilbourn A, Bergfeld J. Value of EMG examination with sports related nerve injury. EEG Clin Neurophys 1983;55:42P–54P.
25. Woodward JL, Weinstein SM. Epidural injections for the diagnosis and management of axial and radicular pain syndromes. Phys Med Rehabil Clin North Am 1995;6:691–714.
26. Wroble RR, Albright JP. Neck and low back injuries in wrestling. Clin Sports Med 1986;5:295–325.

OTHER NEUROLOGIC DISORDERS IN THE ATHLETE

CHAPTER
21

Convulsions in Contact and Collision Sports

Paul McCrory

Convulsive episodes are rare but dramatic events in sports. Traditionally these episodes have been assumed to represent a form of posttraumatic epilepsy; however, recent studies have demonstrated that most, if not all, convulsive episodes seen acutely in a sporting situation are nonepileptic in nature.[1] Although true posttraumatic epilepsy may certainly be seen following severe or penetrating head injury, these forms of head injury are virtually unknown in most collision sports.

CLASSIFICATION

At the present time, there is no classification system that encompasses all the potential causes of posttraumatic convulsions. Because of the widely held view that all convulsive episodes were epileptic, the separation of seizures caused by alternative pathophysiologic mechanisms has not been attempted. From a conceptual standpoint, it may be appropriate to consider posttraumatic convulsions as set out in Table 21–1.

Is it Epilepsy?

When a patient presents with an event that is thought to be a possible epileptic seizure, the history from the patient and eyewitnesses, in addition to a knowledge of the circumstances surrounding the episode, are the crucial factors in establishing a correct diagnosis. Nonepileptic seizures represent the most common problem in the differential diagnosis of these events. A detailed firsthand account of what actually happened during the episode is essential. If videotape is available, the tape may provide invaluable objective data in the assessment of such events.[1, 2]

Differential Diagnosis

The differential diagnosis of convulsive episodes is extensive and well documented in the various comprehensive textbooks on epilepsy.[3, 4] With regard to sports, there are many potential causes of nonepileptic convulsive events that deserve particular discussion, in addition to the entity of posttraumatic epilepsy. These are listed in Table 21–2.

For the team physician involved in collision sports, the tonic posturing and concussive convulsions seen after a concussive brain injury would represent the most common differential diagnosis (Fig. 21–1). Apart from the causes mentioned, consideration should also be given to whether the seizure represents an isolated epileptic seizure.

Table 21–1. Conceptual Approach to Convulsive Episodes in Sport

Classification	Timing of Convulsive Event	Usual Seizure Phenomenology	Likely Etiology
Immediate	Seconds to hours postinjury	Generalized/myoclonic	Non-epileptic
Early	Hours to 7 days postinjury	Focal	Epileptic
Late	> 7 days postinjury	Generalized	Epileptic

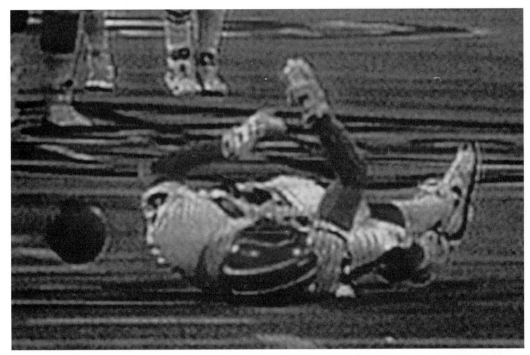

Figure 21–1. American professional football player who suffered a helmet to helmet contact while receiving the ball during a play. Duration of unconsciousness was approximately 60 seconds. As he fell to the ground, a 30-second period of tonic posturing occurred with versive head movement to the right, a "bear hug" posture of his upper limbs, and extension/adduction of his lower limbs.

Specific Syndromes

CONCUSSIVE CONVULSIONS

Concussive convulsions are an infrequent but dramatic accompaniment of concussive brain injury in sports. These convulsive events, although described anecdotally for over a century,[5] have only recently been studied in detail.[1] Concussive convulsions are a distinct entity, which represents a non-epileptic posttraumatic convulsive phenom-

Table 21-2. Differential Diagnosis of Convulsive Events in Sport

Specific Syndromes

Concussive convulsions
Posttraumatic epilepsy
Tonic concussive posturing
Idiopathic epilepsy

Less Common Causes

Syncope
Cardiac rhythm disturbances
Movement disorders
Metabolic disturbance
Illicit drug use/alcohol
Pseudoseizures

enon, somewhat akin to convulsive syncope that has a universally good outcome.

Concussive convulsions are defined as a convulsive episode that begins within 2 seconds of impact associated with concussive brain injury. Following impact, there is typically a phase of brief tonic stiffening followed by myoclonic jerking. The motor phenomena are usually bilateral, but often asymmetric. The convulsive movements may be transient, but can last up to 3 minutes in some cases. There may be some retained awareness of the convulsive movements by some athletes. Following termination of the convulsion, the neurologic and neuropsychologic signs are indistinguishable from typical cases of concussion.[6–9] These episodes are not associated with structural or permanent brain injury and are a nonepileptic phenomenon.

The precise incidence of concussive convulsions has been determined only for Australian football (Fig. 21–2). The total injury incidence rate in that sport is 131 injuries per 1000 player hours, with the concussive incidence rate in elite sporting competition being 4.0 concussions per 1000 player hours.[10] The rate of concussive convulsions

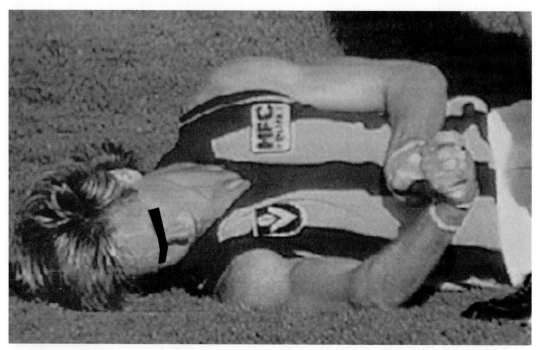

Figure 21–2. Australian professional footballer demonstrating tonic posturing of upper limbs following a concussive injury. Duration of unconsciousness in this case was approximately 3 minutes.

is approximately .06 per 1000 player hours, which gives a crude rate of 1 convulsive episode in every 70 cases of concussion. Although anecdotally reported in other sports, such as American football, Association football (soccer), Rugby union, Rugby league, and horseracing, the overall incidence rate of concussive convulsions is unknown for other sports.[1, 11]

It has been hypothesized that the concussive impact itself creates a transient functional decerebration akin to the corticomedullary dissociation described in convulsive syncope. Early animal research on experimental brain concussion demonstrated immediate and profound disruption of brain stem function associated with vagally mediated vasomotor instability. In some cases, the blows were associated with flexor spasms; however, the animals were anesthetized, which made interpretation of these movements necessarily limited.[12, 13] Thus in concussive convulsions, it is likely that the blow itself initiates transient decerebration, resulting in convulsive movements.

The outcome for athletes with concussive convulsions is universally good. All players returned to professional sport participation within 2 weeks of the episode without aftereffects. In the Australian football study, analysis of match statistics before and after injury did not demonstrate any significant change, further demonstrating that there was no change in functional performance owing to the injury.[1]

POSTTRAUMATIC EPILEPSY

Seizures are common after severe head injury and have been particularly extensively investigated in both military and civilian populations.[14–18] In a community study of epilepsy prevalence, head injuries accounted for 2% of the total cases of epilepsy.[19]

Large epidemiologic studies of posttraumatic epilepsy describe early (within 1 week) and late (after 1 week) convulsions following traumatic brain injury.[14, 15] Other studies have further subdivided the early posttraumatic epilepsy seizures into those occurring within 24 hours of injury and those occurring between 1 and 7 days after injury.[20, 21] Early seizures are more common than late seizures and occur in 2% to 5% of unselected cases admitted to a hospital following head injury.[14, 15, 21, 22]

Early Posttraumatic Epilepsy. As previously mentioned, early seizures refer to

Table 21–3. Head Injury and Early Posttraumatic Epilepsy in Adults

Head Injury Severity	Early Posttraumatic Epilepsy Risk
Mild (No skull fracture/< 30 min PTA)	0.4%
Moderate (Skull fracture or PTA 30 min–24 hr)	2.4%
Severe (ICH, cerebral contusion or PTA > 24 hr)	10.3%

PTA, posttraumatic amnesia; ICH, intracranial hematoma.

Adapted from Annegers J, Hauser W, Coan S, Rocca W. A population based study of seizures after traumatic brain injuries. N Engl J Med 1998;338:20–24.

those events occurring less than 7 days post-injury. Their occurrence is not uniform in that period, however. Approximately one third occur in the first hour, one third between 1 and 24 hours, and one third between 1 and 7 days postinjury. The risk depends on the severity of head trauma. See Table 21–3. The risk factors for early post-traumatic epilepsy reflect increasing severity of brain injury as manifest by prolonged unconsciousness, skull fracture, intracerebral hematomas, hemorrhagic cerebral contusion, and focal neurologic signs. In addition, children have almost three times the risk of early posttraumatic epilepsy as adults for the same severity of brain injury. The predominant clinical seizure type is a focal seizure that may become secondarily generalized. Focal seizures account for 60% to 80% of cases.

Late Posttraumatic Epilepsy. Late post-traumatic epilepsy refers to the development of seizures after 7 days posttrauma.

While some studies of military brain trauma report a decreasing incidence of seizure risk over time, studies in civilian populations suggest that the risk increases at least for the 5 years following the trauma.[21, 22] It is important to note that mild head injury, the predominant form of injury occurring in sports, does not confer any increased risk of late posttraumatic epilepsy. See Table 21–4. The risk factors for late posttraumatic epilepsy include penetrating skull trauma, early posttraumatic epilepsy, intracerebral hematoma, subdural hematoma, Glasgow Coma Scale less than 10, depressed skull fracture, cortical contusion, epidural hematoma, and linear skull fracture.[23] Approximately 50% of late posttraumatic epilepsy victims experienced an early posttraumatic seizure. Unlike early posttraumatic epilepsy, late seizures are typically generalized seizures, which occur in 60% to 70% of cases. Interestingly, the natural history of this condition suggests that 25% to 33% of cases will remit over time.[15, 24]

TONIC CONCUSSIVE POSTURING

In an ongoing research project involving a prospective videometric analysis of 107 cases of acute concussion involving professional Australian football, it was found that approximately 30% of cases demonstrated transient tonic posturing.[25] None of these patients went on to develop a concussive convulsion. The tonic posturing phenomenologically resembled the tonic phase of generalized seizure; see Figures 21–1 and 21–2. Risk factors for these events included loss of consciousness lasting more than 1 minute. The presence of the tonic episodes did not alter the neuropsychologic findings

Table 21–4. Head Injury Late Posttraumatic Epilepsy in Adults

Head Injury Severity	Late Posttraumatic Epilepsy Risk at 1 Year	Late Posttraumatic Epilepsy Risk at 5 Years
Mild (No skull fracture/ < 30 min PTA)	0.1%*	0.6%*
Moderate (Skull fracture or PTA 30 min–24 hr)	0.7%	1.6%
Severe (ICH, cerebral contusion or PTA > 24 hr)	7%	11%

*Not significantly different from general population risk. PTA, posttraumatic amnesia; ICH, intracranial hematoma.

Adapted from Annegers JF, Hauser W, Coon S, Rocca W. A population based study of seizures after traumatic brain injuries. N Engl J Med 1998;338:20–24; Annegers JF, Grabow JD, Kurland LT, Laus ER. The incidence, causes and secular trends of head trauma in Olmstead county, Minnesota, 1935–1974. Neurology 1980;30:912–919.

or clinical signs of the concussive injury when compared with case-matched controls with concussion. The pathophysiologic mechanism of these events is unclear, but speculated to involve brain stem reflex mechanisms stimulated by facial afferent connections. There are also a number of similarities between tonic concussive posturing and the "cerebellar fits" described by John Hughlings Jackson as long ago as the 1860s.[26, 27]

IDIOPATHIC EPILEPSY

The possibility that a seizure episode represents epilepsy unrelated to brain trauma should always be considered. The seizure may represent an episode in a recurring epileptic syndrome or the first presentation of epilepsy. One of the peaks of maximal incidence of epilepsy is in the late teens and early twenties, the time when many men and women are actively involved in athletic pursuits. Given that the prevalence of epilepsy in community populations is approximately 2%, the clinician can expect to encounter athletes with epilepsy. There are many examples of elite professional athletes who have epilepsy, including Tony Lazzeri and Hal Lanier of Major League Baseball, Bobby Jones of the National Basketball Association, Gary Horvath of the National Football League (U.S.) and Tony Greig, former English cricket captain.[28]

Evidence from controlled studies suggests that exercise does not increase either seizure frequency or antiepileptic drug levels or induce epileptiform electroencephalographic (EEG) changes.[29, 30] Furthermore, there is no evidence that epileptics are more prone to seizures after head injury or that epileptics are more prone to injury than other athletes.[31, 32] It would seem, therefore, that epileptic patients may be involved in collision sports without specific restriction or particular risk. Good judgment and common sense should always prevail in individual cases.[33]

Other Less Common Causes of Convulsions in Sport

Syncope. Patients who faint often have convulsive movements of the extremities, and this feature is often under recognized, even by experienced physicians. In fact, the whole spectrum of convulsive manifestations, from myoclonus to generalized seizures, has been reported. Incontinence and tongue biting have been noted as well.[34] These events tend to commence within 10 seconds of the onset of cerebral hypoperfusion and are thought to be caused by a brain stem reflex phenomenon. EEG recording during these episodes has conclusively demonstrated their nonepileptic nature.[35] They require no specific treatment apart from correct diagnosis and patient reassurance.

Cardiac Rhythm Disturbances. The development of an anoxic convulsion may occur when a primary cardiac rhythm disturbance compromises cardiac output and reduces cerebral perfusion. Cardiac disease represents one of the common mechanisms of deaths in sport, and a transient arrhythmia may be due to a large number of causes. The recent deaths in professional basketball in the United States have highlighted this problem. In sports where the so-called "athlete's heart syndrome" is a concern, team physicians need to investigate and manage these athletes correctly.[36]

Movement Disorders. Of a number of episodic involuntary movement disorders, paroxysmal kinesthogenic choreoathetosis is the best known.[37] These episodes are precipitated by movement or exercise, and each episode lasts for seconds to minutes; the episodes often occur in clusters. The movements are mostly choreic with normal consciousness; however, inexperienced observers may describe the observed movements as epileptiform. Presentation is usually in adolescence. Paroxysmal kinesthogenic dystonia is less common, but the attacks of exercise-induced dystonia sometimes last for many hours. It is extremely rare for true epilepsy to be precipitated by movement.

Metabolic Disturbances. Convulsive activity, dystonia, and syncope occur secondary to metabolic disturbances in a number of reported cases. These include hypoglycemia, hyponatremia, hypocalcemia, and hypomagnesemia, all conditions recognized in specific sports, particularly endurance running and ultra marathons.[38] In such cases symptoms usually develop gradually and persist for hours. The exception to this is hypocalcemia, where acute tetany superficially resembling tonic posturing may be precipitated by exercise.[4, 39]

Illicit Drug Use and Alcohol. Increasingly,

attention of team physicians has been drawn to the complications of illicit drug use and alcohol abuse. These complications include seizure episodes as well as cardiovascular collapse. In addition, an athlete under the influence of such agents may be at greater risk of injury, especially head injury, in collision and contact sports. A team physician suspicious of such a cause for the athlete's convulsive episode may consider performing a drug screen to assist with diagnosis.[40]

Pseudoseizures. Pseudoseizure, or nonepileptic attack disorder, is a disorder characterized by prominent nonepileptic convulsive motor phenomena. This disorder is associated with abnormal illness behavior as well as frank psychiatric illness. The diagnosis may be evident on history; however, video-EEG monitoring may be required in difficult cases.[2] Although more commonly seen in hospital epilepsy practice, nevertheless the disorder may appear in athletes.

MANAGEMENT ISSUES

The practical management of convulsions in sports can be divided into broad areas where the issues and treatment priorities differ considerably. In the acute on-field situation, first aid is the main issue, whereas at an emergency facility, accurate diagnosis and exclusion of intracranial pathology are the main priorities.

IMMEDIATE MANAGEMENT

For the clinician in attendance at a sporting event who is called upon to manage an acute injury, the major priorities at this early stage are the basic principles of first aid. The simple mnemonic DR ABC may be a useful memory aid.

D Danger Ensure that there are no immediate environmental dangers that may potentially injure the patient or treatment team. This may involve stopping play in a football match or marshalling cars on a motor race track.

R Response Is the patient conscious? Can he or she talk?

A Airway Ensure a clear and unobstructed airway. Remove any mouthguard or dental device that may be present.

B Breathing Ensure that the patient is breathing adequately.

C Circulation Ensure an adequate circulation.

Once these basic aspects of care have been achieved and the patient has been stabilized, consideration of removal of the patient from the field to an appropriate facility is necessary. At this time, careful assessment for the presence of a cervical spine or other injury is necessary. If the patient is unconscious, a cervical injury should be assumed until proven otherwise. Airway protection takes precedence over any potential spinal injury. In this situation, the removal of helmets or other head protectors should be performed only by individuals trained in this aspect of trauma management.[41]

When no physician is in attendance at the sporting event, the patient should be managed with the same first aid principles and then referred to a medical facility for assessment as soon as possible. It is recommended that all referees, umpires, sports trainers, and sporting officials be trained in first aid management.

EARLY MANAGEMENT

Early management refers to the situation in which an injured athlete has been brought for assessment to the medical room, or, alternatively, to an emergency department or medical facility. Assessment of injury severity is generally best performed in a quiet medical room rather than in the middle of a football field in front of a hundred thousand screaming fans.

In assessment of the acutely injured player, the history and antecedent events, both from the athlete and eyewitnesses, are crucial. A full neurologic examination is important. Because the major management priorities at this stage are to establish an accurate diagnosis and exclude a catastrophic intracranial injury, this part of the examination should be particularly thorough.

Most athletes who have experienced a convulsive episode are likely to have coexistent brain injuries. This situation needs to be assessed specifically. The common symptoms of concussion have been examined in prospective studies and include headache, dizziness, blurred vision, and nausea.[7] It is worth noting that the presence of headache is not confined to concussion, with up to 20% of sporting athletes reporting exercise-related headache.[42]

The use of computed tomography or magnetic resonance imaging to ascertain the presence or absence of cerebral pathology is necessary in most cases of traumatic convulsive episodes. The availability of the various imaging techniques in different countries may influence imaging strategies. The role of EEG is controversial in such situations. If the event is clearly nonepileptic in origin, an EEG will not aid diagnosis or management. If the episode is suspected to be epileptic in nature, early (within 24 hours) EEG is recommended to assist in diagnosis.

RETURN TO SPORTS

Following the full recovery of the injured athlete, a decision must be made regarding the timing of return to sports. The guiding policy should be that until *completely* symptom free, injured athletes should not resume any training or competition. All athletes sustaining a convulsive episode require a medical clearance, which may include neuropsychologic testing, before resumption of their sports.

If the athlete has sustained a concussive convulsion or tonic concussive episode, then antiepileptic therapy is not indicated, and prohibition from collision sport is unwarranted. The treating clinician can reassure the patient that concussive convulsions are benign, and overall management should center on the appropriate treatment of the concussive injury itself.

When the convulsion is due to a nonepileptic mechanism, correction or removal of the underlying problem is necessary. At times, no specific therapy is required beyond a correct diagnosis. If game videotape is available, it should be reviewed prior to making a final diagnosis. When the event is epileptic in nature, therapy with antiepileptic medication may be considered, depending upon the individual circumstances. Apart from posttraumatic epilepsy, restriction should not be placed upon driving licensing, nor should there be any mandatory follow-up required.

If a nonepileptic condition, such as a concussive convulsion, is misdiagnosed as epilepsy, then there may be medicolegal implications for the treating physician or neurologist over and above the risk of medication side effects and the unnecessary restriction from sport. When the patient is a professional athlete, an inappropriate restriction of sport (or trade) based upon an incorrect diagnosis or negligent management could conceivably result in a legal action to overturn such restrictions. Key sporting bodies must take care in establishing formal guidelines for medical conditions, particularly where mandatory exclusion periods are utilized in the absence of scientific support.

No specific recommendations for prevention of concussive convulsions are possible at this time. In general terms, reducing the number and severity of concussions in sports should reduce the incidence of convulsive sequels. There are a number of suggested means by which this may be achieved; however, the evidence for effect is theoretical rather than scientifically proven. These measures include rule changes to avoid head impact, neck muscle conditioning, mouthguard use, and the use of helmets or head protectors. There is, however, no conclusive evidence that wearing a helmet will prevent either concussive brain injury or convulsive episodes in collision sports. Several reviews have recently addressed this issue.[43, 44]

CONCLUSION

Convulsions are a dramatic aspect of medical care in all collision sports, and a team physician needs to be aware of the possible causes and appropriate management of these entities. In the acute on-field setting, convulsive events are most likely to be due to nonepileptic phenomena. In severe or penetrating head injury, which might be seen in motorcar racing, posttraumatic epilepsy is the more likely diagnosis. The confusion and lack of understanding of concussive or impact convulsions and the assumption that these represented a form of posttraumatic epilepsy have led to a number of athletes being inappropriately restricted from their sports and often treated with antiepileptic medication. Furthermore, the social stigma of being diagnosed as epileptic may have implications in terms of occupation and driving restrictions. Athletes who suffer these episodes can be reassured that concussive convulsions are benign, not associated with a long-term risk of epilepsy, and do not require specific pharmacotherapy, and that the overall management should center on the correct management of the associated concussive injury. Appropriate management in all cases must be preceded by an accurate diagnosis.

References

1. McCrory P, Bladin P, Berkovic S. Retrospective study of concussive convulsions in elite Australian rules and rugby league footballers: Phenomenology, aetiology and outcome. BMJ 1997;314:171–174.
2. Samuel M, Duncan J. The use of the hand held video camcorder in the evaluation of seizures. J Neurol Neurosurg Psychiatry 1994;57:1417–1418.
3. Engel J, Pedley T (eds). Epilepsy: A comprehensive textbook. Philadelphia, Lippincot-Raven, 1998, pp 52–56.
4. Duncan J, Shorvon S, Fish D. Clinical epilepsy. London, Churchill-Livingstone, 1995, pp 1–23.
5. Gowers WR. Epilepsy and the chronic convulsive diseases: Their causes, symptoms and treatment. London, J & A Churchill, 1881, pp 224–240.
6. Maddocks D, Saling M. Neuropsychological sequelae following concussion in Australian rules footballers. J Clin Exp Neuropsychol 1991;13:439.
7. Maddocks DL, Dicker GD, Saling MM. The assessment of orientation following concussion in athletes. Clin J Sport Med 1995;5:32–35.
8. Maddocks DL. Neuropsychological recovery after concussion in Australian rules footballers. [PhD thesis]. Melbourne, University of Melbourne, 1995.
9. McCrory P. Were you knocked out? A team physician's approach to initial concussion management. Med Sci Sports Exerc 1997;29:S207–212.
10. Orchard J, Wood T, Seward H, Broad A. Comparison of injuries in elite senior and junior Australian football. J Sci Med Sport 1998;1(2):83–89.
11. Chadwick D. Wrong diagnosis may deprive people of their livelihood (letter to the editor). BMJ 1997;314:1283.
12. Westphal CFO. Artificial production of epilepsy in guinea pigs. Berliner Klinische Wochenschr (quoted in BMJ 1872;1:399) 1871;1:39.
13. Denny-Brown D, Russell WR. Experimental cerebral concussion. Brain 1941;64:93–163.
14. Jennett B. Early traumatic epilepsy. Arch Neurol 1974;30:394–398.
15. Jennett B. Epilepsy after non-missile head injuries, 2nd ed. London, Heineman, 1975.
16. Caveness WF. Post traumatic sequelae. In Caveness WF, Walker AE (eds): Head Injury. Philadelphia; JB Lippincott, 1966, pp 76–90.
17. Walker AE, Caveness WF, Critchley M (eds). The late effects of head injury. Springfield, IL, Charles C Thomas, Publisher, 1969, p 103.
18. Phillips G. Traumatic epilepsy after closed head injury. J Neurol Neurosurg Psychiatiatry 1954;17:1–10.
19. Sander J, Hart Y, Johnson A, Shorvon S. The national general practice study of epilepsy: newly diagnosed epileptic seizures in a general population. Lancet 1990;336:1267–1271.
20. Annegers JF, Grabow JD, Groover RV, et al. Seizures after head trauma: A population study. Neurology 1980;30:683–689.
21. Annegers J, Hauser W, Coan S, Rocca W. A population based study of seizures after traumatic brain injuries. N Engl J Med 1998;338:20–24.
22. Annegers JF, Grabow JD, Kurland LT, Laws ER. The incidence, causes and secular trends of head trauma in Olmstead county, Minnesota, 1935–1974. Neurology 1980;30:912–919.
23. Narayan R, Wilberger J, Povishlok J. Neurotrauma. New York, McGraw-Hill, 1996, pp 611–619.
24. Caveness WF. Onset and cessation of fits following craniocerebral trauma. J Neurosurg 1963;20:570–583.
25. McCrory P, Berkovic SF. Videoanalysis of acute motor and convulsive manifestations of sport-related concussion. Neurology (in press).
26. Jackson J. Epileptiform seizures (unilateral) after an injury to the head. Medical Times & Gazette 1863;ii:65.
27. McCrory P, Bladin P, Berkovic S. The cerebellar seizures of Hughlings Jackson. Neurology 1999; 52:1888–1890.
28. Lang D. Seizure disorders and physical activity. Your Patient & Fitness 1996;10:24–27.
29. Nakken K, Bjorholt P, Johannessen S. Effect of physical training on aerobic capacity, seizure occurrence and serum level of anticonvulsant drugs in adults with epilepsy. Epilepsia 1990;31:88–94.
30. Korczyn A. Participation of epileptic patients in sports. J Sports Med 1979;19:195–198.
31. Aisenson M. Accidental injuries in epileptic children. Pediatrics 1948;2:85–88.
32. Berman W. Sport and the child with epilepsy (letter). Pediatrics 1984;74:320–321.
33. Bennett D. Epilepsy and the Athlete. In Jordan B, Tsaris P, Warren RF (eds): Sports Neurology. Rockville, MD, Aspen Publishers, 1989, pp 116–126.
34. Lempert T, Bauer M, Schmidt D. Syncope: A videometric analysis of 56 episodes of transient cerebral hypoxia. Ann Neurol 1994;36:233–237.
35. Gastaut H, Fisher-William M. Electroencephalographic study of syncope: Its differentiation from epilepsy. Lancet 1957;2:1018–1025.
36. Mueller FO, Cantu RC, Van Camp SP. Catastrophic injuries in high school and college sports. Champaign, IL, Human Kinetics, 1996, pp 23–36.
37. Fahn S. Paroxysmal Dyskinesias. In Marsden C, Fahn S (eds): Movement disorders 3. London, Butterworth Scientific, 1994, pp 310–345.
38. Brukner P, Khan KM. Clinical Sports Medicine. Sydney, McGraw-Hill, 1993, pp 627–633.
39. Soffer D, Licht A, Yaar I, Abramsky O. Paroxysmal choreoathetosis as a presenting symptom in idiopathic hypoparathyroidism. J Neurol Neurosurg Psychiatry 1977;40:692–694.
40. Alldredge B, Lowenstein D, Simon R. Seizures associated with recreational drug abuse. Neurology 1989;39:1037–1039.
41. Patel MN, Rund DA. Emergency removal of football helmets. Phys Sportsmed 1994;22:57–59.
42. McCrory P. Exercise related headache. Phys Sportsmed 1997;25:33–43.
43. Cantu R. Head injuries in sport. Br J Sports Med 1996;30:289–296.
44. Roos R. Guidelines for managing concussions in sports. Phys Sportsmed 1996;24:67–74.

22

Stroke in Athletes

Paul McCrory

The occurrence of stroke in sports is a rare phenomenon. Unlike older age groups, in which stroke represents one of the commonest neurologic diseases, stroke in young people, who tend to be more involved in sports, is an uncommon event. Of course, both young and older athletes, whether performing at a recreational or elite level, may develop the same stroke syndromes as non-athletes. In some cases, the athlete may have unsuspected risk factors that increase the risk of stroke during exercise, whereas in other cases the sporting activity itself may confer an intrinsic stroke mechanism. A sports physician, therefore, needs background knowledge of stroke risk factors at all ages as well as specific knowledge of stroke syndromes associated with sports.

EPIDEMIOLOGY OF STROKE

Stroke is the third leading cause of death in the Western world. In the United States alone, at least 500,000 people experience a new stroke each year, and, of these, 150,000 die. The prevalence of stroke, according to the U.S. National Health Interview Survey, is 720 per 100,000 in the white population, and 910 per 100,000 in the nonwhite population.[78] Community studies demonstrate that the annual incidence rate of stroke is 102 per 100,000 population.[52] In the 15- to 44-year-old age group, the overall incidence of stroke is 9 cases per 100,000 population.[69]

ETIOLOGY OF STROKE

Ischemic strokes can be due to intrinsic vascular occlusions (thrombus) or an occlusion of a vessel by material that originates elsewhere in the vascular system (embo-lism). An overview of published studies of ischemic stroke in young people suggests that the common causes of stroke are large artery atherosclerosis, migraine, lacunae (small vessel, deep infarctions), and cardiac embolism. Less commonly, hematologic disease and illicit drug abuse are recognized. Finally, in many patients, the cause of the stroke remains undefined.[79] A number of rarer causes of stroke in young populations also may need to be considered.[70]

Approximately 70 published case reports in the medical literature report stroke in a sports setting (Table 22–1). These reports demonstrate that arterial dissection is the predominant pathophysiologic mechanism of sports-related stroke, occurring in approximately 80% of cases.

Preparticipation Physical Examination (PPPE)

Recognizing that a variety of underlying conditions may predispose to stroke, the team or family physician who performs routine PPPEs is in an ideal place to look specifically for these risk factors. In sporting populations, the causes of stroke fall into a relatively small group of risk factors that should be specifically sought on the PPPE, such as:

(a) Trauma to the extracranial cerebral arterial tree
(b) Exercise-induced hypertension
(c) Pre-existing cardiac or vascular disease
(d) Environmental injuries (e.g., hyperthermia, decompression illness)
(e) Drug and stimulant abuse

A detailed history, physical examination, and judicious use of investigations should

Table 22–1. Reported Cases of Stroke in Sports

Arterial Territory	Sport	Reference	CNS Findings	Proposed Mechanism
Subclavian artery	Baseball pitching	16	R hemisphere infarct	Thrombosis
Internal carotid artery	American football	64	Hemisphere infarct	Unknown
	American football	65	Cerebral infarct	Unknown
	Basketball	38	R hemisphere infarct	ICA dissection
	Bodybuilding/anabolic steroid	2	Basal ganglia infarct	Thrombosis
	Bodybuilding/anabolic steroid	19	Hemispheric infarct	Thrombosis
	Bodybuilding/anabolic steroid	47	Hemispheric infarct	Thrombosis
	Bowling	38	R hemispheric TIAs	Carotid disease
	Cross-country skiing (3 cases)	28	Hemispheric stroke	"exertion"
	Cycling	21	L hemispheric infarct	Embolic disease
	Cycling	21	R lacunar infarct	Small vessel disease
	Jogging	34	Ischemic infarct	Unknown
	Jogging	55	L MCA ischemic infarct	Hyperviscosity
	Judo	36	L thalamic stroke	Unknown
	Karate	3	Hemispheric infarct	Dissection
	Exertion	46	Hemorrhagic infarct	Arterial stenosis
	Scuba diving	49	L hemisphere stroke	ICA dissection
	Skiing (10 cases)	51	Hemispheric infarcts	Unknown
	Squash	60	Hemispheric infarct	Dissection
	Soccer	21	L lacunar infarct	Small vessel disease
	Soccer	21	R lacunar infarct	Dissection
	Swimming	38	L hemisphere infarct	Small vessel disease
	Tennis	21	L hemispheric infarct	Arterial stenosis
	Water skiing	17	R hemisphere infarct	Unknown
	Weightlifting	45a	R hemispheric infarct	Dissection
Vertebral artery	American football	64	Brainstem infarct	Dissection
	American football	63	Cervical cord infarct	Dissection
	American football	63	Cervical cord infarct	Dissection
	American football	63	Brainstem TIAs	Dissection
	American football	38	Brainstem infarct	Dissection
	American football	41	Brainstem infarct	Dissection
	Archery	68	R medullary infarct	Dissection
	Australian football	45a	Brainstem infarct	Dissection
	Australian football	45a	Brainstem infarct	Dissection
	Calisthenics	22	Cervical cord infarct	Dissection
	Calisthenics	48	Cervical cord infarct	Dissection
	Diving	73	R medullary TIAs	Vertebral artery stenosis
	Golf	74	Lateral medullary stroke	Dissection
	Gymnastics	48	Cervical cord infarct	Dissection
	Racquetball	75	L medullary infarct	Dissection
	Rugby football	45a	Medullary infarct	Dissection
	Skating	40	Cerebellar stroke	Unknown
	Soccer	21	Lateral medullary syndrome	Vertebral arterial stenosis
	Swimming	76	R cerebellar infarct	Dissection
	Tennis	59	Brainstem infarct	Dissection
	Tennis	44	R lateral medullary syndrome	Dissection
	Tennis	44	R cerebellar infarct	Dissection
	Tennis	80	L brainstem infarct	Dissection
	Volleyball	4	Brainstem TIA	Unknown
	Wrestling	18	Brainstem TIA	Dissection
	Wrestling	58	R brainstem infarct	Dissection
	Yoga	48	L cerebellar infarct	Dissection
	Yoga	17	L brainstem infarct	Dissection
	Yoga	27	Medullary and cerebellar infarct	Dissection
Other	Bodybuilding/anabolic steroid	31	Sagittal sinus thrombosis	Thrombosis

R, right; ICA, internal carotid artery; TIA, transient ischemic attack; L, left; MCA, middle cerebral artery.

assist the physician in determining the risk profile of the athlete being examined.

History

A history of recurrent syncope or loss of consciousness associated with exercise raises the possibility of occult cardiac disease. Approximately 15% of cases of sudden death in sports are associated with prior syncopal episodes.[42] The traditional cardiac ischemic symptoms of chest pain or dyspnea with exercise should also be sought, as well as a history of congenital heart disease or cardiac valve infection.[13]

A history of headache should also be requested. Migraine is extremely common, with a prevalence of 15% to 20% in community populations.[45] The incidence of migrainous cerebral infarction symptoms is extremely low; however, this mechanism represents one of the causes of stroke in young people, occurring in 2% to 18% of cases.[79] Congenital intracranial aneurysms occur with an incidence of 2000 per 100,000 population and have a rate of rupture of 12 per 100,000 per year.[56] As many as 50% of patients describe a severe sentinel warning headache prior to rupture.[20] Differentiating these from other headache syndromes may be extremely difficult. The presence of an unexplained severe headache, particularly in patients with no headache history or with a family history of aneurysmal rupture, should prompt further investigation. A family history of stroke or unexplained death at young ages may suggest a hereditary blood disorder such as a coagulopathy, bleeding diathesis, or hyperviscosity state.

Drug, alcohol, and stimulant abuse must be specifically sought. A variety of medications and illicit drugs have been associated with stroke in the 15- to 44-year-old age group, as discussed later.[10, 26] Similarly, a history of brain trauma or environmental exposure to altitude, extremes of heat, or scuba diving should raise suspicion of these mechanisms of cerebral injury.

Examination

On general appearance, a marfanoid body habitus should raise the possibility of cardiac valvular disease. The skin should be examined for lesions suggestive of an underlying vascular disease, such as Osler-Rendu-Weber syndrome. A full cardiovascular examination should be performed in all patients. Detailed guidelines for preparticipation examination in young athletes have been published elsewhere.[8]

Investigations

The role of investigations should be limited to athletes whose history or examination findings are suggestive of an underlying disease. If cardiac disease is suspected, then chest radiograph, electrocardiogram (ECG), and echocardiogram are the usual initial screening investigations. If ischemic heart disease is suspected, then an exercise ECG test or thallium scan may be performed. If an intracerebral aneurysm is suspected, then a cerebral computed tomographic (CT) or magnetic resonance (MR) scan should be performed with MR angiography, which is considerably less invasive and carries less morbidity than carotid and vertebral angiography. Coagulopathic disease, bleeding diathesis, hyperviscosity syndromes, or autoimmune disease can be detected on appropriate hematologic and serologic workup. A drug screen may be necessary in some situations.

SPECIFIC STROKE SYNDROMES IN SPORTING POPULATIONS

As can be seen from Table 22–1, stroke in athletes is commonly associated with dissection of the extracranial vessels, presumably secondary to arterial trauma caused either by neck movement or by a blow to the region. Far less commonly, other pathophysiologic mechanisms, such as hyperviscosity states, hemodynamic compromise, exercise-induced hypertension, drug-induced stroke, or atherosclerotic small vessel disease, have been noted.

Vertebral Arterial Dissection (VAD)

VAD is an uncommon and incompletely understood condition. The precise incidence is unknown.[24] Approximately 25 cases have been reported to occur in sport (see Table 22–1). The average age of patients with VAD is 38 years, with a range from 3 to 63 years.[29] Most patients are healthy, without predisposing risk factors for stroke.[72] Failure to make the diagnosis and institute appropriate therapy may result in long-term neurologic sequelae or death, although spontaneous resolution of the condition does occur.[72] The initiating factor for this condition is thought to be a tear in the arterial intima, with subsequent formation of in situ thrombosis. The pathologic injury may involve only the arterial intima or may extend to involve the tunica media. Less frequently, the adventitial layer is breached, with bleeding outside the vessel wall.[43] Spontaneous dissections are rare, and reported cases are often related to other disease states.[67]

A great deal of discussion revolves around the relationship of cervical movement to vertebral artery compression. Anecdotally the presence of cervical abnormalities such as zygapophyseal joint osteophytes, fractures, dislocations, and rheumatoid arthritis may potentially cause symptomatic vertebrobasilar ischemia when the head is turned. From a pathophysiologic standpoint, in order for vertebrobasilar ischemia to occur, there must be contralateral vertebrobasilar artery hemodynamic restriction, either from stenosis, from atherosclerotic disease, or from hypoplasia.[71]

Cases of vertebral artery dissection related to trauma are more commonly reported, often in the presence of major cervical spinal trauma, such as vertebral fracture or subluxation.[83] Most recognized cases, however, occurred following a seemingly trivial traumatic event, such as sneezing, coughing, riding a roller coaster, horseback riding, visiting a hairdresser, or performing yoga exercises.[6, 35, 66] A number of cases have also been reported following chiropractic manipulation.[43, 72] Interestingly, in all of these cases, the arteriographic appearance of the contralateral vertebrobasilar arteries was normal (Figs. 22–1 and 22–2).

A wide variety of clinical neurologic deficits are found in relation to VAD, perhaps related to the variable pathologic mechanisms (thrombosis or embolism), the complexity of neural structures supplied by the posterior circulation, and the variability of the vascular architecture. The most common initial symptoms in VAD are neck pain and occipital headache that may precede the onset of neurologic symptoms from seconds to weeks.[43] It was noted that headache symptoms in the majority of cases were ipsilateral to the vascular injury, and that the pain usually radiated to the temporal region, frontal area, eye, or ear. None of the reported cases had cervical tenderness or objective restriction of neck movement, although a subjective exacerbation of pain did occur with neck movement.[72]

The typical course of untreated VAD is progression in a stuttering fashion over hours to days. This progression is thought to result either from propagation of the thrombus or from distal embolization.[24] This is the rationale for the use of anticoagulation in the treatment of extracranial VAD.

From the standpoint of early recognition of this condition, the combination of unilateral neck pain or headache of abrupt onset following a history of neck trauma should lead to the suspicion of VAD, even in the face of seemingly trivial trauma. The clinical suspicion of VAD should be investigated by transcranial Doppler ultrasound, vertebral artery angiography, or magnetic resonance angiography after neurologic opinion is sought. The history or detection of major neurologic findings such as vertigo, diplopia, ataxia, dysarthria, cranial nerve palsies, or altered mental function should be an absolute indication for urgent neurologic consultation and hospital admission. It is important to emphasize that the neurologic findings may be delayed days or weeks after the onset of neck pain, and optimal management of this condition should involve early recognition, appropriate investigation, and institution of anticoagulation when indicated. A clinical algorithm for the Emergency Department management of VAD has been published.[67]

Carotid Arterial Dissection

Direct trauma to the head or neck during sport can potentially injure the carotid arteries. In addition, forcible hyperextension or lateral rotation may similarly cause arterial injury.[51] Hypertrophy of the posterior belly of the digastric muscle leading to compression of the internal carotid artery and causing transient ischemic episodes with neck rotation has been reported in a retired professional football player.[15] Nonpenetrating neck trauma has been reported to cause

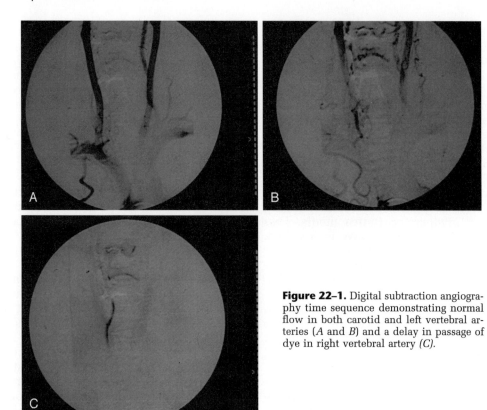

Figure 22–1. Digital subtraction angiography time sequence demonstrating normal flow in both carotid and left vertebral arteries (*A* and *B*) and a delay in passage of dye in right vertebral artery *(C)*.

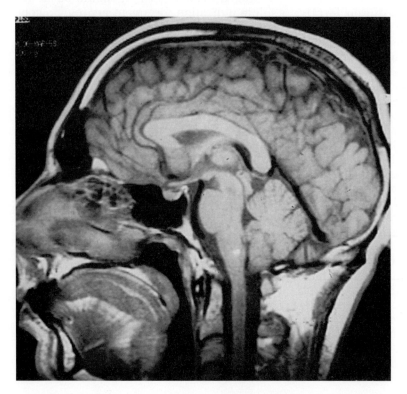

Figure 22–2. Sagittal T2 magnetic resonance image of brain demonstrating small area of increased intensity in medulla consistent with a lateral medullary infarction. (Same patient as Figure 22–1.)

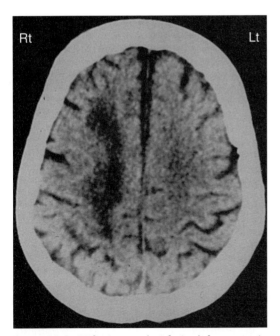

Figure 22–3. CT brain scan (axial view) demonstrating area of decreased attenuation on right side consistent with an area of infarction in a watershed distribution following unilateral carotid dissection.

thrombosis of both the external carotid and, more importantly, the internal carotid artery with associated ischemic hemispheric injury (Figs. 22–3 and 22–4).[16]

Clinically, apart from the history of trauma and ipsilateral hemispheric stroke symptoms, tenderness of the carotid vessels, oculomotor palsies, and ipsilateral Horner's syndrome may alert the examiner to the carotid injury. In addition to stroke episodes, trauma to the carotid arteries may induce a severe unilateral headache associated with profound autonomic symptoms. This entity, known as traumatic dysautonomic cephalgia, may be successfully treated with propranolol.[81]

Anecdotally about half of all carotid dissections result in stroke, which is in keeping with the age profile of most cases and presumably intact collateral circulation.[61, 70] Recurrence is unusual and does not typically affect the same segment or artery as the initial presentation.[62] Most authors recommend anticoagulation therapy for carotid dissection, although there are no prospective trials demonstrating the efficacy of such treatment.

Subclavian Artery Stenosis

One case of subclavian artery stenosis has been reported in a baseball pitcher who developed an acute hemispheric stroke due to thrombus propagated into the carotid artery. The putative lesion was thought to be caused by compression of the subclavian artery at the level of the thoracic outlet and first rib.[17] More typically, subclavian vessel disease causes acute upper limb ischemia.

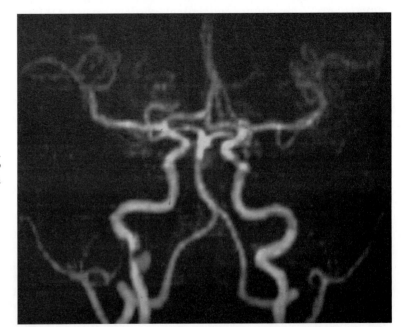

Figure 22–4. Magnetic resonance angiogram seen in AP view demonstrating dissection of right internal carotid artery.

Migraine

Migraine is often an etiologic consideration in young stroke patients.[82] Because there is no diagnostic marker for migraine, the clinician must rely on the patient's history.[30] Because exercise-related headache is common to many sports, differentiating migrainous events from other causes of headache may be clinically difficult.

Migraine without aura is associated with a threefold increase in stroke in young women, and a sixfold increase in stroke is associated with migraine with aura. In addition, the risk of stroke in migrainous women is markedly increased in those using oral contraceptives (odds ratio = 14) or who are heavy smokers (odds ratio = 10).[77] Oral contraceptives have been implicated in some studies as a cause of stroke, but this remains extremely controversial.[53]

Decompression Sickness

The clinical symptoms of decompression sickness develop rapidly and appear during or immediately after ascent. They usually occur within 3 hours of surfacing, but may, in some cases, take as long as 24 to 36 hours to manifest. The symptoms are mainly seen in persons who have experienced pressures greater than 2 absolute atmospheric pressure (diving to depths greater than 10 meters of seawater). The neurologic manifestations may comprise symptoms from the cerebral hemispheres, cerebellum, and spinal cord as well as vestibular disturbances. Memory loss, convulsions, and even coma can occur in the absence of focal symptoms.

The clinical syndrome of ischemic stroke associated with decompression sickness can be directly due to bubble formation or indirectly due to endothelial damage and coagulopathic disturbance.[32, 54] The therapy for decompression sickness is hyperbaric recompression. The aim of the treatment is to reduce bubble growth, promote the clearance of gas, and counteract ischemia and hypoxia in the affected tissues. Therefore, it is extremely important that the treatment be initiated early, before the pathologic changes have become irreversible.[32]

Heat Stroke

Although the pathogenesis of hyperthermia and heat stroke is distinctly noncerebral in origin, these conditions nevertheless can present with florid neurologic features.[57] Alterations in cerebral metabolism have been demonstrated with core temperatures above 43°C.[50] Heat stroke occurs in young people who exercise in the heat when they are unacclimatized and in older people exposed to high ambient temperatures.[23] It is a particular threat in people taking anticholinergic medications, which interfere with heat dissipation.

Clinically, heat stroke may begin with stupor or coma, or the patient may pass through a stage of agitated delirium. The diagnosis is made by recording a core body temperature in excess of 42°C. This is a medical emergency, and treatment must be instituted urgently. Patients who survive heat stroke are often left with permanent neurologic sequelae. The treatment of heat stroke is rapid correction of hyperthermia and restoration of circulating blood volume. Fluid balance must be carefully monitored in the face of potential myocardial and renal tubular damage.

Cardiogenic Embolism

Cardiogenic embolism leading to focal cerebral ischemia may occur during activity-induced cardiac dysrhythmias. Sinus bradyarrhythmias in athletes have been associated with atrial fibrillation and thrombus formation with secondary embolization to the brain.[1] Athletes who experience stroke episodes secondary to cardiogenic embolism or arrhythmias are at risk for repeated episodes unless the underlying problem can be corrected. In many cases this is not possible, and long-term anticoagulation may be considered as a preventative therapy; however, this form of treatment may preclude athletes from participation in contact and collision sports.

Stimulant and Drug Abuse

Stroke can occur during the first minutes of acute intoxication with a drug, in the hours following ingestion, or weeks following intoxication.[33] Recognition of the role of drug use in the pathogenesis of stroke requires familiarity with the acute effects of commonly used recreational drugs and a high index of suspicion. The physician must question for a history of substance abuse from the patient, friends, and family. Suspicion of drug use can be confirmed through prompt urine toxicology screening.

Stroke can occur as both a direct and an indirect medical complication of the recreational use of several drugs. The direct complications related to cerebrovascular disease are ischemic stroke, intracerebral hemorrhage, and subarachnoid hemorrhage. The drugs typically associated with these complications include cocaine, methamphetamine, MDMA (ecstasy), ephedrine, phenylpropanolamine, methylphenidate, and heroin.[5]

Indirect complications are related to the means of the drug's administration or to contaminants mixed with the drug. For example, cardioembolic stroke can be secondary to bacterial endocarditis in an intravenous drug user who employs unsterile needles. Additionally, cocaine has been reported to cause myocardial infarctions and cardiomyopathies, creating the potential for cardioembolic stroke.[7] Similarly, several drugs intended for intravenous use are mixed with talc or cornstarch. These substances have been found to occlude arteries, leading to stroke.[9]

Strokes have also been reported in several bodybuilders who were consuming anabolic steroids.[2] The duration of anabolic use in these cases ranged from 6 weeks to 4 years. Clinical presentations included hemispheric stroke and sagittal sinus thrombosis. Stroke has also been reported in patients using the same agents for medical indications, suggesting that this risk is not wholly unexpected.[14]

Drug use should be suspected in any young person who presents with a stroke. It should be remembered that drug use encompasses not only illegal substances like cocaine, methamphetamine, and heroin, but also diet pills, over-the-counter decongestants, methylphenidate (Ritalin), and asthma medications. A detailed history should be sought from the patient, friends, and family, and urine toxicology screens used where necessary.

Fat Embolism

Fat embolism is a common complication of severe bone trauma, particularly to the extremities, occurring in up to 15% of such cases.[37] Given that long bone trauma is common in many contact and collision sports, fat embolism needs to be considered in this setting. The neurologic presentation may be delayed by hours to days after trauma. Neurologic symptoms such as hemiparesis, altered mental status, seizures, and coma are common. Associated hypoxia secondary to pulmonary infarction may complicate the presentation. The treatment of fat embolism is improvement of the oxygen-carrying capacity by eliminating the cause of the hypoxia and, if necessary, red blood cell transfusion. Even in cases of coma, patients may still recover completely.[57]

Intracerebral Hemorrhage

Systolic blood pressure increases during exercise, and the peak pressure rise correlates with the intensity of the exercise and the age of the patient and inversely with the patient's fitness.[11] When a vascular malformation or arterial wall defect such as an aneurysm exists, the risk of rupture is increased during exercise. Given the high peak arterial pressures that occur with sports such as weightlifting, with systolic pressures exceeding 400 mmHg and diastolic pressures above 300 mmHg, it is surprising that intracerebral hemorrhage does not occur more frequently.[39] In cases of stroke, approximately 50% of aneurysms and 25% of vascular malformations present with bleeding during physical exertion or emotional strain.[80] Alcohol intoxication has been reported as an additional risk factor for aneurysm rupture.[25] In addition, two cases have been reported of bleeding into occult intracerebral tumors while the patients were jogging.[12]

SUMMARY

Immediate recognition of a central nervous system injury, institution of cardiopulmonary support where required, and immobilization of the head and neck are the cornerstones of initial management of sport-related neurologic injury. More definitive investigation and treatment of specific stroke syndromes requires an understanding of the etiology, underlying pathogenesis, and temporal profile of the various causes of stroke in sport. The understanding of stroke risk factors in an athletic population may assist the clinician in instituting an appropriate preparticipation screening program to minimize the occurrence of such conditions.

References

1. Abdon N, Lasdin K, Johannson B. Athlete's bradycardia as an embolising disorder. Br Heart J 1984;52:660–666.
2. Akhter J, Hyder S. Cerebrovascular accident associated with anabolic steroid use in a young man. Neurology 1994;44:2405–2406.
3. Almer S. Infarctus cérébral à la suite d'un combat de karate. Presse Med 1985;14:2299.
4. Behnke D, Brady W. Vertebral artery dissection due to minor neck trauma (whilst playing volleyball). J Emerg Med 1994;12:27–31.
5. Bendixen B. Stroke Associated With Drug Abuse. In Gilman S, Goldstein G, Waxman S (eds). Neurobase, 3rd ed. San Diego, Arbor Publishers, 1999.
6. Biousse V, Chabriat H, Amerenco P, Bousser M. Roller-coaster–induced vertebral artery dissection [letter]. Lancet 1995;346:767.
7. Brown E, Prager J, Lee H-Y, Ramsey R. CNS complications of cocaine abuse: Prevalence, pathophysiology, and neuroradiology. AJR Am J Roentgenol 1992;159:137–147.
8. Brukner P, Khan KM. Clinical Sports Medicine. Sydney, McGraw-Hill, 1993, pp 45–48.
9. Brust J, Richter R. Stroke associated with cocaine abuse. NY State J Med 1977;77:1473–1475.
10. Caplan L, Hier D, Banks G. Stroke and drug use. Stroke 1982;17:9–14.
11. Carlstein A, Grimby G. The Circulatory Response to Muscular Exercise in Man. Springfield, IL, Charles C Thomas Publisher, 1966, pp 1–141.
12. Downey R, Antunes J, Michelsen W. Hemorrhage within brain tumors during jogging. Ann Neurol 1980;7:496.
13. Driscoll D. Cardiovascular evaluation of the child and adolescent before participation in sports. Mayo Clin Proc 1985;60:867–873.
14. Einhaupl K, Villringer A. Heparin treatment in sinus venous thrombosis. Lancet 1991;338:597–600.
15. Etheridge S, Effeney D, Ehrenfield W. Symptomatic extrinsic compression of the cervical carotid artery. Arch Neurol 1984;41:672–673.
16. Fields W. Neurovascular syndromes of the neck and shoulders. Semin Neurol 1981;1:301–309.
17. Fields W. Non-penetrating trauma of the cervical arteries. Semin Neurol 1981;1:284–290.
18. Ford F. Syncope, vertigo and disturbances of vision resulting from intermittent obstruction of the vertebral arteries due to defect in the odontoid process and excessive mobility of the second cervical vertebra. Bull Johns Hopkins Hosp 1952;91:168–173.
19. Frankle M, Eichberg R. Anabolic androgenic steroids and stroke in an athlete: Case report. Arch Phys Med Rehabil 1988;69:632–63.
20. Gillingham F. The management of ruptured intracranial aneurysms. Scott Med J 1967;12:377–383.
21. Giroud M, Chague F, Guard O, Dumas R. Accident vasculaire cérébral ischémique et activité sportive. 6 observations. Rev Med Interne 1987;8:373–378.
22. Grinker R, Guy C. Sprain of the cervical spine causing thrombosis of the anterior spinal artery. JAMA 1927;88:1140–1142.
23. Hanson P, Zimmerman S. Exertional heatstroke in novice runners. JAMA 1979;242:154–157.
24. Hart R. Vertebral arterial dissection. Neurology 1988;38:987–989.
25. Hillbom M, Kaste M. Does alcohol intoxication precipitate aneurysmal subarachnoid haemorrhage? J Neurol Neurosurg Psychiatry 1981;44:523–526.
26. Hillbom M, Kaste M, Rasi V. Can ethanol intoxication affect hemocoagulation to increase the risk of brain infarction in young adults? Neurology 1983;33:381–384.
27. Hilton-Jones D, Warlow C. Non-penetrating arterial trauma and cerebral infarction in the young. Lancet 1985;i:1435–1438.
28. Hoffman A, Herold G, Minder E. Internistiche Zwischenfaelle beim Langlaufen. Todesfalle und Hopitalisationen im oberengaden. Schweiz Med Wochenschr 1978;108:1126–1128.
29. Horowitz I, Niparko N. Vertebral artery dissection with bilateral hemiparesis. Pediatr Neurol 1994;11:252–254.
30. International Headache Society. Headache Classification Committee of the International Headache Society: Classification and diagnostic criteria for headache disorders, cranial neuralgias and facial pain. Cephalgia 1997;18(Suppl):43–110.
31. Jaillard A, Hommel M. Venous sinus thrombosis associated with androgens in a healthy young man. Stroke 1994;25:212–213.
32. Jain K. Textbook of Hyperbaric Medicine, 3rd ed. Seattle, Hogrefe & Huber Publishers, 1998, pp 221–321.
33. Kaku D, Lowenstein D. Emergence of recreational drug abuse as a major risk factor for stroke in young adults. Ann Intern Med 1990;113:821–827.
34. Kelly W, Roussak J. Stroke while jogging. Br J Sports Med 1980;14:229–230.
35. Krentz M, Hopkins E, Moore J. Panic with a twist: an unusual presentation of combined psychiatric and neurological symptoms in a tactical jet aviator. Aviat Space Environ Med 1997;68:217–220.
36. Lannuzel A, Moulin T. Vertebral artery dissection following a judo session: Case report. Neuropediatrics 1994;25:106–108.
37. Lepisto P, Alho A. Diagnostic features of the fat embolism syndrome. Acta Chirop Scand 1975;141:245–250.
38. Luken M, Ascher G, Cornell J. Spontaneous dissecting aneurysms of the extracranial internal carotid artery. Clin Neurosurg 1979;26:353–375.
39. MacDougall J, Tuxen D, Sale B. Arterial blood pressure response to heavy resistance exercise. J Appl Physiol 1985;58:785–790.
40. MacGowan D, Caronna J. Stroke in Sports. In Jordan B, (ed): Sports Neurology, 2nd ed. Philadelphia, Lippincott-Raven, 1998, pp 289–299.
41. Marks R, Freed M. Non-penetrating injuries of the neck and cerebrovascular accident. Arch Neurol 1973;28:412–414.
42. Maron B, Roberts W, McAllister H. Sudden death in young athletes. Circulation 1980;62:218–229.
43. Mas J, Henin D, Bousser M, et al. Dissecting aneurysm of the vertebral artery and cervical manipulation. Neurology 1989;39:512–515.
44. McCrory P. Cervical headache in tennis players: An uncommon cause. Med Sci Sports Exerc 1994;26(Suppl 1):S519.

45. McCrory P. Exercise related headache. Phys Sportsmed 1997;25:33–43.
45a. McCrory P. Vertebral arterial dissection in sport. J Clin Neurosci 2000;7: (in press).
46. Milder D, Lauce J. Intermittent claudication of one cerebral hemisphere. Neurology 1984;34:692–694.
47. Mochizuki R, Richter K. Cardiomyopathy and cerebrovascular accident associated with anabolic-androgenic steroid use. Phys Sportsmed 1988; 16:109–114.
48. Nagler W. Vertebral artery obstruction by hyperextension of the neck: Report of three cases. Arch Phys Med Rehabil 1973;54:237–240.
49. Nelson E. Internal carotid artery dissection associated with scuba diving. Ann Emerg Med 1995;25:103–106.
50. Nemoto E, Frankel H. Cerebral oxygenation and metabolism during progressive hyperthermia. J Appl Physiol 1970;219:1784–1788.
51. Noelle B, Clavier I. Cervicocephalic arterial dissections related to skiing. Stroke 1994;24:526–527.
52. Orencia A, Biller J. Epidemiology and Natural History of Adult Ischemic Cerebrovascular Disease. In Zieler R (ed): Surgical Management of Cerebrovascular Disease. New York, McGraw-Hill, 1995, pp 101–125.
53. World Health Organization. WHO Collaborative Study of Cardiovascular Disease and Steroid Hormone Contraception. Ischaemic stroke and combined oral contraceptives: results of an international, multicentre, case-control study. Lancet 1996;348:498–505.
54. Palmer A, Calder I, Yates P. Cerebral vasculopathy in divers. Neuropath Appl Neurobiol 1992;12:113–114.
55. Phillips J, Horner B, Doorly T. Cerebrovascular accident in a 14 year old marathon runner. BMJ 1983;286:351–352.
56. Phillips L, Whisnant J, O'Fallon W. The unchanging pattern of subarachnoid hemorrhage in the community. Neurology 1980;30:1034–1040.
57. Plum F, Posner JB. The Diagnosis of Stupor and Coma (3rd ed.) Philadelphia, F. A. Davis Co., 1987, p 259.
58. Rogers L, Sweeney P. Stroke: A neurological complication of wrestling. Am J Sports Med 1979; 7:352–354.
59. Ronaldes G, Lartigue C, Bondigue M, et al. Dissection de l'artère vertébrale dans sa portion extra-cranienne après un match de tennis. Presse Med 1985;14:102–108.
60. Roux J. Hémiplegie après une partie de squash chez un adolescent. Conc Med 1985;107:167.
61. Schievink W, Mokri B. Internal carotid artery dissection in a community, Rochester, Minnesota. Stroke 1993;24:1678–1680.
62. Schievink W, Mokri B. Spontaneous dissections of cervicocephalic arteries in childhood and adolescence. Neurology 1994;44:1607–1612.
63. Schneider R, Gosch H, Norrell H. Vascular insufficiency and differential distortion of the brain and cord caused by cervico-medullary football injuries. J Neurosurg 1970;33:363–375.
64. Schneider RC. Serious and fatal neurosurgical football injuries. Clin Neurosurg 1966;12:226–236.
65. Schneider RC, Reifel E, Crisler HO, Oosterbaan BG. Serious and fatal football injuries involving the head and spinal cord. JAMA 1961;177:362–367.
66. Shimura H, Yuzawa K, Nozue M. Stroke after visit to a hairdresser. Lancet 1997;350:1778.
67. Showalter W, Esekogwu V, Newton K, Henderson S. Vertebral artery dissection. Acad Emerg Med 1997;4:991–995.
68. Sorenson B. Bow hunter's stroke. Neurosurgery 1978;2:259–261.
69. Stern B, Wtiyk R. Stroke in Young Adults. In Gilman S, Goldstein G, Waxman S (eds): Neurobase, 3rd ed. San Diego, Arbor Publishing, 1999.
70. Sturzennegger M, Huber P. Cranial nerve palsies in spontaneous carotid artery dissection. J Neurol Neurosurg Psychiatry 1993;56:1191–1199.
71. Sturzennegger M, Newell D. Dynamic transcranial Doppler assessment of positional vertebro-basilar ischemia. Stroke 1994;25:1776–1783.
72. Sturzennegger M. Headache and neck pain: The warning symptoms of vertebral artery dissection. Headache 1994;34:187–193.
73. Suechting R, French R. Posterior inferior cerebellar artery syndrome following fracture of the cervical vertebrae. J Neurosurg 1955;12:187–189.
74. Tanaguchi A, Wako K. Wallenberg syndrome and vertebral artery dissection probably due to trivial trauma during golf exercise. Rinsho Shinkeigaku 1993;33:338–340.
75. Tramo M, Hainline B. Stroke in Sports. In Jordan B, Tsaris P, Warren R (eds): Sports Neurology. Rockville, MD, Aspen Publishers, 1989, pp 101–115.
76. Tramo M, Hainline B, Petito F. Vertebral artery injury and cerebellar stroke while swimming: Case report. Stroke 1985;16:1039–1042.
77. Tzourio C, Tehindrazanarivelo A, Iglesias S, et al. Case-control study of migraine and risk of ischaemic stroke in young women. BMJ 1995;310:830–833.
78. U.S. Department of Health and Human Services Task Force on Black and Minority Health, 1984–1985. National Health Interview Survey. Washington, DC: U.S. Department of Health and Human Services, 1992, pp 1–2.
79. van den Berg J, Limburg M. Ischemic stroke in the young: Influence of diagnostic criteria. Cerebrovasc Dis 1993;3:227–230.
80. van Gijn J, van Dongen K. Computed tomography in sub-arachnoid haemorrhage: Difference between patients with and without aneurysms on angiography. Neurology 1980;30:538–539.
81. Vijayan N. A new post traumatic headache syndrome: Clinical and therapeutic observations. Headache 1977;17:19–22.
82. Welch K, Levine S. Migraine-related stroke in the context of the International Headache Society classification of head pain. Arch Neurol 1990;47:458–462.
83. Willis B, Greiner F, Orison W, Benzel E. The incidence of vertebral artery injury after mid-cervical fracture or subluxation. Neurosurgery 1994;34:435–441.

23

Epilepsy and Athletics

Robert V. Cantu

At the beginning of spring, the boy ought to be purged and his life ordered as follows: He should rise early and take a moderate walk to the gymnasium . . . where the exercise would be calculated to warm up the body in order to expel excess material and should aim at strengthening the head and the cardia.[1]

The Greek physician Galen gave this advice to the father of a child with epilepsy circa A.D. 180. Likely to be phrased a little differently today, these words remain true for most patients with epilepsy. Modern medicine, however, has not always encouraged physical activity for epileptics.

Little more than 20 years ago, many physicians believed that epileptic patients should not enter any sport, let alone collision sports such as football and hockey. Epilepsy was viewed as "an illness and illnesses require rest."[2] In a 1968 American Medical Association (AMA) publication, it was advised that individuals with "a convulsive disorder not completely controlled by medication" should avoid not only collision (e.g., football and hockey) and contact (e.g., baseball and basketball) sports, but even noncontact sports such as tennis.[3] In 1974 the AMA amended its stance, agreeing that epileptics with reasonable control of seizures should be allowed to play any sport except activities where chronic head trauma may occur. In 1983 the American Academy of Pediatrics allowed for further individual consideration, stating, "Epilepsy per se should not exclude a child from hockey, baseball, football, basketball, and wrestling."[4]

The debate regarding epileptic patients and their participation in sports, especially contact and collision sports, is understandable. With neither firm and consistent guidelines nor data from the medical literature, physicians often turned to anecdotal reports. Growing evidence suggests that most patients with epilepsy benefit from regular exercise, while there is little evidence to show that contact and collision sports place epileptics at increased risk for injury compared with athletes without epilepsy. Substantial evidence indicates that severely limiting a child's participation in physical activities has harmful psychological consequences.

DEFINITION AND EPIDEMIOLOGY OF EPILEPSY

A seizure is an abnormal electrical discharge within the brain. More specifically, "convulsive disorders (epilepsy) are states characterized by sudden, brief, repetitive and stereotyped alterations in behavior which are presumed to be due to a paroxysmal discharge of cortical and subcortical neurons."[5]

Epilepsy is a common neurologic disorder. Studies have shown that about 3% of the population will develop epilepsy by the age of 70, and 10% of the population will have a seizure at some point in their lifetime.[6] Most people who develop epilepsy experience their first seizure before the age of 30. In 1981 it was estimated that 375,000 people between the ages of 5 and 24 years had epilepsy. About 25% of these people were institutionalized, severely handicapped, or attended schools with restricted activities. The remaining 277,000 were attending conventional schools.[7]

Given the relatively high incidence of epilepsy and its early onset, one might expect a proportionate number of elementary, high school, and college athletes with the disorder. Surveys show that few epileptics play competitive sports. In one survey of 6000 high school students, 17 were found to have epilepsy, of whom none played sports. Of

3000 Division 1 National Collegiate Athletic Association (NCAA) athletes, only one, a gymnast, had epilepsy.[8]

An outdated and protective attitude on the part of some parents and physicians plays a large role in the lack of athletic participation by children with epilepsy. In many developing countries, epilepsy carries a stigma that "may rank with leprosy and mental illness."[9] In a study among rural Tanzanian residents, only 3.9% of those questioned believed that epileptics have normal intelligence. Additionally, 62% of responders would not let their child attend school if he had epilepsy, and 11% feared another child with epilepsy could infect their child. The Tanzanian with epilepsy is "ostracized, rejected, and isolated, remaining an outcast from the community."[10] This ostracism is due in part to the lack of a known cause in many cases of epilepsy. Of Tanzanians questioned, 68% did not know the cause, 3.4% blamed brain infection, and 2.2% brain injury. Other explanations included dog bite, malaria, bangi (marijuana), and whooping cough. It is interesting to compare these responses with the findings of a study in Rochester, Minnesota, where in 68.7% of epilepsy cases, the cause was unknown, 13% were due to cerebral vascular disease, 5.5% to developmental deficits, 4.1% to brain trauma, 3.6% to brain tumors, 2.6% to infection, and 1.8% to degenerative changes.[11]

Types of Seizures

Seizures can be divided into two main categories: generalized and partial (Table 23–1). Generalized seizures include at least eight subtypes, all of which are of abrupt onset and involve alteration in consciousness. Partial seizures include both simple and complex types. Simple partial seizures do not alter consciousness, and the only manifestation may be an olfactory, visual, or auditory hallucination. Complex partial seizures involve an alteration or loss of consciousness and frequently involve automatisms (semipurposeful inappropriate movements) and amnesia of the event. Partial seizures tend to have a focal onset, often owing to structural brain disease. Either type of partial seizure can become secondarily generalized. Generalized seizures are often bilateral and symmetric.

Table 23–1. Classification of Epileptic Seizures

I. **Partial Seizures**
   A. Simple partial seizures
      1. motor signs
      2. sensory signs
      3. autonomic signs
      4. psychic symptoms
   B. Complex partial seizures
      1. Simple partial seizure that develops alteration in consciousness
      2. With impairment of consciousness at onset
   C. Partial seizures that become generalized seizures
II. **Generalized Seizures**
   A. Absence seizures
   B. Clonic seizures
   C. Myoclonic seizures
   D. Tonic seizures
   E. Tonic-clonic seizures
   F. Atonic seizures
   G. Infantile spasms
   H. Akinetic seizures
III. **Unclassified Epileptic Seizures**

From van Linschoten R. Epilepsy and sports. Sports Med 1990;10:11.

DIAGNOSIS AND TREATMENT

After a single seizure, the individual should be evaluated by a neurologist to help determine the etiology of the seizure and the likelihood of future attacks. Assessment includes a careful history and physical examination, with detailed neurologic examination, blood tests to rule out a metabolic cause, electroencephalogram, and often brain imaging (magnetic resonance imaging or computed tomographic scan).

Medications referred to as antiepileptic drugs (AEDs) are the cornerstone of epilepsy treatment. Good nutrition with adequate sleep and rest are also important. Surgery is rarely needed. The more common AEDs include phenytoin (Dilantin), carbamazepine (Tegretol), phenobarbital (Luminal), ethosuximide (Zarontin), valproic acid (Depakene), primidone (Mysoline), and clonazepam (Klonopin).[12] About half of patients on AEDs will remain seizure free. In prescribing AEDs for athletes, potential side effects should be considered (Table 23–2). Phenobarbital and primidone, for example, have a sedative effect, which may be detrimental to athletic participation. Phenytoin and carbamazepine can cause ataxia, which makes them less desirable for athletes. Most AEDs are approved by the NCAA and the

Table 23–2. Common Antiepileptic Drugs and Potential Side Effects for Athletes

Drug	Side Effect
Dilantin	Ataxia
Tegretol	Ataxia
Luminal	Sedation
Klonopin	Sedation
Mysoline	Sedation
Depakene	Sedation/weakness

International Olympic Committee, with some restrictions in sports involving firearms.

Exercise and Drug Metabolism

Because medications remain the primary treatment for epilepsy, how exercise affects drug metabolism deserves study. This question is significant, given the low therapeutic index for many AEDs. It is generally thought that exercise induces liver enzymes, "increasing with increasing physical fitness."[13] Nakken and colleagues monitored daily levels of phenobarbital, phenytoin, and carbamazapine in 21 adult patients during a 4-week period of daily exercise, followed by a 2-week period of relative inactivity. They did not find a statistically significant fluctuation in serum drug levels with physical training. They postulate that since several AEDs are themselves strong inducers of liver enzymes, further activation by exercise may be limited.[14]

Exercise and Seizure Activity

In 1941 the epilepsy pioneer W.G. Lennox wrote that "physical and mental exercises seem to be an antagonist of seizures. Epilepsy prefers to attack when the patient is off-guard, sleeping, resting, or idling."[15] Lennox's claim has since been confirmed. Experiments on electrical brain activity have shown that abnormal discharges that trigger seizures often disappear during exertion and return at rest. Clinical studies have shown a decreased number of seizures during exercise.[16]

How exercise inhibits seizure activity is still debated. One common theory is that lowered blood pH due to lactic acidosis is responsible, as acidosis is known to reduce cortical irritability and alkalosis to increase it. Gotze and coworkers postulated that acidosis during exercise increases the concentration of gamma-aminobutyric acid (GABA), which suppresses electrical activity in the nervous system.[17] Others contend that exercise does not change blood pH sufficiently to affect electrical activity. They maintain that the release of beta-endorphins during physical activity results in the decreased number of seizures, as beta-endorphins do inhibit epileptic activity.[18] Finally, the increased mental alertness and attention during exercise may help reduce seizure activity.

EPILEPSY AND SPORTS

Participation in many sports, particularly contact (e.g., basketball, soccer, baseball) and collision sports (e.g., football, rugby, hockey), carries inherent risks. Witness the late Vince Lombardi, who stated, "Pro football is a violent, dangerous sport. To play it other than violently would be imbecilic."[19] Despite advances in prevention and treatment, the potential for serious and permanent injury remains. An essential question is whether athletes with epilepsy assume greater risk for themselves and towards other competitors. With a few exceptions, there is little data to show that epileptics and their fellow athletes are at increased risk of injury.

Contact and Collision Sports

In 1974 the AMA Committee on Medical Aspects of Sports declared: "There is ample evidence to show that patients with epilepsy will not be affected adversely by indulging in any sport, including football, provided the normal safeguards for sports participation are followed, including adequate head protection."[20] For contact and collision sports, the author knows of no data to contest the AMA's statement. Investigations into seizure control following repetitive minor head injuries in athletic competition failed to show any deterioration.[21] Although more data is needed, it does not appear that epileptics are at greater risk for immediate or early seizures after head injury. Berman studied 301 children who suffered blunt head injury, 9 of whom were previously known to have epilepsy. Of the nine epileptic patients, one suffered a seizure 1 week after injury. Berman concluded that "a history of epilepsy does not indicate a predisposition to a seizure after a blunt head injury."[22]

Some authors who have approved participation in collision sports for athletes who have epilepsy have singled out boxing as a sport to be avoided. To the author's knowledge, no data exists to show that fighters with epilepsy are at greater risk for seizure than nonepileptic boxers. Livingston and colleagues reported on hundreds of athletes participating in contact and collision sports, including some in boxing. They did not find "a single instance of recurrence of epileptic seizures related to head injury in any of these athletes."[23] While penetrating head injuries are known to cause seizures, Livingston concluded that "the relationship of the adverse effect of blunt head injuries on the course of pre-existing epilepsy has been completely exaggerated and probably does not exist."[24]

Swimming

Swimming is acceptable for people with epilepsy, provided there is close supervision, preferably by a trained lifeguard who has been notified of the swimmer's condition. Recreational swimming does carry a fourfold increased risk of drowning for epileptics compared with the general population, but the absolute risk is still small.[25] In a 10-year study of all drownings in King County, Washington, 89% of the victims did not have adequate supervision. Among adolescents who drowned in lakes or rivers, alcohol was by far the most common denominator (25% of cases). Epilepsy posed the greatest risk for children more than 5 years old who were bathing alone. Of five children who drowned while bathing, four had a seizure history and none had detectable levels of drugs or alcohol.[26] In another study over a 5-year period in Hawaii, no epileptic child drowned in the sea or in a swimming pool.[27]

Motor Sports

For individuals with regular seizures (>1–2 seizures per year), sports such as auto racing, motorcycle racing, and boat racing should likely be avoided. In the Netherlands, requirements for participation in these sports are similar to those for obtaining a driver's license, that is, drivers must be free of seizures for 2 years and undergo a yearly checkup.[28] Given the potential for catastrophic injury if an athlete has a seizure behind the wheel, it seems reasonable that the Netherlands' guidelines should be the minimum requirement for participation.

Falls

Participation in sports where falls could result in serious injury (e.g., cycling, gymnastics, horseback riding) should be judged on an individual basis. Seizure frequency and type of seizure are important considerations. A seizure during sports such as rock climbing, hang-gliding, and skydiving would place the athlete, fellow participants, and spectators at great risk. Nonetheless, epileptics have attempted, via litigation, to participate in these activities. The legal and ethical issues in this area preclude any strict guidelines, but physicians should use common sense when discussing the risks with patients.

Children

Concerned parents and team physicians have limited the athletic pursuits of many epileptic children. The evidence does not support this protective stance. Aisenson followed 1000 children, of whom 28% had epilepsy. The children participated in sports including soccer, football, and boxing. Over a 16-year period, the injury rate was identical for children with epilepsy and those without.[29] Another study looked at the number of "accidents" in epileptic and nonepileptic children during sports participation. A total of 16 seizures occured, 14 of which did not result in an accident. Overall there was no significant difference in accident rates among children with epilepsy and those without.[30]

Morbidity and Mortality

The overall risk of injury or death does not appear higher in athletes with epilepsy who compete in organized sports. One exception is swimming in open water. The type of injury caused by a seizure itself is no different whether the person is at rest or exercising. The most common serious injuries from generalized tonic-clonic seizures include fractures of the humeral neck, femoral trochanter, clavicle, and ankle. Shoulder and hip dislocations have also been reported.[31] Falls during seizures can cause cervical spine and head injury. There is no evidence that the sudden death syndrome in epileptics is related to activity. An investigation into this subject by Jay and Leetsma found that most patients had died presumably while sleeping.[32]

PHYSICAL BENEFITS OF EXERCISE

People with epilepsy enjoy the same benefits of exercise as anyone else: increased aerobic capacity, increased work capacity, increased lean body mass, and increased self-esteem. In Nakken's study of 21 adult epileptics who entered a 4-week exercise program, objective gains were measured. Participants exercised at least 45 minutes, three times a day, 6 days a week. Sports included aerobics, swimming, jogging, hiking, volleyball, horseback riding, bicycling, and rowing. The intensity of exercise was aimed to produce a minimum of 60% of maximal oxygen uptake ($\dot{V}O_2$ max). The maximal $\dot{V}O_2$ increased by a mean of 19% after 4 weeks. Only six patients had a seizure while exercising, with one injury; a bicyclist without a helmet (despite instruction) sustained a "minor cutaneous head injury."[33]

As a group, patients with epilepsy tend to lack physical fitness compared with age- and sex-matched controls. Steinhoff and colleagues compared 136 patients with epilepsy to 145 controls and demonstrated significant differences in aerobic endurance, muscle strength, and flexibility.[34] This difference may stem from the fact that the control group spent more of their leisure time in sports and athletic pursuits. When questioned about their attitudes toward sports, the two groups answered similarly regarding sports being fun, healthy, and suitable. Interestingly, when asked, "Are sports dangerous?" 89% of the controls answered affirmatively compared with 75% of the patients

with epilepsy. These numbers suggest that some other factor, be it overprotection by family or physician, reduced access to facilities, or fear of having a seizure while exercising, is preventing many epileptics from attaining better levels of physical fitness.

The decreased incidence of seizures while exercising has been well documented. The U.S. Commission for the Control of Epilepsy and its Consequences reported that "physical activity also appears to play a role in seizure prevention."[35] Whether a regular exercise program improves overall seizure control is not well known, but certainly merits further study.

PSYCHOLOGICAL BENEFITS OF EXERCISE

Epilepsy often leads to psychosocial disturbances. The suicide rate among epileptics is estimated at five times that for the population as a whole.[36] Unemployment is twice that of the general population. Thompson and Oxley examined 92 patients with poorly controlled epilepsy. They found that 68% had no close personal friends, 34% never formed true friendships, and only 8% were married or cohabiting.[37] The seemingly random nature of epilepsy, with sudden and unpredictable seizures, often generates a loss or "externality" of control in the epileptic. This loss of control contributes to the self-imposed isolation of many epileptics.

In 1978 Livingston wrote, "The most serious hazard of epilepsy is often not the seizures per se but the associated emotional aberrations that are prone to develop in patients with this disorder."[38] Livingston added that many patients under his care had suffered "severe emotional disturbances" when team physicians or parents forbade their participation in sports. The psychosocial gains of exercise and sports should not be underestimated for patients with epilepsy. The benefits are greatest, perhaps, for young children who are developing a sense of identity and personal ability. The feeling of accomplishment children with epilepsy can derive from sports may improve their sense of control over their disease, and just allowing children a chance to participate removes some of the stigma they bear.

References

1. Bennett DR. Sports and epilepsy: To play or not to play. Semin Neurol 1981;1:345–357.
2. Simmons RW. Epilepsy: The implications for the teacher of physical education. Br J Phys Ed 1973;4:75–76.
3. Livingston S. Epilepsy and sports [editorial]. Am Fam Physician 1978;17:67–69.
4. American Academy of Pediatrics Committee on Children with Handicaps. Sports and the child with epilepsy. Pediatrics 1983;72:884–885.
5. Bennett DR. Epilepsy and the athlete. *In* Jordan BC (ed): Sports Neurology. Aspen Publishers, 1989, pp 116–126.
6. Gates JR, Spriegel RH. Epilepsy, sports, and exercise. Sports Med 1993;15:1–5.
7. Bennett DR. Epilepsy and the athlete. *In* Jordan BC (ed): Sports Neurology. Aspen Publishers, 1989, pp 116–126.
8. Bennett DR. Sports and epilepsy: To play or not to play. Semin Neurol 1981;1:345–357.
9. Rwiza HT, Matuja HL, Kilonzo GP, et al. Knowledge, attitude, and practice toward epilepsy among rural Tanzanian residents. Epilepsia 1993;34:1017–1023.
10. Rwiza HT, Matuja HL, Kilonzo GP, et al. Knowledge, attitude, and practice toward epilepsy among rural Tanzanian residents. Epilepsia 1993;34:1017–1023.
11. Annegers JF. Epidemiology and genetics of epilepsy. Neurol Clin 1994;12:15–29.
12. Gates JR. Epilepsy and sports participation. Phys Sportsmed 1991;19:98–104.
13. Nakken KO, Bjorholt PG, Johannessen SI, et al. Effect of physical training on aerobic capacity, seizure occurrence, and serum levels of antiepileptic drugs in adults with epilepsy. Epilepsia 1990;31:88–94.
14. Nakken KO, Bjorholt PG, Johannessen SI, et al. Effect of physical training on aerobic capacity, seizure occurrence, and serum levels of antiepileptic drugs in adults with epilepsy. Epilepsia 1990;31:88–94.
15. Bennett DR, Sports and epilepsy: To play or not to play. Semin Neurol 1981;1:345–357.
16. van Linschoten R, Backx PJG, Mulder OGM, et al. Epilepsy and sports. Sports Med 1990;10:9–19.
17. Gotze W, Kubicki ST, Munter M, et al. Effect of physical exercise on seizure threshold. Dis Nerv Sys 1967;28:664–667.
18. van Linschoten R, Backx FJG, Mulder OGM, et al. Epilepsy and sports. Sports Med 1990;10:9–19.
19. O'Brien M. Vince—A personal biography of Vince Lombardi. New York, Morrow, 1987, p 16.
20. Corbitt RW, Cooper DL, Erickson DJ, et al. Epileptics and contact sports [editorial]. JAMA 1974;229:820–821.
21. van Linschoten R, Backx FJG, Mulder OGM, et al. Epilepsy and sports. Sports Med 1990;10:9–19.
22. Berman W. Sports and the child with epilepsy [letter to the editor]. Pediatrics 1984;74:520–521.
23. Livingston S, Berman W. Participation of epileptic patients in sports. JAMA 1973;224:236–238.
24. Livingston S, Berman W. Participation of epileptic patients in sports. JAMA 1973;224:236–238.
25. Gates JR, Spriegel RH. Epilepsy, sports, and exercise. Sports Med 1993;15:1–5.
26. Quan L, Edmund JG, Wentz K, et al. Ten year study of pediatric drownings and near drownings in Kings County, Washington: Lessons in injury prevention. Pediatrics. 1989;83:1035–1040.
27. Gates JR. Epilepsy and sports participation. Phys Sportsmed 1991;19:98–104.
28. van Linschoten R, Backx FJG, Mulder OGM, et al. Epilepsy and sports. Sports Med 1990;10:9–19.
29. Aisenson MR. Accidental injuries in epileptic children. Pediatrics 1948;2:85–88.
30. van Linschoten R, Backx FJG, Mulder OGM, et al. Epilepsy and sports. Sports Med 1990;10:9–19.
31. Bennett DR. Epilepsy and the athlete. *In* Jordan BC (ed): Sports Neurology. Aspen Publishers, 1989, pp 116–126.
32. Jay GW, Leetsma JE. Sudden death in epilepsy. Acta Neurol Scand 1981;82:1–66.
33. Nakken KO, Bjorholt PG, Johannessen SI, et al. Effect of physical training on aerobic capacity, seizure occurrence, and serum levels of antiepileptic drugs in adults with epilepsy. Epilepsia 1990;31:88–94.
34. Steinhoff BJ, Neususs K, Thegeder H, et al. Leisure time activity and physical fitness in patients with epilepsy. Epilepsia 1996;37:1221–1227.
35. Bennett DR. Epilepsy and the athlete. *In* Jordan BC (ed): Sports Neurology. Aspen Publishers, 1989, pp 116–126.
36. Gehlert S. Perceptions of control in adults with epilepsy. Epilepsia 1994;35:81–88.
37. Meador KJ. Research use of the new quality-of-life in epilepsy inventory. Epilepsia 1993;34(suppl 4):534–38.
38. Livingston S. Epilepsy and sports [editorial]. Am Fam Physician 1978;17:67–69.

24

Headaches in the Athlete

Robert J. Dimeff

Chronic headaches may affect up to 20% of the population, and it is estimated that 42 million Americans each year present to physicians for evaluation and treatment of headache.[27, 50] Over 40% of active men and women admit to headache related to sports participation.[79] Headache is the most common neurologic disorder and is one of the most common entities to affect mankind. Headache often interferes with the sufferer's entire lifestyle, including work, play, exercise, sleep, social interactions, and sexual activity. Athletes suffering from headache disorders may have deterioration of their training, practice, and performance. High-level athletes suffering from chronic headache syndromes have been forced to retire from their sports.

Several mechanisms may be responsible for the pain experienced during a headache. All extracranial tissues are sensitive to pain, including skin, scalp, fascia, muscles, mucosa, and arteries. The intracranial structures most sensitive to pain are the great venous sinuses, afferent veins, dura mater, arteries within the dura, arachnoid and pia mater, and cerebral arteries at the base of the brain. Pain is elicited if any of these structures is distended, compressed, distorted, dilated, irritated, or inflamed. The trigeminal nerve, which contains the pain pathways for structures above the tentorium, refers pain to the frontal, temporal, and parietal areas. The glossopharyngeal, vagus, and upper cervical nerves, which contain the pain pathways for structures below the tentorium, refer pain to the occipital area.[20, 59, 62]

The list of potential causes of headache is extensive. In addition to headaches seen in the general populace, there are numerous headaches related to physical activity and sport participation. Significant diagnostic confusion exists because in the past, headache disorders were ill defined, diagnoses varied widely from country to country, and the pathophysiology of these disorders was poorly understood.[11] Recent advances in headache research and the publication of the Headache Classification System (Table 24–1) by the Headache Classification Committee of the International Headache Society (IHS) in 1988 have allowed a more scientific approach to the evaluation and treatment of headache syndromes.[51] Epidemiologic, pathophysiologic, and therapeutic research has progressed rapidly since the publication of the IHS headache classification system, and as a result, a second edition of the classification is due to be published soon.[11]

In evaluating and treating the athlete with a headache, it is important to be aware of the most common headache syndromes, as well as the common headaches associated with exercise, sports, and physical activity (Table 24–2). While the IHS classification system allows a logical approach in evaluating the patient with headache, there are a number of headache syndromes described in the athlete which do not fit easily into this system. In the past, if a particular headache was associated with a specific sport or exercise, it was named after that activity. Thus, diagnoses of weight lifter's cephalgia, swimmer's migraine, and roller coaster headache appear in the literature. This review will attempt to classify exercise- and activity-related headaches into the IHS classification system. The purposes of this chapter are to discuss the evaluation of the athlete with headache, to review the common causes of headache by following the IHS headache classification system, and to review headaches related to physical activity and sport participation.

EVALUATION

History

As is the case with most medical conditions, the medical history is the most im-

Table 24–1. International Headache Society Headache Classification System

1. Migraine

1.1 Migraine without aura
1.2 Migraine with aura
   1.2.1 Migraine with typical aura
   1.2.2 Migraine with prolonged aura
   1.2.3 Familial hemiplegic migraine
   1.2.4 Basilar migraine
   1.2.5 Migraine aura without headache
   1.2.6 Migraine with acute onset aura
1.3 Ophthalmoplegic migraine
1.4 Retinal migraine
1.5 Childhood periodic syndromes that may be precursors to or associated with migraine
   1.5.1 Benign paroxysmal vertigo of childhood
   1.5.2 Alternating hemiplegia of childhood
1.6 Complications of migraine
   1.6.1 Status migrainosus
   1.6.2 Migrainous infarction
1.7 Migrainous disorder not fulfilling above criteria

2. Tension-type Headache

2.1 Episodic tension-type headache
   2.1.1 Episodic tension-type headache associated with disorder of pericranial muscles
   2.1.2 Episodic tension-type headache unassociated with disorder of pericranial muscles
2.2 Chronic tension-type headache
   2.2.1 Chronic tension-type headache associated with disorder of pericranial muscles
   2.2.2 Chronic tension-type headache unassociated with disorder of pericranial muscles
2.3 Headache of the tension-type not fulfilling above criteria

3. Cluster Headache and Chronic Paroxysmal Hemicrania

3.1 Cluster headache
   3.1.1 Cluster headache periodicity undetermined
   3.1.2 Episodic cluster headache
   3.1.3 Chronic cluster headache
      3.1.3.1 Unremitting from onset
      3.1.3.2 Evolved from episodic
3.2 Chronic paroxysmal hemicrania
3.3 Cluster headache-like disorder not fulfilling above criteria

4. Miscellaneous Headaches Unassociated With Structural Lesion

4.2 External compression headache
4.3 Cold stimulus headache
   4.3.1 External application of a cold stimulus
   4.3.2 Ingestion of a cold stimulus
4.4 Benign cough headache
4.5 Benign exertional headache
4.6 Headache associated with sexual activity
   4.6.1 Dull-type
   4.6.2 Explosive-type
   4.6.3 Postural-type

5. Headache Associated With Head Trauma

5.1 Acute posttraumatic headache
   5.1.1 With significant head trauma and/or confirmatory signs
   5.1.2 With minor head trauma and no confirmatory signs
5.2 Chronic posttraumatic headache
   5.2.1 With significant head trauma and/or confirmatory signs
   5.2.2 With minor head trauma and no confirmatory signs

6. Headache Associated With Vascular Disorders

6.1 Acute ischemic cerebrovascular disease
   6.1.1 Transient ischemic attack (TIA)
   6.1.2 Thromboembolic stroke
6.2 Intracranial hematoma
   6.2.1 Intracerebral hematoma
   6.2.2 Subdural hematoma
   6.2.3 Epidural hematoma

Table continued on following page

Table 24–1. International Headache Society Headache Classification System *Continued*

6.3 Subarachnoid hemorrhage
6.4 Unruptured vascular malformation
   6.4.1 Arteriovenous malformation
   6.4.2 Saccular aneurysm
6.5 Arteritis
   6.5.1 Giant cell arteritis
   6.5.2 Other systemic arteritides
   6.5.3 Primary intracranial arteritis
6.6 Carotid or vertebral artery pain
   6.6.1 Carotid or vertebral dissection
   6.6.2 Carotidynia (idiopathic)
   6.6.3 Postendarterectomy headache
6.7 Venous thrombosis
6.8 Arterial hypertension
   6.8.1 Acute pressor response to exogenous agent
   6.8.2 Pheochromocytoma
   6.8.3 Malignant (accelerated) hypertension
   6.8.4 Preeclampsia and eclampsia
6.9 Headache associated with other vascular disorder

7. Headache Associated With Nonvascular Intracranial Disorder

7.1 High cerebrospinal fluid pressure
   7.1.1 Benign intracranial hypertension
   7.1.2 High pressure hydrocephalus
7.2 Low cerebrospinal fluid pressure
   7.2.1 Post-lumbar puncture headache
   7.2.2 Cerebrospinal fluid fistula headache
7.3 Intracranial infection
7.4 Intracranial sarcoidosis and other noninfectious inflammatory diseases
7.5 Headache related to intrathecal injections
   7.5.1 Direct effect
   7.5.2 Due to chemical meningitis
7.6 Intracranial neoplasm
7.7 Headache associated with other intracranial disorder

8. Headache Associated With Substances or Their Withdrawal

8.1 Headache induced by acute substance use or exposure
   8.1.1 Nitrate/nitrite induced headache
   8.1.2 Monosodium glutamate induced headache
   8.1.3 Carbon monoxide induced headache
   8.1.4 Alcohol induced headache
   8.1.5 Other substances
8.2 Headache induced by chronic substance use or exposure
   8.2.1 Ergotamine induced headache
   8.2.2 Analgesics abuse headache
   8.2.3 Other substances
8.3 Headache from substance withdrawal (acute use)
   8.3.1 Alcohol withdrawal headache (hangover)
   8.3.2 Other substances
8.4 Headache from substance withdrawal (chronic use)
   8.4.1 Ergotamine withdrawal headache
   8.4.2 Caffeine withdrawal headache
   8.4.3 Narcotics abstinence headache
   8.4.4 Other substances
8.5 Headache associated with substances but with uncertain mechanism
   8.5.1 Birth control pills or estrogens
   8.5.2 Other substances

9. Headache Associated With Noncephalic Infection

9.1 Viral infection
   9.1.1 Focal noncephalic
   9.1.2 Systemic
9.2 Bacterial infection
   9.2.1 Focal noncephalic
   9.2.2 Systemic (septicemia)
9.3 Headache related to other infection

Table 24–1. International Headache Society Headache Classification System *Continued*

10. Headache Associated With Metabolic Disorder

10.1 Hypoxia
    10.1.1 High altitude headache
    10.1.2 Hypoxic headache
    10.1.3 Sleep apnea headache
10.2 Hypercapnia
10.3 Mixed hypoxia and hypercapnia
10.4 Hypoglycemia
10.5 Dialysis
10.6 Headache related to other metabolic abnormality

11. Headache or Facial Pain Associated With Disorder of Cranium, Neck, Eye, Ears, Nose, Sinuses, Teeth, Mouth, or Other Facial or Cranial Structures

11.1 Cranial bone
11.2 Neck
    11.2.1 Cervical spine
    11.2.2 Retropharyngeal tendinitis
11.3 Eyes
    11.3.1 Acute glaucoma
    11.3.2 Refractive errors
    11.3.3 Heterophoria or heterotropia
11.4 Ears
11.5 Nose and sinuses
    11.5.1 Acute sinus headache
    11.5.2 Other diseases of nose or sinuses
11.6 Teeth, jaws, and related structure
11.7 Temporomandibular joint disease

12. Cranial Neuralgias, Nerve Trunk Pain, and Deafferentation Pain

12.1 Persistent (in contrast to tic-like) pain of cranial nerve origin
    12.1.1 Compression or distortion of cranial nerves and second or third cervical roots
    12.1.2 Demyelination of cranial nerves
        12.1.2.1 Optic neuritis (retrobulbar neuritis)
    12.1.3 Infarction of cranial nerves
        12.1.3.1 Diabetic neuritis
    12.1.4 Inflammation of cranial nerves
        12.1.4.1 Herpes zoster
        12.1.4.2 Chronic postherpetic neuralgia
    12.1.5 Tolosa-Hunt syndrome
    12.1.6 Neck-tongue syndrome
    12.1.7 Other causes of persistent pain of cranial nerve origin
12.2 Trigeminal neuralgia
    12.2.1 Idiopathic trigeminal neuralgia
    12.2.2 Symptomatic trigeminal neuralgia
        12.2.2.1 Compression of trigeminal root or ganglion
        12.2.2.2 Central lesions
12.3 Glossopharyngeal neuralgia
    12.3.1 Idiopathic glossopharyngeal neuralgia
    12.3.2 Symptomatic glossopharyngeal neuralgia
12.4 Nervus intermedius neuralgia
12.5 Superior laryngeal neuralgia
12.6 Occipital neuralgia
12.7 Central causes of head and facial pain other than tic douloureux
    12.7.1 Anesthesia dolorosa
    12.7.2 Thalamic pain
12.8 Facial pain not fulfilling criteria in groups 11 or 12

13. Headache Not Classifiable

From Oleson J, Lance JW. Classification and diagnostic criteria for headache disorders, cranial neuralgias, and facial pain by the Headache Classification Committee of the International Headache Society. Cephalalgia 1988;8(Suppl 7):9–96.

Table 24-2. Headaches Related to Physical Activity, Exercise, and Sports Participation

Headache Associated With Head Trauma

Tension-type
Migraine
Mixed
Traumatic dysautonomic cephalgia
Second impact catastrophic
Local headache

Physical Activity, Exercise, and Sports Participation Headaches

Exertional headache
Effort headache
Acute effort migraine
Weight lifter's headache
Water-skier's headache
Luger's headache
Altitude headache
Ischemic headache
Swimmer's, diver's, and surfer's headaches
Racquet sports headache
Roller coaster headache
Sexual activity headache
Cervical neuralgia

---

portant component in the clinical examination of a patient suffering from headaches. The age and sex of the patient should be noted. Age at onset of headache, headache frequency and duration, time and mode of headache onset, headache intensity and quality, and location and radiation of pain should be determined. Precipitating and aggravating factors should be identified. These may include emotional or physical stress; fatigue or lack of sleep; skipped meals; specific food or drink such as alcohol, caffeine, chocolate, or nitrate-containing foods; exposure to cold air, fluid, or foods; changes in altitude, ambient temperature and barometric pressure; or change in activity. For headaches that are associated with change in activity, detailed information should be obtained regarding the nature and type of activity, and any special equipment used during the activity. A search should be made for any history of head or neck trauma. Previous treatment should also be reviewed, noting therapies which have been successful, unsuccessful, or associated with adverse effects.

A thorough review of associated symptoms is necessary. Migraine aura symptoms may include scintillating scotomas (blind spots), teichopsia (fortification spectra), photopsia (flashing lights), hemianopsia, blurred vision, nausea, paresthesias, weak-ness, vertigo, ataxia, aphasia, and syncope.[14, 17, 59, 80] Some migraine patients without aura describe symptoms 2 to 72 hours before the attack that may include hunger, anorexia, drowsiness, irritability, tension, energy surge, or a sense of well-being.[17] Athletes suffering from headache related to trauma may experience symptoms of dizziness, lightheadedness, nausea, vomiting, vertigo, fatigue, tinnitus, irritability, memory impairment, lack of concentration, personality changes, alcohol intolerance, weakness, sensory and balance disturbance, and loss of libido.[17] Infectious symptoms should be reviewed, such as fever, chills, night sweats, malaise, fatigue, myalgias, gastrointestinal complaints, stiff neck, sore throat, earache, toothache, nasal congestion and rhinorrhea, cough, sputum production, anorexia, and weight loss.[20, 59] Cardiovascular symptoms and risk factors should be reviewed; chest pain or pressure, palpitations, dyspnea, dyspnea on exertion, exercise-induced syncope or near-syncope, previous myocardial infarction, claudication, hypertension, tobacco use, diabetes mellitus, hypercholesterolemia, and family history of coronary artery disease or sudden death in young relatives may assist in determining the cause of headache.[7, 41, 77]

The history should also include information regarding the general health status of the athlete; current and previous medical diseases; previous surgeries and hospitalizations; allergies; current and previous pregnancies; menstrual patterns; previous concussions; caffeine, alcohol, and drug use; social and living situation; psychological disturbances, traits and disorders; and occupational or environmental exposures. Current medication use, abuse, and withdrawal should be determined; nonsteroidal anti-inflammatory drugs, analgesics, antibiotics, antihypertensives, H_2 blockers, corticosteroids, nitrazepam, oral contraceptives, sympathomimetics, theophyline, vasodilator agents, and other medications may cause headache syndromes.[11, 51] A review of headache disorders and other medical and psychiatric diseases in family members should also be performed.

Physical Examination

All patients presenting with headache should have a complete general physical examination. Vital signs, general appearance, and head, eye, ear, nose, mouth, dental, and throat examinations may assist in determining a diagnosis. The neck may be checked for range of motion, nuchal rigidity, tenderness, bruits, adenopathy, and masses. Chest, breast, cardiopulmonary, peripheral vascular, and abdominal examinations should be performed. Genitalia, pelvic, and rectal examinations may be necessary based on pertinent, positive history. Examination of the skin may reveal rashes, hemangiomas, café au lait spots, neurofibromas, and other dermatologic manifestations of headache producing diseases. A full neurologic evaluation is essential. This should include evaluation of speech, mental status, cranial nerve function (including visual acuity, visual field, and funduscopic examinations), sensory and motor systems, cerebellar function, and gait.

Laboratory and Radiographic Investigations

Laboratory testing may be required as part of the headache evaluation. Testing should be performed based on the medical history and examination. Blood testing may include complete blood count and differential, erythrocyte sedimentation rate, C-reactive protein, electrolyte, blood urea nitrogen, creatinine, glucose, liver enzyme, thyroid stimulating hormone, iron studies, ferritin, bacterial cultures, toxicology screening, and arterial blood gas.[20, 22, 23, 59] Lumbar puncture and fluid analysis is helpful in confirming cases of headache due to high or low cerebrospinal fluid pressure, infection, and hemorrhage.

Numerous radiographic studies may be necessary to evaluate the athlete with a headache.[3, 8, 10, 25, 26, 37, 65, 68, 71] Plain radiographs may reveal fractures, abscesses, sinus infection, and foreign bodies. Computed tomographic (CT) scan with contrast and magnetic resonance imaging (MRI) scan of the brain assist in the evaluation of intracranial pathology. Limited CT scan of the head may also be used to evaluate the orbits, sinuses, and dentition. Magnetic resonance angiography and angiography are useful in the investigation of vascular anomalies, hemorrhage, tumor vascularity, and cerebral vasospasm. Technetium-99m single photon emission computerized tomography (SPECT) has been used to document brain hypoperfusion in cases of exertional headache.[3] Electroencephalography (EEG) may be useful in the evaluation of the younger athlete in whom seizure disorders may mimic headache syndromes. Cardiac exercise stress–thallium testing has been used to evaluate headache syndromes in patients with suspected cardiovascular disease.[7, 39, 41, 77]

COMMON HEADACHE SYNDROMES

Migraine

Migraine headaches affect 17.6% of women and 5.7% of men and usually begin in the second to fourth decades of life.[73] The frequency and intensity of the attacks tend to decrease with advancing age. Ninety percent of migraine sufferers have a positive family history. Migraines are typically divided into classes based on the presence or absence of an aura and on the area of brain involved (see Table 24–1). Migraine without aura (1.1) was previously known as the common migraine, and migraine with aura (1.2) was known as the classic migraine. The migraine variants are more specifically defined by structure involved, for example, ophthalmoplegic migraine (1.3) or retinal migraine (1.4).

Migraine headaches are believed to be due to cerebrovascular dilatation; recent studies have identified an area of brain stem nerves that may actually be the generator of migraine attacks. Neurotransmitter alteration may be responsible for the pain associated with migraine.[14, 17, 19, 40, 59] Migraine attacks occur in clear-cut episodes that may last from 4 to 72 hours; between attacks the patients are normal. The pain is usually unilateral, pulsating, or throbbing, and of moderate to severe intensity. Attacks may be accompanied by nausea, vomiting, photophobia, and phonophobia. Some patients describe premonitory symptoms that occur 2 to 72 hours before an attack; these include mood disturbance, hunger, anorexia, drowsiness, irritability, tension, energy surge, or feeling a sense of well-being. Migraine attacks may be triggered by dietary factors (alcohol, aspartame, avocado, caffeine, cheese, chocolate, monosodium glutamate, nitrates and nitrites, nuts, onions, red grapes, skipped meals, smoked or pickled fish or meats, yeast), medications (antibiotics, anti-hypertensive agents, erythropoietin, estrogens, histamine-2 blockers, isotretinoin, nicotine, NSAIDs, oral contraceptives, and vasodilators), and other factors (altitude change, exercise, menstruation, perfume, sleep pattern changes, stress, trauma, and weather changes).[6, 14, 15, 17, 19, 20, 29, 45, 55, 56, 59, 74, 75]

Migraines with aura are preceded about 1 hour before the onset of headache by a prodrome of brisk, clear neurologic symptoms that typically lasts 15 to 20 minutes. This may include visual disturbances such as scotomata (blind spots), teichopsia (fortification spectra), photopsia, (flashing lights), hemianopsia, or complex hallucinations. Other symptoms include paresthesia, weakness, vertigo, ataxia, aphasia, and syncope. The aura is due to cerebrovascular vasoconstriction with decreased cerebral blood flow; this phase is followed by cerebrovascular dilatation and increased blood flow, which results in the contralateral headache.[17, 19, 59] Complications of migraine (1.6) occur when the neurologic deficits outlast the headache.

The migraine sufferer is easy to recognize if there is a history of recurrent similar headaches and a positive family history. The patient is generally alert, oriented, and afebrile, with a normal neurologic examination and supple neck. New onset migraine headache and patients who do not fit these criteria require further investigation, including lumbar puncture and CT or MRI scan.

Nonpharmacologic treatment can reduce the frequency and intensity of migraine attacks; this may include hot or cold therapy, massage, biofeedback, relaxation techniques, and regular aerobic exercise.[14, 15, 16, 38, 74] Abortive therapy for migraine headaches may include sublingual or inhaled ergotamine tartrate, oral or rectal ergotamine preparations with caffeine (Cafergot) or caffeine and pentobarbital (Cafergot PB), intravenous or intramuscular dihydroergotamine mesylate (D.H.E. 45), oral or injectable sumatriptan succinate (Imitrex), oral rizatriptan benzoate (Maxalt), isometheptene mucate/dichloralphenazone/acetaminophen (Midrin), intranasal lidocaine, nonsteroidal anti-inflammatory agents (NSAIDs), intramuscular analgesics such as meperidine (Demerol), antiemetics such as metoclopramide (Reglan), promethazine hydrochloride (Phenergan) and prochlorperazine (Compazine), and oral or parenteral dexamethasone. Prophylactic therapy for frequent or severe migraine suffers includes beta-blockers such as propranolol (Inderal) and timolol maleate (Blocadren), divalproex sodium (Depakote), ergotamine tartrate/phenobarbital/ belladona combination (Bellergal Spacetabs), methysergide maleate (Sansert), cyproheptadine (Periactin), clonidine (Catapres), monoamine oxidase (MAO) inhibitors, nonsteroidal anti-inflammatory agents, tricyclic antidepressants such as amitriptyline (Elavil) and doxepin (Sinequan), selective serontonin reuptake inhibitors, calcium channel blockers such as verapamil (Isoptin, Calan) and nifedipine (Procardia), danazol, angiotensin-converting enzyme inhibitors, and lithium carbonate. Therapy must be individualized, should begin with the least toxic agents, and should be reviewed on a regular interval with the patient.[5, 16, 17, 19, 20, 36, 40, 65, 74]

Tension-Type Headache

Tension-type headache, previously referred to as muscle contraction or tension headache, is the most common type of headache. It is estimated that up to 70% of all headaches are of this type. The most common cause of tension-type headache is increased muscle contraction caused by anxiety, stress, and depression. Temporal mandibular joint dysfunction, head or cervical trauma, cervical arthritis, inflammatory conditions of the eyes and sinuses, or general eye strain may be the cause of tension-type headache.

Tension-type headache may be classified as episodic or chronic. Episodic headache occurs less than 15 days a month, and chronic headache occurs more than 15 days a month, often on a daily basis. Both episodic and chronic tension-type headache can be further divided into headache with and without pericranial muscle symptoms. Increased contraction and tension of cervical and scalp muscles may result in loss of cervical motion and areas of soft tissue tenderness.[11, 51]

The pain of tension-type headache tends to be continuous, of variable intensity, and may last for weeks, months, or years. There is often a seasonal variation and periods of months or years when there are few or no attacks. The pain is characterized by a mild to moderate, dull, nonthrobbing, steady, aching pain that spreads to both sides of the head and may last for hours to days. It is constant and often described as pressure or band-like. It generally begins in the cervical or occipital areas, and a patient may have a stiff, painful neck. The discomfort tends to increase over the course of the day and is often provoked by fatigue and nervous strain. Other associated symptoms include generalized muscle aching, chronic fatigue, decreased libido, disturbance of memory and concentration, and irritability. These individuals are often depressed, anxious, and suffering from insomnia.[20, 50, 59, 74]

Nonpharmacologic treatment includes use of warm or cold compresses, soft tissue massage, instruction on flexibility, posture, isotonic, and progressive resistance exercises; relaxation techniques such as biofeedback training and stress management; alteration in exercise training schedules; psychosocial counseling; and use of physical therapy modalities such as transcutaneous electrical nerve stimulation and ultrasound.[16, 19, 20, 27, 74] Pharmacologic treatment includes use of mild analgesics such as acetaminophen, NSAIDs, and muscle relaxants. For the severe acute headache attack, the use of oral or parenteral ketorlac (Toradol), tramadol (Ultram), or nasal butorphanol (Stadol NS) may be helpful; however, abuse may occur with the use of tramadol and butorphanol. Butalbital and caffeine-containing compounds such as Fioricet (with acetaminophen) and Fiorinal (with aspirin) should be avoided, as they may lead to rebound headache and can perpetuate ongoing daily pain. Chronic tension-type headache may respond to anxiolytic agents, sedating tricyclic antidepressant medications such as amitriptyline (Elavil) or doxepin (Sinequan), or the serotonin reuptake inhibitors, such as fluoxetine (Prozac) and sertraline (Zoloft). It is also important to treat the depression that is commonly associated with chronic tension-type headache.[16, 17, 19, 50, 59, 74]

Cluster Headache and Chronic Paroxysmal Hemicrania

Cluster headaches occur four times more commonly in men than in women. Attacks usually begin in the second to fourth decades of life. Unlike migraine headaches, there is little hereditary influence. Physical stress, emotional stress, alcohol, and cigarette smoking may trigger cluster headache attacks.[50, 59]

Cluster headaches occur in a series which may last for weeks to months. During a series, the patient may have one to eight acute headaches per day. Fifty percent of the headaches occur at night. Attacks are brief in duration, lasting from 15 minutes to 3 hours; these tend to occur daily for several weeks or months. These clusters are often followed by symptom-free intervals, during which the patient may remain asymptomatic for many years. Cluster headaches are characterized by intense, severe, unilateral pain in the supraorbital, orbital, or temporal area and always occur on the same side during a series. The pain is often described as nonthrobbing, stabbing, deep, boring, burning, or gnawing. Lacrimation, conjunctival injection, unilateral nasal congestion followed by rhinorrhea, forehead and facial diaphoresis, miosis, ptosis, and flushing and edema of the cheek and eyelid often occur during the attack. The patient is typically agitated and restless, unable to lie or sit owing to the excruciating pain. Patients may be suicidal because of the pain, and often awaken at night because of the pain. Ten percent of cluster headache sufferers have chronic symptoms continuing for more than a year without remission, or with remission periods lasting less than 2 weeks.[9, 17, 20, 21, 59, 74]

The use of abortive therapy for cluster headaches must involve an agent that is rapidly effective because the pain generally lasts for a short period of time. Inhalation of 100% oxygen at 5 L/min to 8 L/min, sublingual or rectal ergotamine preparations, parenteral DHE-45, parenteral sumatriptin, intranasal topical 4% lidocaine or capsaicin, and high-dose oral corticosteroids may all be effective abortive treatment. Prophylactic treatment options include the use of methysergide, cyproheptadine, prednisone, calcium channel blockers, lithium carbonate, ergotamine tartrate, and the combination of ergotamine-phenobarbital-belladonna.[9, 16, 17, 35, 74]

Miscellaneous Headaches Unassociated With Structural Lesion

Headaches in this category include stabbing and compression headaches, and headaches associated with cold stimulation, cough, exertion, and sexual activity. A specific headache cannot be diagnosed until systemic diseases, organic cranial and intracranial diseases, and structural lesions have been excluded as a cause. Many of these headache patterns may be related to participation in sports, exercise, and other activities. This section will provide an overview of these headaches, with a further detailed discussion of sports-related headaches provided in the section Headaches Related to Physical Activity, Exercise, and Sports Participation.

Idiopathic Stabbing Headache

Idiopathic stabbing headache, previously termed *ice-pick headache*, refers to brief, sharp, moderate to severe, stabbing pains that occur as single episodes or in brief, repeated volleys. The pain is confined to the head, usually in the first division of the trigeminal nerve, and lasts for a fraction of a second to 10 seconds. Headaches recur at irregular intervals from hours to days, with up to 50 attacks per day. This is likely a vascular phenomenon, as over 40% of migraineurs experience this type of headache compared with only 3% of nonmigraine controls. Many migraineurs experience this headache regularly with their migraine, as a herald to a migraine attack, or with associated scintillating scotomas, acroparesthesias, facial paresthesias, or syncope. Indomethacin 75–150 mg a day is recommended for patients with frequent headache recurrences; propanolol may also be helpful.[11, 34, 51, 60, 61, 66]

External Compression Headache

Continued stimulation of forehead or scalp cutaneous nerves by the application of direct pressure may cause pain in the area of compression. This dull, boring, constant pain is prevented by avoidance of the precipitating cause. Migraine attacks may occur if the external compression is prolonged.[11, 20, 30, 51, 55]

Cold Stimulus Headache

Application of a cold stimulus to the head or ingestion of cold substances may produce

a headache.[11, 28, 37, 52, 66, 72] The first type of cold stimulus headache is due to exposure of the unprotected head to low air temperature or cold water, which produces a generalized, bilateral headache that varies in intensity with the severity and duration of the cold stimulus, and is prevented by avoidance of cold exposure. Because of the rapid development of headache after cold exposure, it has been suggested that this headache is due to a cutaneous sensory response.[28] The second type of cold stimulus headache is due to the passage of a cold solid or liquid over the palate and posterior pharynx, which causes a short-duration headache previously known as ice cream headache. A nonpulsatile, deep-seated pain is produced, which reaches a crescendo 25–60 seconds after exposure and lasts for several seconds to several minutes; it is usually located in the middle forehead, anterior temporal area, orbit, palate, throat, or ear. It occurs more commonly in individuals overheated from exercise or exposed to a hot environment. Ninety percent of migraineurs and 30% of controls experience this headache, suggesting cerebral vasoconstriction as the etiology. Middle cerebral artery flow velocity has been shown to decrease in affected individuals following the application of cold stimulus.[72] The cold stimulus may be anatomically specific in sufferers; ice applied to the roof of the mouth or posterior pharynx causes headache, but ice applied to gastric and esophagus mucosa does not elicit pain. This headache is prevented by avoiding the rapid ingestion of cold food and drink and stirring ice cream to a semisolid consistency.

Benign Cough Headache

Coughing may produce a bilateral headache of sudden onset that resolves in less than 1 minute.[11, 37, 51, 52, 60, 66] Headache is of moderate to high intensity, sharp, bursting, or splitting, and may be located in the temporal, frontal, or occipital areas. Usually there is no headache between attacks; however, some sufferers have a dull headache that may last from minutes to hours. This headache is probably due to increased intracranial pressure; cough increases intrathoracic and intra-abdominal pressure, which decreases right atrial venous return, leading to increased central venous pressure, which is ultimately transmitted to the epidural venous plexus. Headache onset is later in life, usually between age 35 and 77, is four times more common in males, resolves within 2 months to 2 years, and is improved with indomethacin. Ten percent to 65% of cough headaches may be due to serious underlying conditions such as Arnold-Chiari malformation type I, tumor, brain cyst, or basilar impression.[37, 52, 63] These patients tend to be younger, with an average age of 39; report headache associated with laughing, weightlifting, bending over, stooping, and acute head or body position changes; and are not improved with the use of analgesics.

Benign Exertional Headache

This category includes headache due to any form of exercise and accounts for 50% of sports-related headaches in males and 75% of sports-related headaches in females.[80] Numerous different headache patterns have been reported; these different subvarieties are described, which leads to confusion in the literature. By definition, benign exertional headache is brought on specifically by physical exercise, is bilateral and throbbing at onset, lasts from 5 minutes to 24 hours, may cause migraine features in those susceptible to migraine, and is prevented by avoidance of excessive exertion, particularly in hot weather or at high altitude.[11, 51] It typically affects men, is prompt in onset, of moderate to severe intensity, has a rapid peak, and then fades to a dull ache that may persist for hours after the activity. The pain is usually throbbing, variable in location but consistent for each patient, and increased with physical effort or neck movement; nausea and vomiting are rare. The physical examination is normal.

Benign exertional headache has been described in runners, weight lifters, cyclists, swimmers, rugby and hockey players, and aerobics participants.[80] The average age at onset is 24 years, with a frequency between one per day and one every 2 months, appearing for a variable period of time, ranging from 15 days to 10 years.[52] High altitude, hot weather, dehydration, hypoglycemia, poor fitness level, extreme or exhaustive exercise, and alcohol and caffeine use are associated with attacks. The etiology is uncertain; however, it may be similar to benign cough headache, and indeed, some experts describe these conditions together.[60, 66] Proposed mechanisms include increased intrathoracic pressure leading to increased intracranial pressure; external compression of blood vessels by muscle tension; vasodilation or vasoconstriction of cerebral blood vessels; neck muscle tension or strain; neurogenic factors; and a combination of these factors. The most commonly accepted mechanism is increased intrathoracic pressure that causes increased intracranial venous sinus pressure, leading to increased intracranial pressure and decreased cerebral blood flow, resulting in the development of a headache.[3, 18, 19, 33, 34, 37, 46, 50, 53, 58, 76, 80] However, given the various presentations of individuals with benign exertional headaches, it is likely that different mechanisms have a role in causing these attacks. Exertional headache may be prevented by ingestion of indomethacin, ergotamine tartrate, methysergide, and propranolol before exercise.[11, 18, 37, 51, 52, 66] Gradual endurance training, biofeedback techniques, and modification of activity may be helpful.[18, 37, 54]

Exertional headaches are usually benign. In Rooke's[63] series of 103 consecutive patients with exertional headache, 93 had no significant pathology, 30 had complete relief within 5 years, and 73 within 10 years. Of the 10 patients with pathology, there were two tumors, two subdural hematomas, three Arnold-Chiari malformations, and three other lesions. In Sands'[66] review of 219 cases of cough and benign exertional headache, 48 had organic pathology; primarily space-occupying posttrauma or postcraniotomy lesions, or basilar impression. In Pascual's[52] series of 28 patients with exertional headache, 12 had significant pathology, 10 with subarachnoid hemorrhage, 1 with brain metastasis, and 1 due to sinusitis. These patients were older, with an average age of 42 (compared with age 24 in the benign group), had acute severe headache attacks, and often had associated nausea, vomiting, and photophobia. Other causes of symptomatic exertional headache include subdural hematoma, arteriovenous malformation, leaking or vasospasm of cerebral aneurysm, chronic central nervous system infection, pheochromocytoma, myxedema, thyrotoxicosis, Cushing's disease, hypoglycemia, glaucoma, dental abscess, TMJ dysfunction, chronic obstructive pulmonary disease, acute anemia, and anabolic-androgenic steroid use.[18, 37, 60, 74]

Headache Associated With Sexual Activity

Sexual activity may produce three distinct headache patterns, dull-type, explosive-type, and postural-type. These different headache types actually overlap other described headache patterns. This category includes any headache precipitated by masturbation or coitus. Headache usually starts, as sexual excitement increases, as a dull, bilateral ache that suddenly becomes intense at orgasm and is prevented or eased by ceasing sexual activity.[11, 51] Sexual headache is four times more common in males, usually occurs between ages 20 and 60, and has a variable and unpredictable course.[37, 52, 60, 66, 70] Dull-type sexual headache, Type I, affects about 25% of sufferers. It begins early in the course of sexual activity, occurs in the neck and head (usually occipital but may be diffuse), is dull and aching but may be severe and explosive, and increases at orgasm. The headache lasts from less than 1 minute to 3 hours, although it may last for days; it mimics tension-type headache. It may be caused by excessive facial and neck muscle contraction or cerebral vascular alterations.[21, 37, 52, 60, 66, 70, 71] Explosive-type sexual headache, Type II, affects about 70% of sufferers. It occurs at or shortly before orgasm, is frontal or occipital in location, is explosive or throbbing, lasts for a few minutes to a few hours (generally less than 15 minutes), and may be followed by a mild, dull headache lasting up to 48 hours. It appears to be a migraine-like headache. It is probably due to alterations in cerebral vascular blood flow; 25% of patients have a history of migraine headaches, 28% have a family history of migraine headaches, and the headache has been treated successfully with ergotamine tartrate, Bellergal-S, atenolol, propranolol, and indomethacin.[37, 52, 60, 66, 70, 71] Postural-type sexual headache, Type III, occurs after orgasm and resembles a low–cerebrospinal fluid (CSF)-pressure headache. This extremely rare condition is due to a tear in the arachnoid membrane with CSF leak, resulting in decreased CSF pressure. The headache is variable in intensity, increased with upright posture, and may last for weeks or months. Following natural repair of the tear, usually within 2 to 3 weeks, the symptoms resolve.[37, 52, 60, 66, 70, 71] Risk factors for the development of sexual headaches include obesity, hypertension, fatigue, poor physical condition, personal or family history of migraine headaches, and peripheral vascular disease. Potentially serious causes of headache during sexual activity include leaking or vasospasm from cerebral aneurysm, arteriovenous malformation, subarachnoid hemorrhage, peripheral vascular disease, cerebral hemorrhage, meningitis, hydrocephalus, encephalitis, pheochromocytoma, glaucoma, sinusitis, Cushing's disease, myxedema, hypoglycemia, chronic obstructive lung disease, acute anemia, use of oral contraceptives, and recreational drug use.[66]

Headache Associated With Head Trauma

Direct trauma to the head and neck area may lead to the occurrence of headache; this is a common cause of headache in collision and contact sports. Posttraumatic headaches begin within 14 days of the trauma or of regaining consciousness if the athlete lost consciousness. Posttraumatic headaches are classified as acute, if the headache resolves within 8 weeks, and chronic, if the headache lasts longer than 8 weeks. Posttraumatic headaches are further divided into those associated with significant trauma or neurologic findings and those with minor trauma and no neurologic findings.[11, 51]

Significant intracranial injuries may occur as a result of direct trauma during sports participation. Epidural and subdural hemorrhage and hematoma, intracranial artery dissection, cerebral contusion, and severe concussion cause severe headaches and may be fatal. Nausea, vomiting, focal neurologic findings, and mental status changes may be present. CT or MRI scan and prompt neurosurgical consultation are required.[20] Further details of these injuries are discussed in Parts III and IV.

Within the context of acute and chronic posttraumatic headache with minor head trauma, at least six forms have been described (see Table 24–2).[19, 20, 47] These include chronic tension-type headache; migraine; mixed migraine and tension-type headache; dysautonomic headache; second-impact catastrophic headache; and superficial pain at the site of head or skull trauma.

The first posttraumatic headache resembles chronic tension-type headache. The pain is described as a constant, nonthrobbing, dull ache, of variable intensity, in the bifrontal and occipital regions. It is often present upon awakening and tends to worsen later in the day. This should be treated as a chronic tension-type headache. Unfortunately for the athlete, this type of headache may last for months or years.[19, 42]

The second posttraumatic headache is clinically indistinguishable from a migraine headache. Initially described by Matthews[45] as footballer's migraine, head trauma from playing English football or soccer resulted in a player sustaining a migraine with aura. This has been reported in other sports such as American football, basketball, rugby, wrestling, and boxing. Visual disturbances, at times requiring cessation from sports participation, occur within minutes of relatively minor head trauma. Vision complaints usually resolve after a period of 30 minutes to 4 hours and are followed by the onset of a unilateral, throbbing, severe headache that is often retro-orbital. Nausea, vomiting, photophobia, paresthesia, and hemiplegia may occur. The migraine symptoms usually resolve within 24 hours. Many athletes with posttraumatic migraines do not have a personal or family history of migraine. Standard treatment for migraine should be administered; however, prophylaxis has not been consistently effective.[2, 6, 7, 32, 45, 56, 69, 80]

The third type of posttraumatic headache is a mixed headache. This syndrome is characterized by chronic tension-type headache with muscle contraction with superimposed episodic migraine attacks. Routine treatment of migraine and tension-type headache should be instituted to alleviate and control the symptoms.

As described by Vijayan,[78] the fourth type of posttraumatic headache is traumatic dysautonomic cephalgia. This condition may be due to damage to the sympathetic fibers near the carotid vessels in the cervical area. Headache attacks are accompanied by ipsilateral pupillary dilatation and excessive facial diaphoresis. A partial ipsilateral Horner's syndrome with ptosis, meiosis, and excessive perspiration often occurs between attacks. Propranolol is the drug of choice for this condition.

Second-impact catastrophic headache is the fifth type of posttraumatic headache.[67] This rare syndrome occurs after a mild concussion in which the athlete returns to participation before complete resolution of symptoms. Following a second minor blow to the head, the athlete develops rapid cerebral hyperemia with an increase in blood volume in the white matter of the brain. This causes an increase in brain volume, leading to an increase in intracranial pressure, resulting in brain herniation and death. This syndrome may be due to loss of autoregulation of blood flow to the brain. Since it was initially described in 1984, there have been reports of fatal and nonfatal cerebral edema in similar clinical situations. Additionally, Torg[76] described two cases in which youngsters with infectious mononucleosis sustained relatively minor head trauma that caused malignant cerebral edema and death.

The sixth type of posttraumatic headache results in superficial pain and tenderness at the site of trauma. This is perhaps the most common type of posttraumatic headache. Treatment depends on site of injury and may include local measures such as ice and massage, mild analgesics, and protective headgear or facemask.

The athlete suffering from posttraumatic headache requires complete evaluation to detect any underlying organic pathology that may be associated with the injury. CT or MRI scan should be performed if the neurologic examination, including mental status examination, is abnormal; if the headache is not readily categorized; if it is the first posttraumatic migraine; or if there is prolonged loss of consciousness. The athlete with posttraumatic headache may return to competition when significant headache relief has been achieved if there is no exacerbation of the headache with increased activity, and if the neurologic abnormalities are resolved. If brain imaging is normal but minor neurologic complaints persist, it is prudent to withhold the athlete from competition until the symptoms resolve.[19, 20]

Headache Associated With Vascular Disorders

Vascular disorders causing headache include: ischemic cerebrovascular disease such as transient ischemic attack (TIA) and cerebrovascular accident (CVA or stroke); intracranial hematoma; subarachnoid hemorrhage; vascular malformation; arteritis; pain from carotid or vertebral artery disease; venous thrombosis; hypertension; and other vascular disorders.[11, 51] Most of these conditions are uncommon in the young athlete. However, owing to the morbidity and mortality associated with significant bleeding, these conditions must be considered in the athlete and active patient with severe headache and neurologic deficits.

Intracranial Hemorrhage

Intracranial hemorrhage may be traumatic or atraumatic. Traumatic intracranial hemorrhage and hematoma related to sports participation are reviewed in detail in Chapter 13. Atraumatic intracerebral hemorrhage into the brain substance and subarachnoid hemorrhage due to small vessel rupture near the brain surface are usually associated with underlying intracranial pathology such as cerebral aneurysm, arteriovenous malformation (AVM), and malignant hypertension. These conditions occur most commonly in athletes over 35 years of age and may be precipitated by exercise and physical activity.[37, 43, 52, 60, 66] Vascular malformations may slowly leak, causing symptoms that develop insidiously over a period of days to weeks. Many patients experience a sudden, severe headache that lasts for only a few minutes without associated neurologic signs due to a small vascular bleed; this is referred to as a "sentinel headache" and may precede a massive hemorrhage.[16, 37, 60, 66] A large hemorrhage due to traumatic or atraumatic causes will result in a rapid increase in intracranial pressure, with loss of consciousness, collapse, and death. The athlete may present with catastrophic headache, nausea, vomiting, visual changes, photophobia, aphasia, nuchal rigidity, and weakness.[16, 37, 52, 59] While the diagnosis of acute intracerebral hemorrhage is usually quite obvious, CT scan with contrast, MRI scan, MRA scan, angiography, and lumbar puncture may be necessary to confirm and determine the source of the hemorrhage.[20, 37, 52, 60, 66] Because most intracranial hemorrhages occur in older individuals, it may be appropriate to observe the young athlete with a severe headache. If the headache did not begin abruptly or during exertion; if the individual is alert, oriented, and afebrile without nuchal rigidity or neurologic abnormalities; and if the headache is easing, it may be appropriate to follow the athlete closely without extensive workup.[10, 17, 20] However,

immediate neurosurgical evaluation is required of patients with intracerebral hemorrhage.

Hypertension

Headache occurs with equal frequency in hypertensive individuals and age-matched controls. Chronic hypertension, with diastolic blood pressures over 120 mmHg, may cause mild headaches that occur upon awakening and clear with activity.[4] Acute hypertension may lead to headache without causing intracranial hemorrhage.[11, 22, 48, 51] The most common causes of acute severe hypertension are drugs such as amphetamines, cocaine, and monoamine oxidase inhibitors; preeclampsia and eclampsia; neurogenic factors; and pheochromocytoma. Acute hypertensive encephalopathy may lead to multiple focal neurologic deficits, seizure, cerebral edema, obtundation, and death. Aggressive blood pressure reduction is necessary; the drug of choice is intravenous sodium nitroprusside; intravenous nitroglycerin, labetalol, and esmolol may also be used.[22, 48]

Headache Associated With Nonvascular Intracranial Disorder

The class of headaches associated with intracranial disorders unrelated to vascular abnormalities includes high cerebrospinal fluid pressure (CSF) states with intracranial pressure greater than 200 mm water (such as benign intracranial hypertension [previously referred to as pseudotumor cerebri], high-pressure hydrocephalus, or posttraumatic hydrocephalus), low CSF pressure states (such as after lumbar puncture or due to cerebrospinal fluid leak), intracranial infections (such as brain abscess, meningitis, encephalitis, or subdural empyema), intracranial sarcoidosis and other inflammatory disorders, postintrathecal injection headache, intracranial neoplasm, and other disorders.[11, 51]

Intracranial Infection

Intracranial infections may result from hematogenous spread or by extension from surface structures. Bacterial meningitis, infection of the pia and arachnoid mater and CSF, is most commonly caused by *Haemophilus influenzae, Neisseria meningitides, or Streptococcus pneumoniae.* Aseptic meningitis or encephalitis, infection of the meninges, spinal cord, or brain, is usually of viral etiology.[59] Severe headache, nuchal rigidity, delirium, fever, and seizures are common in cases of severe meningitis. If the examination reveals no papilledema or focal neurologic deficits, a lumbar puncture should be performed, and intravenous antibiotic therapy should be initiated. If papilledema or focal neurologic deficits are present, the patient should have a CT scan performed prior to lumbar puncture to evaluate for the presence of brain abscess, subdural empyema, septic emboli, or other masses; it is often prudent to administer empiric antibiotics prior to obtaining the CT scan. Viral encephalitis, which tends to occur in seasonal outbreaks, may be difficult to differentiate from early or partially treated bacterial meningitis. Fever, headache, nuchal rigidity, myalgias, and delirium are common. Lumbar puncture will generally reveal a mononuclear pleocytosis, negative Gram's stain, and negative culture; administration of intravenous antibiotics until culture results are known should be considered.[20] During an encephalitis outbreak, it may be appropriate to observe and symptomatically treat the exposed, infected athlete.[49]

Intracranial Neoplasm

The cranial cavity contains brain tissue, vascular structures, and CSF, all of which are relatively incompressible substances. Brain mass is increased by the presence of an intracranial neoplasm that may alter cerebral blood supply and CSF pressure. Depending on neoplasm type and location, the patient may present with a general decline in neurologic function, signs of increasing intracerebral pressure, or focal neurologic defects.[59] Sixty percent of patients with brain tumor experience headache; 2% to 4% have headache related to physical exertion.[52, 63] Headache in the tumor patient tends to be deep-seated, dull, mild to severe, throbbing, periodic, bifrontal, and occipital; it is usually present upon awakening and awakens the patient during the night. Headache is probably due to a shift in the brain tissue with subsequent traction on pain-sensitive structures.

MRI scan is considered the screening modality of choice for determining the location and extent of the tumor mass; CT scan with enhancement also provides the location of the tumor, shows any calcification, and may be helpful in determining probable diagnosis. Angiography evaluates tumor vascularity and is a guide for presurgical embolization of meningiomas.[10]

Headache Associated With Substances or Their Withdrawal

Headaches associated with the use of medication, alcohol, and tobacco, and illicit drugs are classified as due to acute or chronic use or withdrawal.[11, 51] The headache is often moderate to severe, diffuse, and throbbing.[20] An accurate medical history, physical examination, and appropriate use of laboratory testing will usually allow for an accurate diagnosis. Treatment depends on the cause of the headache, and prevention is by avoidance of the substance. In addition to the headache syndrome, other associated conditions may be diagnosed, including acute intoxication, harmful use, dependency syndrome, withdrawal state, withdrawal state with delirium, psychotic state, amnestic syndrome, residual and late-onset psychotic disorder, and other mental and behavioral disorders; these conditions may require psychiatric evaluation and treatment.[11]

The acute use of or exposure to nitrates and nitrites, monosodium glutamate, carbon monoxide, alcohol, opioids, cannabinoids, sedatives, hypnotics, cocaine, stimulants including caffeine, hallucinogens, tobacco, volatile solvents, or other psychoactive substances may cause an acute headache syndrome. There should be a temporal connection between the onset of headache and substance intake, headache should occur in at least half the exposures and at least three times, and symptoms should resolve when the substance is eliminated. Headache due to nitrite and nitrate exposure should occur within 1 hour of consumption. Headache due to monosodium glutamate occurs within 1 hour of ingestion and is associated with chest pressure; facial pressure or tightness; burning of the chest, shoulder, and neck; facial flushing; dizziness; and abdominal discomfort. Acute alcohol-induced headache occurs within 3 hours of alcohol ingestion. When two or more substances are involved, it may be impossible to determine which are contributing to the headache.[11, 51]

The chronic use of ergotamine preparations, analgesics, NSAIDs, oral contraceptive agents or estrogens, and other substances may actually cause headache. The headache occurs after daily doses of a substance for at least 3 months, occurs at least 15 days per month, and disappears within 1 month after the substance has been withdrawn. Ergotamine-use headache is diffuse, pulsating, and distinguished from migraine by the absence of an attack pattern or associated symptoms. Analgesic abuse headache requires the ingestion of at least 50 grams of aspirin per month or the equivalent, or the ingestion of 100 tablets per month of analgesic combined with barbiturates or nonopioid compounds.[11, 51]

Headache associated with withdrawal from acute substance abuse is most commonly due to alcohol withdrawal (the "hangover"); however, other substances can produce a similar headache syndrome. Withdrawal from chronic use of barbiturates, benzodiazepines, caffeine, ergotamine preparations, narcotics, and other compounds may cause headache. Ergotamine withdrawal headache occurs within 48 hours after cessation of ergotamine intake in a patient who has used ergotamine daily for 3 months. Caffeine withdrawal headache is diagnosed if a headache develops within 24 hours of last caffeine intake that is relieved within 1 hour by the ingestion of 100 mg caffeine, and if the patient has consumed at least 15 g caffeine per month for the preceding 3 months.[11, 51]

Headache Associated With Noncephalic Infection

Headaches due to noncephalic infections are divided into those of viral or bacterial etiology, and those due to other infectious agents. This type of headache is further divided into infections due to a focal, noncephalic location and those due to septicemia. Diagnosis is based on the presence of signs and symptoms of infection and may be confirmed by laboratory and radiographic findings. The headache is a new symptom or a new type of headache that occurs with the onset of the infection and resolves within 1 month after successful treatment or remission of the infection.[11, 51]

Viral syndromes, regardless of the presence of encephalopathy or encephalitis, often present with headache as a constitutional symptom. These headaches tend to be global, throbbing in nature, and relieved with simple analgesics. Low-grade fever, generalized malaise and fatigue, myalgias, and gastrointestinal symptoms are common complaints. The headache of noncephalic bacterial infections may be moderate to severe, diffuse, sharp, stabbing, throbbing, or pressure like. Other symptoms depend on the site of infection, pathogenic organism, and host response. Patients with systemic bacterial infections may be febrile, toxic, hypotensive, and suffer from delirium; aggressive evaluation and treatment are necessary. The reader is referred to other sources for a more detailed discussion.[48, 59]

Headache Associated With Metabolic Disorder

Headache may result from numerous metabolic disorders. Hypoxia, hypercapnia, hyperventilation, respiratory acidosis, hypoglycemia, hypothyroidism, Cushing's disease, Addison's disease, hyperaldosteronism, anemia, and other metabolic abnormalities may cause headache.[11, 20, 51] The headache may be variable; it is often of mild to moderate intensity, diffuse, and throbbing. Headache frequency and intensity correlate with variations in the metabolic disturbance, and headache disappears within 7 days of normalization of the metabolic state. The history and physical examination may detect symptoms and signs of an underlying metabolic disturbance. Appropriate laboratory tests to determine the etiology may include complete blood count, electrolytes, blood glucose level, thyroid studies, cortisol levels, dexamethasone suppression tests, ACTH stimulation tests, and arterial blood gas analysis. CT or MRI scan of the head may be required to exclude other possible serious intracranial lesions.[12, 13, 21–23, 27, 50, 59] Simple analgesics and mild narcotics are generally adequate to control headache pain.

Perhaps the most common headache associated with a metabolic disorder in the athlete is due to acute altitude change. This headache occurs within 24 hours after sudden ascent to altitudes above 3000 m and is associated with Cheyne-Stokes respiration at night, the desire to overbreathe, and exertional dyspnea.[1, 11, 19, 51, 56] This unique syndrome in its benign form results in acute mountain sickness, which is characterized by headache, malaise, nausea, vomiting, insomnia, anorexia, palpitations, dim vision, and anxiety. The headache is usually frontal or generalized, with throbbing in the occipital area, and increases with maneuvers that increase intracerebral pressure, such as reclining, coughing, straining, and physical exertion. The headache varies in intensity and characteristics among different individuals. It does tend to recur in an individual when returning to altitude.[1, 12, 19, 66] High altitude cerebral edema is a severe form of mountain sickness which occurs above 4500 m. After a few days of increasing headache, psychological changes such as memory loss, irritability, delusions, and hallucinations occur. If unrecognized or untreated, truncal ataxia, wide-based gait, stupor, seizures, paralysis, coma, and death may occur. This condition most commonly occurs in individuals who are involved in a strenuous, rapid ascent, who are poorly conditioned, and who neglect or minimize their symptoms.[1, 12, 19, 20, 66] Acute mountain sickness and high altitude cerebral edema appear to be due to hypoxia-induced cerebrovascular vasodilatation causing increased cerebral blood flow, increased CSF pressure, and cerebral edema. Increased P_{CO_2} that occurs during sleep may also cause cerebrovascular vasodilatation, exacerbating the cerebral edema.[1, 12, 19, 66] The headache of mountain sickness may improve with use of mild analgesics, avoidance of exhaustive exercise, and oral intake of cold fluids and carbohydrates. Headache usually resolves within several days with acclimatization; descent may be necessary. The treatment of cerebral edema requires immediate rapid descent to at least 5000 m, oxygen, and corticosteroids; portable hyperbaric bags and positive airway pressure may stabilize the patient in the event that descent is prevented by poor weather, poor planning, or other conditions. These altitude-related disorders may be prevented by the use of acetazolamide (Diamox) 250 mg three times per day for 3 days prior to ascent and continued for 3 days after ascent, and gradual acclimatization.[1, 12, 19, 20, 66]

Headache or Facial Pain Associated With Disorder of Cranium, Neck, Eyes, Ears, Nose, Sinuses, Teeth, Mouth, or Other Facial or Cranial Structures

Headaches due to disorders of anatomic structures in the head (skull, eyes, ears, nose, sinuses, throat, teeth, jaw, and temporomandibular joint) and neck are included in this category. Headache is localized to the affected structure and often radiates to adjacent tissues. Headaches due to these conditions disappear within 1 month of successful treatment or with remission of the underlying disorder.[11, 51] Any extracranial tissue infection may cause a headache that is usually localized and may be sharp, stabbing, throbbing, or pressure-like; associated symptoms depend on the source of infection. Extracranial tissue abscesses are uncommon but will present with local tenderness, erythema, warmth, swelling, induration, and low-grade fever; treatment includes antibiotics and incision and drainage.[20]

Except for osteomyelitis, multiple myeloma, and Paget's disease of the skull, most disorders of the cranium do not cause headache. Cervical spine anomalies, arthritis, fracture, tumor, and other disorders may cause cervical and occipital pain that radiates to the forehead, orbits, temples, and vertex and is precipitated by neck position and movement. Active and passive neck movements are limited, and the patient has neck muscle tenderness. Retropharyngeal tendinitis causes uni- or bilateral posterior neck and head pain that is aggravated by neck extension, is associated with retropharyngeal soft tissue swelling, and resolves with NSAID therapy. Eye disorders such as glaucoma, refractive errors or improper corrective lenses, heterophoria, or heterotropia may cause mild to moderate frontal headache with pain in, behind, or above the eyes. Ear disorders such as otitis externa, otitis media, auricular hematoma, eustachian tube dysfunction, and mastoiditis cause various headache patterns with associated ear symptoms and physical findings. The most common nasal disorder causing headache is acute sinusitis. True sinus headache is uncommon; most of these patients actually experience tension-type or migraine headaches. In the case of acute purulent sinusitis, patients will usually present with abrupt onset of severe headache localized to the area of the infected sinus. The patient appears ill, is febrile, and has purulent nasal drainage with tenderness to palpation in the frontal or maxillary areas. Diagnosis can be confirmed by transillumination, paranasal sinus radiographs that show mucosal thickening and air fluid levels, or limited CT scan through the sinuses that clearly delineates these abnormalities. Treatment includes local compresses, analgesics, antibiotics, decongestants, and possible referral to an otolaryngologist for further evaluation. Untreated acute sinusitis may result in meningoencephalitis, brain abscess, empyema, or septic intracranial venous thrombosis; more extensive investigations, including CT scan and lumbar puncture, may be required to make these diagnoses.[20, 24, 48] Chronic sinusitis does not cause headache unless acute relapse occurs. Tooth disorders may cause facial pain, referred pain, and diffuse headache. Periodontitis and pericoronitis around embedded and impacted wisdom teeth are common causes of headache. Dental abscesses are also common and cause localized, dull, throbbing pain. These dental diagnoses are confirmed with radiographs and are treated with antibiotics and dental referral. Temporomandibular joint (TMJ) dysfunction may cause a local or generalized headache or mild to moderate intensity. Jaw motion is painful, limited, and associated with crepitus and tenderness of the TMJ.

Cranial Neuralgias, Nerve Trunk Pain, and Deafferentation Pain

Headache syndromes that are due to cranial and upper cervical nerve disorders are included in this category. Any condition that results in compression, distortion, demyelination, inflammation, infarction, or other insult to cranial or cervical nerves may produce a specific headache syndrome. Additionally, central lesions may cause head and facial pain. Headache pain due to nerve lesions is typically located in the anatomic distribution of the affected nerve. Headache is often precipitated by maneuvers that use the innervated muscles or put stress on the specific nerve, such as chewing, swallowing, eating, talking, yawning, coughing,

voice straining, face washing, teeth cleansing, and sudden head turning. Pain may be of mild to severe intensity; it is often sudden, superficial, sharp, stabbing, or burning. Pain may be seconds to minutes to hours in duration, intermittent or constant, and associated with paralysis. The affected nerve is often tender to palpation. The duration of symptoms and treatment depends on the underlying etiology; local or systemic corticosteroids are prescribed for many of these conditions.[19, 20, 67]

Headache not Classifiable

Headaches that cannot be classified using published criteria are placed in this category.

HEADACHES RELATED TO PHYSICAL ACTIVITY, EXERCISE, AND SPORTS PARTICIPATION

Based on the IHS headache classification system, headaches related to physical activity, exercise, and sports participation are often difficult to classify. Moreover, these headaches may meet criteria for one or more diagnosis. Because the pathophysiology of many headaches has not been established, different headache presentations and patterns may actually represent the same disease process. Earlier reports suggested that acute mountain sickness and benign exertional headache were of the same etiology.[13, 44] Benign cough headache and benign exertional headache have been proposed as having the same pathophysiology.[18, 19, 31, 33, 37, 47, 52, 60, 66, 70, 71, 80] All three types of headaches associated with sexual activity have proposed mechanisms that are similar to other headache patterns.[21, 37, 52, 60, 66, 70, 71] Some authors have described short-duration benign exertional headache and prolonged benign exertional headache as a continuum of disease state, while others describe these as different disorders.[11, 18, 19, 37, 51, 66, 70, 80] Even migraine headache and tension-type headache are viewed by some as representing different manifestations of the same pathophysiology, whereas others believe these conditions are entirely unrelated.

Historically, many authors have described headache syndromes related to a specific activity or exercise and named the headache after the activity with which it was associated.[1, 7, 12, 13, 21, 29, 30, 44, 53–55, 58, 64, 76] These headaches have been referred to as benign exertional or effort-induced headaches and have also been referred to by the specific activity that caused the headache, such as swimmer's migraine[29] or weight lifter's cephalgia.[58] It is apparent when reviewing activity-related headaches that there have been numerous presentations reported since Tinel's initial description of cough headache in 1932.[20] Headaches related to sports trauma have been easier to classify, and are discussed in further detail in the previous section, Headache Associated With Head Trauma.

Williams[80] attempted to organize sports headaches into four major categories using the IHS classification system, differentiating traumatic from nontraumatic headache, and migraine from nonmigraine headache. Thus, the categories of sport and exercise headache are effort migraine, trauma-triggered migraine, effort-exertion headache, and posttraumatic headache. Of the 129 sports-related headaches in this series, 9% were effort migraines, 6% were trauma-triggered migraines, 63% were effort-exertion headaches, and 22% were posttraumatic headaches. Unfortunately, effort-exertion headaches were further divided into acute exertion headache (lasting seconds or minutes) and gradual effort headache (lasting over 1 hour), which implies different etiology and treatment. The remainder of this chapter focuses on specific headaches related to exercise and activity.

Exertional Headache

Exertional headache, which by IHS definition includes any headache due to any form of exercise or activity, is included in the category of benign exertional headache. See the section, Miscellaneous Headaches Unassociated With Structural Lesion. This is the most common headache related to activity. The headache is prompt in onset, has a rapid peak, and then resolves within a few minutes. It may be followed by a dull ache that may last for hours after the activity. Pain is usually moderate to severe, bilateral and throbbing at onset, variable in location but often in the cervical or occipital area, consistent in location for each patient,

and increased with physical effort or neck movement. This headache pattern may be isolated or may recur for many years. Numerous etiologic mechanisms have been proposed, the most commonly accepted being increased intrathoracic pressure from Valsalva maneuver causing increased intracranial venous sinus pressure leading to increased intracranial pressure and decreased cerebral blood flow, resulting in the development of a headache.[3, 19, 33, 34, 37, 38, 46, 50, 53, 58, 60, 66, 80] This headache has been reported in runners, weight lifters, cyclists, swimmers, rugby and hockey players, aerobics participants, and other athletes exercising at high intensity. The physical examination is normal, but a CT or MRI scan may be required to rule out intracranial pathology. Indomethacin, 50 mg three times per day, has been found to be quite beneficial; however, activity modification may be necessary.[16, 18, 31, 33, 37, 54, 58, 66]

Effort Headache

Effort headache, which develops gradually after prolonged low-intensity exercise, is part of the benign exertional headache category of the IHS classification. See Miscellaneous Headaches Unassociated With Structural Lesion. This headache is of moderate intensity, throbbing or aching, unilateral or bilateral, and may last for hours. It may be vascular in origin, as the patient often has associated nausea, visual disturbances, and neurologic changes. This headache is commonly seen in poorly conditioned athletes and is also associated with high altitude, excessive heat load, dehydration, hypoglycemia, poor acclimatization, and alcohol and caffeine use. Physical examination is generally unremarkable; CT or MRI scan may be necessary, however, to rule out significant organic pathology. Treatment consists of NSAIDs, a general conditioning program, and avoidance of the causative factors.[19, 37, 44, 60, 66, 80]

Acute Effort Migraine

Athletes involved in short, intense, maximal exertion activity may develop a migraine syndrome referred to as acute effort migraine. These headaches are often severe but brief, and may be associated with caffeine use, poor nutrition, dehydration, heat load, hypoglycemia, and the use of alcohol. Most sufferers have a personal or family history of migraine. Exertional migraines have been reported in weight lifters, runners, cyclists, hockey players, and swimmers.[13, 14, 19, 29, 34, 44, 55, 80] Additionally, migraine prodrome without headache has been reported in runners.[75] The exact mechanism of effort migraine is uncertain, but the headache may be due to Valsalva maneuver causing increased intracranial pressure and decreased cerebral blood flow, or to hyperventilation causing decreased cerebral P_{CO_2}, leading to vasoconstriction; decreased cerebral blood flow causes the migraine aura, which is then followed by vasodilatation and headache. The evaluation and treatment of this type of headache should be identical to any other patient with a migraine headache. Improved overall physical conditioning and a gradual warm-up period may be beneficial in the prevention of exercise-induced migraine.[14, 15, 38, 59]

Weight Lifter's Headache

Weight lifter's headache was initially reported in an individual doing leg press exercises who had only recently begun a weightlifting program.[58] The headache was described as severe and explosive, and the patient also reported explosive-type sexual headache; thus, it appears that this description better fits the exertional headache category. Paulson first described the more common headache pattern associated with trained athletes involved in intense weightlifting.[53] Maximal exertion during weightlifting may lead to abrupt onset of intense, severe pain that begins in the occipital and upper cervical region and extends into the parietal areas. The pain is described as steady, burning, or boring; it gradually subsides, leaving a residual aching type of headache that may last days or weeks. Nausea, vomiting, and neurologic signs are absent. This headache is believed to be due to stretching or forceful contraction of the pericranial soft tissues, with the development of a tension-type headache. It may be due to Valsalva maneuver causing venous obstruction, leading to increased intracranial pressure, which would make this condition a variant of exertional headache.[3, 19, 33, 37, 46, 50, 53, 58, 60, 66, 70, 80] Examination may reveal

cervical spasm; cervical spine radiographs, CT or MRI scan, and lumbar puncture may be required for evaluation. Treatment includes cryotherapy, indomethacin, naproxen or other NSAIDs, relative rest, and cervical muscle rehabilitation.[16, 18, 20, 58, 74]

Water-skier's Headache

Exertional headache has been described in experienced, aggressive water-skiers.[31] Water-skiers who pull hard across the wake on a slalom ski have reported the sudden onset of headache. It is suggested that the increased trunk and upper- and lower-extremity muscle contraction necessary to perform this activity, coupled with Valsalva maneuver, is the cause of these headaches. Two different headache patterns have been reported. The first pattern is similar to the weight lifter's headache. The pain is sudden in onset, bilateral, diffuse, intense, and throbbing, lasting for about 1 hour; this has been followed by 6 weeks of nearly daily, less severe headaches related to mild exercise and activity. The second pattern results in the sudden onset of unilateral, throbbing pain with associated vision disturbances, nausea, and lightheadedness; this may be followed by several days or weeks of dull, unilateral headache aggravated by exertion. Physical examination is usually normal; CT or MRI scan should be performed to evaluate for intracranial pathology. Relative rest and NSAIDs are recommended until headaches resolve, which is usually within 3 months. It has been suggested that a trial of ergot alkaloids, beta blockers, or calcium channel blockers be used for the athlete with frequent or resistant headaches.[31] The etiology of this headache is probably similar to that of weight lifter's headache, that is, stretching or forceful contraction of the pericranial soft tissues, with the development of a tension-type headache, or Valsalva maneuver causing venous obstruction, leading to increased intracranial pressure. These headaches may also represent other variations of exertional or effort headache, acute effort migraine, or cervical neuralgia.

Luger's Headache

Luge participation may produce a headache syndrome similar to weight lifter's headache. The athletes describe a bilateral, throbbing or constant, mild to severe headache that may last for minutes to days. The symptoms are more frequent and worse early in the training season and exacerbated by fast and rough tracks. Treatment and prevention may include cervical muscle strengthening exercises, moist heat, cryotherapy, soft tissue massage, NSAIDs, and use of a cervical brace. This headache is likely due to cervical muscle contraction; other theories include vascular etiology exacerbated by the high altitude where luge runs are located, and enhancement or diminution of the monoamine transmission pathway.[46, 50, 64]

Altitude Headaches

Any athlete exposed to acute altitude change may suffer from headache as part of the syndrome known as acute mountain sickness. See the section Headache Associated With Metabolic Disorder. This headache occurs 6 to 96 hours after exposure to 3500 m of elevation in unacclimatized individuals. It is characterized by a mild throbbing, frontal or generalized headache that increases with maneuvers that increase intracerebral pressure, and is accompanied by malaise, nausea, vomiting, insomnia, and anorexia. Gradual acclimatization, analgesics, fluids, carbohydrates, and rest are helpful; the use of acetazolamide for 3 days prior to and after ascent may prevent this syndrome. High altitude cerebral edema is a severe form of mountain sickness characterized by increasing headache and progressive neurologic deterioration that may lead to coma and death if unrecognized or untreated. Treatment requires immediate rapid descent, oxygen, and corticosteroids.

Ischemic Headache

Cardiac cephalgia, or walk headache, is an activity-related headache that is a manifestation of ischemic heart disease. This headache has been reported primarily in males in the fifth and sixth decades of life who report headache related to physical exertion; some had previously documented coronary vessel disease and surgical intervention.[7, 39, 41, 76] Based on the IHS criteria, this would be classified as *6.9 Headache*

associated with other vascular disorder[11, 51]; however, some authors include it in *4.0 Miscellaneous headache unassociated with structural lesion.*[41] Patients have no or minimal cardiac symptoms, but do have headache associated with ST segment depression and reversible perfusion defects during stress thallium electrocardiogram (ECG) testing. The headache may be mild to severe, unilateral or bilateral, sharp shooting or squeezing in nature. While the headache presentation may be quite variable, it is consistent within the individual during exercise. Resolution of symptoms and ECG changes occur following rest; good long-term success has been reported with the use of isosorbide dinitrate, nitroglycerin, diltiazem, nifedipine, angioplasty, and coronary artery bypass grafting.[41] The actual cause of headache in these patients is uncertain, but a number of theories have been postulated.[39, 41] First, the cervical and thoracic ganglia supply cardiac sympathetic fibers and structures of the eye, face, neck, and cerebrovasculature; thus, headache may be referred pain. Second, cardiac ischemia decreases cardiac output, which increases left ventricular and right atrial pressure, which in turn causes a decrease in venous return from the brain, leading to increased intracranial pressure and headache. Third, cardiac ischemia may cause the release of pain mediators such as serotonin, bradykinin, histamine, or substance P, which act on brain pain-sensitive structures, or vasodilators such as atrial natriuretic protein or brain natriuretic protein, which produce headache by cerebrovasculature dilation.

Swimmer's, Diver's, and Surfer's Headaches

There are numerous types of headaches described in athletes participating in water sports. Headache diagnoses specific to this group of athletes are generally evident with a thorough history and physical examination. Recognition of these headaches is necessary, as most are improved or prevented by correction of the underlying cause.[19, 20]

Swimming is a sport frequently reported as causing exertional headache, effort headache, and acute effort migraine. Swimmers may suffer from goggle headache, which presents with facial and temporal pain due to a tight mask compressing the supraorbital and supratrochlear nerves.[30] Tight goggles may also cause goggle migraine, which may present with a reversible full homonymous hemianopsia.[55] Loosening and periodic adjustment of the goggles generally will prevent goggle-induced headaches. The use of tight eyewear, headgear, or helmets during other sports activities may produce similar headache patterns.[74]

A variety of different headache patterns have been reported in scuba divers.[19, 20, 74] Divers who practice skip breathing gradually develop hypercapnia, which leads to cerebral vasodilatation. This vasodilatation produces a mild to moderate, diffuse, throbbing vascular type of headache. Dental caries and chronic sinusitis may lead to severe sinus headaches due to the change in barometric pressure. The tight facemask and increased pressure resulting from deeper dives may produce the goggle headache and goggle migraine reported in swimmers. A tension-type headache may be caused by the strain of facial and cervical muscle contraction associated with gripping the mouthpiece. Divers may also suffer from TMJ dysfunction headache from use of the mouthpiece. The patient will have a dull, boring, throbbing temporal headache with pain, tenderness, and crepitus of the TMJ joint. Any athlete wearing a poorly fitted mouth guard may experience this headache pattern; use of a frequently replaced, custom mouth guard is recommended.

Winter surfers report a specific, moderate to severe, nauseating frontal headache of 20 to 30 seconds duration that occurs within seconds of diving through a cold, breaking wave.[28] Exposure of the face to the cold water probably causes a cutaneous sensory response that leads to the development of this headache pattern. Any swimmer or diver whose face is exposed to cold water may experience this phenomenon. See the section on Cold Stimulus Headache under Miscellaneous Headaches Unassociated With Structural Lesion.

Racquet Sports Headache

A specific headache pattern caused by participation in tennis, squash, or other racquet sports has been described.[26] Athletes participating in aggressive racquet sports may develop a continuous, moderate to severe, occipital, or generalized headache 6 to 12 hours after the activity. The headache is relieved by lying down and increased by sitting or standing, and may be associated with concomitant or delayed onset of diplopia. Patients have very low CSF pressure (0–25 mm H_2O), which increases in the sitting position. The headache resolves with conservative management within 6 weeks. It is postulated that repetitive brachial plexus traction during participation disrupts nerve root sleeves, leading to a transitory CSF leak and gradual decrease in CSF pressure; concomitant dehydration from exercise would further decrease CSF pressure.[26] Racquet sport headache is similar in presentation to headache related to low CSF pressure states, such as headache after lumbar puncture or due to CSF leak; see the section Headache Associated With Nonvascular Intracranial Disorder.

Roller Coaster Headache

Roller coaster riding has been associated with a number of headache syndromes due to structural injuries.[8, 25, 68] Subdural hematoma may result from riding roller coasters, especially those with sudden rotational direction changes and those that swing riders upside down. Patients will usually present with weeks to months of moderate to severe, constant, generalized headache that developed after riding a roller coaster. Headache is often worse with sitting, standing, and head shaking, and in the morning, and improved with lying down. Nausea, vomiting, photophobia, hearing loss, vertigo, and other neurologic symptoms may be present; an acute rebleed may be associated with sudden neurologic deterioration. CT or MRI scan will confirm the diagnosis. Treatment may be conservative or surgical and is determined by the neurologic status of the patient. Roller coaster riding applies sudden rotational, positional, and acceleration forces to the head. Subdural hematoma then results from these tensile and shearing stresses, which rupture bridging veins that connect the pia and dura mater or tear small cortical arterial vessels.[8, 25] Carotid artery dissection, vertebral artery dissection, subarachnoid hemorrhage, and cerebral thromboembolic events have also been associated with roller coaster riding.[25, 68]

Roller coaster riding has also been associated with headache related to intracranial hypotension due to a CSF leak; this syndrome has been reported in white-water rafters, jet skiers, volleyball players, and weight lifters.[68] Patients may present with moderate to severe headache exacerbated in the upright position and improved by lying down; nausea, vomiting, photophobia, and paravertebral pain may be present. Physical examination and CT scan are usually normal. MRI scan may reveal diffuse meningeal enhancement, decreased volume of prepontine cistern, flattening of the pons, and low-lying cerebellar tonsils.[68] Lumbar puncture opening pressure is low, suggestive of a CSF leak, and myelography may define the actual site of CSF leakage. Most leaks occur from a meningeal diverticulum or from a simple tear and are usually located in the cervical or thoracic spine. Treatment includes analgesics and rest; an epidural blood patch may be considered. Symptoms resolve when the dural tear heals, usually within 2 to 3 months. This type of roller coaster headache is similar in presentation to headache related to low CSF pressure states, such as headache after lumbar puncture or due to CSF leak; see Headache Associated With Nonvascular Intracranial Disorder.

Sexual Activity Headache

Three distinct patterns of headache are associated with sexual activity; dull or tension-type headache, explosive or migraine-like headache, and postural or low CSF pressure headache. See Miscellaneous Headaches Unassociated With Structural Lesion; Headache Associated With Sexual Activity.

Cervical Neuralgia

Headaches as a result of traumatic injuries to cervical nerves have been reported in a number of sports.[57, 67] The athlete presents with a continuous, fluctuating, dull, boring, unilateral, or bilateral headache in the cervical region that spreads to the occipital, parietal, and frontal areas. A history of forceful neck and shoulder extension is usually elicited. Pain is aggravated by sudden head and neck movements, head positioning, and neck extension; nausea, vomiting, dizziness, photophobia, blurred vision, and swal-

lowing difficulties may be present. Restricted cervical motion and nuchal and occipital tenderness are present; a positive Tinel sign may be present. Cervical radiographs, CT and MRI scans are normal. Occipital neuralgia is due to irritation of the C2 nerve, which pierces the semispinalis and trapezius muscles to supply sensation to the posterior scalp. The pathophysiology is uncertain, but the headache is likely caused by entrapment of the occipital nerve as it exits the spine or in the suboccipital region as it courses through the musculature.[67] Other cervical nerves may be involved. Treatment options include rest, ice, NSAIDs, carbamazepine, phenytoin, and surgical neurolysis. Injection of a local anesthetic with a corticosteroid preparation may be diagnostic and therapeutic.[62]

Although the review of headache syndromes in this section reinforces the fact that most headaches related to physical activity, exercise, and sports participation are benign, it also emphasizes the fact that the athlete with an activity-related headache must undergo careful evaluation to exclude organic disease. Once organic pathology has been excluded, an individualized therapeutic program can be initiated.

References

1. Appenzeller O. Altitude headaches. Headache 1972;12:121–129.
2. Ashworth B. Migraine, head trauma and sport. Scott Med J 1985;30:240–242.
3. Basoglu T, Ozbenli T, Bernay I, et al. Demonstration of frontal hypoperfusion in benign exertional headache by technetium-99m-HMPAO SPECT. J Nucl Med 1996;37:1172–1174.
4. Badran RH, Alir RJ, McGuiness JB. Hypertension and headaches. Scott Med J 1970;15:4851.
5. Bender WI. ACE inhibitors for prophylaxis of migraine headache. Headache 1995;35:470–471.
6. Bennett DR, Fuenning SI, Sullivan G, et al. Migraine precipitated by head trauma in athletes. Am J Sports Med 1980;8:202–205.
7. Blacky RA, Rittelmeyer JT, Wallace MR. Headache angina. Am J Cardiol 1987;60:730.
8. Bo-Abbas Y, Bolton CF. Roller-coaster headache. N Engl J Med 1995;32:1585.
9. Bracker MD, Rothrock JF. Cluster headaches among athletes. Phys Sportsmed 1989;17:147–158.
10. Cacayorian ED, Petro GR, Hochhauser L, et al. Headaches in the athlete and radiographic evaluation. Clin Sports Med 1987;6:739–749.
11. Olesen J, Göbel F (eds). ICD-10 Guide for Headaches. Cephalalgia 1997;17:1–82.
12. Clarke C. High altitude cerebral oedema. Int J Sports Med 1988;9:170–174.
13. Dalessio DJ. Effort migraine. Headache 1974;14:53.

14. Darling M. Exercise and migraine, a critical review. J Sports Med Phys Fitness 1991;31:294–302.

15. Darling M. The use of exercise as a method of aborting migraine. Headache 1991;31:616–618.

16. Diamond S. Exercise and headaches: When pain hinders athletic gain. Phys Sportsmed 1991;19:78–86.

17. Diamond S. Treating athletes who have posttraumatic headaches. Phys Sportsmed 1992;20:166–168.

18. Diamond S, Medina JL. Prolonged benign exertional headache: Clinical characteristics and response to indomethacin. Adv Neurol 1982;33:145–149.

19. Diamond S, Solomon GD, Freitag FG. Headache in sports. In Jordan BC, Tsairis P, Warren RF (eds): Sports Neurology. Rockville, MD, Aspen Publishers, 1989, pp 127–132.

20. Dimeff RJ. Headaches in the athlete. Clin Sports Med 1992;11:339–350.

21. Edis RH, Silbert PL. Sequential benign sexual headache and exertional headache. Lancet 1988;1:993.

22. Edmeads J. The worst headache ever: 1. Ominous causes. Postgrad Med 1989;86:93–104.

23. Edmeads J. The worst headache ever: 2. Innocuous causes. Postgrad Med 1989;86:107–110.

24. Fauci AS, Braunwald E, Isselbacher KJ, et al. (eds). Harrison's Principles of Internal Medicine, 14th ed. New York, McGraw-Hill, 1998, pp 749–1227.

25. Fernandes CM, Daya MR. A roller coaster headache: Case report. J Trauma 1994;37:1007–1010.

26. Garcia-Albea E, Cabrera F, Tejeiro J, et al. Delayed postexertional headache, intracranial hypotension and racket sports. J Neurol Neurosurg Psychiatry 1992;55:975.

27. Hammill JM, Bood TM, Rosecrance JC. Effectiveness of physical therapy regimen in the treatment of tension-type headache. Headache 1996;36:149–153.

28. Harries M. Ice cream headache occurred during surfing in winter. BMJ 1997;315:609.

29. Indo T, Takahaski A. Swimmer's migraine. Headache 1990;30:485–487.

30. Jacobson RL. More "goggle headache": Supraorbital neuralgia. N Engl J Med 1983;308:1363.

31. Joy EA, Belgrade MJ. Exertional headache. Phys Sportsmed 1993;21:94–100.

32. Kalenak A, Petro DJ, Brennan RW. Migraine secondary to head trauma in wrestling: A case report. Am J Sports Med 1978;6:112–113.

33. Katchen MS. Exertional headaches with multiple triggers. Aviat Space Environ Med 1990;61:49–51.

34. Kinsella FP. Exercise induced migraine. Ir Med J 1990;83:126.

35. Kudrow L. Response of cluster headache to oxygen inhalation. Headache 1981;21:1–4.

36. Kudrow L, Kudrow DB, Sandweiss MA. Rapid and sustained relief of migraine headache attacks with intranasal lidocaine: Preliminary findings. Headache 1995;35:79–82.

37. Kumar KL, Reuler JB. Uncommon headaches: Diagnosis and treatment. Gen Intern Med 1993;86:333–341.

38. Lambert RW, Burnet DL. Prevention of exercise induced migraine by quantitative warm-up. Headache 1985;25:317–319.

39. Lance JW, Lambros J. Unilateral exertional headache as a symptom of cardiac ischemia. Headache 1998;38:315–316.

40. Landy SH. Divalproex sodium for migraine prevention. Natl Headache Found Headlines 1998;106:3.

41. Lipton RB, Lowenkopf T, Bajwa ZH, et al. Cardiac cephalgia: A treatable form of exertional headache. Neurology 1997;49:813–816.

42. Lombardo JA, McKeag DB. Football player with a persistent headache. Phys Sportsmed 1987;15:75–79.

43. Mandy LM, L'Ecuyer PB. Treatment of infectious diseases. In Carey CC, Lee HH, Woeltje KF (eds): The Washington Manual of Medical Therapeutics, 29th ed. Philadelphia, Lippincott-Raven, 1998, pp 260–287.

44. Massey EW. Effort headache in runners. Headache 1982;22:99–100.

45. Matthews WB. Footballer's migraine. BMJ 1972;2:326–327.

46. McCarthy P. Athletes' headaches: Not necessarily "little" problems. Phys Sportsmed 1988;16:169–173.

47. McCrory P: Recognizing exercise-related headache. Phys Sportsmed 1997;25:33–43.

48. McKenzie CR. Hypertension. In Carey CC, Lee HH, Woeltje KF (eds): The Washington Manual of Medical Therapeutics, 29th ed. Philadelphia, Lippincott-Raven, 1998, pp 61–80.

49. Moore M, Baron FC, Filstein MR, et al. Aseptic meningitis in high school football players. 1978 and 1980. JAMA 1983;244:2039–2043.

50. Mullally WJ. Headache in winter sports: Benign exertional headache. In Casey MJ, Foster C, Hixson E (eds): Winter Sports Medicine. Philadelphia, F.A. Davis, 1990, pp 167–175.

51. Olesen J, Lance JW. Classification and diagnostic criteria for headache disorders, cranial neuralgias, and facial pain by the Headache Classification Committee of the International Headache Society. Cephalalagia, 1988;8(Suppl 7):9–96.

52. Pascual J, Ilgesias F, Oterino A, et al. Cough, exertional, and sexual headaches: An anlysis of 72 benign and symptomatic cases. Neurology 1996;46:1520–1524.

53. Paulson GW. Weightlifters headache. Headache 1983;23:193–194.

54. Perry WJ. Exertional headache. Phys Sportsmed 1985;10:95–99.

55. Pestronk A, Pestronk S. Goggle migraine [letter to the editor]. N Engl J Med 1983;308:226–227.

56. Plager DA, Purvin V. Migraine precipitated by head trauma in athletes. Am J Ophthalmol 1996;122:277–278.

57. Pollman W, Keidel M, Pfaffenrath V, et al. Headache and the cervical spine: A critical review. Cephalalgia 1997;17:801–816.

58. Powell B. Weight lifter's cephalalgia. Ann Emerg Med 1982;11:449–451.

59. Raskin NH. Headache. In Fauci AS, Braunwald E, Isselbacher KJ, et al (eds): Harrison's Principles of Internal Medicine, 14th ed. New York, McGraw-Hill, 1998, pp 68–72.

60. Raskin NH. Short-lived head pains. Neurol Clin 1997;15:143–152.

61. Raskin NH, Schwartz RJ. Icepick-like pain. Neurology 1980;30:203.

62. Rifat SF, Lombardo JA. Occipital neuralgia in a football player: A case report. Clin J Sports Med 1995;5:251–253.

63. Rooke ED. Benign exertional headache. Med Clin North Am 1968;52:801–809.

64. Roos R. Luge participation is hard on the head. Phys Sportsmed 1986;14:185–188.
65. Ryan RE. Maxalt, the newest drug for migraine treatment. Natl Headache Found Headlines 1998;106:1–2.
66. Sands GH, Newman L, Lipton R. Cough, exertional and other miscellaneous headaches. Med Clin North Am 1991;75:733–747.
67. Saunders RL, Harbaugh RE. The second impact in catastrophic contact sports head trauma. JAMA 1984;252:538–539.
68. Schievink WI, Ebersold MJ, Atkinson JL. Roller-coaster headache due to spinal cerebrospinal fluid leak. Lancet 1996;347:1409.
69. Shadel RF, Puffer JC. Managing traumatic headaches in a football player. Phys Sportsmed 1989;18(8):81–84.
70. Silbert PL, Edis RH, Stewart-Wynne EG, et al. Benign vascular sexual headache and exertional headache: Interrelationships and long term prognosis. J Neurol Neurosurg Psychiatry 1991;54:417–421.
71. Silbert PL, Prentice DA, Hankey GJ, et al. Angiographically demonstrated arterial spasm in a case of benign sexual headache and benign exertional headache. Aust N Z J Med 1989;19:466–468.
72. Sleigh JW. Ice cream headache: Cerebral vasoconstriction causing decrease in arterial flow may have a role. BMJ 1997;315:609.
73. Stewart WF, Lipton RB, Celentano DD, et al. Prevalence of migraine headaches in the United States. Relation to age, income, race, and other sociodemographic factors. JAMA 1992;267:64–69.
74. Swain RA, Kaplan B. Diagnosis, prophylaxis, and treatment of headaches in the athlete. South Med J 1997;90:878–888.
75. Thompson JK. Exercise-induced migraine prodrome syndrome. Headache 1987;27:250–251.
76. Torg JS, Beer LA, Begso J. Head trauma in football players with infectious mononucleosis. Phys Sportsmed 1980;8:107–110.
77. Vernay D, Deffond D, Fraysse P, et al. Walk headache: An unusual manifestation of ischemic heart disease. Headache 1989;29:350–351.
78. Vijayan N. A new posttraumatic headache syndrome, clinical and therapeutic observations. Headache 1977;17:19–22.
79. Williams SJ, Nukada H. Sport and exercise headache: Part 1. Prevalence among university students. Br J Sports Med 1994;28:90–95.
80. Williams SJ, Nukada H. Sport and exercise headache: Part 2. Diagnosis and classification. Br J Sports Med 1994;28:96–100.

SPORT-SPECIFIC CONCERNS

Fatalities from Brain and Cervical Spine Injuries in Tackle Football: 54 Years' Experience

Frederick O. Mueller

The purpose of this chapter is to discuss the etiology of football brain and cervical spine fatalities that have occurred in the United States since 1945. Historical information and a review of the related literature are presented in order to show the evolution of football and its association with fatalities to participants.

Fifty-four years of data collection, 1945–1998, point out the incidence of football brain and cervical spine fatalities. In addition to incidence of injury, the data also reveal the type of injury, activity at time of injury, level of play (e.g., college, high school), and whether the injury was incurred in a game or at practice (Tables 25–1—25–7).

On establishing the incidence and etiology of brain and cervical spine fatalities from 1945 through 1998, the data are divided into 10-year spans of time (with the

This research was supported by the American Football Coaches Association, the National Collegiate Athletic Association, the National Federation of State High School Associations, and the University of North Carolina at Chapel Hill.

exception of 1995–1998) and concentrate on the variables that have either increased or decreased fatalities. The chapter concludes with a discussion of the major preventive measures that have been given credit for the reduction of brain and cervical spine

Table 25–2. Brain and Cervical Spine Fatalities, 1945–1998: Level of Play

Level of Play	Brain		Cervical Spine	
	Frequency	%	Frequency	%
College	34	7.0	19	16.4
High School	365	74.9	76	65.5
Professional	13	2.7	12	10.3
Sandlot	75	15.4	9	7.8
Total	487	100.0	116	100.0

Data from Mueller FO, Diehl JL. Annual Survey of Football Injury Research, 1931–1998. American Football Coaches Association, National Collegiate Athletic Association, and National Federation of State High School Associations, 1999.

Table 25–3. Brain and Cervical Spine Fatalities by Decade

Years	Brain		Cervical Spine	
	Frequency	%	Frequency	%
1945–1954	87	18.6	32	27.6
1955–1964	115	24.7	23	19.8
1965–1974	162	34.8	42	36.2
1975–1984	69	14.8	14	12.1
1985–1994	33	7.1	5	4.3
Total	466	100.0	116	100.0

Data from Mueller FO, Diehl JL. Annual Survey of Football Injury Research, 1931–1998. American Football Coaches Association, National Collegiate Athletic Association, and National Federation of State High School Associations, 1999.

Table 25–1. Football Brain and Cervical Spine Fatalities, 1945–1998

Body Part	Frequency	%
Brain	487	68.8
Cervical Spine	116	16.4
Other	105	14.8
Total	708	100.0

Data from Mueller FO, Diehl JL. Annual Survey of Football Injury Research, 1931–1998. American Football Coaches Association, National Collegiate Athletic Association, and National Federation of State High School Associations, 1999.

Table 25–4. Brain and Cervical Spine Fatalities by Decade: Game vs. Practice

	1945–1954	1955–1964	1965–1974	1975–1984	1985–1994
Brain					
Game	59	59	108	40	26
Practice	12	41	46	27	6
Unknown	16	15	8	2	1
Cervical Spine					
Game	26	16	30	10	4
Practice	1	5	10	4	1
Unknown	5	2	2	0	0

Data from Mueller FO, Diehl JL. Annual Survey of Football Injury Research, 1931–1998. American Football Coaches Association, National Collegiate Athletic Association, and National Federation of State High School Associations, 1999.

Table 25–5. Brain and Cervical Spine Fatalities by Decade: Level of Play

	1945–1954	1955–1964	1965–1974	1975–1984	1985–1994
Brain					
College	5	8	11	4	4
High School	52	82	127	58	27
Professional	9	3	1	0	0
Sandlot	21	22	23	7	2
Cervical Spine					
College	4	5	8	2	0
High School	16	14	30	11	5
Professional	9	2	1	0	0
Sandlot	3	2	3	1	0

Data from Mueller FO, Diehl JL. Annual Survey of Football Injury Research, 1931–1998. American Football Coaches Association, National Collegiate Athletic Association, and National Federation of State High School Associations, 1999.

Table 25–6. Brain and Cervical Spine Fatalities by Decade: Type of Injury

Type Injury	1945–1954	1955–1964	1965–1974	1975–1984	1985–1994
Brain					
Fracture	7	8	2	1	0
Subdural	70	89	118	60	15
Aneurysm	0	1	2	2	2
Other	1	4	0	0	16
Unknown	9	13	40	6	0
Totals	87	115	162	69	33
Cervical Spine					
Fracture	26	13	28	11	4
Dislocation	3	3	6	1	0
Fracture-Dislocation	3	6	5	2	1
Other	0	0	2	0	0
Unknown	0	1	1	0	0
Totals	32	23	42	14	5

Data from Mueller FO, Diehl JL. Annual Survey of Football Injury Research, 1931–1998. American Football Coaches Association, National Collegiate Athletic Association, and National Federation of State High School Associations, 1999.

Table 25–7. Brain and Cervical Spine Fatalities by Decade: Activity at Time of Injury

Activity	1945–1954	1955–1964	1965–1974	1975–1984	1985–1994
Brain					
Tackling	27	26	44	16	7
Tackling Drill	1	10	13	9	0
Tackled	13	16	24	11	6
Blocking	4	8	8	3	3
Blocked	1	2	3	1	0
Collision	15	7	11	17	13
Other	5	4	12	1	1
Unknown	21	42	47	11	3
Totals	87	115	162	69	33
Cervical Spine					
Tackling	17	13	26	10	5
Tackled	6	1	3	2	0
Blocking	0	2	2	0	0
Blocked	1	0	2	0	0
Collision	1	0	0	2	0
Other	1	1	2	0	0
Unknown	6	6	7	0	0
Totals	32	23	42	14	5

Data from Mueller FO, Diehl JL. Annual Survey of Football Injury Research, 1931–1998. American Football Coaches Association, National Collegiate Athletic Association, and National Federation of State High School Associations, 1999.

fatalities since 1975, and makes recommendations for continued prevention.

HISTORICAL BACKGROUND

The game of football had a rough beginning since that first Princeton versus Rutgers game in 1869. There were no uniforms; the players actually participated in their street clothing.[3] Football helmets were not worn until 1896, and in those early years strategy played little part in the outcome of the game. Brute force, physical conditioning, and endurance were the determining factors. The 1905 season ended in protest against the brutality of play, and the *Chicago Tribune*'s compilation of injuries showed 18 dead and 159 seriously injured.[3] In midseason, President Theodore Roosevelt met with representatives from Yale, Harvard, and Princeton and told them it was time to save the sport by removing every objectionable feature. The president of the University of California also stated to football officials that the game must be made over or abolished. About the same time, Columbia University abolished the game and did not resume it until 1915. In 1906 rules were initiated to eliminate roughness of play and the danger of injury for the player.[3]

REVIEW OF RELATED LITERATURE

In 1961 Schneider and colleagues[9] published a neurosurgical review of direct fatalities in the 1959 football season. Three case reports were reviewed, and one of the mechanisms of cervical injury was vascular insufficiency of the vertebral arteries following severe cervical hyperextension that resulted in acute central cervical spinal cord injury. On the basis of their research, they suggested changes to the football helmet to help reduce injury.

For the 5-year period from 1959 through 1963, Schneider[10] documented a number of craniocerebral and spinal cord fatalities in football. Craniocerebral fatalities included 4 skull fractures, 4 extradural hematomas, 28 subdural hematomas, 8 intracerebral and intraventricular hemorrhages, and 16 pontine lesions. In addition, there were 16 fatalities to players with cervical fracture-dislocations. Schneider concluded that the football helmet was not adequate and suggested that much more research was needed in this area.

In 1969 Snook[11] reviewed the common head and neck injuries and presented a classification of them. He also discussed early management of head and neck injuries, both on and off the field. The frequency of head and spinal cord injuries at the University of Massachusetts was also presented.

Between 1971 and 1975 the National Football Head and Neck Injury Registry registered 59 intracranial football injuries that resulted in death.[12] This research by Torg later led to the concept of axial loading, and played a significant role in the reduction of head and cervical spine fatalities.

In 1980 Carter and Frankel[2] published the results of a study that was designed to examine the guillotine mechanism of injury proposed by Schneider in his earlier research. Static-free body analyses were undertaken to determine the forces imposed on the cervical spine when the football helmet face guard is struck in a manner to create hyperextension of the cervical spine. They concluded that the proposed guillotine mechanism of injury is invalid.

The notion of the posterior rim of the helmet striking the cervical spine about the C4-to-C5 level was considered to be without foundation by Virgin[13] in 1980. Virgin studied 16 football players using cineradiography to evaluate the possible roles of the posterior rim of the football helmet in causing neck injury. Five different helmets from different manufacturers were used, and no contact existed at any time between the posterior rim of any helmet and the fourth cervical vertebral spinous process.

Maroon and colleagues[5] published a football head and neck injury update in 1980. They discussed the decrease in football deaths and the increase in serious spinal cord injuries. Preconditioning and strengthening of the head and neck musculature were presented as being essential for the prevention of catastrophic head and neck injury. Proper blocking and tackling techniques were also presented as playing a major role in reducing head and neck injuries.

In a 1982 publication, Bruce and coworkers[1] stated that accidental injury to the brain and spinal cord in children under 15 years of age occurs at the rate of 230 per 100,000 children per year; such injuries requiring hospitalization affect 1 per 100,000 children per year. The rates are slightly higher in the 15-to-24 age group. In children under 15 years of age, 70% of the head injuries and nearly 100% of the spinal injuries are the result of automobile accidents. The authors state that, from these figures, it is clear that the frequency of children receiving these types of injuries in sports participation is very low. The rate does increase dramatically in the 15-to-18 age group.

Hodgson and Thomas[4] stated that all the advantage in football rests with the head-up players, and that playing with the head up when blocking and tackling will greatly reduce the risk of serious head and neck injury.

In 1984, Mueller and Blyth[6] questioned whether it were possible to continue to improve the fatality statistics in football. The number of fatalities continued to decline from 1968, when there were a total of 36 fatalities. Their latest figures, for 1982, had shown a total of nine direct fatalities. A number of experts in the field stated that football fatalities will never be eliminated owing to the nature of the sport and the increased size of the participants. Mueller and Blyth stated that fatalities may never be eliminated, but that additional research should be emphasized in order to continue the reduction of fatalities.

Mueller and Schindler[8] and Mueller and Diehl[7] in their annual reports of football fatalities show that the number of fatalities has decreased dramatically since 1968, and in 1990, for the first time since 1931, there were no fatalities in football. For the period 1989–1998, there was only one cervical spine fatality, and the total number of annual fatalities has been in single digits since 1987. These reports also show the average number of football participants in the decade 1985–1994 to be 1.8 million players annually.

HEAD AND CERVICAL SPINE FATALITY DATA

Since 1931 the American Football Coaches Association has collected football fatality data annually, with the exception of 1942.[7, 8] The original survey was chaired by Marvin Stevens of Yale University, and since 1980 Frederick O. Mueller of the University of North Carolina at Chapel Hill has continued this research. The primary purpose of the Annual Survey of Football Injury Research is to make the game of football safer for the participants. Football has benefited from these surveys because the research results have been the basis for football rule changes and equipment improvement.

Data Collection

Data are collected on a national level from all organized football programs—public schools, college, professional, and youth programs—through personal contact and questionnaires on each football fatality. Information collected includes demographic data on the injured player, equipment data, injury type and body part, and pertinent information on the exact circumstances of the accident. Fatalities that resulted from participation in the fundamentals of football—blocking and tackling—are considered direct, whereas fatalities that were caused by systemic failure as a result of exertion during participation in a football activity or by a complication that was secondary to a nonfatal injury are considered indirect. Heat stroke injuries are an example of indirect fatalities. For the purpose of this report, the data will use only direct fatality information.

1945–1998

Each year from 1945 through 1998, with the exception of 1990, has produced a brain or cervical spine fatality in football. Data from 1945 through 1998 are reviewed and discussed in this section; data covering 10-year spans of time (with the exception of 1995–1998) are presented and discussed in the sections that follow.

Football fatalities from 1945 through 1998 totaled 708. Brain injuries accounted for 487, or 68.8%, cervical spine injuries accounted for 116, or 16.4%, and other injuries accounted for 105, or 14.8%. Brain and cervical spine fatalities combined accounted for 85.2% of the total (see Table 25–1).

The type of injury associated with the majority of brain fatalities was the subdural hematoma, numbering 363; skull fractures numbered 18. Almost all of the cervical spine fatalities were fractures, dislocations, or fracture-dislocations.

A majority of the brain fatalities happened during participation in games (63.4%), and as shown in Table 25–2, 74.9% were to high school players. A majority of the cervical spine fatalities also happened in games, and 65.5% were to high school players. It should be noted that there are greater numbers of football players at the high school level than in either the college or professional ranks.

Most of the players who died as a result of either a brain or cervical spine injury were either tackling or being tackled when they received their injuries. A detailed analysis of the activity at the time of injury appears in the sections that follow.

1945–1954

In 1945 an important rule change eliminated the requirement that passes be thrown from 5 yards behind the line of scrimmage, and declared that they could be thrown from anywhere behind the line. Improvement took place in the football helmet during the late 1940s, and the plastic-shelled helmet was introduced. A single-bar facemask was introduced in the early 1950s. The fundamentals of football play an important role in injury prevention, and during this decade the techniques of blocking and tackling used the shoulder as the initial contact point. Participation during this time averaged approximately 700,000 players per year.

During this decade there were 87 brain fatalities and 32 cervical spine fatalities in all levels of football. Other injuries accounted for 34 fatalities. Brain and cervical spine injuries in 1945–1954 accounted for 77.7% of the fatalities in that decade and 17.4% of the fatalities from 1945 through 1994 (16.8% of the fatalities in 1945–1998).

Sixty-seven percent of the brain fatalities and 81% of the cervical spine fatalities took place in games. As mentioned earlier, a majority of the injured players, 57.1%, participated at the high school level.

Subdural hematomas were related to 80% of the head fatalities, and fractures were shown to be the cause of 81.2% of the cervical spine fatalities.

To help prevent serious football injuries and fatalities, it is important to know the exact activity the individual was involved in at the time of the injury. Tackling and being tackled led to 47% of the brain fatalities and 71.8% of the cervical spine fatalities. For evaluation of this area it is important to know exactly how the individual executed the skill—head down, head-to-head, head-to-knee, and so forth. These data are difficult to investigate and were not available in some of the earlier surveys.

1955–1964

In the late 1950s the techniques of blocking and tackling used the shoulder as the main area of initial contact. Players were told to keep their heads up, aim at their opponents' midsection or chest, and at the last second slide their head to one side and make contact with their shoulder. Toward the end of this decade there was a move to make initial contact with the head and face. The football helmet continued to improve, and the one-bar facemask was replaced by the two-bar. Some players had full facemasks to prevent a fractured nose or other facial injury.

From 1955 through 1964, there were 115 brain fatalities, 23 cervical spine fatalities, and 37 other fatalities. Brain and cervical spine injuries in 1955–1964 accounted for 78.8% of the fatalities during this decade and 20.2% of the fatalities from 1945 through 1994 (19.5% of the fatalities in 1945–1998). On average, approximately 850,000 players participated in football annually during the decade from 1955 through 1964.

Fifty-one percent of the brain fatalities and 69% of the cervical spine injuries took place in games, and a majority of the injured players, 70%, participated at the high school level.

Seventy-seven percent of the brain fatalities were subdural hematomas, and 56% of the cervical spine fatalities were fractures.

As was the case in the preceding decade, tackling and being tackled caused a major share of the fatalities. Forty-five percent of the brain fatalities and 60% of the cervical spine injuries were due to tackling or being tackled. There was a significant increase in the number of tackling drill fatalities in 1955 through 1964 when compared with the 1945–1954 data.

The 1955–1964 data show an increase in the percentage of brain fatalities, when compared with data from the previous decade, and a decrease in the percentage of cervical spine fatalities.

1965–1974

The period from 1965 through 1974 in football became well known for terms like "spearing," "butt blocking and tackling," "face to the numbers," "face to the chest," and a number of others. Tackling and blocking techniques involved placing the face of the tackler or blocker into the chest of the individual being tackled or blocked. The initial contact was now being made with the head. Players were wearing full facemasks and felt well protected when striking with their heads. It was also a time when cervical spine injuries were causing permanent disability to football participants, and injury data collection systems were being initiated.

The decade starting in 1965 and ending in 1974 produced 162 brain fatalities, 42 cervical spine fatalities, and 19 other fatalities. The sum of 204 brain and cervical spine injuries in 1965–1974 amounted to 91.5% of all fatalities during that decade and to 29.8% of the fatalities from 1945 through 1994 (28.8% of the fatalities in 1945–1998). The 1965–1974 figures show a dramatic increase over those of the two previous decades. During the decade from 1965 through 1974, annual participation figures ranged from a low of 1.1 million players to a high of 1.3 million.

Sixty-seven percent of the brain fatalities and 71% of the cervical spine fatalities took place in games, and a majority of the injured players, 77%, participated at the high school level.

Seventy-two percent of the brain fatalities were subdural hematomas, and 66% of the cervical spine fatalities were fractures.

A majority of football brain and cervical spine fatalities have always resulted from tackling and being tackled. Owing to incomplete data collection during the early years of this research, the type of activity that resulted in many of the fatalities was listed as "unknown." If the type of activity had been known, tackling and being tackled would have been associated with a much higher percentage of brain and cervical spine fatalities. Brain fatalities associated with tackling drills increased again from 1965 through 1974.

The 1965–1974 data reveal a dramatic percentage of increase in both brain and cervical spine fatalities when compared with the data from the two previous decades. The 1968 football season was also associated with 36 fatalities, the greatest number since 1931, and all were brain and cervical spine fatalities.

1975–1984

Many important changes were made in football during the decade 1975–1984, and these changes have helped to reduce the number of head and cervical spine fatalities. Data collection indicated a serious problem with head and neck injuries prior to 1975, and in 1976 a change in the football rules made it illegal to butt block, face tackle, or spear. These techniques involved using the frontal area or top of the helmet or the facemask to make initial contact with the opponent. The National Operating Committee on Standards for Athletic Equipment (NOCSAE) developed a safety standard for the football helmet that went into effect during the 1978 season for colleges and the 1980 season for high schools.

From 1975 through 1984, there were 69 brain fatalities, 14 cervical spine fatalities, and 9 other fatalities. Brain and cervical spine injuries during this decade were associated with 90.2% of the fatalities in that period and accounted for 12.1% of all fatalities from 1945 through 1994 (11.7% of the fatalities in 1945–1998). The number of brain and cervical spine fatalities decreased dramatically when compared to the previous decade.

Fifty-eight percent of the brain fatalities and 71% of the cervical spine fatalities took place in games, and a majority of the injured players, 83%, participated at the high school level.

Eighty-seven percent of the brain fatalities were subdural hematomas, and 78% of the cervical spine fatalities were fractures.

A majority of the fatalities again involved tackling and being tackled. These activities were associated with 52% of the brain fatalities and 85% of the cervical spine fatalities. The number of football participants during this decade numbered approximately 1.3 million players each year.

1985–1994

The many changes that took place during the decade 1975–1984 were again emphasized in 1984–1994 as the reasons for the dramatic decrease in brain and cervical spine fatalities, and there was a great effort by those in the football family—coaches, administrators, athletic trainers, physicians, national organizations, and researchers—to get this information out to schools, colleges, recreation departments, and others. The information was well received, and the number of brain and cervical spine fatalities con-

tinued to decline, even though the number of football players continued to increase. The average number of football players during this decade was approximately 1.8 million per year.

From 1985 through 1994 there were 33 brain fatalities, 5 cervical spine fatalities, and 4 other fatalities. Brain and cervical spine fatalities in 1985–1994 accounted for 90.5% of the fatalities during this decade and 5.5% of all fatalities from 1945 through 1994 (5.4% of the fatalities in 1945–1998).

Eighty-one percent of the brain injuries and 100% of the cervical spine injuries were to high school players. Forty-five percent of the brain injuries were subdural hematomas, and 80% of the spine injuries were fractures. Tackling and being tackled were related to 47.4% of the brain and cervical spine fatalities. Tackling accounted for all of the cervical spine fatalities.

1995–1998

The first four years (1995–1998) of data collection for the next decade (1995–2004) revealed 21 brain fatalities, no cervical spine fatalities, and 2 other fatalities. Nineteen of the injuries were at the high school level and two at the college level. Seventeen fatalities took place in games, three in practice, and one was unknown. Subdural hematomas numbered 11, and the others were listed as brain trauma. If the current numbers continue during the final 6 years of this period, there may be a slight increase in brain and cervical spine fatalities. The seven brain injuries in 1998 are the largest number since the nine in 1986. It will be important to monitor these figures during 1999–2004.

DISCUSSION

Brain and cervical spine fatalities accounted for 85% of all football fatalities from 1945 through 1998, and the decade with the highest percentage was 1965 through 1974. There was a dramatic decrease in both numbers and percentages of head and cervical spine fatalities for the decades 1975–1984 and 1985–1994. This section presents preventive measures that were responsible for this reduction and will make recommendations for the next decade.

Data collection plays an important role in

the prevention of injuries. The fatality data collected by the American Football Coaches Association since 1931, brain and neck surveys that began in the late 1960s and early 1970s, and data collected by the National Collegiate Athletic Association (NCAA) and the National Federation of State High School Associations have all contributed to the reduction of fatalities. There is no question that the beneficial changes are the result of reliable data collection and the publication of the results in the athletic and medical literature. Persistent surveillance of sports injury data is mandatory if progress is to continue in the prevention of fatalities. Continuous data are needed in order to observe the development of specific trends, to implement in-depth investigation into areas of concern, and to carry out preventive measures. If continued progress in football injury prevention is to be made, reliable data are a must.

Rule changes made since 1969 to help prevent injuries in football have played an important role in reducing fatalities. The rule change that has played a major role in reducing head and cervical spine fatalities is the 1976 rule that prohibits a player from making initial contact with the helmet or facemask when tackling or blocking. These now illegal techniques are called butt blocking and face tackling. Both techniques involve driving the facemask, frontal area, or top of the helmet directly into an opponent as the primary or initial point of contact. There is no doubt in the minds of sports medicine researchers that this 1976 rule change has made a major contribution to the reduction of brain and cervical spine fatalities. The American Football Coaches Association Ethics Committee also went on record opposing this type of blocking and tackling.

To help offset the trend of increasing brain and neck injuries and fatalities, the National Operating Committee for Standards in Athletic Equipment (NOCSAE) was founded in 1969 to establish safety standards for athletic equipment. The initial research effort was directed at head protection for the football player. A safety standard for football helmets was achieved in 1973, and the first helmets were tested against the NOCSAE Standard in 1974. The NOCSAE Standard was accepted by the NCAA for the 1978 football season and by the National Federation of State High School Associations for the 1980 football season. It is mandatory for all student athletes in both college and high school to wear a NOCSAE-certified helmet. When helmets are sent to a reconditioner, only those helmets that have passed the NOCSAE test when manufactured may be certified by the NOCSAE recertification procedures. The development of the NOCSAE research program points out the major role played by everyone interested in athletic injury research in making athletic activity safer for the participants.

The education of coaches and the proper techniques for tackling and blocking being taught by coaches have also played an important role in decreasing the number of brain and cervical spine fatalities. Research has shown that the safest way to tackle and block is with the head up, but not as the initial point of contact. Head-up hitting has been proven safer both in laboratory research and on the field of play. A large majority of high schools and colleges made special efforts to coach their players into keeping their heads up, and the heads up technique is helping to reduce brain and neck fatalities and serious injuries.

Coaches are also doing a better job getting their players into good physical condition, and physical conditioning is a major factor in reducing injuries. In addition, coaches are purchasing improved protective equipment and are spending more time fitting their players with their equipment. Helmet manufacturers all stress the importance of proper fit to help reduce head injuries.

Improved medical care of athletes is also an area that is important in prevention. Physicians and athletic trainers continue to increase in numbers on the football fields, and their presence has been a positive factor in injury prevention. Most major college programs have a physician at all games and practices, and some of the smaller programs have athletic trainers. It is important that all schools and colleges have athletic trainers. Many states are also setting goals that will have a qualified trainer at each high school, but this goal is far from being achieved. Physicians and trainers have the ability to prevent injuries, and immediate care may prevent an injury from developing into something more serious.

RECOMMENDATIONS

There was a definite decline in the number of football brain and cervical spine fatalities during the 24 years from 1975 through 1998, when compared with the number of fatalities in preceding decades. An all-out effort must be made to continue this trend and to avoid another increase in these types of fatalities. The following are suggestions for reducing brain and cervical spine fatalities.

1. Mandatory medical examinations and a medical history should be taken before allowing an athlete to participate in football. The NCAA recommends a thorough medical examination when the athlete first enters the college athletic program and an annual health history update with use of referral examinations when warranted. If the doctor or coach has any questions about the athlete's readiness to participate, the athlete should not be allowed to play. High school coaches should follow the recommendations set by their state high school athletic associations.

2. A physician or National Athletic Trainers Association certified athletic trainer should be present at all games and practice sessions. If this is not possible, emergency measures must be well planned and provided for.

3. Athletes must be given proper conditioning exercises that will strengthen their necks, enabling them to hold their heads firmly erect when making contact.

4. Coaches should drill the athletes in the proper execution of the fundamental football skills, particularly blocking and tackling. **KEEP THE HEAD OUT OF FOOTBALL.**

5. Coaches and officials should discourage players from using their heads as battering rams when blocking and tackling. The rules prohibiting spearing should be enforced in practice as well as in games. Players should be taught that the helmet is a protective device and should not be used as a weapon.

6. Strict enforcement of the rules of the game by both coaches and officials will help reduce serious injuries.

7. When a player has experienced or shown signs of brain trauma (loss of consciousness, visual disturbance, headache, inability to walk correctly, obvious disorientation, memory loss), he should receive immediate medical attention and should not be allowed to return to practice or the game without permission from the proper medical authorities. A number of players whose deaths were associated with brain trauma complained of headaches or had previous concussions prior to their deaths. Players should be made aware of these signs by the physician, athletic trainer, or coach. Players should also be encouraged to notify the team physician, athletic trainer, or coach if they are experiencing signs of brain trauma.

8. Coaches should never make the decision to allow a player to return to a game or to active participation in a practice if that player experiences brain trauma.

The following case study indicates the importance of proper supervision and medical care.

CASE STUDY

A 21-year-old college football player received a blow to the head while tackling in the first quarter. The player lost consciousness. He was allowed to return to the game in the fourth quarter, when he received another blow to the head while tackling. He collapsed on the sidelines, went into a coma, and died 10 days later from a subdural hematoma.

SUMMARY

Football brain and cervical spine fatalities have been related to 85% of all football fatalities from 1945 through 1998. The decade from 1965 through 1974 saw the greatest number and percentage of brain and cervical spine fatalities, and the two decades from 1975 through 1994 were associated with the smallest numbers and percentages. The data reveal that the majority of brain and cervical spine fatalities are related to high school football players either tackling or being tackled in a game. The majority of brain fatalities are caused by subdural hematomas, and almost all of the cervical spine fatalities are fractures, dislocations, or fracture-dislocations. There has been a dramatic reduction in these types of fatalities during the two decades from 1975 through 1994, and the preventive measures that have received most of the credit have been the 1976 rule change that prohibits initial contact with the head and face when blocking and tackling, the NOCSAE helmet standard that went into effect in colleges in 1978 and high schools in 1980, better coaching in the techniques of blocking and tackling, and improved medical care. There has been a reduction in brain and cervical spine fatalities, but the analysis of data for the next decade, 1995 through 2004, will be important if continued progress is to be made. Additional preventive measures and continued research efforts are critical. A number of researchers have stated that in order for brain and cervical spine fatalities to continue decreasing, there must be increased research, with an emphasis on concussions.

References

1. Bruce DA, Schut L, Sutton LN. Brain and cervical spine injuries occurring during organized sports activities in children and adolescents. Clin Sports Med 1982;1:175–194.
2. Carter DR, Frankel VH. Biomechanics of hyperextension injuries to the cervical spine in football. Am J Sports Med 1980;8:302–308.
3. Danzig A. The History of American Football. Englewood Cliffs, NJ, Prentice-Hall, 1956, pp 1–42.
4. Hodgson VR, Thomas LM. Play head-up football. Natl Fed News 1985;2:24–27.
5. Maroon JC, Steele PB, Berlin R. Football head and neck injuries—An update. Clin Neurosurg 1980;27:414–429.
6. Mueller FO, Blyth CS. Can we continue to improve injury statistics in football? Phys Sportsmed 1984;12:79–82.
7. Mueller FO, Diehl JL. Annual Survey of Football Injury Research, 1931–1997. Waco, TX, American Football Coaches Association, 1998, pp 1–23.
8. Mueller FO, Schindler RD. Annual Survey of Football Injury Research, 1931–1994. Waco, TX, American Football Coaches Association, 1995, pp 1–24.
9. Schneider RC, Reifel E, Crisler HO, et al. Serious and fatal football injuries involving the head and spinal cord. JAMA 1961;177:362–366.
10. Schneider RC. Serious and fatal neurosurgical football injuries. Clin Neurosurg 1965;12:226–235.
11. Snook GA. Head and neck injuries in contact sports. Med Sci Sports Exerc 1969;1:117–123.
12. Torg JS, Truex R, Quendenfeld TC, et al. The National Football Head and Neck Injury Registry. JAMA 1979;241:1477–1479.
13. Virgin, H. Cineradiographic study of football helmets and the cervical spine. Am J Sports Med 1980;8:310–317.

26

Head, Neck, and Spine Soccer Injuries

Harry Nafpliotis

It is not certain exactly where, when, or how the game of soccer originated. There are several very different versions of its origin. According to one soccer historian, the game began about the time the Vikings attempted to invade Saxony. In order to celebrate the capture of a Viking, the Saxons would play a game of football—or soccer, as it is called in the United States—using the prisoner's decapitated head as the "football"! Another historian reports that the game originated in Ancient Greece and was, at that time, called "Harpaston." A form of this ancient Greek game was adopted by the Romans, who used the sport not only for recreation, but also as one aspect of military training.

The United States developed its own soccer organization, the United States Soccer Federation, in 1913, but only two states participated at that time. The popularity of soccer has grown in this country since 1980 as a result of the formation of professional leagues, the public relations done by these leagues, and the establishment of fine coaching schools.

Regardless of its origin, at the present soccer is the only true international sport. In many countries it is the national sport. Its popularity throughout the world may, in part, be attributed to the Romans, who introduced the game of soccer (or football, as it is called in most countries) to the modern civilizations. However, the major credit for its popularity should go to the sport itself, for several reasons. Its simplicity of rules and strategy makes it easy for both the participant and the spectator to understand. Even a novice can master the sport without too much difficulty. Age is not a limiting factor in soccer—the only prerequisite is conditional stamina.[1]

Through the 1990s soccer gained popular-ity in the United States. This popularity is attributable to a general interest in the sport itself, the impression by the general public that soccer is safer than other sports, and the arrival of the World Cup in the United States in 1994.

Soccer is the most popular sport in the world, according to the registrations recorded by the Federation International Football Association (FIFA). There are approximately 200 million players in 186 countries registered. Further, there is estimated to be an equal number of unregistered soccer players. The nature of soccer is characterized as a vigorous, high-intensity, intermittent ball and contact sport. Such characteristics, obviously, place great demands on the technical and physical skills of individual players. A direct blow from a soccer ball or a stray kick may result in fractures, bruising, or even death. Soccer players can also suffer from a range of overuse injuries associated with running, jumping, pivoting, heading, and kicking of the ball.[2] The majority of soccer injuries, however, can be classified as impact injuries.

EPIDEMIOLOGY

The statistical investigation of soccer injuries is difficult. On a national level, the few studies that are available are mostly derived from 1- or 2-day soccer tournaments in different parts of the country. This is largely owing to two factors: (1) The development of soccer in the United States has fluctuated in relation to the popularity of the sport. Consequently, few investigators are interested in studying a sport that is changing continuously. (2) Statistics can only be considered valid if they reflect data collected during previous years.[3]

Sports medicine as a specialty has only come into existence since 1970. Therefore, any statistics on specific neurologic injuries resulting from soccer are available only from personal experience and from a review of the international literature of the past 30 years. Statistics are essential to developing a sense of perspective. As Sperryn has stated, "The relative risks of death from various activities show 4 in 100,000 to be at risk per year from playing football (soccer), compared with 2 in 100,000 from taking contraceptives, 6 in 100,000 from being run over, 20 in 100,000 from influenza, and 500 in 100,000 from smoking 20 cigarettes a day."[4]

The clinical and statistical investigation of injuries that has been carried out on Italian athletes engaged in strenuous sports under the supervision of the Italian Olympic Committee during the years 1955 and 1959 included 457,957 athletes, one fifth of whom were soccer players.[3] The overall figures showed 910 sprained knees and 843 sprained ankles; of these, soccer players alone accounted for 726 sprained knees and 620 sprained ankles. The statistics, however, differed for soccer goalkeepers. Goalkeepers accounted for the greatest number of serious injuries to the upper extremities, head, neck, and shoulders. Of injuries suffered by goalkeepers, 49.4% were severe, as compared with 15% for other players.[3]

In the United States, the Consumer Products Safety Commission has determined through the National Electronic Injury Surveillance System that between 1989 and 1992 there were 647,368 injuries secondary to soccer, as documented through emergency room admissions. It should be noted that this figure is an underestimation of the actual number of injuries that have occurred nationwide, as this figure does not include nonhospitalization physician visits. Among those injuries, 71% were sustained by males and 29% by females. Ankle injuries comprised 19.2%, knee injuries 12.7%, and head and facial injuries 11.3%. In addition, 18% of all injuries occurred to the goalkeeper. It should be noted that goalkeepers comprise 6% of the total soccer population. Over a period of 13 years, the Consumer Products Safety Commission has identified 18 individuals who have died secondary to impacts with goal posts. This is the most common mechanism of injury within the sport of soccer.[5]

The nature of the game of soccer, an intense contact with the ball and other players along with the essential underlying components of running and kicking, indicates the vulnerability of the lower extremities. The epidemiologic soccer literature clearly indicates that the majority of soccer injuries occur to the lower extremities. Lower extremity injuries account for from 58% to 93% of all injuries for adults, and 39.1% to 89% for children. The predominant injuries occur to the knees, ankles, and shins.[2] The results of a similar statistical study reporting the types and frequencies of injuries sustained in the 1984 Norway Cup—the largest soccer tournament in the world—paralleled those documented almost 30 years ago by the Italian Olympic Committee.

In the 1984 study, 60% of the injuries overall involved the lower extremities, 17% involved the head and neck, and 14% involved the upper extremities.[6] Similar statistics were reported by Metrany's 1986 study[7] of soccer injuries between 1960 and 1985. This study reported that 89% of the soccer players injured sustained injury to the lower extremities and 11% to the upper extremities. Most of the lower extremity injuries involved the ankle (68%), and only 21% involved the knee. These findings are the reverse of those reported by the Italian Olympic Committee study between 1955 and 1959. Metrany reported that in the last 25 years "only one footballer sustained a severe neck injury (C6 disk herniation) which caused severe weakness of his arm. Many head concussions were reported within these years, but all of them recovered without any complications."[7] Investigations of the Middlesbrough soccer teams in England between 1963 and 1968 showed in two independent surveys the similarity in the type and incidence of injuries occurring in professional players. Of 224 injuries, 75% were soft tissue injuries, 0.8% were head injuries, and 1.4% were low back injuries.[8]

One of the most extensive statistical studies, undertaken during the period 1970 to 1974, was reported by the Norwegian Football Association.[9] During this five year period 3616 injuries were recorded among 550 soccer players (480 adolescents and 70 adults) (Table 26–1). This study showed a much higher incidence of injuries to the head and neck (22%) than previously reported. The investigators, however, did not describe the extent of these injuries but mentioned that the injury rate of adult play-

Table 26–1. Major injuries in Norwegian Football

Injury Location	Number	Percentage
Head and Neck	785	22
Upper Extremities	633	17
Trunk	132	4
Lower Extremities	1872	52
Unclassified	194	5
Total	3616	100

From Roaas A, Nillson S. Major injuries in Norwegian football. Br J Sports Med 1979;13:3–5.

ers was ten times higher than the injury rate of adolescent players. They suggested that the reason for the disparity was that the adolescent players spent less time playing soccer and had less frequent training periods.

Perhaps the best statistical study of deaths from soccer was undertaken in Czechoslovakia in 1962. Between 1938 and 1948, there were six deaths out of 98,900 registered soccer players, or 0.61 deaths per 100,000 players.[10] During the period 1950 to 1959, there were 17 deaths out of 167,500 players, or 1.2 per 100,000 players.[10]

HEAD AND NECK INJURIES

While the vast majority of soccer injuries occur to the lower extremities, injuries to the head and neck may also occur. From the international literature, the proportion of reported injuries to the head, spine, and trunk areas ranges from 4% to 22% in adults, and 9% to 26% in youths. The neck is particularly vulnerable because of its extreme mobility. It can be sprained by vigorous pulls to the side or when forced up, forward, or backwards into hyperflexion and hyperextension (Fig. 26–1). These movements, combined with rotation or lateral flexion in either direction, may result in soft tissue injury to muscle or ligamentous structures (Figs. 26–2 and 26–3). Repetitive injuries of this nature over a period of many years may lead to degenerative disease of the cervical spine. Pain resulting from the current soft-tissue neck injury can also lead to chronic discogenic disease. Multiple minor trauma to the cervical spine may lead to degenerative changes much sooner among soccer players than among nonsoccer players of the same age group.[11]

In soccer, the head is quite vulnerable and cannot be protected as in other sports, such as football or hockey. Smodlaka[12] reported that the average number of headings, a move in soccer in which a player attempts to redirect the ball by hitting it with his forehead, for each player is five per game. If this number were multiplied by 70 games per year, at the end of 15 years the total would be 5250 headings per player. These figures exclude practice sessions, which further increase the number of headings. Thus, multiple blows to the head from a soccer ball, which weighs between 14 and 16 ounces (or 396 to 453 g) and travels at the speed of 60 to 120 km per hour, creates a force of approximately 200 to 212 joules.[12] This, indeed, is traumatic to the head and cervical spine, even if the proper technique for heading the ball is applied.[12]

One way of minimizing this trauma would be a rule change in the distance the ball may be kicked during a foul from 10 yards to 15 yards. This would protect the soccer player from head or other vital organ injury. Injuries to the head or neck can, at times, be severe or fatal. Table 26–2 shows the type of head and neck injuries sustained during soccer matches.

Acute cervical disk herniation was reported in a 29-year-old fullback.[13] He complained of pain and stiffness in the neck during a game and experienced radiating pain and numbness corresponding to the left seventh cervical disk, with paresthesia of

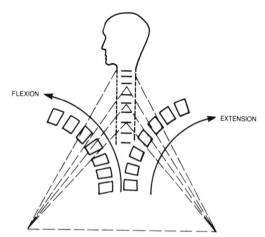

Figure 26–1. Mechanisms of cervical spine injury in soccer. A hyperflexion or hyperextension injury can be avoided if the flexors and extensors demonstrated by the triangle are well balanced. Courtesy of the Physical Therapy Center of Teaneck, NJ.

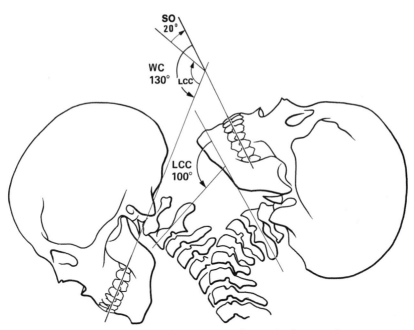

Figure 26–2. Cervical flexion/extension mechanics in degrees of movement.

the second and third fingers. Myelography revealed disk herniation compressing the nerve root. After an interbody fusion, the patient was immediately relieved of pain, with a gradual increase of muscle strength. The injury, however, ended his career.[13]

From a statistical perspective, as quoted earlier by Dr. Sperryn,[4] it appears that soccer is relatively one of the safer sports. How-

ever, the death of a 13-year-old boy in Pennsylvania, who suffered a brain injury after heading a soccer ball, poses the question, Well, is it?[14] Dr. Robert Contiguglia, who has served on the Sports Medicine Committee of the United States Soccer Federation, stated, "The types of injuries that occur in soccer are usually minor, and when there is serious injury, it is extremely rare."[14] The 13-year-old player died from a brain hemorrhage. The injury occurred when the boy's head was hit by the ball. He died five days later at the Pennsylvania State University's Hershey Medical Center.

Between 5 million and 6 million boys and girls in the United States play soccer with the youth division on a regular basis, according to the United States Soccer Federa-

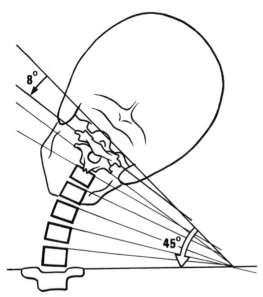

Figure 26–3. Cervical lateral flexion mechanics in degrees of movement.

Table 26–2. Types of Severe or Fatal Head and Neck Injuries in Soccer*

Diagnosis	Number
Fractured skull	5
Subdural hematoma	5
Cerebral hemorrhage	2
Epidural hematoma	1
Spinal cord transection	1

*Over a 15-year period.
From Smodlaka VM. Death on the soccer field and its presentation. Phys Sportsmed 1981;9:101–107, with permission of McGraw-Hill, Inc.

tion (USSF). Although experts say that soccer is safer than football, the rate of injury increases as soccer players grow into teenagers, and the game becomes rougher and more competitive. The Pennsylvania boy's death, although clearly an unusual occurrence, has added fuel to the ever-growing debate regarding the safety of heading.[14]

In the late 1980s there appeared several studies to suggest that cumulative effects of repeated headings may cause chronic brain damage. Simultaneous studies of Norwegian soccer players found that a special proportion of them demonstrated deficits in tests measuring mental skills. In another study of teenaged, young adult soccer players, Dr. Adrian Witol, a neuropsychologist at Virginia Commonwealth University's Medical College of Virginia, found that players who headed the ball most frequently had, on average, a lower IQ than players who did not head as often.[14] Similar studies were undertaken in the Netherlands involving 53 male professional soccer players in a cross-comparison with 27 male elite swimmers and track athletes. Both groups underwent 14 neuropsychologic tests that generated 27 scores. The performance of the soccer players was significantly lower than that of controls on verbal and visual memory, planning, and visual perceptual processing tasks. Players who headed the ball most frequently—forwards and defenders—had significantly lower scores than players who headed the ball less often—mid-fielders and goalkeepers. Such results, the authors cautioned, did not apply to amateur players, who had less exposure to heading than professionals.[15]

This ongoing debate continued to March 1996 from researchers at the University of California, Los Angeles. They compared a group of elite male United States national team soccer players to elite track athletes to see whether the repetitive heading of the ball caused either symptoms of brain injury or changes in the brain that could be detected by magnetic resonance imaging (MRI) scans. They found no differences between the two groups. Thomas Toppino, a psychology professor at Villanova University who was studying more than 200 students who played organized sports, stated, "The studies to date which pointed to potential problems, were unconvincing unto themselves and show no cause for immediate alarm."[14] There is some evidence that heading might

be an issue that should be treated seriously and requires more research, he said.

Another study, by David Janda, an orthopedic surgeon from the Institute of Preventive Sports Medicine in Ann Arbor, Michigan, of 9- to 11-year-olds, revealed concern about the possible dangers of heading the ball when he observed several children staggering around the field. He wondered whether heading might be a bad idea for children, who reportedly "developed headaches and feeling sick to the stomach." Janda has been researching with a lightweight soccer helmet that will lessen the impact of the ball hitting the head. "We are not trying to change the game," he said. "We are trying to make it safer."[14]

While the debate continues over the danger of repetitive heading, there is clearly some danger of suffering a head injury while playing soccer. Two players can knock heads when both go to head the ball, or a player might crash into the goal post, or get kicked in the head (especially if the player is the goalkeeper). Such collisions can cause a concussion, a temporary loss of consciousness, with such symptoms as confusion, dizziness, blurred vision, or vomiting. A severe blow to the head may cause bleeding and nerve damage.[14]

At this time, the use of helmets by young soccer players is not anticipated, but the author does encourage correct coaching for heading the ball by well-qualified, experienced coaches. Good coaching, in realistic training programs, should stress correct body mechanics in teaching proper heading techniques. Helmets, according to Janda, "have gained popularity in recent years."[16] However, the author has not seen any study reporting the use of helmets, either nationally or internationally. Perhaps there is some merit to the use of helmets, although the author cannot see it at this time, unless the entire sport of soccer is modified to accommodate a very low percentage of head injuries.[17]

Perhaps a metaphoric example related to helmets for preventing head injuries is the prophylactic knee brace used in American football. J. C. Hughston, who did a study in prophylactic knee bracing in college football, stated, "The only sure way to prevent knee injuries is to play football with casts on both legs and to change the rules in football prohibiting tackling below the waist."[18] In the meantime, realistically, soccer players

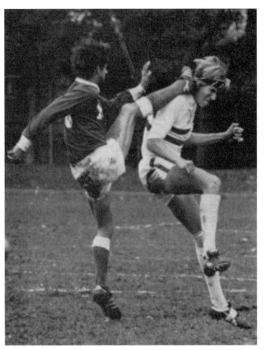

Figure 26–4. Courtesy of the Physical Therapy Center of Teaneck, NJ.

must be educated in safe techniques of heading by a knowledgeable coaching staff. To this end good soccer coaching schools must be established.

Although head injuries in soccer are rare,

as illustrated by the above statistics, the development of cervical spondylosis, however, is quite common in older soccer players. These players sustain multiple strains to the neck, exceeding the normal mobility of the cervical spine and resulting in degeneration of the articulations, capsules, and disks.[10] Torn neck muscles are caused by extreme neck rotation or extreme lateral flexion. Initially, patients may have an appearance of traumatic torticollis, or "wryneck."[13] Figures 26–4, 26–5, and 26–6 illustrate head, neck, and face injuries.

The muscles most often injured are the upper and middle fibers of the trapezius, which are neck extensors, and the sternocleidomastoids, which are neck flexors and rotators. Partial tears of one or the other are usually seen. Both muscles are rarely injured simultaneously. Disability from torn neck muscles lasts between 5 days and 3 weeks, depending on the degree of the tear and the muscle groups involved (Fig. 26–7).

Dr. Edward E. Williams, a Philadelphia dentist specializing in sports dentistry, has identified another injury in soccer, known as athlete's jaw disorder.[19] Those who are familiar with this term are also familiar with the effects of injury to the temporomandibular joint (TMJ), which surrounds the delicate structures in the head. Dr. Williams states, "This is, perhaps, the most misunderstood

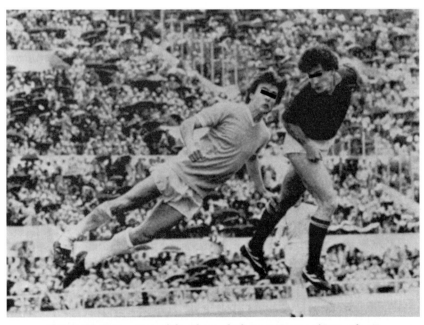

Figure 26–5. Courtesy of the Physical Therapy Center of Teaneck, NJ.

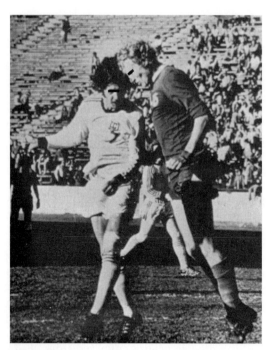

Figure 26–6. Courtesy of the Physical Therapy Center of Teaneck, NJ.

and unreported injury in soccer and occurs with alarming frequency." There are many players suffering many symptoms from the jaw joint injury. Dr. Williams is working on a device known as WIPSS mouth and jaw joint protector. In his studies and work with athletes of all ages, Dr. Williams has developed this new equipment to prevent damaging injuries to the areas that are protecting the delicate bones of the TMJ, ear, and face of the brain. This patented appliance has been developed after years of research and treatment of hundreds of athletes, many of whom were soccer players.[20]

In summary, the epidemologic data clearly indicate that soccer-induced head and neck injuries are infrequent and do not occur as often as injuries to the rest of the body. In the most extensive report of soccer injuries that was presented in a sports medicine convention in Cincinnati, Ohio, in June 1985, Dr. Frank Noyes reported that out of 50,000 teenage soccer players, there was an average injury rate of seven cases per 1000 hours of playing. There was one head injury that resulted in a subdural hematoma, which was treated successfully with no further disability.[21] Although serious injuries of the head and neck occur at a low rate during the 15 active years of a professional or semi-

professional soccer player's career, the cervical spine is exposed to repetitive trauma through heading a ball, head-on collisions with an opponent, or falls. About 5% of soccer players sustain brain injuries as a result of their sport. This may occur from head to head contact, from falls, or from being struck by the ball on the head.[22]

Degenerative changes to the cervical spine were found to be significantly higher in soccer players and a control group of the same age.[10] Radiologic and clinical examination of 43 young soccer players revealed degenerative changes to the cervical spine corresponding to those of 50- or 60-year-old individuals who had not played soccer.[10]

Murphey and Simmons reported on "trivial" injuries to the neck in a number of adult soccer players and discovered several with fracture-dislocations of the cervical spine without neurologic deficit. They concluded that all players who complain of cervical pain and stiffness should have roentgenograms with lateral flexion and extension views.[10]

CARE OF THE INJURED ATHLETE

In minor neck injuries not accompanied by head injuries, the player may be allowed to return to the game if no neurologic signs are present, and if the range of neck movements is painless and unrestricted. In severe neck injuries, the head and neck should be stabilized on the field with sandbags or foam cushion positioners. In the head-injured athlete with neck pain or sensory or brachial symptoms, the head should not be moved or manipulated. If the injured player is incoherent, he or she should be observed for any obvious skeletal abnormalities or any limitations of limb movement. The injured athlete should remain immobile until a physician's instructions are obtained.

Head Injury Without Unconsciousness

The athlete may complain of a headache, nausea, or light-headedness, and may also turn pale or vomit. There may or may not be transient loss of memory. Athletes should stop playing immediately and should be

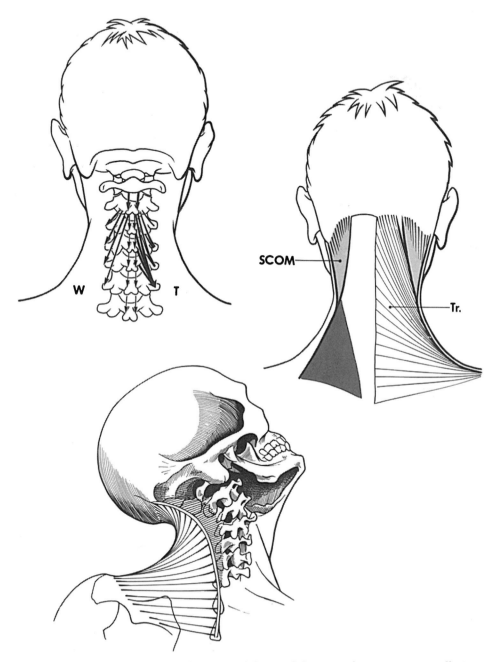

Figure 26–7. Posterior muscles of the neck act as stabilizers of the cervical spine synergistically in extension, lateral flexion, and rotation.

kept under observation and serially tested for orientation and memory functions. A physician should be consulted before return to play.

Head Injury with Unconsciousness of Short Duration

If the athlete lies unconscious for a brief time (less than 2 minutes), is complaining of headache, nausea, vomiting, or dizziness, and shows memory dysfunction, then a serious brain injury probably occurred. The player should be removed from the field and transported to a hospital for further diagnostic tests. A 24-hour observation period is recommended.

Head Injury With Unconsciousness of Long Duration

The athlete who is unconscious for more than 2 minutes should be removed by stretcher, with minimal movement of the head, and taken to a hospital as soon as possible for diagnostic tests and treatment. It is important to ensure immediately that an unconscious athlete has free air passage. If an injured athlete is breathing, he or she should be placed on his or her side (recovery position). While waiting for transport, the athlete should be kept covered and a blanket placed beneath him. If there is suspicion of a neck injury, the head should *not* be bent backward to free the air passages. Instead, the airway should be cleared by raising the lower jaw.

Recently there have been injuries reported where neurologic impairment has been caused by damage to the jaw joint. According to Dr. Williams,[19] there has been a misconception in the United States that the jaw joint of the head is not important, as evidenced by the anthropomorphic test device commonly known as the crash test dummy. As Figure 26–8 shows, however, the dummy has no jaw joint. When jaw joint damage does exist, the result appears to be a neurologic impairment at the nerve trunk that affects the athlete's strength.[20] In many cases, continues Dr. Williams, the seasoned athlete can lose as much as 35% of arm

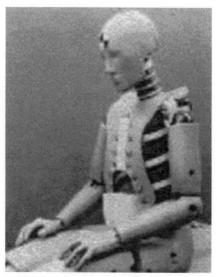

Figure 26–8. Anthropomorphic crash test dummy without jaw joint.

(deltoid) and leg (quadriceps and hamstring) strength owing to jaw joint injury.[20]

As reported earlier, the amount of force, when the soccer ball hits the head, at times exceeds 208 joules, the impact causing the lower jaw to crash against the base of the skull. Such forces account for a large percentage of jaw joint injuries among soccer players.

Serious jaw joint injuries occur with an alarming rate in soccer. According to Bill Whitney, Olympic Development soccer coach, the primary reasons for injuries are: (1) getting hit in the jaw by the ball, (2) the aggressive action of the opponent, and (3) heading the ball[20] (Fig. 26–9).

Head injuries with unconsciousness should be considered serious and are usually associated with complications. For example, intracranial bleeding may occur, causing herniation of brain tissue. Bleeding from the ear or bleeding associated with leakage of cerebrospinal fluid from the nose suggests a basal skull fracture.

Return to Play

Before an injured player is allowed to return to the game, he or she must be fully alert and oriented, be free of headache and dizziness, and have no mental dysfunction. Players may return to contact soccer activity when they are asymptomatic and neurologically normal and have full cervical motion.

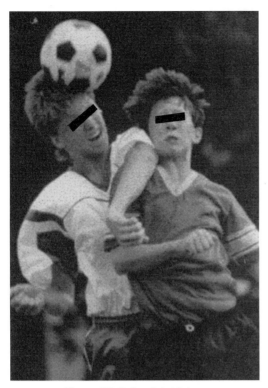

Figure 26–9. Jaw joint injury.

the muscles surrounding the cervical spine must be integral parts of the athlete's training.

"Use your head" is usually good advice. For an experienced soccer player, however, taking that advice literally could cause neurologic problems, according to Dr. Adrian Witol, a psychologist, who presented a study at the American Psychological Association's annual meeting during the summer of 1995. At that meeting, she presented a study of 60 soccer players between the ages of 18 and 29. Those who headed the ball at least 10 times per match did not score as well on tests that measured attention and mental flexibility as those who headed the ball less frequently. They also posted somewhat lower IQ scores. Though these findings do not prove cause and effect, similar evidence of subtle, impact-related brain injury in other sports attest that the connection is real.[23] Although such findings appear to be worrisome, one must consider that the players' scores were in the normal range, and none of the players had difficulties in doing work at home or at school. Additionally, the researchers did not report whether the minor neurologic problems lasted beyond the soccer season.

Good coaching techniques, therefore, in every aspect of the game (and especially in heading the ball) are essential in reducing the risk for injury. In heading the ball, certain criteria must be observed. In a defensive play, heading the ball involves strength to displace the ball for distance. In an offensive play, heading the ball requires accuracy. In heading balls from the ground, the power should originate from the lower trunk, legs, and feet, while the neck remains rigid. As the ball approaches, the body must be bent backward while the full forehead faces squarely toward the ball and the neck muscles remain rigid. Just before the ball hits the forehead, the feet, hips, and trunk simultaneously drive upward, throwing the forehead toward the ball while the body is straightening[24] (Fig. 26–10).

In heading the ball in the air, the same technique applies, with the exception that the timing must be such that the ball does not strike when the player is unprepared[25] (Fig. 26–11). The eyes must be kept on the ball at all times during a heading.

Proper rehabilitation of the injured athlete is essential if he or she is to return to the sport with full function. It is unproductive

All injuries must be carefully attended, but evaluation and management of injuries involving the cervical spine and head require particular attention. In severe head injury with transient unconsciousness, the player should not be allowed to return to the game. The player should be carefully observed for 24 hours, with serial examination, and should not be allowed to return to activity for two weeks, subject to physician's approval. The trainer should keep a record of all head injuries or concussions. Such a record is essential in establishing a medical history for future care of the athlete.

PREVENTION AND PHYSICAL THERAPY

For an athlete returning to soccer activity, following a program of rehabilitation exercises is crucial. Injury prevention through preseason calisthenics to develop strength for anterior and posterior neck and shoulder muscles is the best method of preventing most neck injuries. Methods designed to improve range of motion, to prevent atrophy from disuse, and to increase the strength of

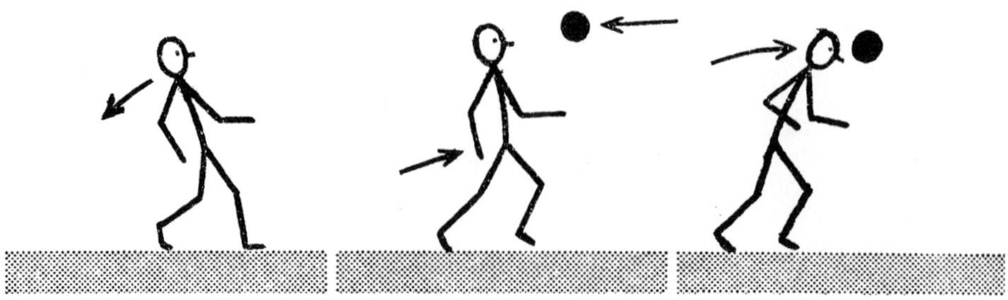

Figure 26–10. Illustration of body mechanics used when heading the ball from the ground. From Wade A. Soccer to Training & Coaching. Heinemann Educational Books Ltd., 1977, p 69, with permission.

for the rehabilitation specialist simply to repair the injured part and then to allow the athlete to resume playing without outlining a specific exercise program to maintain the repaired part in good condition. Injuries need to be properly managed to reduce the possibility of further damage. Overall the treatment goals are pain relief, promotion of healing, decreased inflammation, and return to functional and sports activities as soon as possible.

The procedure, as far as the trainer is concerned, may involve first aid, taping or bracing, and referral and general rehabilitation at a physical therapy center specializing in sports training. This individualized program in rehabilitation should include exercises in range of motion (for normal joint mobilization), muscle strengthening—both static (isometric) and dynamic—and subsequent coordination training in all the tasks necessary for the athlete's specific activity. The soccer player should not participate in a soccer match before training with a soccer ball and regaining coordination.[26]

A considerable amount of time may be

necessary before the player is completely ready to resume play. Sports medicine and rehabilitation centers must be able to provide simulated testing conditions, indoors or outdoors, with particular attention to the correct procedures required for the soccer player's position. The exchange of information among all those involved in the rehabilitation of the injured player is of the utmost importance. To paraphrase an old Greek proverb, every day that is gained in the rehabilitation of an injured player is worth gold, and every week is worth diamonds.

SOFT TISSUE NECK INJURIES

Significant differences exist between child and adult soccer players; therefore, the prevention program strategies for children should be considered separately from those for adults, despite the fact that the injuries may be attributed to many of the same factors associated with injuries in adult soccer players. Knowledge of the circumstances of the injuries is invaluable in evaluation and immediate treatment. When fractures have been ruled out, the following treatment modalities should be applied: (1) Ice packs should be applied to reduce blood flow and to decrease the damage to injured tissues. (2) A soft foam splint or soft cervical collar that inhibits movement should be worn for 24 to 48 hours, or for as long as is necessary, depending on the degree of pain. (3) The application of helium neon heat to relieve soft tissue pain has been established and has been useful during the first 24 hours following injury. (4) Adequate periods of rest are essential in reducing the initial stages of injury.

In the treatment of soft tissue injuries of the neck after 48 hours (Table 26–3), a physical therapy program should include the fol-

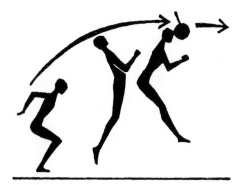

Figure 26–11. Illustrations of body mechanics used when heading the ball in the air. From Scholich M. Soccer: Circular Training and Coaching, p 213, with permission. See reference #25.

Table 26–3. Treatment of Soft Tissue Injuries After 48 Hours

1. Heat (hydrocollator packs for 20 minutes)
2. Ultrasound
3. Pulsating high-voltage stimulation (90 to 120 pulses/sec, usually for 20 minutes after day 3 postinjury) to fatigue muscles and to reduce spasms
4. Massage in the form of effleurage (mild, milking strokes) around the upper trapezius
5. Mobilization rather than manipulation (gentle mobilization techniques are more successful than violent manipulations, which result in painful aftereffects and further tissue damage)
6. Intermittent traction after full range of motion has been restored (usually around day 5 or 6 postinjury, starting with 12 lb and increasing gradually to 30 lb or as tolerated) to be applied horizontally
7. Progressive resistance exercises after complete range of motion has been restored, beginning with isometric exercises and progressing to dynamic exercises with increased resistance

lowing procedures: (1) Exercise and massage for prevention of muscle atrophy. (2) Improvement of joint range of motion through exercise. (3) Elimination of pain by use of ultrasound or moist heat, or Dynatron 200, to be applied manually, and 400 in the form of electrical stimulation. (4) Cervical traction, preferably horizontally rather than vertically, using the Hill Anatomotor Traction Table.

Electrical stimulation, using the Dynatron 200 and 400, appears to be the most popular form of treatment at this time, not only for psychological but also for physical reasons. Psychologically, it is the author's personal experience that electrical stimulation gives the athlete a sense that "something is being done" when he or she observes the involuntary movement of the muscle. Physically, stimulation of an injured muscle may retard disuse atrophy. In injuries to the extremities, the athlete can combine voluntary movements with the involuntary movements stimulated by the pulsating current. The most sophisticated unit at this time is the Dynatron 400, which gives a variety of protocols in current delivery, including the pulsed current.

Intermittent or static traction is usually applied after full range of motion has been restored, starting with 12 pounds and progressively increasing to 30 pounds, or to pain tolerance level. The author prefers, throughout cervical traction, to use a hori-

zontal position rather than a vertical position because, according to the patients, it provides relief sooner and does not allow the painful gravitational force to impede the pain relief process. Traction is used to reduce the spasms of the cervical paraspinal musculature.

At this time, the staff of the Physical Therapy Center of Teaneck, P.A., has also been very successful in using magnet therapy with an infratonic unit, and also in applying magnets to painful areas. Research issued to us, as well as our own data for 1994–1999, has shown magnets to have been very successful in postinjury rehabilitation of tissue, especially of the paraspinal musculature. Our protocol delivers static magnetic fields over 500 Gauss over the trigger points of the cervical spine. The reference includes the most recent research in magnet therapy.[27]

EXERCISE TECHNIQUES FOR NECK REHABILITATION

When complete range of motion of the cervical spine has been restored (Fig. 26–12), and the pain has dissipated, then progressive resistance exercises are employed to obtain total rehabilitation and to promote early comeback. Because frequent treatments speed the results, the athlete should be participating in as many as four sessions per day.

Initially, isometric exercise should start with slow contractions to avoid pain. Subsequently, increased resistance should be used so that the degree of tension on the exercised muscle includes more forceful contraction. Once maximum resistance has been reached isometrically without pain, dynamic exercises may begin. Dynamic exercise is started gradually, initially using only the weight of the part involved, and eventually the resistance can be increased by adding weights to the injured parts, as well as proprioceptively to the proximal and lateral joints.

Postural muscle assessment is important in view of the action of opposing muscle groups and the injured part, such as the cervical spine flexors and extensors. As Sahrman has stated, "Maintenance of muscular and mechanical balance helps to prevent the development of painful musculoskeletal conditions, particularly those that are from repetitive activity."[28]

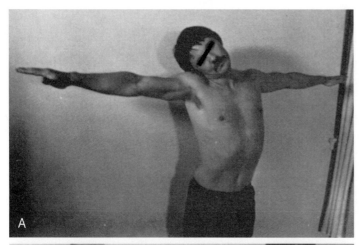

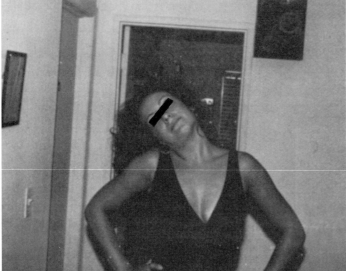

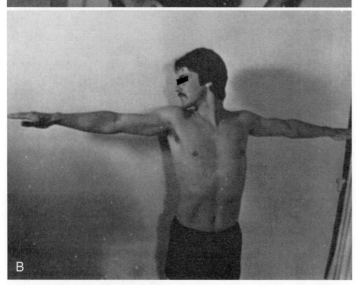

Figure 26–12. *(A)* Neck. Lateral flexion and rotation as well as forward flexion and extension; *(B)* rotation.

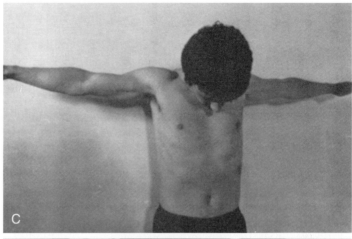

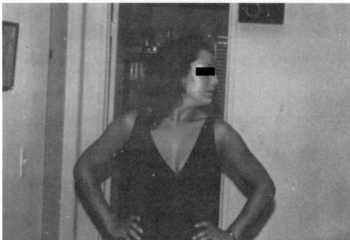

Figure 26–12 *Continued. (C)* flexion; *(D)* extension.

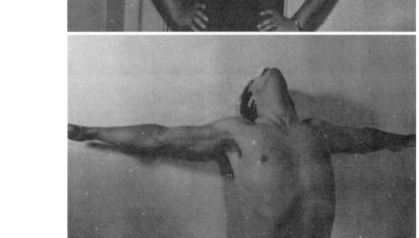

Individualized Fitness Programs

Assuming the fact that the vertical integrity of the spine will counteract gravity, the neck's limited musculature is designed to handle a comparatively modest task: to move the head from front to back and from side to side. Modern, relaxed, limited-motion life encourages the spine to move into forward flexion, distorting its "S" curve into a "C" curve and forcing the mechanics of the neck "to hard labor in order to keep us from losing our heads. With the head tilted forward, gravity has us by the nose and is pulling."[29] As a consequence, the cervical spine may well be doing the most strenuous work of any part of the musculoskeletal system with the fewest resources. The price is neck pain and stiffness, dizziness, vertigo, headaches, TMJ disorder, and more.[29] Therefore, the final task in rehabilitating a soccer player is to test the athlete for specific skills. These skills include jogging, sprinting, kicking, heading, and other tasks of agility, coordination, and balance.

At a sports physical therapy facility, such testing is possible with the use of electric treadmills, ergometers, isokinetic systems, and dynamic exercise units related to testing strength in heading and kicking. For a specific technique such as heading, however, the athlete must be tested on the soccer field with careful and controlled drilling.

The postoperative procedure will follow the same protocol as posttraumatic procedures, making sure that the protocols applied in improving the range of motion and strength, as well as reducing the pain, will precede the resistance exercises. (Such postoperative rehabilitation procedures must be discussed at length with the neurosurgeon and orthopedic surgeon to assure the safety and the future potential of the injured athlete.) Expectations of total and permanent relief from pain after an operation are likely to be disappointed. Most operations are successful, and the pain is dramatically reduced. An individual, however, must follow the advice of the surgeon and the physiotherapist postoperatively in order to realize the greatest benefit.[30] Exercises produced with a theraband at the Physical Therapy Center of Teaneck for strengthening neck musculature are illustrated by Figures 26–13 through 26–16.

Finally, at the Physical Therapy Center of Teaneck, P.A., a study has been conducted using biomechanical body suits to enhance muscle balance for posttraumatic injuries of the spine, especially those occurring in soccer players. A posttraumatic body is one that carries an unstable load that is out of line (compensation) with gravity, and is loaded with extra strain.

The goal of stretching and strengthening regularly is to balance the opposing muscle pulls at every joint so that the body gradually and involuntarily lines up with the force of gravity. Stretching and strengthening the muscles involved balances the body at all its joints, automatically improving body stability and consequently conserving

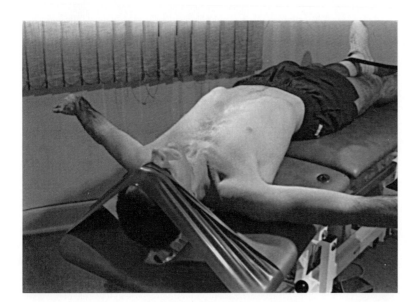

Figure 26–13. Neck flexor strengthening assisted by shoulder protractors.

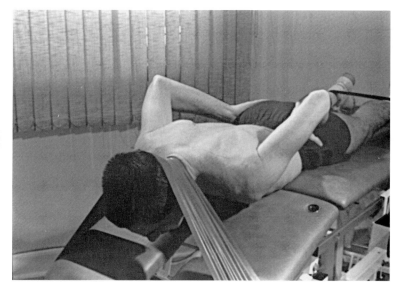

Figure 26–14. Strengthening with elastic band resistance for neck extensor muscles.

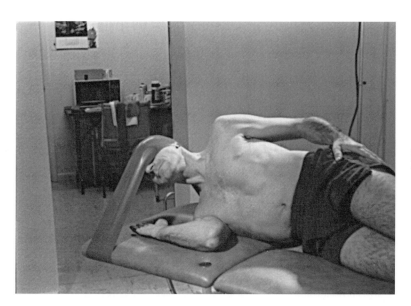

Figure 26–15. Strengthening for lateral flexor muscles.

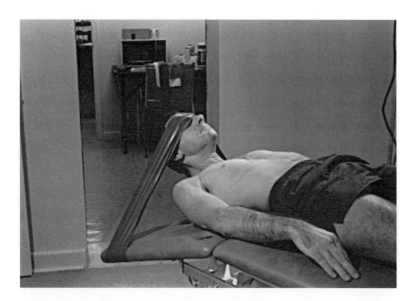

Figure 26–16. Strengthening for neck flexor muscles.

valuable energy needed for performances in jogging, running, and jumping.[31]

The body suits used in the study included weighted pockets, as well as elastic suspenders, located posterolaterally for enhancing muscle balance and for effectuating good posture, resistance exercises, and among others, also cardiovascular fitness (see Figs. 26–17, 26–18, and 26–19—patent pending). The preliminary results for pretraumatic and posttraumatic, as well as for pre- and postoperative procedures, have been very promising (especially for those with neck and spine injuries).

RECOMMENDATIONS

There is significant risk of head, neck, and spine injury from playing soccer. The research presented seems to indicate so. The question is, how much damage? And how can players be protected? The following are some of the recommendations that appear in the current literature.

1. Padding systems should be used on stationary goal posts to decrease the force of impact.

2. Helmets should be used for heading the ball (David Janda, orthopedic surgeon).

3. The WIPSS jaw joint protector should be used (Edward D. Williams, D.M.D.)[20]

4. Children should be encouraged to play with smaller-sized soccer balls.

5. A campaign aimed at increasing soccer players' awareness of the injury conse-

quences of training errors should be developed and promoted.

6. More biomechanical and epidemiologic research into the mechanisms of injury should be conducted, protective equipment should be developed and tested, and education for both players and coaches, especially in the United States, emphasizing correct techniques in heading the ball, particularly in coaching children, should be improved.

CONCLUSION

Head and neck injuries among soccer players are rare, but can be fatal. The goalkeeper is more at risk than any other player (18% of all injuries—see the aforementioned statistics). Improper training and misjudgment in heading powerfully driven balls can produce cranial-cervical damage. Degenerative changes to the cervical spine are a common outgrowth of a current neck injury and may become debilitating. Coaching techniques should focus on the negative effects of heading the ball. On an international level, the exchange of safety information should be encouraged. Pressuring FIFA officials to change certain rules, for example to increase the distance in kicking fouls, will also improve the game's safety. Nevertheless, risk-taking in any sport is directly related to reward. The greater the reward, the greater the risk the player is willing to take.[32]

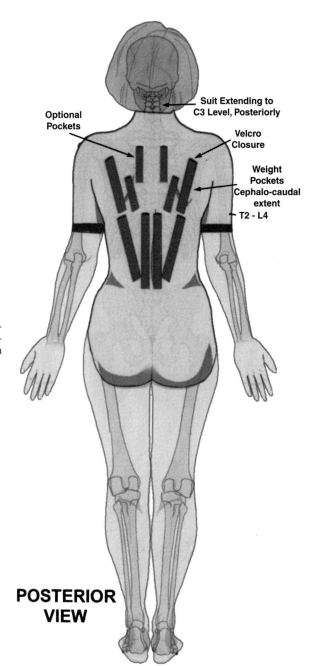

Figure 26–17. Biomechanical suit posteriorly extends from the C3 level to wrap around an individual's buttocks and connect with the forward portion through the crotch.

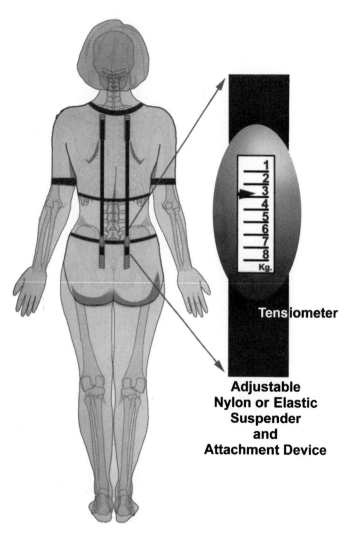

1
2
3
4
5
6
7
8
Kg.

Tensiometer

**Adjustable
Nylon or Elastic
Suspender
and
Attachment Device**

Figure 26–18. Biomechanical suit with suspenders. Posterior view comprises a mini-shirt and shorts connected front and rear by suspenders, which are adjustably mounted and include tension measuring means to provide the necessary tension for resistance through the Tensiometer.

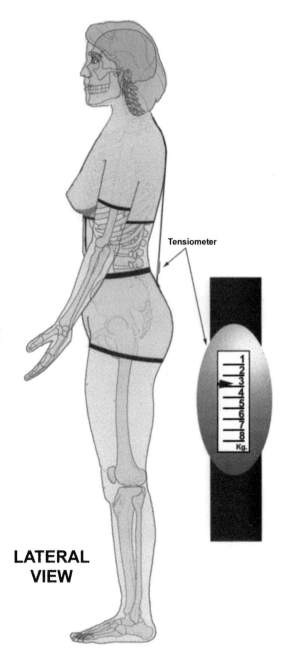

Figure 26-19. Biomechanical suit with suspenders, lateral view. Accentuates the suspension system as well as the Tensiometer, which provides resistance from 1 kg to 8 kg.

Tensiometer

LATERAL
VIEW

References

1. Nafpliotis H. Soccer Injuries: A Physical Therapy View in Care and Prevention. New York, Anthe Publishers, 1981.
2. McGrath CA, Smith OJ. Heading Injuries Out of Soccer. Monash University Accident Research Center, 1997.
3. Jokl EJ, Simon E. International Research in Sports and Physical Education. Springfield, IL, Charles C Thomas Publisher, 1964.
4. Sperryn PN. Sport and Medicine. Boston, Butterworth, 1983, p3.
5. Janda DH, Bir C, Wild B, et al. Goal post injuries in soccer. Am J Sports Med 1995;23:340–344.
6. Maehlum S, Dahl E, Daljord O. Frequency of injuries in a youth soccer tournament. Sports Med 1986;14:78.
7. Metrany R. Personal written communication, Wingate Institute of Physical Education, Tel Aviv, 1986.
8. Phillips N. Medical aspects of professional association football. J R Coll Gen Pract 1970;19:349–352.
9. Roaas A, Nillson S. Major injuries in Norwegian football. Br J Sports Med 1979;13:3–5.
10. Smodlaka VM. Death on the soccer field and its presentation. Phys Sportsmed 1981;9:101–107.
11. Sortland O, Tysvaer A, Sorti O. Changes in the cervical spine in association football players. Br J Sports Med 1982;16:80–84.
12. Smodlaka VM. Medical aspects of heading the ball in soccer. Phys Sportsmed 1984;12:127–131.
13. Tysvaer AT. Case report: Cervical disc herniation in a football player. Br J Sports Med 1985;19:43–44.
14. Fitzgerald S. Heads up on soccer safety. Philadelphia Inquirer. September 16, 1996.
15. Matser JT, Kessel AGH, Jordan BD, et al. Chronic traumatic brain injury in professional soccer players. Neurology 1998;51:791–796.
16. Janda D, in Feeney T. (1995). Keeping soccer safe. Adv Phys Therapists 1995;32:22, 62.
17. Nafpliotis H. Further research suggested in preventing soccer injuries. Adv Phys Therapists 1995;12:20, 54.
18. Eftimiadis J. Anatomy, etiology and treatment of patellofemoral dysfunction. Adv Phys Therapist (October 1991).
19. Williams ED. Jaw joint disorders in contact-sports athletes: Diagnosis and prevention. In Hoerner EF (ed): Head and Neck Injuries in Sports, ASTM 1229, Philadelphia, American Society for Testing and Materials, 1994.
20. Williams ED. Jaw joint disorders in contact sports athletes: Diagnosis and prevention. In Hoerner EF (ed): Head and Neck Injuries in Sports, ASTM 1229, Philadelphia, American Society for Testing and Materials, 1994.
21. Noyes F. Sports injuries: Neurologic and musculoskeletal injuries and their prevention. Tape presented at the Sports Medicine Convention, Cincinnati, OH, June, 1985.
22. Bruce DA, Schut L, Sutton LN. Brain and cervical spine injuries occurring during organized sports activities in children and adolescents. Prim Care 1984;11:175–194.
23. Witol A. Heading soccer balls safely. Health News, N Engl J Med, September 1995.
24. Wade A. Soccer, Guide to Training and Coaching. New York, Heinemann Educational Books Ltd., 1977, pp 67, 69–71.
25. Scholich M. Soccer: Circular Training and Coaching. Kreis Training Sportverlag, Berlin, Thessaloniki, SALTO Publishers, 1989, p 213.
26. Peterson L, Renstrom P. Sports Injuries. Chicago, Martin Dunitz Publishers, 1986, pp 165, 198–199.
27. Vallbona C, Hazelwood CF. Response of pain to static magnetic fields in post-polio patients. Arch Phys Med Rehabil 1997;78:1200–1203.
28. Sahrman S. The Shirley Sahrmann Exercise Series I. St. Louis, Videoscope, Inc., 1991.
29. Egoscue P. Pain Free: A Revolutionary Method of Stopping Chronic Pain. New York, Bantam Books, 1998, p 186.
30. Tanner J. Beating Back Pain. London, Dorling Kindersley Publishers Limited, 1987, p 117.
31. Balaskas A. Soft Exercises. London, Unwin Hyman Limited, 1983, p 108.
32. Wilkinson WHG. A practical view of soccer injuries. Br J Sports Med 1978;12:43–45.

27

Neurologic Injuries in Alpine Skiing

John B. Harris

When our three young children began to show downhill ski racing promise, we ordered two dozen bamboo slalom gate poles with red and blue flags and promptly relocated our neurosurgical practice to Lake Tahoe.

A solo practice in a rural setting with an emphasis on Alpine ski trauma was a feasible proposition in 1975, inasmuch as neurosurgical specialization was still in its adolescence. At once we became aware of the unappreciated magnitude of neurologic injury occurring in and among the trees, chair lifts, and ski runs at the 18 ski resorts ringing Lake Tahoe.

It was clear that an unusual opportunity existed to undertake America's first on-the-spot daily neurosurgical study of brain and spinal cord trauma within this ski injury arena, with the advantage of immediate memorializing of all details of the accident and ambient factors—most importantly, in a prospective manner. Being on site furnished the unusual and invaluable opportunity to include, at the very outset, simultaneous details of injury mechanism, skier experience, age and skill level, equipment use, hill difficulty, and coexistent daily meteorological and snow conditions, and the contribution of these factors to the severity of neurologic injury.

In this chapter we review head and spine neurologic injuries in Alpine skiing from the perspective of both the recreational and the competitive skier. The observations are drawn from America's first prospective study of neurologic ski and winter sports injuries, initiated in 1975.

Contemporary insight and observations were made by one race neurosurgeon with experience as a ski instructor, as a racer, and as a ski patroller with appointments to the Olympic Ski Patrol and Professional Ski Patrol. Over the space of 2 decades, the data was gathered immediately at the time of injury, either from a site on the hill or at the receiving hospital, located at the epicenter of 18 ski resorts. Our 1983 and 1989 reports were the first to relate such observations to neurologic head and spine injury in American skiing.[25, 26]

Unique situations that one may encounter as a race physician are highlighted by relevant case reports. Our series includes 430 hospitalized winter sports patients, including 347 neurologically injured skiers. Concluding comments touch upon demographic, technical, patroller, equipment, and ski resort trends since 1990 as well.

For most of us, the goal of becoming a good skier is achieved after a fairly long epoch of trial and error, composed of lessons and falls, until the nuances of ski edge turning pressure and release are mastered through complex yet subtle combinations of lower extremity weight-shifting and timing. Mastery of these skills enhances the act and grace of a satisfying controlled downhill ski descent that is a beauty to witness yet difficult to describe.

To summarize, the skier must bring to the sport the favorable physical attributes of fitness, agility, strength, and endurance, and apply these prerequisites moment-by-moment while instantaneously integrating numerous stimuli. That being accomplished, the skier must then transmit correct forces and angulation to the ski edge(s) with precise timing. Otherwise, the incorrect integration of the sensory stimuli and the necessary motor responses, if coupled with significant speed, may result in musculoskeletal and even neurologic injury. Little wonder that many of us have known skiers who always seem to be off somewhere taking a lesson.

HISTORICAL BACKGROUND

America's most popular winter sports activity, skiing, arose from the humble, basic need of Europeans to eat. The earliest skis were made from animal tusks some 4000 years ago, with the basic objective of enhancing success in nomadic winter hunting.[52] It was not long until skiing was adapted to Scandinavian tribal winter mountain warfare, and then on a larger scale for Nordic geopolitical expansion. It seems logical, therefore, that the first organized ski competition was held by the Norwegian army in 1767.

The first Winter Olympic Games were held at Chamonix, France, in 1924; the competition was limited to the traditional Nordic events, cross-country and ski jumping. Alpine events were added 12 years later, in 1936. In the period prior to World War II, head injury made up 2.5% of the injuries reported by Petitpierre, presumably because at the time of that study (1939) there were fewer skiers, and they were skiing at slower speeds than later.[48] The work of later European contributors Unterharnscheidt,[60] Oh,[46] Reudi,[47] and, more recently, Furrer and colleagues[19] as well as Blankstein and coworkers[3] added to the study of neurologic injuries in skiing.

Primitive competition was known on the American continent by the late 19th century, but it was not until the first Lake Placid Winter Olympics in 1932 that skiing as an American winter sport was officially launched. The completion of the Union Pacific Railroad line to Ketchum, Idaho, and the Sun Valley "Dollar Mountain" single chair lift, brought winter sports to the Westerner's front door.

ALPINE SKIING

In earlier days, Alpine (downhill) skiing amounted to packing a lunch and climbing a mountain in the morning. Perhaps two runs in a day were possible if favorable conditions existed. Unprecedented worldwide popularity of skiing had to await the coming of mountain mechanization, first the drag lifts, then the gondola cable Seilbahn and the chairlift, with all its recent permutations.

Technique

The simplest form of Alpine skiing is sliding downhill in a controlled manner while avoiding obstacles, either recreationally or in competition. Alpine competitive skiing is subdivided into four groups: slalom, giant slalom, super giant slalom ("Super G"), and downhill. The four divisions represent a graduation from the shortest, slowest, most precise, most closely set slalom gates, requiring numerous direction changes, to the longest, fastest, least controlled, with fewest turns, and more dispersed gates of the downhill.

In the slalom, the entire course and its flagged gates may be totally visible from the start, while in the case of the downhill course, the start to finish distance is extraordinarily long and serpentine, with the bulk of the course unseen from its starting gate. For example, the FIS* guidelines for minimum vertical drop for a World Cup downhill course is 800 m for men, and 500 m for women. In contrast, for slalom, the minimum vertical drop is 140 m for men, and 120 m for women.[35]

Downhill Ski Injuries

Two basic types of acute ski accidents occur in Alpine skiing, falls and collisions.

Falls. Falls are of two general types: twisting (rotational) and nontwisting (nonrotational). Falls occur in fairly predictable patterns. Rotational falls involve the lower extremity at knee and ankle level, whereas nonrotational falls often involve a forward fall component, leading to boot top fractures or rupture of the Achilles tendon.

Collisions. Collisions occur in a wide variety of mechanisms that may injure any part of the body. These mechanisms are the source of most head and spinal injuries observed in the management of winter sport neurologic trauma.

Early anecdotal observations date from our early 1950s ski resort patrol experiences, both on the hill and in the ski area First Aid room. Then, injuries ordinarily involved the lower extremity, most often distal to the

---

*Federation Internationale de Ski, founded in February 1924, during the first winter Olympic Games, in Chamonix, France. Today, 100 national ski associations comprise the membership of FIS.

knee, induced by primitive boots and bindings. Low skier density, drag lifts, primitive bindings, and the often less challenging recreational slopes (usually ungroomed) characteristically induced low-velocity accidents, commonly falls, and less frequently, collisions.

EPIDEMIOLOGY

About 1970, roughly 10% of the American population would ski 5 or more days per year, reportedly producing a total of 500,000 ski injuries annually. Now total accidents are far fewer (though numerous authorities claim more severe), with a range of 165,000 to 600,000 injuries being reported yearly, according to industry group figures.[28] This is somewhat speculative because only 25% to 50% of injuries are reported to ski patrols.[21] A complicating aspect in the difficulty of accurately evaluating the statistics is the difficulty in collection of a good denominator at ski resorts; therefore, ski injury data are mostly presented in skier-days, estimated from the use of the transport system.[11] A 1992 Munich study of medical professionals who ski was in this regard illuminating. It revealed an incidence of 4.2 injuries per 1000 skiing days, compared with a frequently cited value of 2.7 injuries from current literature. Thus, it has been asserted, every epidemiologic study clearly underestimates the actual rate of skiing injuries.[51] With such handicaps, the incidence of neurologic injury in skiing can be obscured. Most mild to moderate ski injuries require emergent general and predominantly orthopedic care,[13] but moderate to severe injuries often involve neurosurgical problems as well.

In America, the first analysis of ski injuries in the United States, in its overall entirety, was done in 1943 by Moritz, whose 3-year study covered 1372 injuries. Of these, 20% were to extremities, of which more than 50% were sprains and strains. The average disability time of 4 days suggested that many minor accidents were included. In Moritz's record keeping system, 334 injuries were classified as "miscellaneous," including 11 brain concussions. Moritz noted that the incidence of these "miscellaneous" injuries varied greatly with the terrain and the type of skiing.[38] A subsequent 8-year linear study of the New Hampshire Waterville Valley ski area, surveying general ski injuries, was published by Young in 1976. It featured a stable ski population, generous control population, and, importantly, was first to suggest American trends in overall accident type and number.[62]

The prospective study of Alpine skiing neurologic trauma, however, is relatively recent. America's first consecutive extended series specifically targeting neurologic injury in skiing and winter sports was published in 1983.[25] Our cautious warnings contained in that report were later echoed by Morrow's publication, in 1988, describing 16 downhill ski fatalities between 1980 and 1986 that were retrospectively studied.[39] In the interval, Blitzer and coworkers had retrospectively reviewed 8 years of Sugarbush North (Warren, VT) child and adult overall injuries, noting the presence of pediatric head and spine injuries with an incidence of 6.2%,[4] and Shealy, also in 1985, cataloged fatal injuries as well, mentioning speed as a lethal factor.[49] It was also during this time that Ambach, Tributsch, and Henn had concurrently reported an increase in fatal skiing accidents in the Tyrol.[1]

First U.S. Neurologic, Prospective, On-Site Ski Study

The initial data covering the first 126 patients were reported by Tahoe Neurosurgery in 1983. The updated and expanded data prospectively collected for neurologic ski injuries during the Tahoe winter seasons of 1975 to 1987 are summarized in Table 27–1. More proximate years' data are undergoing further analysis. In summary, Tahoe neurologic ski injuries were found to be twice as common in men as in women, and head

Table 27–1. Data Collected for Winter Sports Injuries, Commencing 1975

Head Injury	393
Spine Injury	182
Concussion	368
Skiers, with concussion	347

Note: The study group consisted of 285 males, 145 females, 430 total hospitalized patients with neurologic injuries. Cohort of skiers: 347.

From Harris JB. Neurologic Injuries in Skiing and Winter Sports in America. *In* Jordan BD, Tsaris P, Warren RF (eds): Sports Neurology. Rockville MD, Aspen Publishers, 1989, p 296.

injury was more than twice as common as spine injury.

In this detailed prospective and consecutive study, 347 skiers in a 430-patient study of skiers, snowboarders, and toboggan injured, the frequency of neurologic head injuries tended to correlate with ascending skier skill level. Beginners had 44 injuries (22.9%), Intermediates had 92 (26.5%), Advanced had 79 (22.9%), and Experts had 80 head injuries (23.1%). The combined total of racer, ski patrol, and instructor neurologic injury was almost 15%. These figures combined with other data acquired suggest that as skier skill advances, total injuries may decline, but the severity of head and spinal neurologic injury increases.

The data invite questions about fatigue factors, equipment, and speed, and also about the education of those who provide initial care to the neurologically injured skier.

Skiers were classified by age and sex, as is seen in Table 27–2. As might be suspected, the age group of 21 to 30 sustained the highest number of neurologic traumas, with men predominating (85 vs. 39 women, total, 135). The next highest was the 11- to 20-year-old group, with males again predominating more than 2:1 in frequency (85 vs. 39 females, total, 124).

In addition to the 347 patients sustaining neurologic injury during Alpine skiing, the study chronicled an array of 83 other ski resort neurologic injuries, on or adjacent to the ski slope, related to various mechanisms.

Alpine (Downhill) Skiing

Americans flocked to skiing in ever-increasing yearly totals up to the beginning of the 1990s, when skier starts decelerated and ski lift ticket sales plateaued. Simultaneous with technologic advances in personal ski equipment, limb injuries shifted from the ankle up the leg, first to lower extremity spiral fractures, later to boot top fractures, and most recently to internal derangement of the knee.

Comparing the 1990s with earlier decades, a dramatic change in the frequency of certain injury types is apparent. The 1939–1976 general Alpine skiing injury rate, which fell toward 3 cases per 1000 skier-days over two decades,[56] remained static until more recently; however, the incidence of serious, often multiple injuries began to climb, frequently involving head and spinal injury as well as internal chest and abdominal injury, with instances of traumatic death reported as well.[2, 3, 20, 41]

Paradoxically, measures designed to reduce overall minor to moderate injuries and to improve the quality of the skiing experience may have unintentionally increased the risk of lethal or serious injury requiring neurologic care. Among these are improvements in hill grooming and the combined advances in ski boot-, ski binding-, and associated technology.

Technologic improvements in both hill grooming and ski equipment have created the possibility of the skier with intermediate or advanced skill exceeding safe speeds with ease, and plunging downhill with a false sense of confidence and self-control. For example, since 1975, ski base plastics technology, which relates to the gliding surface of the ski, has increased attainable downhill ski speeds by 15% to 20%.

The growing tendency toward more seri-

Table 27–2. Skiers, 1975–1988, vs. Any Type Surgery (Any Mechanism)

Age of Skier	Number of Surgeries					Total
	1	2	3	4	5	
5–10	3	0	0	0	0	3
11–15	4	1	0	0	0	4
16–20	16	6	3	0	0	25
21–25	7	8	3	0	1	19
26–30	9	2	1	0	1	13
31–35	7	2	1	0	0	10
36–40	3	1	0	1	0	5
41–45	2	1	0	0	0	3
46–50	1	1	1	0	0	3
51–55	1	0	0	0	0	1
56–60	2	0	0	0	0	2
Totals	55	23	9	1	2	89

ous injuries suggests that the kinetics of recent ski injuries are now similar to that of automobile accidents.[6] Certainly this appears to be an outgrowth of improved ski equipment, ski technique, hill grooming, and the resultant increased skier speed.

At high speeds, skiing becomes essentially a contact sport because the skier acts as a missile.[15] Accidents at high speeds, with abrupt deceleration on impact, shift toward neurologic injury. Furthermore, the collision mechanism of injury at high speed specifically suggests being out of control or close to the limits of control.

Collision: Experience at Tahoe

Collisions occur in a wide variety of mechanisms that may injure any part of the body. Collisions were the source of most head and spinal injuries that we observed in winter sports neurologic trauma. Collisions caused 176 of 347 skier concussions studied. Thirteen skiers struck lifts, 25 struck boulders, 69 struck trees, and 67 struck other skiers (12 of these 67 skier-skier collisions required major surgery).

Collision with various objects (skiers, trees, boulders, moguls, lifts, aerial landing zones) had a bearing upon just how many surgical procedures would be required. Table 27–3 depicts this distribution; skiers experiencing collisions with trees required more than twice as many surgical procedures compared with skiers who suffered the second most common mechanism, skier-skier collision. Twenty-five percent of the skiers sustained combined head and spinal injuries.

Skier collision mortality was 1.7% (discussed later). Permanent radiculopathy was seen in 13 patients, and permanent myelopathy was seen in 4 patients. Transient quadriplegia was seen in 13; diplegia was seen in 10. Transient paraplegia and hemiplegia were seen in 3 each. Most plegic patients were either expert recreational skiers, instructors, or racers, and, as such, all commonly skied at extreme speeds.

Of the 347 skiers sustaining concussion, 34 required major cranial surgery. Most patients undergoing one or more craniotomy or cranioplasty were found within the age group of 21 to 25, with the next largest subset in the 16-to-21 age group.

Fifty-five of all series patients required a single surgical procedure of varying complexity, 51 of whom required major surgery. Two skiers required no less than five separate surgical procedures of various complexities. The severity of these identified cases speaks to the factor of speed involved at the time the injury was sustained, and of peak acceleration at time of impact in production of the injury. The extent to which this type of trauma, specifically American neurologic ski injury, may have been sustained earlier (prior to this study) is without known record, but undoubtedly must exist, as well as an unknown element of mortality.

The interval between airborne helicopter VHF radio announcement of the impending arrival at the hospital of an injured skier and the operating room emergency induction of an injured skier, at times, was no more than 30 minutes. Immediate emergency open craniotomy was performed on 19 skiers, one of whom required a second craniotomy in the acute postoperative period. All received benefit from wide decompression technique, as well as evacuation of severely pulped brain, compounded bone fragments, and intracerebral, subdural, and epidural hematomas. Surgical technique emphasized the use of generous dimensions in surgical exposure. We are confident that such technique was often instrumental in saving skiers' lives and enhancing the skiers' subsequent quality of life.

Table 27–3. Common Skier Collision Mechanisms vs. Number of Surgical Procedures, 1975–1988

Mechanism	One	Two	Three	Four	Five	Total
Skier-skier	10	3	1	0	0	14
Tree	20	6	3	0	2	31
Aerial	3	3	5	1	0	12
Boulder	2	3	5	1	0	11
Mogul	3	1	0	0	0	4
Lift	2	1	0	0	0	3

Many of the injured skiers in this group returned for elective cranioplasty. Twelve of these skiers underwent one cranioplasty, and three required bilateral cranioplasties. The procedures were performed as much for safety as for cosmesis, since these life-saving craniotomies were often as much as 10 to 14 cm in anteroposterior dimension. In each case, methyl methacrylate cranioplasty was required, since bone flap storage facilities were not consistently available.

Collision: Skier Age vs. Surgery

If skiers undergoing surgery for neurologic injuries (irrespective of the complexity) are viewed by age, the Tahoe statistics revealed that the 16-to-25-year-old group underwent surgery most frequently. This same age cohort of neurologically injured skiers required 49.4% of all surgery completed. Its chronologic predecessor, the 16-to-20-year-old skiers, ranked second in frequency of surgical treatment.

Skier mortality was 1.7%. Six skiers died. No sudden death of vague or unexplained nature occurred; all were related to trauma. The mean time of skier injury resulting in death was 12:48 P.M. Male skier deaths outnumbered female skiers 5:1. The average age at death was 26, but only one skier death did not fall within the 19-to-26-year-old age span. Over the last 5 years, by comparison, 187 fatalities have been reported countrywide, a 21% increase over the preceding five ski seasons. At Tahoe, collisions with trees and boulders were the most common fatal impact mechanisms. According to Brinkhous, to cause death from impact, striking velocity to head or chest must typically exceed 6.7 m/s.[7]

ANATOMY OF SKIING NEUROLOGIC INJURY

Skull Fracture

In the Lake Tahoe study, skull fractures were generally confined to one fossa. The most commonly involved area was the frontal cranial fossa. Basal skull fractures were next in frequency, and parietal fractures were the least frequent.*

---

*Fractures: n = 82. Fracture areas distribution: vault: 53, basal: 48, frontal: 23, temporal: 21, occipital: 17, depressed: 19, compound: 13, bilateral: 14.

Closed blunt trauma most often was the cause of skull fracture. The less frequent yet more unusual injuries involved open penetration of the skull, by either ski tip, ski tail, or ski pole.

Some of these skier skull fracture accidents are tragically grotesque. One involving skull perforation and brain self-impalement was reported. A 23-year-old "excellent" skier attempted to arrest his accelerating slide with the handle of his ski pole following a fall on an icy, undulating slope. When he did so, the ski pole handle encountered an icy protuberance, causing the ski pole's point to penetrate his right temporal squama, impaling the brain to the midline.

He was transported from the hill accident site by helicopter and promptly underwent right-sided exploratory craniotomy. Shortly thereafter a ski patrol officer arrived at the hospital operating room and presented the impaling ski pole. Dried blood and brain matter covered the ski pole from tip to basket.

The postoperative diagnoses included (1) brain laceration, (2) right acute subdural hematoma, (3) intracerebral hematoma, (4) laceration of the vascular radicals of the sylvian triangle of the middle cerebral artery, (5) compound depressed skull fracture, (6) encephalomalacia adjacent to an expanding intracranial hematoma, (7) left acute traumatic hemiplegia resolving to hemiparesis, (8) cerebral concussion, and (9) facial laceration.

In the postoperative recovery phase he developed posttraumatic jacksonian seizures, which were successfully controlled with medication. Physical therapy restored him to virtually full function, despite moderate spastic hemiparesis, evident at infrequent intervals, only to close friends, and only when fatigued. Medication-free since 1978, he now has a successful real estate business with 15 employees.

Neck and Spine Injury

Spinal injuries are customarily regarded to be a small percentage of total ski accidents, but for surviving patients, they may be the most devastating. Overall general ski spine injury rates, from recreational beginner to experienced competitor, are variously reported from 1.8% to 4.7% of the total ski injuries sustained.[14, 18, 32] The number of Tahoe series cervical spine injuries related to the cervical segments was greater than all other skier spinal levels combined (81 vs. 76).

Thoracic, lumbar, and sacral injuries were often seen with aerial and freestyle maneuvers. In contrast, cervical injuries were generally associated with coexistent head injuries, ordinarily sustained in high-speed downhill skiing impacts. Nevertheless, at times a relatively low-force and seemingly innocuous mechanism may produce serious spinal injury and marked neurologic impairment.

One such incident involved a 33-year-old second-year female skier who fell while debarking from a lift chair, striking her head in a marked flexed and right-rotated fashion on the off-loading ramp. She was immediately examined by a neurosurgeon, who fortuitously happened to be in the next chair, and found to be initially unresponsive, then stuporus, unable to move any limb, and totally flaccid.

The neurosurgeon applied traction to the head. Partial function was restored, and the patient was transported by ambulance to the hospital as the neurosurgeon maintained continuous manual traction. Examination and spinal imaging were completed at once. With cervical immobilization, significant progress was seen during her acute hospitalization. On discharge the patient's diagnosis included (1) traumatic quadriplegia (severe and transient); (2) residual quadriparesis with persistent right upper extremity monoplegia; (3) probable cervical spine fracture-dislocation with spontaneous closed reduction, associated with higher cervical spine neurologic motor deficit, (4) cerebral concussion; and (5) shock, presumed neurogenic hypotension, secondary to apparent transient spinal cord ischemia.

No positive evidence of cervical spine fracture or frank dislocation was noted on acute roentgenographic studies. It was believed that the absence of severe persistent quadriplegia was due to serendipitous prompt and resourceful treatment rendered on the scene by the visiting skier-neurosurgeon.

Downhill skiing spinal injury, much like head injury, primarily stems from collision. In collision the cervical segments are commonly involved, not surprisingly usually with concurrent head injuries. As mentioned earlier, this relationship appears to be constant except for those skiers involved in inverted aerials, in whom thoracolumbar and lumbosacral injuries are seen. Simultaneous fractures of the skull and cervical spine present at other times as well, particularly in collisions with boulders and trees, and fatal outcome in such a combination is not unusual.

Although rapid deceleration with boulder impact may rarely induce atlantoaxial dislocation, the general spectrum of Alpine skiing cervical spine traumatic ligamentous instability and cervical fracture-dislocation seen at Tahoe was consistent with the customary cervical distribution of neurosurgical injury reported elsewhere. In the cervical segments of the spine, C4–C5 was most commonly involved, as described by Yashon.[61]

Falls in mogul fields often induced cervical spine flexion injuries because they usually occur on steep slopes, and loss of control in a mogul field often pitches the skier forward, bending the head and neck in a posture vulnerable to the initial impact.

The study raised this question: Is there a relationship between severity of cervical spine injury in the Tahoe skiers and their skill levels? Some degree of correlation did indeed exist between the severity of cervical spine injury and the skill level of Tahoe non-professional skiers ($R = .172$, $P = .0037$).

Eight skiers underwent laminectomy or fusion.

Nerve and Plexus Injuries

Shoulder dislocation in fall or collision mechanisms occasionally induced brachial plexus injury. Noninverted aerials compounded by poor landings, on rare occasions, have produced sacral plexus and sciatic axonotmetic injuries of extended morbidity. These were seen most frequently when the freestyle aerialist poorly executed a "daffy" (a daffy is a noninverted aerial jump accompanied by an exaggerated leg stride while the skier is above the snow).

Peripheral Nerve Injuries

It is now uncommon for the neurologic specialists engaged in ski injury to see pure peripheral nerve injuries, because the majority of such peripheral nerve injuries stemmed from the earlier use of the "ski leash," which has largely been abandoned as an after-fall ski retention device.* This device was superseded by the now-ubiquitous "ski brake." The ski brake is a spring-loaded pair of prongs attached to the ski sides that serves to arrest the ski by projecting from the ski-binding area once the ski boot separates from the ski. Thus freed in the fall, the separated ski customarily exits the fall perimeter of the skier, but remains safely nearby.

Seizures

Ten of the 347 victim skiers in the Tahoe study experienced major seizures during skiing. In five of these skiers sustaining seizure, the trauma sustained appeared to incite or contribute to the appearance of a seizure. The other five revealed a preexisting history of seizures. The current consensus suggests that with few exceptions, scant current data exist to suggest an increased risk of injury to epileptics involved in sports.[8] On the other hand, the participation of such seizure-susceptible patients in sports with significant levels of physical exertion depends largely on the degree of seizure control. It is important to recognize that in skiing, as in participation in other sporting events, it may be possible that such exertion could result in metabolic or psychological mechanisms that precipitate seizure.[36]

SPECIFIC NEUROLOGIC CONSIDERATIONS OF DOWNHILL COMPETITION

The Equipment

In the area of formal Alpine competition, the severity of injuries to today's competitors is in part reduced by the quality of the equipment, particularly the introduction and use of the downhill helmet, without which many more downhill racers would undoubtedly die. Haid, the Austrian physician at Innsbruck, evaluated fatal Tyrolean ski accidents treated in 1995 and was the first to suggest that injury might have been less severe if a helmet had been worn.[24]

Since the introduction of the helmet in downhill skiing, study of the competitive skier fatality rate has continued, and by 1980 the rate had been reduced to approximately 1 case per year.[50]

Helmet padding density and padding thickness have profound influence on the brain's ability to accommodate the g-forces absorbed at the time of collision. The effects of various thicknesses of polyurethane padding and of velocity on peak head acceleration have been studied comprehensively by Gurdjian.[22] For instance, in Gurdjian's experiments, increasing zygomatic padding from $\frac{1}{2}$ in to 2 in was found to attenuate a 1.1 lb Stryker force impact of 10.5 ft per second from 100 g down to less than 5 g.

The benefit of such protection seems intuitive; yet, contrasting opinions are voiced; to wit: "Helmets don't seem to prevent serious head injury when a skier is traveling more than a relatively leisurely 12 miles an hour," according to a ski industry affiliate when interviewed by the Wall Street Journal.*[16] This in essence suggests that head injury in many cases may not be preventable. However, the results of Gurdjian's research clearly suggests that protective head padding (1) attenuates the effect of the impact over a larger area, and (2) significantly reduces the g forces absorbed by the brain, with the potential to attenuate cerebral contusion to concussion, and concussion to perhaps an innocuous impact.

Through the various combinations of padding density and padding thickness, significant attenuation of the initial raw g force velocity can be achieved by extending the time during which the force is applied by several milliseconds, which directly mitigates the total kinetic energy absorbed.

The Downhill Course

Downhill racers currently descend iced and frozen courses at speeds as high as 60 to 80 mph, and only recently, briefly at 90 mph.† The skier is visually guided primarily by paired high-visibility flags, steering between two trails of closely spaced pine

---

*Perhaps this type of injury may experience a resurgence, inasmuch as there is now casual talk of using the same type of device for snowboards.

*The ski industry apparently has not enthusiastically embraced the idea of ski helmets. Perhaps the presence of helmets might send the subtle implication to customers that danger could exist.

†In the 1998 ski season a new speed skiing record was set: 155 mph!

boughs that are seen, at racing speed, as a twin green blur. These cues are intended as guidance to assist the racer in preparing for the next turn and in gauging alterations in the course pitch or hill steepness. Fractional miscalculation of these cues can lead to failure to negotiate a curve and to consequent collision with a fence, boulder, tree, or (if the skier is fortunate) a protective net.

At the point of collision the protective design of the downhill helmet is tested. Forces sufficient to produce concussion have been inferred from Gurdjian's plots of acceleration time tolerance curves. Skull fractures generally occur at 112 g to 160 g and concussion at 90 g, but usually little or no skull vault injury occurs at 80 g or less. For example, one World Cup competitor, on a typical downhill course, wearing an approved official downhill helmet, hit a Tahoe snow fence, sustained severe generalized brain injury, and remained in a traumatic coma for a month. Unquestionably, this injury would have been lethal without the helmet. Her miraculous recovery was marred only by her inability to return to international competition owing to a subtle organic brain syndrome that thereafter caused her, as ski coaches have suggested, "to read gates slowly."

Almost half the injuries in Alpine ski races occur in the last third of the course, which emphasizes the important contribution of fatigue to the occurrence of injuries.[29]

Neurospecialists in Sports and Skiing

The neurosurgeon's appearance in the field of sports injury as well as the appearance of head protection both date from the work of Gurdjian, Norrell, and Schneider,[53, 54] whose efforts improved the design of football helmets. Norrell was the first neurosurgeon to expand significantly the application of sports neurology beyond football players.[44]

Our experience as a race physician at downhill races in America and Europe has presented the twin challenges of immediate racer assessment on the downhill course, and the formulation of reasonable criteria for resumption of Alpine skiing competition for neurologically injured racers. The timing of return to downhill ski competition relates to the mechanism of injury, the degree of injury, and whether or not cerebral concus-

sion was accompanied by (1) additional craniocerebral mechanisms or (2) involvement of spinal injury associated with the head insult.

Where the race physician has identified cerebral concussion, prompt immediate termination of the activity followed by rest and observation is the rule. This is not always easy to enforce, and coaches often have the most influence and, surprisingly (to physicians), usually the last word, particularly where expressed pain or obvious injury is absent.*

The decision regarding the presence or absence of cerebral concussion, specifically in a ski accident victim on the course, can be either straightforward or obscure. In the case of a skier who is obviously confused and demonstrates the typical repetitive question, "What happened?" while being loaded into the ski patrol sled, the presence of cerebral concussion is obvious, as well as the potential hazard to the victim and to others if the skier were to continue. It is in the assessment of injuries of lesser, more obscure, degree where exact quantification of commotio cerebrii can at times be elusive.

The timing and advisability of return to Alpine skiing participation can be related to certain well-known guidelines relating to cerebral concussion that were initially applied to football. In football, the coach may define mild cerebral concussion as obvious when the injured player "cannot remember the plays"[37] because concussion is characterized by such amnesia. These guidelines have been advanced by experts such as Cantu,[9] Torg,[57] Maroon and colleagues,[33, 34] Hugenholtz and Richard,[27] Norrell,[45] and others. See Chapters 6 and 7.

FACTORS PREDISPOSING TO NEUROLOGIC SKI INJURY

Major ski injury risk factors for the recreational skier can be classified on the basis of relation to (1) collision with chair lifts, (2)

---

*This can raise troubling issues regarding professional liability where the attending sports physician is concerned. Such volunteer work is not covered by the Good Samaritan laws in certain states. As of 1998, states that have a "Volunteer Statute" appear to include Arkansas, Colorado, Georgia, Illinois, Indiana, Maryland, Massachusetts, Mississippi, Nevada, New Hampshire, New Jersey, New Mexico, North Dakota, Pennsylvania, Rhode Island, and Tennessee. Davis, McKelvey. Clin Sports Med 1998;1:71–82.

collision with trees, (3) collision on landing after aerial maneuvers, and (4) skier-skier collisions.

Collision With Chair Lifts

The Lake Tahoe study noted that 20 accidents were related to traditional, continuously moving chair lifts. Those in the lift-related accidents were injured as they dismounted, were struck by the chair lift, ran into the towers supporting the lifts, or were working as lift attendants.

The lift crews are particularly vulnerable to being struck by the conventional lift equipment because they are in the path of an oncoming chair as they assist a fallen lift rider. Some crew members working at such lifts have confided that head trauma is not at all uncommon for chair-loading employees.

A tram gondola accident was witnessed as well; however, it is not included in this series because personal involvement was delayed hours by avalanches. Three immediate deaths occurred when a hauling cable apparently jumped the "sheave" wheels,* causing the counterweight cable to crash through the cabin holding 80 skiers and drop the gondola 120 ft. Electric gondola winches had to lower survivors hundreds of feet to the surface in a wind-swept blizzard darkness. The rescue continued until 11:00 P.M., during which time great heroism was exhibited by the ski patrol and by the physicians immediately present, who were successful in saving many more from death. Gondola (Seilbahn) engineering and safety features have undergone progressive improvement through the succeeding years since 1978.

Collision With Trees

Of the 347 patients in the neurologically injured skier study, 69 (19.8%) collided with trees while skiing, resulting in two deaths. Surgery was required in 31 cases. None of the tree collision skiers was wearing a helmet. All required hospitalization for serious injuries or prolonged morbidity. Medical observations undertaken in this study suggest that if a careful examination is

completed on a tree-strike skier, it is almost axiomatic that a serious yet possibly subtle injury will be found involving some organ system. A surprising 5% to 10% have cardiac injuries.

This series appears to grossly under-reflect the number of fatal tree-strike incidents because some skiers are pronounced dead at the scene or shortly thereafter. For example, in one season alone, four nonhospitalized tree-strike skier fatalities occurred in the entire Lake Tahoe area. In contrast, our study's figures relate only to skiers personally seen and hospitalized after collision during this study period.

Our earlier reported observations regarding the lethal nature of collision with trees compared with other skier collision mechanisms were independently corroborated in a 1992 report by Friermood and colleagues in Colorado. Their Injury Severity Scores for tree collisions compared with other collision mechanisms were, respectively, 14.7 compared with 9.1. The comparative death rate was higher in skier-tree collisions as well.[17]

Aerial Skiing Collision Injuries

As the years passed since the inception of this study, organizations that evolved to regulate freestyle skiing undertook efforts to minimize accidents in formal freestyle competition. Efforts were made to ensure prior adequate dry-land training for all aerialists, and, in formal freestyle competitive events, to increase landing hill angles for inverted maneuvers from 23 or 27 degrees to a much steeper 38 degrees.[43] This change has lessened somewhat the tendency toward head-first or "pancake" landings, because a portion of the landing impact force is dissipated in an increased oblique down-slope vector. The initial need to ensure adequate snow cover in the landing areas goes without saying. Regrettably, amateur activities are mostly undertaken without these safeguards.

Aerial maneuvers caused an impressive array of neurologic injuries in the study. Should an aerial maneuver include a forward or backward flip, inducing a transient inverted attitude, the potential hazard is increased in respect to landing. If body position in the landing is not ideal, the vulnerable areas of the spine can be subject to

---

*A pulley wheel over which a "haul cable" passes, carrying chairs for the skiers.

abrupt flexion deformity. These injuries are generally focused at the cervicothoracic or thoracolumbar junctions or, rarely, simultaneously at both.

Of 59 Tahoe aerial neurologic injuries, 17 victims sustained noninverted cervical spine injuries, but nearly half of this group (7) were of severe fracture-subluxation types. The other most common serious aerial injuries at Tahoe were compound depressed skull fractures with intracranial hematoma, and lumbar (4) and sacral (3) spine injuries, with cervical and/or terminal cord injury, responsible for paraplegia or quadriplegia. Permanent disability and one aerial fatality occurred.

These activities require constant surveillance and perhaps should be prohibited at traditional recreational ski resorts, as dramatized by the following example.

A 21-year-old man executed an unsupervised aerial jump at a facility not formally outfitted for such maneuvers, and went over a 40-ft vertical drop, landing headfirst in a boulder formation. He was brought by helicopter to the hospital, where he immediately underwent bilateral decompressive craniotomy with evacuation of a right epidural hematoma, and simultaneous surgery for abdominal injuries. Despite these efforts, the patient died 7 hours after admission. Findings at autopsy included kidney, liver, and spleen laceration, as well as generalized cerebral edema with tentorial and foramen magnum pressure cones.

Skier-Skier Collisions

Skier-skier collisions are more common than ordinarily appreciated, and as downhill skiing speed has increased owing to the factors described earlier, collision fatalities now occur. Of the six skiers who died in skier-skier collisions, the mean age was 26.

One instance involved a skier in a formal ski lesson group. She was positioned stationary on the side of a trail, absorbed in the instructor's verbal critique. A speeding skier performing an aerial burst from the wooded boundary area and lost control while attempting to land on the occupied, groomed ski trail. His ski tip penetrated the student skier's skull in a fatal through-and-through head-blow mechanism.

Another case, that of Mr. H.P., a 48-year-old Chicagoan, is very troubling. He was struck down on a broad intermediate run by a skier who did not assist, but who instead skied away. While Mr. H.P. still sat dazed at the point of impact, he was struck by yet another skier, who skied away as well. Discovered by the patrol, he was transported immediately to the hospital by the ski area helicopter. Our view upon opening the helicopter door suggested an in extremis condition. He died as our group conveyed him quickly through the emergency room entrance.

PREVENTION OF NEUROLOGIC INJURIES IN RECREATIONAL SKIING

Alpine Skiing

Skiers themselves must accept responsibility for proper conditioning, yearly adjustment of equipment, skiing within the limits of ability, and honest recognition of the need for additional instruction when more challenging, yet more dangerous terrain beckons. In addition, the skier must accept responsibility for realizing when each ski day should come to a close because of fatigue.[5] The obscure but important contribution of fatigue to the occurrence of downhill ski injuries is reflected in the recreational injury rate, which increases during the late afternoon, when fatigue, poor lighting, and deteriorating snow conditions come into play together with increased numbers of skiers on the hill, compared with hours earlier in the ski day.[29]

One essential measure effective in reducing overall ski injuries, both in Europe and in America, has been the advancement of a basic code of skiing safety rules, in pamphlets and posted conspicuously at the base terminus where skiers board the lift, including, for example, the maxim that the downhill skier always has the right of way. The observed benefits of these rules multiplied as the decades passed, until the 1990s, when a new challenge surfaced, the increasing numbers of amateur (and often immature) snowboarders, all of whom are anxious to use the lift systems.

A dispassionate observer viewing this skier-boarder heterogeneous ski slope mix might conclude that the cultural disharmony of skiers and skateboard migrants is undisputed, aggravated by the obvious difference in their usual techniques of hill utilization (skiers ski down the hill fall line in short-radius turns, whereas boarders employ broad, curving traverses). Formal lessons in board riding given to beginners at the resorts, as well as the patient guidance of the ski patrol, will likely restore the necessary hill discipline of the past, so painstakingly achieved. The fundamental difference in hill utilization between the two disciplines, as well as the nonoptimal current chair-lift seat configuration (for snowboarders) may ultimately resegregate the respective enthusiasts seeking hill descent by their respective equipment. The need for more study in this area is obvious.

The incidence of serious preventable ski injuries can be favorably influenced at the ski school participant level, incorporating safety instruction, especially at the ski school entry A, B, and C level classes. The Tahoe Neurosurgical Ski Foundation suggests two innovative approaches for consideration:

1. Many skiers exploit the advantages of riding the ski area buses to the base of the hill, thus avoiding traffic congestion, cost, and frequent personal chain-up inconvenience. At modest cost, buses could be outfitted with monitors for showing instructional safety educational videos similar to music videos for riders in transit to the ski area slopes.

2. A less cost efficient (but for youngsters more motivational) pragmatic approach: At sign-up, prior to ski or snowboarding school, the young student would have the option of viewing music video-like safety educational videos, at the conclusion of which an innocuous paper examination is provided. A satisfactory score could later be exchanged upon presentation at the resort cafeteria for a soft drink or a hamburger. Then at lesson line-up, such lesson safety points covered earlier in the video could be easily reinforced by the instructor.

Another, broader preventive measure might be somehow to raise general public awareness about environmental risks that appear during winter, and to educate the children about these risks while still in the home environment, especially at play.

One natural spot for such prewinter sports orientation would be at the school, in physical education classes.[30, 55] Another potential site is the ski or snowboard shop, with in-

creased focus on children's equipment and its use, through improved education of ski shop personnel, as has been done in Sweden.[59]

Since neurologic ski injuries are so devastating, prevention is obviously the key, and this should include a skier's daily personal commitment to efforts at prevention, as outlined in our 1983 plea: The use of the helmet for (a) children, and (b) for skiers who ski through wooded areas, without question. A simple "catching an edge" can violently slam the descending skier's head into a tree. In such circumstances, the helmet not only can reduce the seriousness of injuries but also may save the skier's life. By the midpoint in the 1998–99 season, the reported Tahoe ski area death toll was six. Perhaps lift crew members should also consider wearing helmets (modified to limit peripheral vision as little as possible) because they are constantly exposed to oncoming chairs while helping downed skiers.* They would also set a visible good example for their patrons.

Free Style Skiing

These activities require constant surveillance and perhaps should be prohibited at traditional recreational ski resorts.

PREVENTIVE PRACTICES RELATED TO SCHEDULED COMPETITION

Tandem Slalom Racing

In tandem slalom competition, courses might be safer if set farther apart, but if this is not feasible because of television coverage requirements, then increased use of helmets would be desirable.

Alpine Formal Downhill Events

One simple prophylactic measure of potentially immeasurable value is suggested by the Tahoe Neurosurgical Ski Foundation for

---

*The potential minimal reduction of side peripheral vision must be balanced against the advantage of protecting the exquisitely vulnerable thin bone of the temporal skull and its underlying middle meningeal artery.

inclusion in the yearly prescreening physical assessment of aspiring national team members: A simple lateral spine radiograph of the cervical spine. This one study could identify any candidate potentially at excessive risk for catastrophic injury by virtue of an asymptomatic but latently hazardous spine anatomy. Similarly, those who in the last racing season sustained severe falls and collisions could be reassessed simultaneously for evidence of any progressive yet asymptomatic pathology. Borderline cases in either instance could undergo follow-up magnetic resonance imaging of the spine or computed tomographic scan and consultation.

Helmet use is mandatory for downhill events, and its use is desirable as well for "Super G." This is mentioned only because at one time it was indeed optional.[31]

Although the downhill injury rate is customarily low,[12] competitive Alpine downhill courses are venues of significant potential danger. They are conducive to neurologic injury for participants who are essentially without protection other than their own elite conditioning and downhill helmet. As such, recent efforts to modify such courses to achieve optimal neurologic safety objectives must continue.

At the risk of stating the obvious, downhill courses at all course areas should have a sufficient clear area surrounding them so that racers are not seriously injured by hitting objects, course personnel, or spectators. The growing use of nets strung in trees and "Willy Bags,"* filled with polyethylene fragments, adjacent to fixed poles and tree trunks addresses this area of concern.

This study suggests the need for prompt identification and correct management of the increasing neurologic aspects of the ski injuries and anticipation of their occurrence at formal events. Now, with the Tahoe Neurosurgical Foundation prospective 2-decade study, along with other recent work mentioned, we have sufficient knowledge that debilitating and even catastrophic neurologic ski injuries are to be expected in America. This, coupled with any elective plans to hold a formal downhill event, inescapably leads us to the following conclusion:

Because half the fatalities in all athletes result from trauma to the head and neck,[40] ski areas or race sponsors must provide a way to evacuate the neurologically injured competitor promptly to a facility with advanced neurologic diagnostic equipment, related medical care, and affiliated personnel.

SUMMARY AND CONCLUSIONS

Neurologic injuries in recreational Alpine skiing, although less frequent than orthopedic injuries, induce such morbidity and mortality that PREVENTION is the only rational manner of managing this present and, with the influx of young snowboarders, probably expanding epidemic.[10, 26] Public awareness regarding the serious nature, number, and social cost (especially among productive young people) of these injuries must be raised through education.[42] Resorts must increase efforts in spotting problem skiers and boarders.

Ski, snowboard, and winter sports play injuries cause severe morbidity. Helmet usage, adequate approved training, resort surveillance, and regulation can reduce mortality, morbidity, and the extreme financial costs.[23]

More prospective, on-site, linear, independent physician study will be helpful as well. Such study will facilitate early detection of temporal injury trends so that timely response in the form of adjustments in injury prevention strategy can be effected.[58] The recent twin tragic deaths of well-known national figures (U.S. Representative Sonny Bono and Mr. Michael Kennedy) also serve to further validate the significance of the findings and the importance of the recommendations derived from ongoing research such as the Tahoe Neurosurgical work, the first focused, extended, consecutive prospective study in the specific realm of American neurologic ski and winter sports trauma.

References

1. Ambach E, Tributsch W, Henn R. Epidemiology of fatalities in alpine skiing (1987–1990). Beitr Gerichtl Med 1992;50:333–336.
2. Ambach E, Tributsch W, Henn R. Epidemiology of fatalities in alpine skiing (1987–1990). Beitr Gerichtl Med 1992;50:333–336.
3. Blankstein A, Salai M, Israeli A, et al. Ski injuries

---

*Named for the innovator, Willy Schaeffler, renowned FIS official.

in 1976–1982: Ybrig region, Switzerland. Int J Sports Med 1985;6:298–300.

4. Blitzer CM, Johnson RJ, Ettlinger CF, et al. Downhill skiing injuries in children. Am J Sports Med 1984;12:142–147.

5. Bouter LM, Knipschild PG, Volovics A. Personal and environmental factors in relation to injury risk in downhill skiing. Int J Sports Med 1989;10:298–301.

6. Bowman WD. Winter First Aid Manual, 4th ed. Denver, National Ski Patrol System, 1984 p 114.

7. Brinkhous KM. Accident Pathology. National Highway Safety Bureau (No. FH-1 1-6595). Washington, DC, US Government Printing Office 1968, p 76.

8. Cantu RC. Epilepsy and sports. Clin Sports Med 1998;17:61–69.

9. Cantu RC. Guidelines for return to contact sports after a cerebral concussion. Phys Sportsmed 1986;14:75–83.

10. Chow TK Corbett SW, Farstad DS. Spectrum of injuries from snowboarding. J Trauma 1996;41:321–325.

11. de Loës M. Epidemiology of sports injuries in the Swiss organization "Youth and Sports," 1987–1989. Injuries, exposure and risks of main diagnoses. Int J Sports Med 1995;16:134–138.

12. Ekeland A, Dimmen S, Lystaad H, et al. Completion rates and injuries in alpine races during the 1994 Olympic Winter Games. Scand J Med Sci Sports 1996;6:287–290.

13. Ellison AE. Skiing injuries. Clin Symp 1977;29:2–40.

14. Ellison AE: Skiing injuries. Clin Symp 1977;29:2–40.

15. Erskine LA. The mechanisms involved in ski injuries. Am J Surg 1959;97:667–671.

16. Fatsis S, Costello D. Down a slippery slope. Wall Street Journal 8 Jan. 1999:W1.

17. Friermood TG, Messner DG, Brugman JL, Brenan R. Save the trees: a comparative review of skier-tree collisions. J Orthop Trauma 1994;8:116–118.

18. Frymoyer JW, Pope MH, Kristiansen T. Skiing and spinal trauma. Clin Sports Med 1982;1:309.

19. Furrer M, Erhart S, Frutiger A, et al. Severe skiing injuries: A retrospective analysis of 361 patients, including mechanism of trauma, severity of injury, and mortality. J Trauma 1995;39:737–741.

20. Furrer M, Erhart S, Frutiger A, et al. Severe skiing injuries: A retrospective analysis of 361 patients, including mechanism of trauma, severity of injury, and mortality. J Trauma 1995;39:737–741.

21. Garrick J. The epidemiology of ski injuries. Minn Med 1971;54:17.

22. Gurdgian ES. Impact Head Injury: Mechanistic, Clinical, and Preventive Correlations. Detroit, Charles C Thomas Publisher, 1975, pp 308–349.

23. Hackman DJ, Kreller M, Pearl RH. Snow-related recreational injuries in children: Assessment of morbidity and management strategies. J Pediatr Surg 1999;34:65–69.

24. Haid B. Todliche skiverletzungen in einzugsgebiet der chirgische universitatsklinik Innsbruck von 1944–1954. Arch Orthop Unfall Chir 1955;47:105–114.

25. Harris JB. Neurological injuries in winter sports. Phys Sportsmed 1983;11:12.

26. Harris JB. First report of snowboard neurological injury. Clin Sports Med 1989;1:45–56.

27. Hugenholtz H, Richard MT. The on-site management of athletes with head injuries. Phys Sportsmed 1983;11:71–78.

28. Johnson RJ, Ettlinger CF, Campbell RJ, et al. Trends in ski injuries: Analysis of a six year study (1972–1978). Am J Sports Med 1980;8.

29. Lamprecht H. Fachgruppe der Seilbahnen in der sektion verkehr der Tiroler handelskammer. Skiunfallerhebung. Winter 1984–85. Innsbruck 1986;2.

30. MacNab AJ, Codman R. Demographics of alpine skiing and snowboarding: Lessons for prevention programs, Inj Prev 1996;2:286–289.

31. Mang WR, Maurer PC. Der todliche Skiunfall. Fortsch Med 1976;3:107–110.

32. Margreiter R, Raas E, Lugger LJ. The risk of experienced alpine skiers. Orthop Clin North Am 1976;7:51–54.

33. Maroon JC, Steele PB, Berlin R. "Burning Hands" in football spinal cord injuries. JAMA 1977;238:2049–2051.

34. Maroon JC, Steele PB, Berlin R. Football head and neck injuries—an update. Clin Neurosurg 1980;27:414–429.

35. Personal communication: McBerty J, Steadman R, Steadman-Hawkins Sports Medicine Foundation, Vail CO, 1998.

36. McLaurin PL. Epilepsy and contact sports. JAMA 1973;3:225–287.

37. Meggyesy D. Out of Their League. Berkeley, CA, Ramparts, 1970, p 125.

38. Moritz JR. Ski injuries: A statistical and analytic study. JAMA 1943;121:97–99.

39. Morrow PL, McQuillen EN, Eaton LA, Jr., Bernstein CJ. Downhill ski fatalities: The Vermont experience. J Trauma 1988;28:95–100.

40. Murphy F, Simmons JCH. Initial management of athletic injuries to the head and neck. Am J Surg 1959;98:379–383.

41. Myles ST, Mohtadi NG, Schnittker J. Injuries to the nervous system and spine in downhill skiing. Can J Surg 1992;35:643–648.

42. Myles ST, Mohtadi NG, Schnittker J. Injuries to the nervous system and spine in downhill skiing. Can J Surg 1992;35:643–648.

43. Myers C. US freestyle: Upside down and out? Ski Mag, February 1987, pp 29–36.

44. Norrell H. Sports injuries. Presented at the 29th annual meeting, Congress of Neurological Surgeons, Las Vegas, NV, Oct. 10, 1971.

45. Norrell H. The neurosurgeon's responsibility in the prevention of sports injuries. Clin Neurosurg 1972;19:208–219.

46. Oh S. Fachgruppe der Seilbahnen, in der Sektion verkher der Tiroler handelskammer, ergebissne unfallerhebung, Winter (1980–1983). In Prevention of head injuries in skiing. Basel, Karger, 1985, pp. 2–3.

47. Oh S, Reudi M. Depressed skull fractures in skiing and their experimental study. Int J Sports Med 1982;3:168–173.

48. Petitpierre M. Die winter sportverletzungen. Stuttgart, F. Enke, 1939, 1:193.

49. Shealy JE: Death in downhill skiing. In Johnson R, Mote CD, Jr. (eds): Skiing trauma and safety. Fifth International Symposium. Philadelphia, American Society for Testing and Materials, 1985, pp 349–357.

50. Schaeffler W. Personal communication, 1980.

51. Scherer MA, Ascherl R, Lechner F. Zur aussagekraft epidemiologischer studen uber verletzungen beim

skisport. Sportverletz Sportschaden 1992;6:150–155.

52. Schneider RC, Kennady IC, Plant ML, et al. Sports injuries—Mechanism, prevention and treatment. Baltimore, Williams and Wilkins, 1985, pp 256–270.

53. Schneider RC. Serious and fatal football injuries. Clin Neurosurg 1964;12:226–236.

54. Schneider RC. Concomitant craniocerebral and spinal trauma with special reference to the cervicomedullary region. Clin Neurosurg 1969;17:300.

55. Shephard RJ. Asphyxial death of a young skier. Am J Sports Med 1996;36:223–227.

56. Tapper EM. Ski injuries from 1939–1976: The Sun Valley experience. Am J Sports Med 1978;6:114.

57. Torg JS. Athletic Injuries to the Head, Neck and Face. Philadelphia, Lea and Febiger, 1982 pp 39–52.

58. Ueland O, Kopjar B. Occurrence and trends in ski injuries in Norway. Br J Sports Med 1998;32:299–303.

59. Ungerholm S, Gustavsson J. Skiing safety in children: A prospective study of downhill skiing injuries and their relation to the skier and his equipment. Int J Sports Med 1985;6:353–358.

60. Unterthamscheidt EJ. Injuries due to boxing and other sports. Handb Clin Neural 1975;23:577–682.

61. Yashon D. Spinal Injury, 2nd ed. East Norwalk, CT, Appleton-Century-Crofts, 1986, p 10.

62. Young LR, Oman CM, Crane H, et al. The etiology of ski injuries: An eight years study of the skier and his equipment. Orthop Clin North Am 1976;7:13–29.

28

Spinal Injuries in Canadian Ice Hockey Players, 1966–1996

**Charles H. Tator, James D. Carson,
and Robert Cushman**

Hockey injuries are a considerable public health problem, both in financial and human terms.[15] We have data that more than 60 hockey players in Canada now require wheelchairs for their activities of daily living owing to a spinal cord injury suffered while playing ice hockey. For decades in Canada, diving has been a leading sport or recreational cause of cervical spine injury,[28] and hockey was a rare cause until 1979. However, since then, cervical spine injuries in hockey have continued to occur at a catastrophic rate despite prevention programs and attempts to educate the public.[25] The cause of spinal injuries in hockey is multifactorial, and violence has been considered a causative factor. There is now widespread public concern about the level of violence in ice hockey.[12] We must continue to document the burden of injury and attempt to identify the causes. Such documentation is essential for the development and monitoring of more effective preventive strategies.

With the increased use of hockey helmets in Canada since the late 1960s, it is perhaps surprising that both spinal injuries and brain injuries have increased.[1, 25] We believe that the same general mechanisms that cause spinal injuries in ice hockey are responsible for what appears to be a significantly increased incidence of head injuries and career threatening concussions among North American professional ice hockey players. In Canada, both the press and physicians have commented about a recent rise in the incidence of concussions in ice hockey. According to a catastrophic sports injury registry, sports that have the greatest chance of causing catastrophic head injury are football, gymnastics, ice hockey, and wrestling.[5] In ice hockey, head injury is often due to striking the boards headfirst, which is the same mechanism for many spinal injuries. The sports that carry a risk for catastrophic head injury pose an even greater risk for minor head injury.[4] Prevention of head injuries and spinal injuries therefore must address the same issues.

METHODS

Since 1981 we have maintained a registry of spinal injuries in Canadian hockey, and, more recently, we have collected information on spinal injuries in other countries. The present report covers Canadian injuries only. All of the data has been collected retrospectively. In 1981 questionnaires were sent to all the neurosurgeons, orthopedic surgeons, and physical medicine and rehabilitation specialists in Canada asking for information about spinal injuries in hockey up to that point. In 1985 and at 2- to 3-year intervals since, these physicians have been asked to report all additional major hockey-related spinal injuries for inclusion in our permanent registry. Our definition of a major spinal injury includes any fracture or dislocation of the spine of a hockey player with or without injury to the spinal cord or nerve roots. The definition includes injuries with or without a permanent neurologic deficit. Cases of transient paralysis or transient sensory loss were also collected beginning in March 1987. We have also included any injury that involved a neurologic deficit. Minor injuries such as strains or whiplash are excluded. The demographic details were augmented in some cases by information obtained from players, coaches, and league officials. Reports published in the media were investigated to ensure that a physician had also reported the case.

Our latest study by questionnaire to 1965 physicians adds cases to the registry from 1994 through 1996. In the present survey, Canadian sports medicine physicians were included as recipients for the first time, and several cases were reported from sources other than physicians. In addition, several cases were identified through a catastrophic recreational injury study that we coordinated utilizing 13 trauma centers in Ontario. The player insurance reporting mechanism of the Canadian Hockey Association also identified a small number of cases that were unreported by physicians.

Statistical analysis was performed by examining the relationship by regression analysis between calendar year and the following variables: total number of injuries per year; number of injuries produced by checking from behind per year; number of spinal cord injuries produced by checking from behind per year; and number of severe injuries per year defined as injuries causing complete motor paralysis. All regressions and descriptive statistics were performed with a SAS statistical package (SAS Institute Inc., Raleigh, North Carolina).

RESULTS

In Canada, a total of 250 major spinal injuries have been reported for the years 1966–1996. Major spinal injuries in ice hockey were rare in the 1960s and 1970s, but beginning in 1980, the annual incidence increased markedly, as shown in Table 28–1, and from 1981 to 1996 averaged 14 cases per year with a maximum of 18 injuries during both 1990 and 1992. Six players are known to have died as a result of their injuries. Complete motor injuries were suffered by 63 players, who would thus require wheelchairs for their activities of daily living. Of the remaining injuries, 166 occurred during organized games, while 10 occurred during practice, and 4 occurred during "shinny" games, with the remainder in unknown circumstances.

The most frequent precipitating event in

Table 28–1. Annual Number of Injuries,* 1966–1996

Year	Total Injuries†	From Behind‡	Cerv/Behind§	CervCord/Behind‖
1966	1	0	0	0
1975	1	1	1	1
1976	2	0	0	0
1977	2	1	1	1
1978	3	0	0	0
1979	2	0	0	0
1980	8	3	3	2
1981	12	2	1	1
1982	14	5	5	3
1983	13	6	4	2
1984	14	0	0	0
1985	11	5	3	1
1986	16	6	5	2
1987	9	2	2	1
1988	17	8	5	3
1989	16	7	4	4
1990	18	6	3	2
1991	17	4	4	3
1992	18	7	6	4
1993	14	3	3	1
1994	7	2	1	0
1995	17	3	2	1
1996	11	3	0	0
Total	**243**	**74**	**53**	**33**

*Includes only those 243 out of 250 injuries for which adequate documentation was available to assess the number of injuries annually and those injuries with checking from behind as a mechanism.
†Total injuries: Number of ice hockey related spinal injuries.
‡From behind: Number of spinal injuries due to a check from behind.
§Cerv/behind: Cervical spine injuries due to a check from behind.
‖CervCord/behind: Cervical cord injuries due to a check from behind.

Table 28–2. Vertebral Level of Spinal Injury,* 1966–1996

	Frequency	Percentage
Cervical		
C1–C7/T1	184	85.2
Thoracic		
T1–T11	9	4.2
Thoracic-Lumbar		
T11/12–L1/2	13	6.0
Lumbosacral		
L2–S5	10	4.6
Total	**216**	**100**

*Includes only those 216 out of 250 injuries for whom adequate documentation was available.

Table 28–4. Age of Injured Players, 1966–1996

Age	Frequency	Percentage
11–15	48	20.8
16–20	116	50.2
21–25	19	8.2
26–30	21	9.1
31–35	14	6.0
36–40	8	3.5
41–45	3	1.3
46–50	2	0.9

Missing information (not supplied by survey respondents): 19.

the total series of injuries was a push or check from behind (Table 28–1). In most instances the injured player was unsuspecting of the impact and was hurled horizontally into the boards, with the cervical spine crushed by an axial loading force applied to the head.[30] Table 28–2 demonstrates the vertebral level of spinal injury, while Table 28–3 demonstrates the type of neurologic injury suffered. Of the 184 cases with adequate documentation, 74, or 40.2%, were due to a push or check from behind. An additional 46 players, or 24.9%, were pushed or checked but not from behind. Thirty-seven players, or 20.1%, tripped on

the ice; 17 injuries, or 9.2%, were due to sliding along the ice; and 10 players, or 5.3%, were tripped by another player. Impacts with the boards accounted for 157 (76.9%) of 204 adequately documented injuries. Impact between players (32 out of 204) was also a frequent mechanism of injury (15.7%), whereas impacts with the ice or goal post were less frequent. The youngest player with a major spinal injury was 11 years of age, and the oldest was 47. The median age was 17, and 20.4 was the mean age. Table 28–4 shows the number of injuries for different age groupings. Of the injured players, only 6 were females. Table 28–5 shows the distribution across Canada of these injuries by province or territory.

Burst fractures and fracture-dislocations were the most frequent types of vertebral injuries recorded. In a burst fracture, the main force is axial compression of the cervical spine, which causes comminution of the vertebral body with diminution in its height. Bony fragments are frequently displaced

Table 28–3. Neurologic Injuries,* 1966–1996

	Frequency	Percentage
Spinal Cord Injury		
‡CM + §CS	53	24.0
‡CM + ¶IS	9	4.1
‖IM + ¶IS	39	17.6
¶IS	4	1.8
‡CM	1	0.5
†Transient Sensory Loss/Transient Paralysis	36	16.3
Subtotal	**142**	**64.3**
Root Injury Only	22	10.0
No Neurologic Deficit	57	25.8
Subtotal	**79**	**35.7**
Total	**221**	**100**

*Includes only those 221 out of 250 injuries for whom adequate documentation was available.
†Transient sensory loss and transient paralysis information was only collected after March 1987.
‡CM = complete motor loss.
§CS = complete sensory loss.
‖IM = incomplete motor loss.
¶IS = incomplete sensory loss.

Table 28–5. Geographic Location of Injuries, 1966–1996

Location	Frequency	Percentage
Ontario	129	51.6
Quebec	23	9.2
British Columbia	23	9.2
Alberta	22	8.8
Saskatchewan	21	8.4
Manitoba	10	4.0
Nova Scotia	9	3.6
New Brunswick	5	2.0
Prince Edward Island	5	2.0
Newfoundland	2	0.8
Yukon	1	0.4
Total	**250**	**100**

Table 28–6. Number of Severe* Injuries per 3–Year Period

Period	Total Injuries	Severe Injuries	Percentage of Severe Injuries
1979–1981	22	7	31.8
1982–1984	41	15	36.6
1985–1987	36	7	19.4
1988–1990	51	14	27.5
1991–1993	49	9	18.4
1994–1996	35	6	17.1

*Severe is defined as complete loss of motor function below the level of the injury.

posteriorly into the spinal canal, causing neurologic deficit.[16] Of the 216 cases with adequate documentation, 37 had a neurologic deficit but no bony injury; 55 had vertebral damage but no neurologic deficit; 124 had both vertebral damage and neurologic deficit. We divided the 18 years from 1979 to 1996 into six 3-year periods, and we defined the most severe injuries to be those with complete loss of motor function below the level of the injury. Table 28–6 shows that the percentage of these most severe injuries is lower over the last two 3-year periods.

With respect to the statistical analysis, it should be noted that the data were not collected uniformly throughout the 30-year period. Also, it is not known whether the number of hockey players or the number of hockey hours played has changed. Thus, the analysis is based on reported data only. The highest R^2 value was .73 for the relationship between year and number of injuries for the entire study period. All other R^2 values were less than .5.

DISCUSSION

Injuries are Common and Costly

Ice hockey injuries accounted for 1.77% of all visits to Canadian hospital emergency departments from October 1985 through March 1986, and 5% of these were minor injuries to the neck area.[6] In a study of 287 adult male recreational ice hockey players, 32% of reported injuries were to the head, neck, and facial area, and 42% of these injuries occurred as a result of penalizable behavior.[31] We previously discussed how costly spinal injuries in hockey can be.[25]

Other authors also address the costs of hockey injury and sports-related spinal injury. Rampton and colleagues estimated that hockey injuries result in approximately 2.7–3.0 million Canadian dollars of direct acute-care medical expenditure per year in emergency departments throughout Ontario.[21] In 1993 the Canadian Paraplegic Association found 583 new spinal cord injuries in Canada, 75% in males and 67% between the ages of 16 and 40. Motor vehicle accidents account for the highest percentage of injuries, while falls and sports were second and third, respectively. These injuries have far-reaching implications, not only for the individual and his or her family, but also for society as a whole. These patients survive their injuries and live longer than patients with such injuries did formerly, and their care has advanced considerably.[9]

DeVivo used a cross-sectional multicenter study to estimate the direct costs for each case of spinal cord injury in the United States. Prospective data were collected during 1 year on all charges for emergency medical services, hospitalizations, attendant care, equipment, supplies, medications, environmental modifications, physician and outpatient services, nursing homes, household assistance, vocational rehabilitation, and miscellaneous items. In 1995 dollars, the first year charges averaged $295,643 for sports-related injuries. Recurring annual charges averaged $27,488. Using average age at time of injury for each case, a 2% real discount rate, and the most recent survival data from the National Spinal Cord Injury Statistical Center, the average lifetime charges for each case were $950,973. Given an estimated 10,000 new cases of spinal cord injury occurring each year (in the United States), of which 7.3% are caused by sports, the annual aggregate direct costs of sports-related traumatic spinal cord injury in the United States are $694 million.[10]

Etiology

Several etiologic factors that contribute to spinal injuries in hockey have been previously identified.[26, 27] Social and psychological factors among young hockey players include increased aggressiveness and willingness to take risks, a feeling of invincibility, and a lack of awareness of the possibility of spinal cord injury in hockey. In many cases, victims were injured during illegal play, especially illegal checking or pushing from behind. Our center was the first to identify checking from behind as a major cause of spinal cord injury in hockey and to suggest specific rules against this mechanism. Physical factors include the increased weight and speed of contemporary players, which increases the force generated by collisions, and poor neck muscle development, especially in younger players. Apparently many hockey coaches have not given their players sufficient instruction about the risks of spinal injury and the methods of protecting the spine from injury. Reynen and Clancy expressed the consensus of opinion that the style of play that is allowed a player with head protection may actually increase the chances of cervical spinal trauma.[23]

Biomechanical studies have not supported the notion that the helmet is an important factor in causing spinal injury.[2] Helmets have been extremely effective in reducing the incidence of brain injuries in hockey players,[11] and facemasks have produced a remarkable reduction in the number of eye and dental injuries.[20] The incidence of concussion can be reduced by helmet usage, and is showing a downward trend for players aged 5 to 14 years.[13] However, there is concern that concussions are increasing in professional players.[1] Laprade and co-workers found no evidence that facemasks are related to an increase in overall head and neck injuries,[17] an opinion offered by some hockey observers.[24] Watson and colleagues confirmed an association between larger ice surface size and decreased rates of injury while at the same time showing the absence of any relationship among surface size, neurotrauma, and penalties for aggressive conduct (checking from behind, body contact, and stick-related penalties).[32]

Prevention Strategies to Date

Prevention programs to reduce catastrophic spinal injuries include improvement in player awareness and conditioning, especially in strengthening neck and back muscles; rule changes and enforcement; and refereeing and coaching techniques.[25] As noted previously, specific rules to curb checking from behind[33] have been instituted largely because SportSmart Canada documented the importance of this mechanism

in the etiology of these injuries. We have also produced a video showing safe maneuvers, especially near the boards ("Smart Hockey with Mike Bossy"), and a brochure informing amateur players about neck muscle strengthening. Despite these measures, a major spinal injury due to ice hockey occurs in Canada almost every 2 weeks during the hockey season. Thus, additional prevention measures are required.

Current Attitudes and Ambiguity

Size and aggression are part of the culture of contemporary hockey, and thus players receive an inconsistent or mixed message regarding the amount of aggressiveness that is tolerated. Brust and colleagues showed that only half of the 12- to 15-year-old players understood the seriousness of checking another player from behind; worse, some of them were still willing to do it after learning of the association with serious injury.[3] The marked disparity in the incidence of these injuries between Ontario and Quebec, Canada's two most populous provinces, in which there were an approximately equal number of players, suggests that attitude and coaching techniques were extremely important etiologic factors. In addition, some organizations in Canada want to lower the age at which body checking begins. However, a study that compared checking with no-checking leagues in Peewee-level players (ages 12 through 13) showed that 88% of fractures were related to body checking, and that fractures were 12 times more frequent in players in leagues that allowed body checking. This study also reported that larger players were able to exert an impact force 70% greater than that exerted by smaller players.[22]

Athletes are evaluated on the basis of physical skills and effort, and aberrant behavior may be promoted. For example, some players may be induced to sacrifice their own safety and well-being for the good of the team. When coaches are dealing with young men, they must understand that players often connect these aberrant behaviors with masculinity. Under these conditions, a willingness to endure and use violence becomes an important means of proving one's worth and demonstrating one's membership on the team itself.[8] The National

Coaching Certification Program teaches that the role of the coach includes the responsibility to instill in participants lifetime values of sportsmanship and fair play.[34] There is no ambiguity in this statement. Coaches and trainers, along with the league and referees, have the power to defuse dangerous attitudes by emphasizing the magnitude and serious nature of injury to players.

A feeling of invincibility has been suggested as partially to blame because players believe that they are well protected by their equipment, and the officials may also take this stance. Therefore, referees may be more hesitant to call penalties. Some coaches may also share this feeling of player invincibility, and may attempt to stretch the rules or instruct players to break them in order to gain an advantage.[18] Although coaches state that they believe sportsmanship is important, Brust and colleagues reported that only 59% of players believe that sportsmanship is very important, with older players believing it less than younger players.[3] In most of the injuries in our series, the injured hockey players were playing under direct adult supervision, and many had an aggressive attitude that was supported by parents and coaches. The Hockey Development Centre for Ontario has developed a parents' guide to the prevention of spinal injuries in hockey. An "attitude adjustment" is recommended. The guide advocates "If every parent would stress the aspects of no hitting from behind, and respect for others, it would go a long way in reducing the number of serious injuries in hockey."[19]

Future Prevention Strategies

Further efforts to prevent spinal injuries should focus on the recipients of the safety message, that is, the players, parents, coaches, trainers, and leagues. Effective dissemination of safety information must include greater emphasis on the magnitude of these catastrophic injuries. Hockey players must be able to understand and relate to this information. Redesigning programs to appeal to the teenager is important because teens do not appreciate the magnitude of potential injury and are willing to assume poorly understood risks. All the messages must reinforce each other and point in the same direction.[14] The reduced incidence of cervical spinal injuries in football in the United States is an excellent example of epidemiologic studies leading to specific prevention programs. Clarke concludes that what the epidemiology of neck injuries in sports has best shown is that sports behavior can be changed through education.[7]

We believe that uncertainty about the interpretation and enforcement of hockey rules leads to serious injury. Safety instruction and lessons on how to take a check should be mandatory during practice at all age levels. A consistent safety message from hockey organizations both professional and amateur to the coaches and referees that is clearly passed along to the players and parents will help reduce serious injuries. For example, checking from behind must be eliminated from the game by increasing the severity of the penalty. Fighting should similarly be eliminated by severe penalties. With regard to safety, there is no room for ambiguity.

Improved Research

Now that the burden of injury has been defined and the importance of the problem highlighted, solutions will only come through more and improved research efforts. The database needs to be improved both in terms of the timeliness and of the quality of reporting. To compile our registry, we have actively sought retrospective data from voluntary reporting by multiple jurisdictions. A more useful method would be to make sports-related spinal cord injury part of hospital discharge coding for each province. Currently the reporting of sports-related spinal cord injuries by hospitals is rudimentary owing to lack of specific, sports-related codes. Surveillance programs should be linked with prevention programs.[29] The identification of high risk events, for example, checking from behind, can lead to the design and evaluation of interventions while simultaneously addressing barriers to safety implementation. Significant behavior change in hockey, as in other injury prevention efforts, will follow increased knowledge of problem recognition and require dramatic shifts in social attitudes about on-ice conduct. A significant obstacle lies in counteracting the culture of violence endemic to hockey in Canada and the United States today.

CONCLUSIONS

Major spinal injuries have been recognized as a problem in Canadian ice hockey only since the early 1980s. The causes of these injuries have been shown to be multifactorial. Prevention programs are now in effect and have resulted in a trend toward a decrease in the number of severe injuries and the number of injuries caused by a check from behind, although there has not been a significant decrease in the total number of injuries reported annually. The problem is now an international concern, with several other nations reporting severe injuries. We must be more vigilant about preventing spinal injuries in hockey and encourage a consistent and early introduction and frequent repetition of upgraded prevention programs for all hockey players. Improved safety is one of hockey's most important challenges. If we can educate, adjust attitudes, and eliminate ambiguity regarding hockey safety, we can conquer the challenge to make the next 30 years of hockey safer than the last 30 years.

ACKNOWLEDGMENTS

The authors would like to thank Lillian Lapczak, Virginia Edmonds, Sandi Amaral, Derek Mackesy, and Risa Crotin for their assistance. Lillian Lapczak was responsible for the statistical analyses. Financial support for the current survey was received from the Dr. Tom Pashby Sport Safety Fund, the Canadian Hockey Association, the NHL Players Association, and Bauer Canada Inc.

References

1. Biasca N, Simmen HP, Bartolozzi AR, et al. Review of typical ice hockey injuries. Survey of the North American NHL and Hockey Canada versus European leagues. Unfallchirurg 1995;98:283–2888.
2. Bishop PJ, Norman RW, Wells RP, et al. Changes in the center of mass and moment of inertia of a headform induced by a hockey helmet and face shield. Can J Appl Sport Sci 1983;8:19–25.
3. Brust JD, Leonard BJ, Pheley A, et al. Children's ice hockey injuries. Am J Dis Child 1992;146:741–747.
4. Cantu RC: Return to play guidelines after a head injury. Clin Sports Med 1998;171:45–60.
5. Cantu RC, Mueller F. Catastrophic spine injury in football, 1977–1989. J Spinal Disord 1990;3:227–231.
6. Carson JD, Reesor D. A survey of hockey injuries in an emergency department. Mod Med Canada 1988;43:145–150.
7. Clarke KS. Epidemiology of athletic neck injury. Clin Sports Med 1998;17:83–97.
8. Coakley JJ. Sport in Society. St. Louis, Times Mirror / Mosby College Publishing, 1990.
9. Cooper ME. Acute care of the spinal cord injured. Axone 1996;17:76–80.
10. DeVivo MJ. Causes and costs of spinal cord injury in the United States. Spinal Cord 1997;35:809–813.
11. Fekete JF. Severe brain injury and death following minor hockey accidents. The effectiveness of the safety helmets of amateur hockey players. CMAJ 1968;99:1234–1239.
12. Grossman S, Hines T. National Hockey League players from North America are more violent than those from Europe. Percept Mot Skills 1996; 83:589–590.
13. Honey CR. Brain injury in ice hockey. Clin J Sport Med 1998;8:43–46.
14. Immen W. Smoking on rise in Ontario, ARF finds. The Globe and Mail (Toronto). Oct. 13, 1995.
15. Janda DH. Prevention has everything to do with sports medicine. Clin J Sport Med 1992;2:159–160.
16. Kaye JJ, Nance EP. Thoracic and Lumbar Spine Trauma. In Dalinka MK (ed): Radiologic Clinics of North America. Philadelphia, WB Saunders, 1990, pp 361–377.
17. LaPrade RF, Burnett QM, Zarour R, et al. The effect of the mandatory use of face masks on facial lacerations and head and neck injuries in ice hockey. Am J Sports Med 1995;23:773–775.
18. Murray TM, Livingston LA. Hockey helmets, face masks, and injurious behavior. Pediatrics 1995;3:419–421.
19. Panathere JM. A parents guide to the prevention of spinal injuries in hockey. Toronto, The Hockey Development Centre for Ontario, 1993.
20. Pashby TJ, Pashby RC, Chisholm LDJ, et al. Eye injuries in Canadian hockey. CMAJ 1975;113:663–666.
21. Rampton J, Leach T, Therrien SA, et al. Head, neck, and facial injuries in ice hockey: The effect of protective equipment. Clin J Sport Med 1997;7:162–167.
22. Regnier G, Boileau R, Marcotte G, et al. Effects of Body-Checking in the Pee-Wee (12 and 13 years old) Division in the Province of Quebec. In Castaldi CR, Hoerner ER (eds): Safety in Ice Hockey. Philadelphia, American Society for Testing & Materials, 1989, pp 84–103.
23. Reynen PD, Clancy WG, Jr. Cervical spine injury, hockey helmets, and face masks. Am J Sports Med 1994;22:167–170.
24. Sim FH, Simonet WT, Melton LJ, III, et al. Ice hockey injuries. Am J Sports Med 1987;15:30–40.
25. Tator CH, Carson JD, Edmonds VE. New spinal injuries in hockey. Clin J Sport Med 1997;7:17–21.
26. Tator CH, Edmonds VE, Lapczak L. Spinal Injuries in Ice Hockey: Review of 182 North American Cases and Analysis of Etiologic Factors. In Castaldi CR, Bishop PJ, Hoerner EF (eds): Safety in Ice Hockey. Philadelphia, American Society for Testing and Materials, 1993, pp 11–20.
27. Tator CH, Edmonds VE, Lapczak L, et al. Spinal injuries in ice hockey players, 1966–1987. Can J Surg 1991;34:63–69.
28. Tator CH, Edmonds VE, New ML. Diving: A frequent and potentially preventable cause of spinal cord injury. CMAJ 1981;124:1323–1324.

29. Thurman DJ, Sniezek JE, Johnson D, et al. Guidelines for Surveillance of Central Nervous System Injury. Atlanta, National Center for Injury Prevention and Control, 1995.

30. Torg JS. Athletic Injuries to the Head, Neck, and Face. Philadelphia, Lea & Febiger, 1982.

31. Voaklander DC, Saunders LD, Quinney HA, et al. Epidemiology of recreational and old-timer ice hockey injuries. Clin J Sport Med 1996;6:15–21.

32. Watson RC, Nystrom MA, Buckolz E. Safety in Canadian Junior Ice Hockey: The association between ice surface size and injuries and aggressive penalties in the Ontario Hockey League. Clin J Sport Med 1997;7:192–195.

33. Watson RC, Singer CD, Sproule JR. Checking from behind in ice hockey: A study of injury and penalty data in the Ontario University Athletic Association Hockey League. Clin J Sport Med 1996;6:108–111.

34. The Coaching Association of Canada. Coaching Theory Level 1, National Coaching Certification Program. Gloucester, Ontario, The Coaching Association of Canada, 1988.

29

Head and Spine Injuries in Martial Arts

Meheroz H. Rabadi, Richard B. Birrer, and Barry D. Jordan

The martial arts have their origins in the Orient and were developed by traveling Buddhist monks for self-defense as they undertook long, perilous journeys. Thus martial arts skills were developed to disable and to kill. Since the 1960s, the martial arts have gained worldwide interest and participation. In the United States alone there are an estimated 1.5 to 2 million participants. Reasons for the recent surge in the popularity of the martial arts include learning self-defense, developing self-esteem; increasing endurance, strength and flexibility (especially tai chi); and participating in a competitive sport. The ages 9 to 12 years have been suggested as an ideal period to learn martial arts, for by this age coordination and concentration have developed.[6] Since the martial arts are contact sports, physical injuries are an inherent and often unavoidable aspect of participation. However, the psychological and physical benefits of participation often outweigh the risk of injury. Although the majority of martial arts–related injuries are musculoskeletal, neurologic injuries do occur and can be associated with significant morbidity and mortality.

The commonly practiced martial arts are aikido, judo, jujitsu, karate, tae kwon do, and tai chi (Table 29–1). Each art emphasizes a different technique; therefore, some of the injuries are martial art-specific. In aikido, where throws and joint-lock techniques are practiced, falls and joint sprains are common. In judo, where the emphasis is on throws, grappling to the ground, and choking techniques, upper extremity injuries are common. Jujitsu is similar to judo in terms of throws, grappling, and choking techniques. It also encompasses joint-lock techniques. Falls and joint sprains are common in jujitsu participants. Karate emphasizes the technique of punches, chops, and kicks. In karate, more injuries have been caused by punches than by kicks. In karate, kicks are delivered via the instep mainly to the side of the head. Most of the injuries are craniocerebral, with cerebral concussion being the commonest as a result of (roundhouse) kicks. Contusions of the head, face, trunk, genitalia, and extremities are also common. Tae kwon do emphasizes the technique of hand strikes and high kicks. In tae kwon do, the kick is delivered by the heel mainly to the face. Tai chi emphasizes circular and flowing movements of hands and feet equally.

Table 29–1. Martial Arts, Technique, and Country of Origin

Martial Art	Technique	Country of Origin
Aikido	Throws Joint locks On dynamics of movement	Japan
Judo	Throws Grappling to the ground Choking techniques	Japan
Jujitsu	Throws and takedowns Grappling Choking and strangulation Joint locking Escaping	Japan
Karate	Punches and chops Kicks—4 basic types *Hands and feet equally used*	Japan
Tae kwon do	Hand strikes Kicks (high) *Feet used more than hands*	Korea
Tai chi	Movements—circular and flowing *Hands and feet equally used*	China

EPIDEMIOLOGY

The cultural and sociopolitical history of the martial arts has not lent itself to the collection of accurate data on the frequency, type, extent, risk factors, or prevention of injuries. Whatever research information is available tends to be case reports or based on retrospective surveys derived from tournament and training hall observations or the analysis of gross hospital emergency records. Overall, the martial arts have been found to be safe sports when compared with other sports commonly participated in by school-age children or professionals (Table 29–2).[3]

Through the 1980s and 1990s, approximately 30,000 injuries have been identified electronically (through the National Electronic Injury Surveillance System of the U.S. Consumer Product Safety Commission) or through national and international martial arts activities. Approximately 6% of the athletes (N = 17,500) have been injured, with a 4-to-1 male-to-female distribution.[4] Seventy percent of the injuries have occurred in nontournament or training conditions and the remainder in a competitive or tournament setting.[4] The incidence of martial arts injuries has been calculated to be 1.71 injuries per athlete per year, with more severe injuries and higher rates of injuries occurring in competitive and tournament settings.[4]

Approximately 40% of injuries in martial arts are to the lower extremities.[3] Since the foot is the main striking area of the kick, it is subject to frequent injury.[5] Upper extremity injuries are also common. In one study, 37.6% of judo participants sustained upper extremity injuries.[15] Most of the injuries affecting the limbs are mild to moderate in severity. Head, face, and neck injuries can be severe and potentially life threatening (Table 29–3).[3] Most mild to moderate injuries are sustained in the noncompetitive setting, as more time is spent in training than in actual competition.[3, 15] Severe injuries are sustained in competitive settings.[3, 36] Injury

Table 29–2. Sports-Related Injuries per 1000 Participants per Year

Sports	Average	Men	Women
Football	74.6	83.3	24.6
Basketball	68.4	69.5	64.3
Skating (ice)	46.8	40.2	48.5
Soccer	40	44.5	32.6
Hockey	36	45.3	18.7
Track and field	32.8	34.8	28.9
Cycling	32.5	41.1	22.7
Baseball/Softball	23.8	26.6	15.9
Wrestling	22.9	25.2	16.8
Volleyball	17.2	20.2	15.7
Skiing	16.2	19.3	12.1
Gymnastics	15.6	12.8	17.3
Dancing	7.3	5.9	9.6
General exercise	6.9	7.2	5.9
Golf	5.4	5.9	3.2
Martial arts	3.5	3.9	2.6
Racquet sports	1.5	1.7	1.1
Bowling	1.2	1.2	1.1
Swimming	0.96	1.1	0.9
Horseback riding	0.9	0.4	1.3

From Birrer RB. Trauma epidemiology in martial arts. The results of an eighteen-year international survey. Am J Sports Med 1996; 24:S72–74, with permission.

Table 29–3. Severe Injuries Encountered in the Martial Arts

Injury Types	N (number)
Pneumothorax	8
Contusion:	
Lungs	2
Brain	7
Heart	2
Spinal cord	3
Renal	4
Laceration:	
Spleen	5
Liver	3
Kidney	3
Pancreas	2
Rupture:	
Diaphragm	1
Bladder	3
Hematoma:	
Brain	4
Spinal cord	1
Pericardium	1
Retropericardium	1
Fractures:	
Cricothyroid/larynx	3
Long bones	79
Epiphysis	14
Skull	42
Spine	9
Cerebral concussion	433
Testicular torsion	9
Eye:	
Hypema	17
Retinal detachment	7
Globe contusion	19
Lens dislocation	4
Miscarriage	0.6
Total:	692 (1.7%)

From Birrer RB. Trauma epidemiology in martial arts. The results of an eighteen-year international survey. Am J Sports Med 1996;24:S72–74, with permission.

rate is found to be inversely proportional to participant experience.[3, 36, 38] The peak age for injury is 15 to 24 years, when training and competition are most intense.[38] Unsupervised activity contributes to twice as many (limb) injuries, compared with supervised activities.[9, 38]

Deaths in the martial arts have occurred as a result of trauma to the head (frontal and temporal contusions, intracerebral and subdural hemorrhage with resultant brain stem herniation), neck (cervical cord trauma from cervical fracture-dislocation, and carotid artery laceration), chest (aspiration and asphyxia), and abdomen (splenic rupture), and from suicide.[3, 36]

BRAIN INJURY

Brain injury is an infrequent but potentially catastrophic complication of martial arts participation. The majority of brain injuries in the martial arts are traumatic in nature. However, anoxic brain injury and stroke have been reported. Traumatic brain injury (TBI) has been reported in judo, karate, and tae kwon do. In judo, TBI is most commonly associated with an impact from a throwing technique, whereas the mechanism of injury in karate is usually secondary to an erroneous kick.[4] Potential brain injuries encountered in the martial arts are listed in Table 29–4.

Acute Traumatic Brain Injury

The most common acute traumatic brain injury (ATBI) encountered in the martial arts is the cerebral concussion. Birrer,[3] in an 18-year international survey of martial arts injuries, reported 433 cases of cerebral concussion. In tae kwon do, which emphasizes the technique of hand strikes and high kicks, the rate of cerebral concussion was observed to be 7.04 per 1000 male athlete-exposures and 2.42 per 1000 in female athlete-exposures.[28] The most common situation in which a concussion was sustained in tae kwon do was an unblocked attack, which accounted for 87.5% of the concussions in men and 100% of the concussions in women. Other situations in which a concussion has been observed include falling and blocking a kick.[28] For 91.7% of the men participants and 100% of the women athletes,[28] the most common injury mechanism that resulted in a concussion was receiving a blow. According to Pieter and Zemper,[28] concussions appeared to be more severe in male tae kwon do participants compared with women participants. Among the men 16.7% of the concussions were of a severe nature, characterized by 21 days or more lost to training or competition. In women athletes all of the concussions were mild, as noted by fewer than 7 days lost to training or competition.

Critchley and colleagues[10] reported 160 injuries sustained during three consecutive British Shotokan karate championships. Among these 160 injuries, 12 cases of ATBI were recorded. Eleven of these were concussions not associated with loss of consciousness. The twelfth victim of ATBI exhibited loss of consciousness and was admitted to the hospital and released the next day. Among the 11 athletes who suffered concussion, 6 "had their bell rung" and, because of rapid recovery, were allowed to return to competition. The other five victims were not allowed to continue. Athletes who were concussed without loss of consciousness were observed in the treatment area for a minimum of 15 minutes.

Although less common, more severe ATBI can be encountered in the martial arts. Koiwai[14] reported five deaths secondary to brain injury during judo participation. These injuries included subdural hematoma (two cases), cerebral hemorrhage (two cases), and a subarachnoid hemorrhage secondary to the rupture of an aneurysm. In Japan the most common cause of death in sports among senior high school students was brain contusion sustained during extracurricular judo.[2] The authors are aware of a karate student who sustained a fall while

Table 29–4. Potential Brain Injuries Encountered in the Martial Arts

Acute traumatic brain injury
  Cerebral concussion
  Cerebral contusion
  Subdural hematoma
  Epidural hematoma
  Intracerebral hemorrhage
  Subarachnoid hemorrhage
  Diffuse axonal injury
Chronic traumatic brain injury
Anoxic brain injury
Cerebral infarction

sparring and suffered a subdural hematoma that was evacuated but later complicated by a subdural empyema. Other brain injuries of serious medical concern in the martial arts include brain lacerations and skull fractures.[14] In an 18-year international survey of martial arts injuries, Birrer[3] reported 42 cases of skull fracture.

The proper evaluation of ATBI in the martial artist is essential. The contestant who sustains an ATBI should be immediately removed from the contest and receive a detailed neurologic evaluation that includes a mental status examination. The Glasgow Coma Scale (GCS)[35] is widely used to assess level of consciousness and provide a guide as to the prognosis (Table 29–5). The total score (i.e., the sum of the individual category scores) varies from a minimum of 3 to a maximum of 15. A GCS score of 3 to 8 is considered severe, between 9 and 12 moderate, and 13 to 15 mild. In the martial arts and most sports, the overwhelming majority of ATBIs will be mild in nature. Since the majority of ATBIs in sports are mild, the GCS may not be sensitive enough to assess subtle cognitive difficulties in areas such as attention, learning, and memory. Accordingly, the Standardized Assessment of Concussion (SAC)[19] may be an appropriate assessment tool.

Once the athlete has been assessed, decisions regarding further evaluation and re-

turn to competition can be established. The two most commonly utilized grading scales for the management of concussion in sports are the Cantu scale[7] and the American Academy of Neurology scale.[29] The proper evaluation of the athlete who has sustained an ATBI is important in preventing the second impact syndrome (SIS) and the cumulative effect of multiple cerebral injuries (i.e., chronic traumatic brain injury). The SIS is the result of a second concussion occurring while the individual is still symptomatic from an earlier concussion.[8] Second impact syndrome has been associated with acute brain swelling with raised intracranial pressure as a result of loss of cerebral autoregulation.[8]

Chronic Traumatic Brain Injury

In addition to ATBI, chronic traumatic brain injury (CTBI) has also been reported in the martial arts. CTBI, which represents the cumulative, long-term consequences of repetitive concussive and subconcussive blows to the head, has been noted primarily among professional boxers with long exposure to the sport.[12, 22, 31] However, Aotsuka and coworkers[1] reported a case of CTBI in a karate participant characterized by cerebellar ataxia, seizure, and dementia. Computed tomography (CT) and magnetic resonance imaging (MRI) demonstrated ventricular enlargement and severe atrophy, especially in the frontal base. They speculated that this case of "punch drunk" syndrome resulted from repeated karate traumas.

Anoxic Brain Injury

Anoxic brain injury has been reported in judo when the choke hold has been employed. The choke hold consists of strangling the opponent's neck with arms or legs until he surrenders or loses consciousness. The choke hold reduces blood supply to the brain by applying pressure on the carotid arteries, resulting in loss of consciousness and possible anoxic brain injury.[26] The syncope obtained by choking has been described as "being preceded by a clouding of the state of consciousness and by a general muscular contraction, accompanied by muscular flaccidity and followed by tonic clonic contractions and irregular breathing."[32] Con-

Table 29–5. Glasgow Coma Scale (GCS)

Activity	Score
Eye Opening	
None	1
To pain	2
To speech	3
Spontaneously	4
Verbal Response	
None	1
Incomprehensible speech	2
Inappropriate words	3
Confused	4
Oriented	5
Motor Response	
None	1
Abnormal extensor	2
Abnormal flexor	3
Withdraws	4
Localizes	5
Obeys	6
Total	3–15

sciousness is typically restored within 10 to 15 seconds.[32] Owen and Ghadiali reported a case of a judo participant who was frequently strangled into unconsciousness during his career. The cumulative effects of repeated strangulation resulted in anoxic brain injury that was documented on psychometric evaluation.[26] Koiwai[14] reported a fatality from damage to the carotids during a hold that resulted in a possible reflexive hypotension, irreversible brain damage, and stoppage of the heart.

Electroencephalograms (EEGs) and regional cerebral blood flow (rCBF) studies (using the 133-xenon inhalation method) were obtained in 10 judo contestants who underwent choking-induced syncope.[32] EEG documentation was undertaken before, during, and after the choke-induced syncope. Baseline EEG was normal in all the contestants. Within 10 seconds of the choke, the EEG showed 2 to 3 Hz delta waves in all cerebral regions, with an anterior predominance. This diffuse slowing on EEG persisted for 5 to 6 seconds and gradually returned to normal. Regional CBF studies were performed on all 10 paricipants at rest, and all were within normal limits. Seven individuals had repeat rCBF studies performed when they recovered physiologic breathing after the choke. The rCBF findings after the choke were variable and did not reach statistical significance. Four cases exhibited a 4% to 6% reduction in rCBF, and 2 cases demonstrated a 15% to 21% decrease in blood flow. One individual experienced an increased CBF that was interpreted as a "rebound" phenomenon, an attempt to compensate for reduced CBF that ocurred during choking. The reason for this variable CBF response to choking is unknown. However, it has been speculated that the variable rCBF changes may be attributable to individual differences in the autonomic innervation of the cardiovascular system.[32] Rau and colleagues,[30] utilizing spectral EEG analysis, also noted subclinical changes in brain function among healthy volunteers undergoing choking in judo.

Stroke

Stroke represents another potential complication of martial arts participation. The internal carotid artery can occlude, dissect, or shower thrombic emboli into the intracranial vessels.[18] Internal carotid artery thrombosis has been reported following a karate blow that traumatized the internal carotid artery in the neck.[37] We are also aware of a case of carotid dissection and resultant hemispheric infarction in a 26-year-old following a karate chop ("shuto") to the neck (E. Potes, B. Volpe, personal communication). McCarron and coworkers[18] reported the development of an embolic stroke without dissection of the carotid artery in a 29-year-old man who experienced a neck-holding procedure in a martial arts class. Vertebral artery dissection has also been reported in the martial arts.[17]

CERVICAL SPINE INJURIES

A variety of neck and cervical spine injuries can be encountered in the martial arts. Cervical spine injuries are seen mostly in inexperienced contestants who land on the front of the head or back of the neck as the result of a throw. Although the majority of neck injuries are soft tissue injuries, more severe injuries can be encoutered. Birrer[3] reported three spinal cord contusions and one case of a spinal cord hematoma in an 18-year international survey of martial arts injuries. It was also noted that there were nine spine fractures, but the location was not specified. In judo, Koiwai[14] reported four deaths attributable to cervical spine injuries. These included three cervical fractures and a case of cervical dislocation. These injuries were associated with a forceful fall on the head or neck after a throw.[14] Freeman and colleagues[11] reported a case of traumatic atlantoaxial subluxation in a 39-year-old man who was thrown and suffered a hyperflexion injury to the neck.

INJURY PREVENTION

The martial arts have been found to be safe, compared with other commonly practiced sports (Table 29–2).[3] Neurologic injuries are rare, but usually severe and associated with increased risk of disability and death. Several measures can be employed to improve the safety of martial arts participation and reduce acute, life threatening incidents and chronic, cumulative brain injuries. For example, headgear can reduce facial injuries such as contusions and lacerations.

However, whether headgear will protect against brain and cervical spine injury remains to be determined. Proper supervision of activities (training and competition) by trained personnel cannot be overemphasized in the reduction of injury. In addition, rule changes that prohibit certain high-risk practices (e.g., blows to the carotid artery, choke holds) could potentially have a profound effect on reducing the numbers of severe neurologic injuries. Efficient medical surveillance and care by qualified health care professionals are also a necessity. Medical personnel should be present at competitions to provide emergent medical care when needed. In addition, contestants should be examined prior to the competition to ensure that they are medically fit to participate.

CONCLUSION

If practiced appropriately, the martial arts can be a relatively safe sport. Nonetheless, neurologic injuries can be anticipated. Considering that the worldwide popularity of the martial arts is likely to increase in the future, it becomes imperative that the sport be made safer during both training and competition. The preventive guidelines as mentioned in the preceding section of this chapter will be necessary to accomplish the goal of making the martial arts safer.

References

1. Aotsuka A, Kojima S, Furumoto H, et al. Punch drunk syndrome due to repeated karate kicks and punches. Rinsho Shinkeigaku 1990;30:1243–1246.
2. Athletes' death. B M J 1970;4:4.
3. Birrer RB. Trauma epidemiology in martial arts. The results of an eighteen-year international survey. Am J Sports Med 1996;24:S72–78.
4. Birrer RB. Martial Arts. In Jordan BD, Tsairis P, Warren RF (eds): Sports Neurology. Philadelphia, Lippincott-Raven, 1988, pp 423–428.
5. Burks JB, Satterfield K. Foot and ankle injuries among martial artists. J Am Podiatr Med Assoc 1998;88:268–278.
6. Buschbaker RM, Shay T. Martial arts. Phys Med Rehabil Clin N Am 1999;10:35–47.
7. Cantu RC. Guidelines for return to contact sports after a cerebral concussion. Phys Sportsmed 1986;14:75–83.
8. Cantu RC, Voy R. Second impact syndrome. A risk in any sport. Phys Sportsmed 1995;23:27–34.
9. Chambers RB. Orthopaedic injuries in athletes (ages 6 to 17): Comparison of injuries occurring in six sports. Am J Sports Med 1979;7:195–197.
10. Critchley GR, Mannion S, Meredith C. Injury rates in Shotokan karate. Br J Sports Med 1999;33:174–177.
11. Freeman BJC, Bisbinas I, Nelson IW. Traumatic atlantoaxial subluxation and missed cervical spine injuries. Hosp Med 1998;59:330–331.
12. Jordan BD. Chronic neurologic injuries in boxing. In Jordon BD (ed): Medical Aspects of Boxing. Boca Raton, FL, CRC Press, 1993, pp 177–185.
13. Kelly JP, Nichols JS, Filley CM, et al. Concussion in sports. Guidelines for prevention of catastrophic outcome. JAMA 1991;266:2867–2869.
14. Koiwai EK. Fatalities associated with judo. Phys Sportsmed 1981;9:61–66.
15. Kujala UM, Taimela S, Antti-Poika I, et al. Acute injuries in soccer, ice hockey, volleyball, basketball, judo, and karate: Analysis of national registry data. BMJ 1995;1311:1465–1468.
16. Kurosawa H, Nakasita K, Nakasita H, et al. Complete avulsion of hamstring tendons from ischial tuberosity: Report of two cases sustained in judo. Br J Sports Med 1996;30:72–74.
17. Lannuzel A. Vertebral artery dissection following a judo session. A case report. Neuropediatrics 1994;25:106–108.
18. McCarron MO, Patterson J, Duncan R. Stroke without dissection from a neck holding manoeuvre in martial arts. Br J Sports Med 1997;31:346–347.
19. McCrea M, Kelly JP, Kluge J, et al. Standardized assessment of concussion in football players. Neurology 1997;48:586–588.
20. McLatchie GR. Karate and karate injuries. Br J Sports Med 1981;15:84–86.
21. McLatchie GR, Davies JE, Caulley JH. Injuries in karate—A case for Medical Control. J Trauma 1980;20:956–958.
22. Mendez MF. The neuropsychiatric aspects of boxing. Int J Psychiatry Med 1995;25:249–262.
23. Shahla N. Female judoists: Their hormones, muscles, and bones. Lancet 1996;347:919–920.
24. Neiman EA, Swan PG. Karate injuries. B M J 1971;1:233–235.
25. Oler M, Tomson W, Pepe H, et al. Morbidity and mortality in martial arts: A warning. J Trauma 1991;31:251–253.
26. Owens RG, Ghadiali EJ. Judo as a possible cause of anoxic brain damage. J Sports Med Phys Fitness 1991;31:627–628.
27. Pieter W. Martial Arts. In Caine DJ, Caine CG, Lindner KJ (eds): Epidemiology of Sports Injuries. Champaign, IL, Human Kinetics Publishers, 1996, pp 268–283.
28. Pieter W, Zemper ED. Incidence of reported cerebral contusion in adult tae kwon do athletes. J R Soc Health 1998;118:272–279.
29. Practice parameters: Management of concussion in sports [summary statement]. Neurology 1997; 48:581–585.
30. Rau R, Raschka C, Brunner K, et al. Spectral analysis of EEG changes after choking in judo (juji-jime). Med Sci Sports Exerc 1998;30:1356–1362.
31. Roberts AH. Brain Damage in Boxers. London, Pittman Publishing, 1969.

32. Rodriguez G, Francione S, Gardella M, et al. Judo and choking: EEG and regional blood flow findings. J Sports Med Phys Fitness 1991;31:605–610.

33. Siana JE, Borum P, Kryger H. Injuries in tae kwon do. Br J Sports Med 1986;20:165–166.

34. Stricivec MV, Patel MR, Okazaki T, et al. Karate historical perspective and injuries sustained in national and international tournament competitions. Am J Sports Med 1983;11:320–324.

35. Teasedale G, Jennett B. Assessment of coma and impaired consciousness: A practical scale. Lancet 1974;1:81–84.

36. Wilkerson LA. Martial arts injuries. J Am Osteopath Assoc. 1997;4:221–226.

37. Wos W, Puzio J, Opale G. Traumatic internal carotid artery thrombosis following karate blow. Pol Przegl Chir 1977;49:12, 1271–1273.

38. Zaricznyl B, Shattuck LJM, Mast TA, et al. Sports related injuries in school aged children. Am J Sports Med 1980;8:318–324.

30

Neurologic Injuries in Equestrian Sport

W. H. Brooks

Few creatures have captured the imagination and awe of humankind as the horse. Prehistoric peoples revered the horse as an animal of mysterious speed and beauty. Displayed as animals of strength in Athens and Rome and later utilized by the bellicose Magyars whose horsemanship resulted in the conquest of much of Europe at the close of the first millennium, this animal has become synonymous with speed, agility, and strength. Replaced as a method of rapid and dependable transport by the advent of the industrial age, the horse has continued to engage humanity's affection as a preferred means of sporting and recreational pleasure. To that end, this species has been selectively bred for its sporting abilities as well as its suitability for riding for pleasure. The number of horses used for riding in the United States in the late 1990s has been estimated to be about 7 million.[11] The numbers that roam the National Parks or are kept in pastures as monuments to bygone eras are not known.

Although the horse is used most commonly for pleasure riding or as an aid in agriculture in remote rural areas of the country, its most notable use is for sport. In sporting endeavors horses may be engaged in functions that range from the elegance of dressage to the rough-and-tumble of rodeo; from racing on a flat oval and jumping fences or other fixed objects in excess of 6 feet high or wide to riding on trails or in the back yard. In no other sporting activity does the outcome depend so much on the combination of two species of such differing strength, size, and speed. This unique and sometimes unpredictable combination, the positions that are assumed during riding phases and the strength, speeds, and heights achieved while riding, makes horseback riding potentially one of the most dangerous of sporting events (Fig. 30–1). Indeed, equestrian sports are associated with significant risk of participant morbidity and mortality. The rate of injury is estimated at 4 injuries per 1000 riders.[3, 14] To underscore this risk, over 200 deaths directly related to equestrian activities are projected annually, with most expected to be the result of neurologic injury.[3, 4]

This chapter examines the types of injuries related to horseback riding, explicates the mechanisms of injuries associated with equestrian sport, and presents current methodologies of risk management. It is anticipated that as these become understood and the awareness of risk reduction methodologies become prevalent in the equestrian community, the numbers and severity of neurologic injury will decrease.

TYPES OF INJURY

Although most equestrian-related injuries involve the extremities, the most catastrophic are those involving the central nervous system.[3, 13, 16] Unfortunately, the actual occurrence of neurologic injuries remains unknown because either deaths from craniospinal injury or mild neurologic injury (Grade 1 concussion) frequently are not reported. Nevertheless, it has been estimated that a neurosurgical service can anticipate 1–2 equestrian-related injuries per month per 1 million population referred. Obviously, this will vary according to the traditional interest in the horse in a particular locale. The basis for the information contained in this chapter is provided by a 10-year neurosurgical experience in a community rich in the traditions of equestrian sport

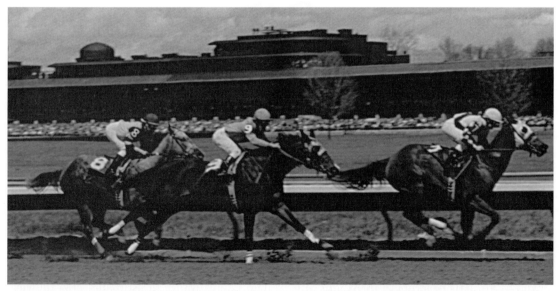

Figure 30–1. Speeds achievable to 40 mph associated with distances from the ground and limited protective equipment make equestrian sports among the most potentially dangerous sporting activities.

and breeding in which most equestrian disciplines are represented (Table 30–1). This group of patients represents a variety of ages (9–83 years; median = 31 years) comprising wide differences in years of riding experience (none to more than 50 years). These data indicate that experience with horseback riding does not provide protection against injury. Indeed, experience and knowledge have differing influences on the risk of riding-related injury. The number of years riding is not correlated with a decrease in injury rate, whereas knowledge and proficiency are related.[12] Furthermore, the risk of repeated injury in this series (98/187) could not be correlated to age or experience. The number of neurologic injuries sustained by an individual was inversely relational to the number of rides or different horses ridden per day. Those individuals who rode more than 1 or 2 horses per day had fewer repeated neurologic injuries than those who rode infrequently. However, this group, which predominantly comprised profes-

sional jockeys, manifested the largest numbers of nonneurologic injuries.

The majority of head injuries sustained by these individuals were concussions ranging from mild to severe (Glasgow Coma Scale [GSC] >13). Nevertheless, alarming numbers of cerebral contusions and intracranial hematomas also were observed (GSC <8) (Table 30–2). The seriousness of these injuries is reflected further in the number of individuals sustaining fatal or persistent neurologic deficits as a result of a riding-related injury (Table 30–3). Head injury accounted for 28% of all equestrian-related injuries reported during this 10-year period. Unfortunately, it is not possible to determine the rate of these injuries among all riders of the various disciplines because the actual number of people engaged in each is unknown. Those data that were available, however, suggest that about 1 head injury, of any severity, will occur per 25 events.

Table 30–1. Equestrian Activities Associated With Neurologic Injury, 1986–1996

1. Recreational	139
2. Fox Hunting	45
3. Combined Training	25
4. Dressage	11
5. Grooming	14

Table 30–2. Classification of Head Injury Associated With Equestrian Activity (N = 187)

1. Concussion	83
2. Cerebral contusion	90
3. Skull fracture	67
4. Intracranial hematoma	
A. Intraparenchymal	20
B. Extracerebral	15

Table 30–3. Neurologic Consequences of Equestrian-Associated Injury

No residual	122
Return to riding with impairment	3
Unable to return to riding	28
Long-term facility care	7
Death	27

Thus, head injury is a concern among healthcare professionals involved in equestrian-related sports. As many as 5% of those patients with head injuries had concomitant spinal injuries; none were associated with spinal cord involvement. Alternatively, no individual sustaining a spinal cord injury secondary to vertebral fracture (17/47) during this period had a head injury, although all (47/47) admitted to having had previous concussions associated with horseback riding.

Skull fractures—linear, basal, or depressed—were seen most commonly in those individuals not wearing protective headgear (60/67), or wearing helmets without a harness (7/67). Unhelmeted riders frequently sustain compound and depressed fractures of the skull after falling or from being kicked or trampled by an uncontrolled horse. Depressed skull fractures were the most common type of head injury observed in those seriously injured while grooming (Fig. 30–2). None of these individuals wore protective headgear. No skull fractures or deaths were seen in individuals wearing appropriate equestrian helmets with a retention harness (0/35). However, intracranial hematomas did occur in these individuals (9/35), supporting the assertion that helmets are most effective in reducing the incidence of skull fracture but provide less protection against inertial loads comprising both impulsive and contact forces. Nevertheless, the occurrence of intracranial hematomas is much more common in those riders who did not wear helmets (24/35). Thus, supporting previous studies,[6] although cerebral injury may occur in spite of appropriate headgear, the overall incidence of serious head injury including skull fracture in those wearing helmets was lessened significantly. Appropriate headgear is effective in reducing the overall incidence of head injury.

Spinal injury occurs with less frequency than head injury, comprising approximately 20% of all neurologic injuries (47/234). For-

tunately, most (30/47) were not associated with spinal cord or nerve root involvement. The thoracolumbar junction (T12–L1) is the most common site of all vertebral fractures associated with horseback riding. These occur when a rider lands on his feet or buttocks subsequent to falling or being thrown (Fig. 30–3). Forced flexion associated with rotation at this level frequently results in neural injury to the conus medullaris or cauda equina (12/17) (Fig. 30–4). Occurring less frequently, fractures of the cervical spine most commonly resulted when the rider's head struck the ground after being thrown forward, causing the neck to be thrust into the extremes of flexion. These fractures typically were unstable and associated with spinal cord injury (4/17). All required stabilization procedures. Cervical fractures rarely occurred in riders who fell with their necks maintained in extension rather than flexion; the few that did occur were unassociated with neurologic deficits and were judged to be stable by flexion/extension radiography or computed tomographic scan. Because riders typically fall with their wrists, arms, and necks extended, axial loading was not observed and has not been substantiated as a mechanism for cervical fracture in equestrian-related neurologic injury.[7]

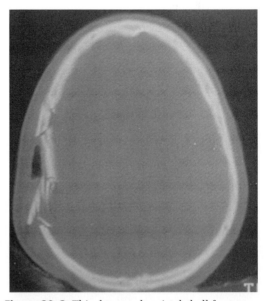

Figure 30–2. This depressed parietal skull fracture occurred as a veterinarian assistant was engaged in delivery of a foal and was kicked by the mare. The individual sustained mild speech dysfunction, which has persisted.

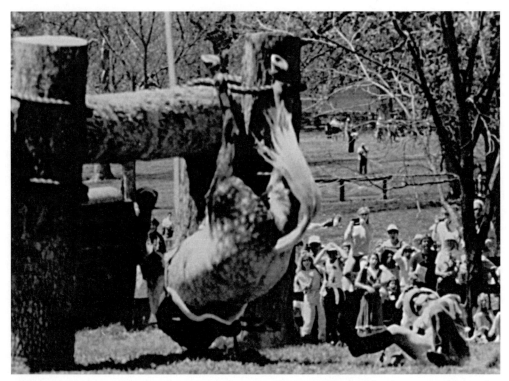

Figure 30–3. This rider sustained a compression fracture of T12 associated with minor reversible cauda equina injury. He returned to riding without dysfunction. (Photo courtesy of V. W. Perry.)

Injuries to the brachial plexus or peripheral nerves are rare. These were observed in only three individuals. These were minor stretch injuries manifesting themselves similarly to those observed in football. Although not represented in these data, compressive median neuropathies may be seen in the elderly equestrian or particularly those engaged in dressage. The necessity for surgical decompression is rare; when necessary, it does not preclude a return to horse-back riding. None has been associated with significant loss of function.

It must be emphasized that neurologic injury can occur in equestrian activities unassociated with riding. Fourteen individuals sustained head injuries while grooming horses or in attendance during foaling; six of these injuries were fatal (Table 30–4). All were the result of being kicked in the head, thereby sustaining a skull fracture associated with further injury to the underlying

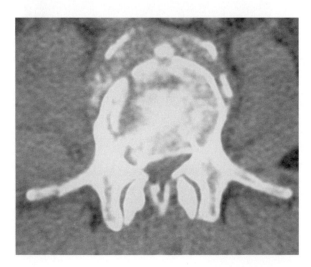

Figure 30–4. Paraplegia secondary to this thoracolumbar fracture resulted from a fall when this rider and her horse slipped and fell over brush while fox hunting.

Table 30–4. Equestrian Activities and Fatalities

	Fatalities/Injuries
1. Recreational	16/139
2. Fox Hunting	3/45
3. Combined Training	1/25
4. Dressage	1/11
5. Grooming	6/14

brain. All required neurosurgical intervention; none returned to work without impairment. Therefore, in relation to all individuals sustaining cranial injuries, this group represented the most hazardous form of equestrian activity. These individuals typically wear no protective headgear, are called on to assist the horse in an unlimited number of circumstances, and frequently are uneducated in safe horse-handling techniques other than those learned through injurious experience. This is further emphasized by the finding that all individuals whose duties were confined to the ground had sustained multiple injuries (average injuries per groom = 9) prior to incurring a neurologic injury.

The number of individuals at risk for neurologic injury associated with riding is directly proportional to the increasing popularity of horseback riding. In the United States, more than 5 million individuals over the age of 12 ride on a regular basis; 59,000 of these people are treated in the emergency department each year.[14] As many as one third of these injuries involve the nervous system, skull, or spine.[10] Therefore, it is important for neurosurgeons to become familiar with the mechanisms involved in these injuries and become acquainted with how they may be averted or lessened.

MECHANISMS OF INJURY

Neurologic injuries may occur subsequent to falling or when a horse kicks or unexpectedly rears. These latter injuries generally take place during horse management (e.g., grooming, loading, shoeing, breeding, or foaling), or when the horse is startled by an unanticipated noise or movement. The force that a horse's shod or unshod hoof is capable of generating is far in excess of the protective potential of the unprotected scalp or skull. Accordingly, these accidents generally result in the most serious of all equestrian-related injuries. Unfortunately, the manner by which these high-spirited animals frequently are handled provides the conditions through which these injuries arise.

The position of the rider coupled with the speeds achievable during riding presupposes significant risks for catastrophic injury (Fig. 30–5). For example, horses are ca-

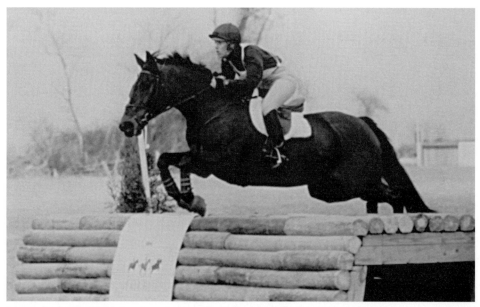

Figure 30–5. The potential for head injury in sport is proportional to the head-forward stance or the energy loads achieved. The classic riding position combined with the speeds associated with equestrian sports presupposes a significant increase in the risks for cerebral injury of all types.

pable of reaching speeds of 40 mph and weigh as much as 2500 lb; thus, a rider perched 9 ft above the ground could receive considerable impact if suddenly dismounted. The unpredictability of the horse-rider relationship combined with the potential biomechanical loads achievable during a fall (dynamic loading) provides more than sufficient energies to result in skull fracture and intracranial hematoma as well as diffuse axonal disruption.

Most head injuries occur after dynamic loading, which includes the head striking the ground or other object (contact loading) and impulsion (inertial loading) imparted by sudden acceleration-deceleration concurrent with an unexpected fall (Fig. 30–6). Although similar mechanisms have been proposed for all contact sports, the loads achievable in equestrian activities far exceed those obtainable in any sport excluding motorcar racing. These forces contribute to the large numbers of concussions that result from horseback riding (Table 30–2). Diffuse, axonal cerebral injuries not associated with skull fracture may be seen in riders choosing to wear helmets. Thus, as with head protective devices commonly used in other contact sports, the risk of skull fracture is lessened;

however, the injurious effects of rotational or angular and translational forces remain unaltered.

Spinal fracture occurs with less frequency than head injury. Most spinal fractures arise in conjunction with a fall in which the rider is forced into extreme lateral flexion by the loads generated with the dismount. Vertebral fractures involving the thoracolumbar area are the most common spinal fractures seen in equestrian-related neurologic injuries. Frequently, the underlying neural elements are involved. These injuries require immediate and appropriate neurosurgical evaluation and treatment, yet usually are associated with persistent paralysis (12/15). Cervical fractures occur less frequently. Typically, they arise when the rider is thrown over the head of the horse with such speed that there is insufficient time to evoke natural protective mechanisms (Fig. 30–7). More commonly, the rider will extend both arms and wrists to absorb the brunt of the fall within the clavicular-shoulder apparatus. Thus, clavicular fracture is common among all riders.

It should be emphasized that riders who are unconscious should be suspected of concurrent spinal injury. Unlike many helmets

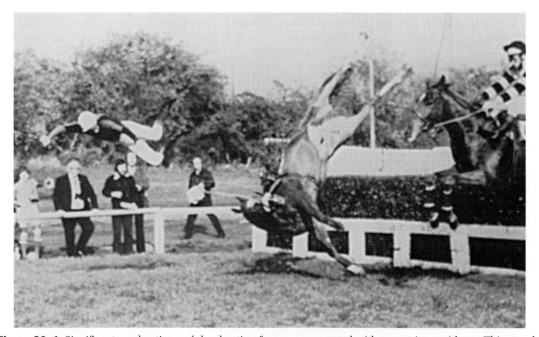

Figure 30–6. Significant acceleration and deceleration forces are generated with equestrian accidents. This steeple-chase jockey died subsequent to massive cerebral injury sustained in this dramatic projectile fall. (From Brooks WH, Bixby-Hammett DM. Head and Spinal Injuries Associated with Equestrian Sports: Mechanisms and Prevention. *In* Torg JS [ed]: Athletic Injuries to the Head, Neck, and Face, 2nd ed. St. Louis, Mosby–Yearbook, 1991, p. 134, with permission.)

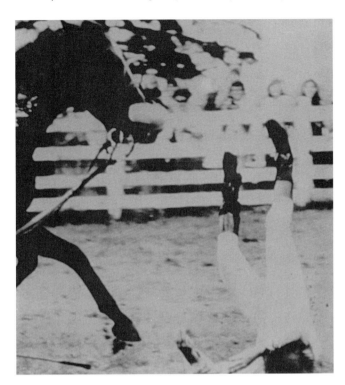

Figure 30–7. Forced flexion resulted in a cervical fracture associated with neurologic involvement. The speed with which this unexpected dismount occurred precluded the more common response to a fall, i.e., extending the arms and wrists and the neck.

used in other sports, equestrian helmets need not be removed in order to obtain access to the airway or to obtain adequate radiographs to determine the presence of a cervical fracture. The airway is easily accessible. Furthermore, these helmets are radiolucent, thereby affording adequate visualization of the cervical spine. Thus, there is little reason to remove an equestrian helmet before radiography or neurologic evaluation.

Brachial plexus and peripheral nerve injuries are rare. However, they can occur when a rider continues to grip the saddle or reins while falling. Attempting to regain balance or prevent falling provides one of the most lethal maneuvers in all sports as the rider pulls the horse down on herself or himself (Fig. 30–8). Fortunately, this mechanism is rare. Brachial plexus and peripheral nerve injuries usually are neurapraxias (rarely, axonotmesis) and resolve rapidly. Compressive median neuropathies may be seen in the older rider or one engaged in frequent and intensive competition or training with resultant thickening of the transverse carpal ligament. Injury to the lumbar plexus has not been reported. Injuries to the common peroneal nerve usually result from direct trauma as the rider strikes the lateral aspect of the upper leg.

Prevention

Certain biomechanical factors are inherent in equestrian sports as noted. However, the overall risks can be lessened by (1) identifying individuals who should not ride; (2) requiring the use of individually fitted and secured protective headgear; (3) developing criteria for permitting resumption of riding after neurologic involvement; and (4) implementing programs that promote education and risk management. The continued cooperation among the biomechanical laboratories devoted to assessing the forces and loads achievable during a fall and those manufacturers developing new materials to absorb and deflect these forces undoubtedly will contribute to the safety and enjoyment of the equestrian community. The American Society for Testing and Materials (ASTM) standards for helmets and protective vests represent one example of these collaborative efforts.[1, 2]

Conditions that absolutely contraindicate horseback riding are shown in Table 30–5. Relative contraindications need to be individualized according to the level of equestrian activity and increase in the risk for serious neurologic injury (Table 30–6). For example, idiopathic epilepsy that is well

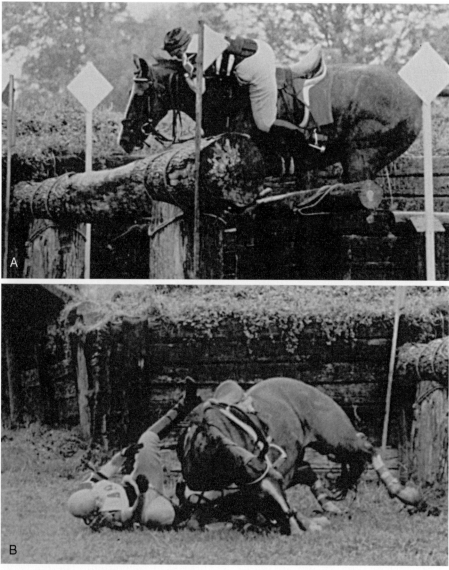

Figure 30–8, *A, B.* Failing to release the reins and pulling the horse resulted in injury to the brachial plexus and cerebral contusion. These injuries also were associated with fracture of the femur. (Photo courtesy of V. W. Perry.)

controlled should not interfere with riding; however, posttraumatic epilepsy warrants concern. Although one may be precluded from competition, riding for enjoyment may be permissible. Nevertheless, it should be underscored that most injuries occur during recreational riding (Table 30–1). Individuals with cervical spinal stenosis should be counseled as to the risks of spinal cord injury should a fall occur (Fig. 30–9). Thorough evaluation is required for all individuals who have sustained neurologic injury before returning to ride. This is particularly true for those engaged in professional or amateur competitions.

Guidelines for resuming horseback riding subsequent to sustaining a head injury are identical to those established for other sports. Riding should not be permitted until all symptoms have resolved. Headache, vertigo, memory loss, or any alteration in cognitive function precludes horseback riding until completely resolved. Moreover, complete evaluation is mandatory before permitting one to ride. It is noteworthy that about one third of riders who suffered a concussion will sustain another within 1 to 3 months of the initial event.[5, 17] This is underscored further by the finding that all professional riders (38/38) admitted to having suffered from at least one concussion previous to the period during which they had sustained

Table 30–5. Conditions That Absolutely Preclude Horseback Riding

1. Any symptomatic (neurologic or pain-producing) abnormalities or spinal anomalies with potential instability.
2. Temporary quadriplegia, paraplegia, or paralysis of any etiology.
3. Permanent cerebral sequel of head injury.
4. Repeated painful injury to the cervical or lumbar spine with radiographic evidence of severe degenerative disease or instability.

another. Thus, repeated concussions are not rare in equestrian sports. Careful examination possibly including advice to curtail riding activity may be justified because of the well-documented consequences of repeated concussion. Distressingly, such advice is rarely heeded.

Tradition is strong in equestrian sport. Unfortunately, this adherence to ritual has retarded the acceptance of protective headgear for various equestrian disciplines,[15] despite the overwhelming data that show that nothing has done more to reduce the number and severity of neurologic injuries than use of appropriate headgear.[8, 9] At present no universal standard is accepted by the entire equestrian community; indeed, not all disciplines require helmets to be worn. Some discourage protective headgear, preferring a traditional hat or bowler. Nevertheless, at present, the best standard for riding helmets is that established by ASTM[1] (Fig. 30–10). The materials and standard design provide protection against penetration as well as distribute impact forces, thereby reducing the risk of head injury. Implementation of this standard has resulted in a steady decline in the incidence of head injuries in riders of the United States Pony Club.[9] Riding helmets adhering to this standard possess a shelf life of about 5–6 years, after which they should be discarded and new helmets purchased. Moreover, helmets must

Table 30–6. Conditions Requiring Evaluation Before Resuming Riding

1. Brachial plexus injury
2. Herniated intervertebral disc with or without surgical treatment
3. Prolonged or repeated postconcussive syndrome
4. Any intracranial or spinal operation
5. Recurrent cervical or lumbar musculoligamentous injuries

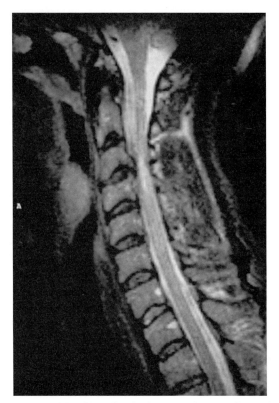

Figure 30–9. This individual sustained a central spinal cord injury after falling from a horse. Notice congenital shallow spinal canal and edema in the spinal cord. Subsequent to cervical laminectomy and recovery, she was permitted to return to recreational riding.

be thoroughly examined or discarded after absorbing a substantial impact. A harness retention system is an integral part of this standard to prevent loss should a fall occur. In this particular series, no individual wearing a helmet with a retention harness sustained a skull fracture; however, five of seven riders wearing helmets without a harness did sustain skull fractures. Despite the abilities of helmets with retention systems to remain in place and reduce impact loading, the ability of the helmet to attenuate rotational forces remains limited. Accordingly, no equestrian helmet is capable of preventing all diffuse axonal injuries that may result from impulsive forces associated with a fall (Fig. 30–11). Notwithstanding this notable limitation, helmets meeting this particular standard should be worn each time one mounts a horse, each time and every time!

Although the acceptance of proper headgear has been limited, the riding community enthusiastically endorses the use of "protective" vests, despite the fact that their effec-

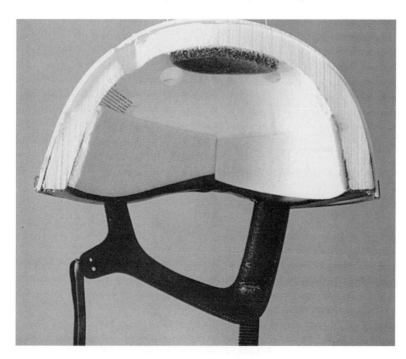

Figure 30–10. ASTM standard equestrian helmets with specially constructed and configured inner and outer shells are designed to reduce skull fracture and reduce the potential for inertia-related head injury. (Lexington Safety) (Photo courtesy of Phil Theobald.)

tiveness primarily is anecdotal; no investigation has ever demonstrated or established their ability to limit neurologic injury (Fig. 30–12). The development of newer materials and standards for vests by ASTM suggests that impact loads may be lessened.[12] These improvements may provide added protection against bruises or abrasions to the skin and, possibly, to the internal organs when compared with commonly utilized, nonstandardized vests. However, because the mechanism of thoracolumbar vertebral fractures associated with riding is primarily rotational and forced flexion, it is unlikely that materials can be sufficiently supportive while, at the same time, allowing a rider to assume the head-forward, flexed position required for equestrian sporting events (Fig. 30–13). At present, these protection devices must be considered investigational and un-

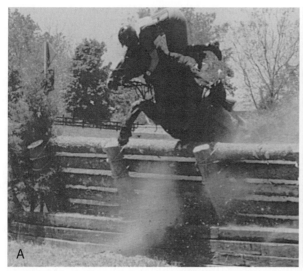
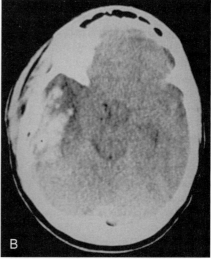

Figure 30–11, *A, B.* A sudden, unexpected refusal of the horse to jump this obstacle resulted in a cerebral contusion to the rider, despite the use of an ASTM/SEI certified helmet. Notice the height from which this individual fell. The concurrence of contact and impulsive loads makes these incidents among the most dangerous in all sports.

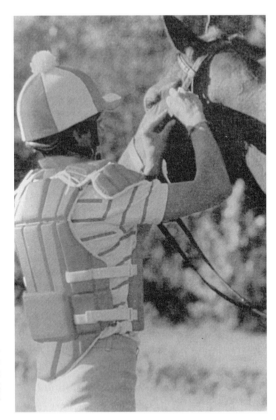

Figure 30–12. This "typical" protective vest must be considered investigational and unproved. Note the extra padding advertised to lessen the risks of spinal fracture. No studies involving equestrian accidents have shown that these garments are helpful in reducing major abdominal or spinal injury.

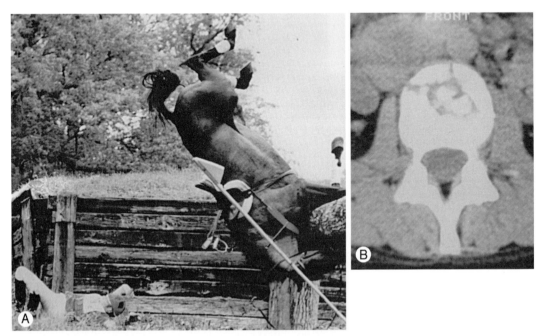

Figure 30–13, A, B. This rider sustained a spinal fracture despite wearing a vest. It is unlikely that directional velocities and loads achievable in falls such as this can be attenuated by vests.

proved in their ability to prevent spinal injury.

Although improvements in the recognition and treatment of neurologic injuries as well as the implementation of requirements for the use of appropriate headgear have lessened the risks attendant upon equestrian sports, few guidelines exist to assure adequate instruction in safe horsemanship. Most adults who ride for pleasure rely on "common sense," yet this may be questioned seriously when 37 of 187 head injuries were associated with intoxication. Because any activity involving the horse entails risk for neurologic injury, it is paramount that neurosurgeons provide the leadership and become involved in educational programs to instruct adults and children in proper and safe horsemanship. This can be accomplished through active involvement in the equestrian community and support for educational organizations such as the American Medical Equestrian Association, the United States Pony Clubs, and 4-H extension programs. Currently, neurologic injuries remain the leading cause of death associated with horseback riding. These risks can be lessened only through knowledge of the risk factors and mechanisms of injury, development and use of head protection against rotational/translational injury, and involvement in the educational process of the entire equestrian community.

References

1. American Society for Testing and Materials. Standard specifications for head gear used in horse sports and horseback riding. Annual Book of ASTM Standards 1988;F1163:1–8.
2. American Society for Testing and Materials. Standard specifications for protective vests used in horse sports and horseback riding. Annual Book of ASTM Standards 1999;F1937–98.
3. Aronson H, Tough SC. Horse-related fatalities in the province of Alberta, 1975–1990. Am J Forensic Med Pathol 1993;14:28–30.
4. Bixby-Hammett DM. Youth accidents with horses. Phys Sportsmed 1985;13:105–117.
5. Bixby-Hammett DM. Accidents in equestrian sports. Am Fam Physician 1987;36:209–214.
6. Bond GR, Christoph RA, Rodgers BM. Pediatric equestrian injuries: Assessing the impact of helmet use. Pediatrics 1995;95:487–489.
7. Brooks WH, Bixby-Hammett DM. Head and Spinal Injuries Associated with Equestrian Sports: Mechanisms and Prevention. In Torg JS (ed): Athletic Injuries to the Head, Neck and Face, 2nd ed. St. Louis, Mosby–Yearbook, 1991, pp. 133–141.
8. Brooks WH, Bixby-Hammett DM. Equestrian Sports. In Jordan BD (ed): Sports Neurology, 2nd ed. Philadelphia, Lippincott-Raven, 1998, pp. 381–391.
9. Brooks WH, Bixby-Hammett DM. Safety Committee annual report. Presented at the annual meeting of the United States Pony Club, Seattle, 1999.
10. Hamilton MG, Tranmer BI. Nervous system injuries in horseback-riding accidents. J Trauma 1993;34:227–231.
11. Horse Industry Directory, 1998. American Horse Council, 1700 K St. NW, Washington, DC 20006.
12. Mahaley MS, Seaber AV: Accident and safety considerations of horseback riding. In Proceedings of the Eighteenth AMA Conference on the Medical Aspects of Sports, Dallas, June 1976.
13. McGhee CNJ, Gullan RW, Miller JD. Horse riding and head injury: Admissions to a regional head injury unit. Br J Neurosurg 1987;1:131–136.
14. National Electronic Injury Surveillance System, US Consumer Product Safety Commission, 5401 Westbard Ave., Washington, DC 20297.
15. Nelson DE, Rivara FP, Condie C. Helmets and horseback riders. Am J Prev Med 1994;10:15–19.
16. Pounder DJ. The grave yawns: Equestrian deaths in South Australia, 1973–1983. Med J Aust 1984;141:632–635.
17. Williams LP, Remmerg EE, Huff SI. The Blue-tail fly syndrome: Horse-related accidents. Presented at the 103rd Annual Meeting of the American Public Health Association, Chicago, 1975.

31

Rugby Injuries to the Cervical Spine and Spinal Cord

Alan T. Scher

Despite ongoing research and changes in rugby laws, serious cervical spinal and spinal cord injuries continue to be a major problem in all countries where rugby is played as an organized sport. The various rule changes in schoolboy rugby have significantly decreased the incidence of serious spinal injury in schoolboys in the United Kingdom,[26] Australia,[30] and South Africa.[14] The situation with regard to injuries to adult rugby players is not satisfying. The true incidence of spinal cord injury in rugby players is still unknown, but only a small decrease, if any, appears to be taking place in adult rugby players. A 1997 publication reviewing spinal injuries in New Zealand rugby from 1976 to 1995[2] reports that contrary to widespread belief, there has not been a decrease in spinal cord injuries in rugby following rule changes in the mid 1980s. A 1998 report from Fiji[10] shows an increase in the incidence of these injuries in adult rugby players.

In South Africa, in common with the rest of world, the true incidence of rugby spinal cord injuries throughout the country is not known. Nevertheless, the incidence of spinal cord injury due to rugby in what was formally known as the Cape Province has been studied for the past 25 years at the Spinal Cord Injury Centre at Conradie Hospital in Pinelands, Cape Town, which is the only specialized spinal unit in the Cape Province. Until recently, this unit received all spinal cord injuries from the former Cape Province, the largest of the four major provinces of South Africa prior to 1994, with a population of approximately 10 million people and an area of 694,000 square kilometers.

A retrospective analysis of all patients with rugby-related spinal cord injuries ad-mitted to the Conradie and Libertas spinal units in Cape Town between 1990 and 1997 was made.[13] There were 67 spinal cord injuries in adult and schoolboy rugby players in the eight seasons studied, an average of 8.4 players per year. This average is very similar to the average of 8.7 players per year recorded in the Cape Province during the period 1981–1987.[23] The finding of a reduced incidence of injury in schoolboys is in keeping with previous analyses in Australia[30] and the United Kingdom,[26] where changes in the rugby rules have been made with gratifying results and a marked decrease in injuries.

Increasing emphasis is being placed on the fact that serious spinal cord injury represents only the tip of the iceberg of all rugby neck injuries. Unpublished evidence suggests that for each serious spinal cord injury in rugby players, there may be as many as 10 severe neck injuries without spinal cord involvement.[8] Calcinai[7] reported 10 near-miss injuries for each spinal cord injury in New Zealand in 1991.

Analysis of only those injuries that cause spinal cord injury, therefore, identifies only a fraction of the total number of cervical injuries in rugby players. Roux[16] and Calcinai[7] have reported that the mechanisms causing near-miss injuries are similar to those causing spinal cord damage, and any measures taken to reduce paralyzing injuries would also reduce the incidence of these injuries.

MECHANISMS OF INJURY

Review of the mechanisms of injury in the study of spinal cord injuries in the Cape Province of South Africa in the 1990s[14] reveals that 52% of injuries for which a mechanism was recorded occurred in the tackle phase of the game. Of these, approximately half were due to vertex impact of the tackler's head with another object or to an illegal high tackle. Twenty-five percent of injuries occurred in the ruck and maul and the remainder (23%) in the collapsed scrum. The playing position of half the injured players was recorded. Front row forwards (props 33%, hookers 9%), locks (12%) and centers (21%) and loose forwards (15%) accounted for 90% of all injuries.

This analysis indicates that the specific mechanisms responsible for injuries as reported in previous studies[20, 23] remain the primary causes for the majority of injuries sustained. As previously reported, the phases of the game responsible for injury are the tight scrum, tackle, rucks, and mauls. The exact mechanisms of injury and associated factors are briefly reviewed in the light of further research into these injuries since publication of previous reviews.

Scrum Injuries

The scrum epitomizes the physical nature of rugby and gives rugby its unique place among contact sports. It is both a powerful offensive skill, affording a base for attacking play, and a defensive skill in denying the opposition clean possession.[12] Because of the great forces generated during a scrum, this phase of play is responsible for a large proportion of serious spinal injuries in rugby.

During a scrum, both packs may generate forces equivalent to 1.5 tons.[29] The front row produces an average forward force during engagement of approximately 1400 lb, and the hooker produces over 700 lb of this force.[12] The forces produced during the scrum exceed the force necessary to cause compression fracture of the vertebral body (1000 lb) or ligamentous injury to the cervical spine (500 lb).[12] Of the players injured in the scrum, the majority sustained anterior dislocation with bilateral locking of facets (Fig. 31-1), while a smaller group sustained dislocation with unilateral locking of facets. The majority of players sustained complete, permanent quadriplegia.

Two important conclusions can be drawn from an analysis of the types of orthopedic injuries sustained. First, the common mechanism of injury is hyperflexion trauma as the major injuring force, with a rotational component in those cases with unilateral facet dislocation. Second, a striking majority of players suffered anterior dislocation with bilateral locking of facets. In cervical spinal cord injury due to causes other than rugby, the percentage of patients with bilateral locking of facets is much lower.[4] This marked preponderance of one particular type of orthopedic injury is of considerable importance because it is indicative of the mechanism of injury, and because of all the orthopedic injuries to the cervical spine, it is one with the most grave prognosis as regards paralysis and death. When complete dislocation and bilateral locking of the articular facets occur, the laminal arch of the upper vertebra at the level of injury comes forward, compressing the dorsal aspect of the spinal cord against the posterosuperior surface of the next lower vertebral body. Injury to the spinal cord is usually severe (Fig. 31-2).

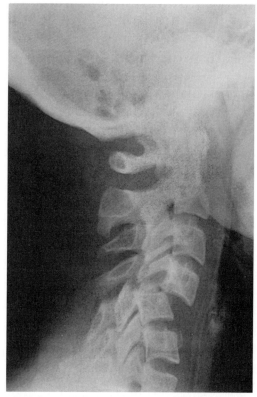

Figure 31-1. Anterior dislocation with bilateral facet dislocation at C4-C5 sustained by a hooker after collapse of rugby scrum.

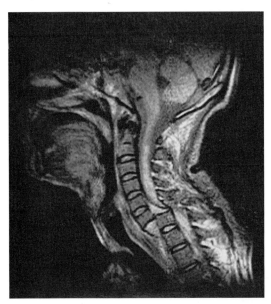

Figure 31–2. Anterior dislocation at C6-C7 with bilateral facet dislocation demonstrating, on magnetic resonance imaging examination, the severe compression of the spinal cord at the site of dislocation. This injury was sustained by a prop after collapse of a rugby scrum.

It has become common practice to utilize magnetic resonance imaging scans of patients with spinal and spinal cord injury. Utilizing this imaging modality in patients who have sustained anterior dislocation with bilateral locking of facets, it has been demonstrated that this injury may be associated with damage to the intervertebral disk and prolapse of damaged disk material into the spinal canal. This extruded disk material may compress the spinal cord when the dislocation is reduced and either aggravate or precipitate spinal cord injury.[9]

The Collapsing Scrum

The collapsing tight rugby scrum would appear to be an ideal mechanism for producing flexion injury to the cervical spine.[20] During engagement, the front-row players slightly flex their cervical spines, thus eliminating the normal lordosis of the cervical spine. If engagement does not properly occur, or should the front row collapse, while the rest of the back continues to push, the front-row players are unable to extricate themselves (Fig. 31–3). The forces thus generated can be transmitted to, and concentrated on, the neck of the front-row player, and a fracture or ligamentous injury of the cervical spine, or both, may result.

This mechanism of injury is clearly described by one patient who was a hooker. The patient states that the scrum collapsed, his forehead struck the ground, the rest of the pack kept on pushing, and he felt his chin being forced onto the chest, at which stage he clearly heard a "snap" and became totally paralyzed.

Injury Due to Crashing of the Scrum

Deliberate crashing in an attempt to intimidate or unsettle the opposing pack is a contravention of the rules, as clearly stated in the Laws of the Game of Rugby Football (1981).[27] Law 20 deals with the scrum and reads: "It is dangerous play for a front row to form some distance from its opponents and rush against them. The force or 'impact weight' exerted as the packs meet is considerable and, if the front rows are not correctly positioned, a dangerous situation leading to severe flexion injuries may arise."[20]

Preventive Measures

To protect the front row and the hooker, several strategies may be adopted.[33] It has

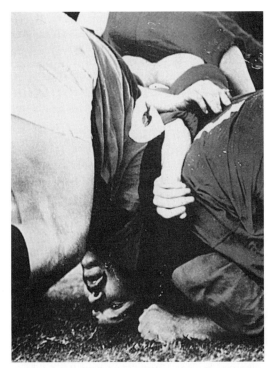

Figure 31–3. Collapsed rugby scrum; note the prop nearest the camera, whose head is pinned against the ground.

been suggested that weight-based categories rather than chronologic age should be used to select players. Use of only chronologic age[33] to select players can result in a mismatch of physical abilities, especially in the front row, and may result in an increased incidence of injuries during the scrum. Another strategy is to "depower the scrum." This can be accomplished by controlling and slowing engagement, so that the props crouch, touch, pause, and then engage.[33] Yet another method to control engagement of the scrum is termed "sequential engagement."[33] The front rows engage separately from the pack, and the rest of the pack joins the front rows once they have engaged, and a stable scrum is established.

TACKLING INJURIES

Tackling means closing both arms around a player carrying the ball and clasping him so that he is not only stopped but also forced to his side or toppled to the ground and effectively put out of action.

Injuries are sustained by both the tackler, because of incorrect technique, and the tackled player, as a consequence of the force of the tackle and the severity of impact on being forced to the ground.

An analysis of the circumstances of and types of injuries sustained reveals three specific mechanisms of injury: (1) injury due to impact of the tackler's head[20]; (2) injury due to the high tackle[17]; and (3) injury due to the double or "sandwich" tackle.[19]

Injury Due to Impact of the Tackler's Head

In this group of injuries, the player, having launched himself through the air to make a tackle, is brought to a halt abruptly when his head strikes either the ground (after missing his opponent) or the tackled player's thigh.

When the neck is slightly flexed, as in the diving position, normal lordosis is lost and the spine straightens. If severe force is applied to the top of the head when the cervical spine is in straight alignment, this force is transmitted down the long axis of the spine, causing compression fractures of the vertebral bodies (Figs. 31–4 and 31–5).[18]

There is a high risk of trauma when the head is the primary point of contact on im-

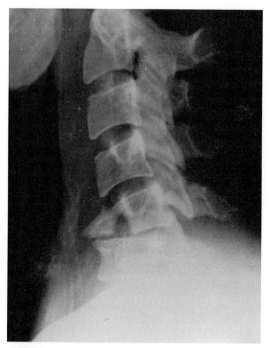

Figure 31–4. "Tear-drop" fracture of the vertebral body of C5 sustained by a player who attempted to dive-tackle an opponent and struck the ground. Note the displacement of the posterior fracture fragment into the spinal canal.

pact. This has been shown in an analysis of American football players with cervical spinal cord injuries due to direct vertex impact.[31]

The force caused by the impact of fit young men running at high speed and colliding abruptly is considerable. With players weighing 150 lb to 250 lb, great forces are generated when the tackler collides with the opponent's body or misses his opponent and strikes the ground headfirst.

Rarely, dislocation can occur with the head and neck in the neutral position on impact. Anterior cervical vertebral dislocation is usually due to forced hyperflexion, but this injury has also been noted after direct trauma to the vertex in swimmers injured by diving into shallow water, as well as in rugby players.[18]

Clinical observations that dislocation can occur with the head and neck in the neutral position have been confirmed experimentally. Bauze and Ardran[3] have shown that vertical compression applied through a lever comprising the head and upper cervical spine is a significant factor in forward dislocation.

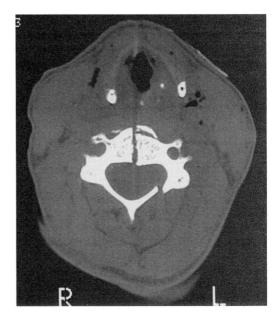

Figure 31–5. Typical sagittal, vertical fracture of the vertebral body associated with the "tear-drop" fracture as demonstrated by computed tomographic scan.

Injuries Sustained While Being Tackled

The High Tackle

The tackle from behind is more difficult than the side tackle, which is the easiest of all tackles. The orthodox tackle from behind, aiming for the waist or thighs, is highly effective (Fig. 31–6) but is likely to be dangerous. This is particularly so if the tackle is made too low when there is a risk of being struck in the face by the heels of the runner.

The spinal injuries sustained by the players subjected to high tackles varied according to the direction of the tackle. Some players were tackled from behind, the tackler wrapping one arm around his opponent's neck and pulling posteriorly and downwards (Fig. 31–7). Force applied in this manner would be likely to produce a hyperextension injury to the cervical spine (Figs. 31–8 and 31–9). Because the tackle is made with one arm, the neck tends to become

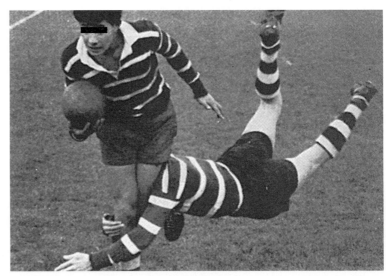

Figure 31–6. Correct method of making a tackle; note that the tackler has his head and neck behind the tackled player's legs.

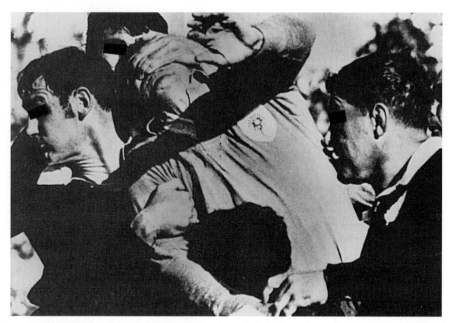

Figure 31–7. Extension force being applied to the tackled player, just after he has passed the ball.

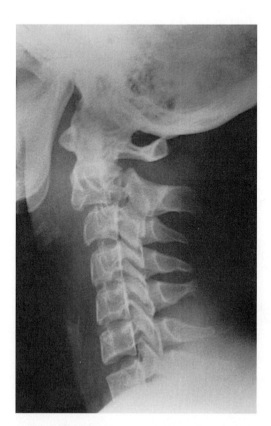

Figure 31–8. Hangman's fracture at C2 sustained during a high tackle. Note the extensive prevertebral hematoma.

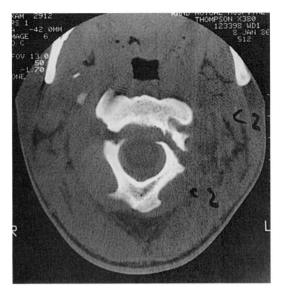

Figure 31–9. Hangman's fracture demonstrated on computed tomographic examination.

twisted as it is forced into hyperextension, thereby adding rotational stress to the hyperextension force.

Other players were tackled from the side, with the tackler wrapping one arm around the neck and forcing it into hyperflexion (Fig. 31–10). Rotational force is also applied to the neck in this type of tackle.

A player running with the ball or attempting to kick it may have one or both feet off the ground when tackled. He is then

less able to withstand the forces being applied to his neck. In addition to being off balance, he is usually unaware of the impending tackle, and therefore unable to tense his cervical muscles against the attack.

The Double Tackle

This is a rare cause of cervical injury. A double tackle occurs when a player is tackled simultaneously by two opponents. This is also sometimes referred to as a "scissors" or "sandwich" tackle.

Double tackles are difficult to avoid owing to the speed at which rugby is played competitively. Sometimes a particular player is so formidable that he is marked by two players who utilize a double-tackle technique deliberately in an attempt to neutralize his potential. More commonly, a double tackle takes place in the heat of the moment, particularly when an opponent is close to the line and about to score a try.

In theory, a correctly made tackle by a single player should not cause injury to either the tackler or tackled player, whereas the double tackle places both the tackled player and tacklers at risk. The tacklers may collide with each other in midair, missing their opponent completely. If the double tackle is made successfully, the tackled player is vulnerable to cervical injury for the following reasons. The tackler nearest to

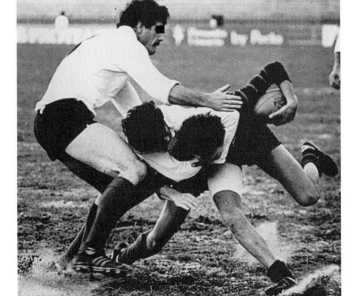

Figure 31–10. Typical high tackle.

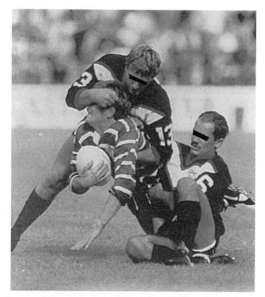

Figure 31–11. A double tackle; note the rotary force being applied to the tackled player's head.

the ball carrier usually tackles low (around the thighs or waist), so that the second tackler is forced to go in high and take the ball carrier around the chest, shoulders, or neck (Fig. 31–11). Because the first tackler often tackles fractionally before the second tackler, the tackled player is actually falling forward, allowing the second tackler to tackle from above, increasing the force applied to the neck at the moment of impact. Further, because the lower body of the tackled player is firmly held, he is unable to move with the momentum of the tackle, and this increases the force dissipated on the cervical spine, particularly regarding rotational stress.

Injuries Sustained in Rucks and Mauls

Rucks and mauls form part of what is termed "loose play" and are often referred to as a "loose scrum." There is an essential difference between a ruck and a maul, defined according to the Laws of the Game of Rugby Football as follows[27]:

A ruck, which can take place only in the field of play, is formed when the ball is on the ground and one or more players from each team are on their feet in physical contact, closing around the ball between them.

A maul, which can take place only in the field of play, is formed by one or more players from each team on their feet and in physical contact closing around the player who is carrying the ball.

These two phases of loose play are not only responsible for spinal injury, but are also an important cause of rugby injuries generally. Illegal play is often generated in rucks and mauls, and many injuries are sustained due to kicking and trampling (Fig. 31–12).

Spinal injuries as a result of loose play occur in three different ways[20]: (1) forced flexion of the ball carrier's neck; (2) forced flexion of the neck of the player at the bottom of the ruck; or (3) head and neck injury due to charging into a mass of struggling players.

SPINAL CORD CONCUSSION IN RUGBY PLAYERS

During an analysis of a group of 40 rugby players who had sustained cervical spinal cord injuries, 9 players were identified who

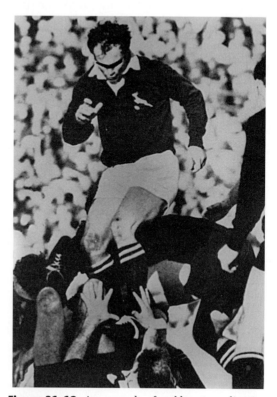

Figure 31–12. An example of reckless trampling in a loose maul.

had sustained only transient paralysis.[22] A retrospective analysis of the clinical and radiologic findings in this group of rugby players was carried out. In addition, the spinal canal diameter was assessed, utilizing the ratio method of assessment.[32]

The analysis showed that in five of the nine players, spinal stenosis was present, with the maximal spinal canal narrowing at C3 and C4. In the remaining four players, one showed evidence of osteoarthrotic change at two levels, while another had congenital fusion of two vertebral bodies.

The study confirmed that cervical spinal cord concussion does occur in rugby players. Spinal cord concussion is a transient disturbance of spinal cord function that results from a rapid alternation in velocity following trauma and resolves in 48 hours. The spinal cord concussion may be in association with bony narrowing in the spinal canal or in association with congenital fusion of the vertebrae or osteoarthrotic change[22] (Fig. 31–13).

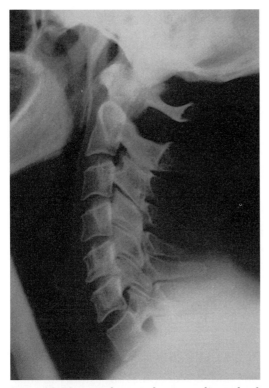

Figure 31–13. Lateral cervical spine radiograph of a rugby player who sustained transient neurapraxia of the spinal cord after a tackle. The spinal canal is narrowed, as demonstrated by the close apposition of the spinolaminal line to the articular masses. Note also the posterior osteophytic spurring at C5-C6.

PREMATURE ONSET OF DEGENERATIVE DISEASE OF THE CERVICAL SPINE IN RUGBY PLAYERS

In an attempt to assess whether rugby players are prone to the development of premature degenerative disease,[21] radiographs of the cervical spines of 150 rugby players were compared with a control group of 150 male hospital patients. The study revealed that rugby players showed premature and advanced changes of degenerative disease when compared with the control group. These changes were most marked in the cervical spines of the tight forwards. Rugby players so affected are therefore more likely to present with the symptoms and signs of cervical osteoarthrosis and are at greater risk of hyperextension injury to the cervical spinal cord.[21]

RISK FACTORS FOR SPINAL CORD INJURIES IN RUGBY PLAYERS

A retrospective study of spinal cord injuries in Cape Province rugby players from 1960 to 1989, undertaken to determine etiologic factors for 117 catastrophic neck injuries in rugby players, identified high risk factors for spinal cord injuries in rugby players.[8] Specific points of interest arising out of these risk factors are briefly discussed.

Match Play

The most obvious risk factor was match play. Ninety-eight percent of all injuries occurred during match play.[8] This finding is especially significant, since considerably more time is spent in practice than in match play. It would seem that the competitiveness and aggression unleashed in match play must be an important factor contributing to these injuries.

Age

It was originally believed that schoolboy rugby players were at greatest risk of spinal cord injury.[30] This and other studies refute this. Sixty-nine percent of all injuries in the study were sustained by adults. The significance of this is that in most rugby-playing countries, far more schoolboys than adults play rugby. In the geographic area of the study, the ratio of schoolboy to adult rugby players may be of the order of 5–10:1. Thus the more than twofold greater number of spinal cord injuries in adult players could indicate a 10–12-fold higher risk for the injury in adults than in schoolboys.

Level of Play

The third risk factor is level of play. Injury risk was greatest at the higher levels of play, as 69% of injuries were suffered by players in either first or age-group A teams. Since there are relatively few such players in the total rugby-playing population, this finding suggests that high levels of both skill and physical fitness, far from protecting against these injuries, must actually make injury more likely. The greater number of injuries in the more skilled players is probably explained by their more aggressive approach to the game and their more dangerous style of play, both of which might be explained by a "win at all costs" attitude associated with "psyching up." This possibility is further supported by the finding that these injuries occur almost exclusively during matches.

Phase of Play

As has repeatedly been shown, four different phases of play contribute to the vast majority of these injuries.[20] In the study[8] the tackling phase of the game, including tackling (21%) and being tackled (30%), accounted for more than half all injuries, with the tight scrum (21%) and the ruck and maul (18%) accounting for the majority (39%) of the remaining injuries.

Interestingly, there appear to be national differences in the proportion of injuries occurring in the different phases of play. Thus, in South Africa and in the recent past in New Zealand,[6] there are fewer injuries in the scrum (<25%) and more in the tackle situation (>50%), whereas in Australia,[30] Canada,[28] Eire,[15] and Northern Ireland,[11] scrummaging accounts for the majority of all injuries. A retrospective study of the cervical spinal injuries sustained in rugby in the United States from 1970 to 1996 reveals that 58% of the 62 documented injured players injured their cervical spines during the scrum.[33] Significantly more injuries occurred during engagement than during collapse.

Playing Position

Back line players suffer most of their injuries in the tackling situation,[24] whereas props and hookers are at risk during scrummaging.[24, 30] Ruck and maul injuries appear to be more common in forwards.[24]

In this study the position that carried by far the highest risk was the hooker.[8] This is a finding common to studies from New Zealand[5] and Australia.[30] In Australia props were the second most frequently injured players,[30] whereas in South Africa props were among the least frequently injured players. This discrepancy could be explained by the large number of injuries caused by "crashing" the scrum in Australia.[30]

Only one previous study has detailed the exact playing positions of injured back line players.[1] In the study, centers and flyhalves were at greatest risk. Virtually all injuries to back line players (85%) occurred during the tackling phase of the game; the rest occurred in the ruck and maul.

Time of Season

The period of greatest risk for both adult and schoolboy rugby players was at the start of the season, and again after the midseason break. This has been reported in numerous other studies of both spinal cord injuries and of all rugby injuries.

CONCLUSION

An editorial in the *British Medical Journal* in 1995[13] draws attention to the fact that the true incidence of spinal cord injury in rugby players is still unknown. Despite numerous pleas for accurate data on cervical spinal injuries from the major rugby-playing countries of the world, this data is still not available. Because of this lack of data, conflicting reports of either decreases or increases in spinal cord injuries in different countries and even within the same country are published. The *BMJ* editorial[13] once again makes a plea for the international community of doctors involved in rugby to persuade rugby administrators in all countries to set up epidemiologically valid surveys of injuries. It is only with accurate data that changes in the rules of rugby and in coaching methods can be instituted to decrease the incidence of these spinal and spinal cord injuries.

References

1. Akpata T. Spinal injuries in US rugby: 1970–1990. Rugby 1990;18:14–15.
2. Armour KS, Clatworthy BJ, Bean AR, et al. Spinal injuries in New Zealand rugby and rugby league—a twenty year survey. N Z Med J 1997;110:462–465.
3. Bauze RJ, Ardran M. Experimental production of forward dislocation in the human cervical spine. J Bone Joint Surg 1978;60B:239–245.
4. Braakman R, Penning L. Injuries of the Cervical Spine. Amsterdam, Excerpta Medica, 1971, p 268.
5. Burry HC, Gowland H. Cervical injury in rugby football—A New Zealand survey. Br J Sports Med 1981;15:56–59.
6. Burry HC, Calcinai CJ. The need to make rugby safer. BMJ 1988;296:149–150.
7. Calcinai C. Cervical spine injuries. NZJ Sport Med 1992;20:14–15.
8. Kew T, Noakes TD, Scher AT, et al. A retrospective study of spinal cord injuries in Cape Province rugby players, 1963–1989. S Afr Med J 1991;80:127–133.
9. Mahale YJ, Silver JR, Henderson NJ. Neurological complications of the reduction of cervical spine dislocations. J Bone Joint Surg 1994;32:442–453.
10. Maharaj JC, Cameron ID. Increase in spinal injury among rugby union players in Fiji. Med J Aust 1998;168:418.
11. McCoy GF, Piggot J, Macafee AL, et al. Injuries of the cervical spine in schoolboy rugby football. J Bone Joint Surg Br 1984;66:500–503.
12. Milburn PD. Biomechanics of rugby union scrummaging. Technical and safety issues. Sports Med 1993;16:168–179.
13. Noakes T, Jakoet I. Spinal cord injuries in rugby union players. BMJ 1995;310:1345–1346.
14. Noakes T, Jakoet I, Koets G. Apparent reduction in the incidence and severity of spinal cord injuries in schoolboy rugby players in the Cape Province since 1990. S Afr Med J (in press) 1999.
15. O'Carrol PF, Sheehan JM, Gregg TM. Cervical spine injuries in rugby football. Ir Med J 1981;74:377–379.
16. Roux CE. The epidemiology of schoolboy rugby injuries. Cape Town, University of Cape Town, South Africa, 1992, pp 307–313.
17. Scher AT. The high rugby tackle—an avoidable cause of cervical spine cord injury. S Afr Med J 1978;53:1015–1018.
18. Scher AT. Diving injuries to the cervical spinal cord. S Afr Med J 1981;59:603–605.
19. Scher AT. The "double" tackle—Another cause of serious cervical spinal injury in rugby players. S Afr Med J 1983;64:595–596.
20. Scher AT. Rugby injuries of the spine and spinal cord. Clin Sports Med 1987;6:87–99.
21. Scher AT. Premature onset of degenerative disease of the cervical spine in rugby players. S Afr Med J 1990;77:557–558.
22. Scher AT. Spinal cord concussion in rugby players. Am J Sports Med 1991;19:485–488.
23. Scher AT. Rugby injuries to the cervical spine and spinal cord: A 10-year review. Clin Sports Med 1998;17:195–206.
24. Silver JR. Injuries of the spine sustained in rugby. Br Med J 1984;288:37–43.
25. Silver JR, Gill S. Injuries of the spine sustained during rugby. Sports Med 1988;5:328–334.
26. Silver JR. Injuries of the spine sustained during rugby. Br J Sports Med 1992;26:253–258.
27. South African Rugby Board. The Laws of the Game of Rugby Football. Cape Town, SARB, 1981, pp 35–36.
28. Sovio OM, Van Petegham PK, Schweigel JF. Cervical spine injuries in rugby players. CMAJ 1984;130:735–736.
29. Stubbs DA. Personal communication, 1981.
30. Taylor TKF, Coolican MRJ. Spinal cord injuries in Australian footballers, 1960–1985. Med J Aust 1987;147:112–118.
31. Torg JS, Truex RC, Marshall J, et al. Spinal injury at the level of the third and fourth cervical vertebrae from football. J Bone Joint Surg 1977;59A:1015–1019.
32. Torg JS, Pavlov H, Genuario SE, et al. Neurapraxia of the cervical spinal cord with transient quadriplegia. J Bone Joint Surg 1986;68:1354–1370.
33. Wetzler MJ, Akpata T, Laughlin W, et al. Occurrence of cervical spine injuries during the rugby scrum. Am J Sports Med 1998;26:177–180.

32

Mountaineering Head and Spine Injuries

Edward G. Hixson

Evolved from primates, man has the ability and urge to climb. The child's jungle gym becomes the high-tech climbing wall. The sport of mountaineering is intimately involved with the wilderness mountain environment. The earth's land mass is 42% mountainous.[1] The dramatic improvements in travel have made most of the world's highest mountains available to adventurous climbers. Mountaineering is an individual sport with personal rewards. One's goal may be reaching a summit, climbing a rock or ice face, or, simply, accomplishing a difficult "move." The challenge is technical, physical, and psychological. Strength, endurance, knowledge, and training are required. Mountaineering is done by individuals, either solo or in groups, in one-day climbs or major expeditions. As in all vigorous athletic activities, injuries occur. The wilderness mountain environment is an injury multiplier. Mortality and morbidity are increased. Risk of injury in mountaineering is similar to that in other sports; however, the mortality is higher.[2] Head and spine injuries account for the majority of deaths and major disabilities. From 1959 to 1968 there were 1521 mountaineering accidents in the United Kingdom; about 20% were fatal.[3]

Mountaineering is increasing in popularity. This is obvious from both media attention, and the crowds at trail heads and popular climbing areas. Grand Teton National Park recorded more than 8000 climbs in 1982. Mount Rainier sees more than 5000 yearly. There are more than 100,000 active climbers in the United States.[4] Very high altitude (18,000 ft) is reached by more than 5000 climbers yearly.[5] As of January 1997, there had been 397 expeditions to Mount Everest (167 of which successfully achieved the summit).[6] In spite of vastly improved equipment and techniques, increased numbers at risk result in increased injuries and deaths. Seventy-seven climbers reached the summit of Mount Everest from 1928 to 1979, with 44 deaths (57%).[7] Through 1997, the summit was attempted by 4400 climbers, 728 successfully, with 148 killed in the effort (20%). Forty people stood on the summit of Mount Everest on May 10, 1993, the most ever on a single day. Relative risk has decreased. The greatest number of deaths occurred in 1996; 15 were killed; however, 95 reached the summit. In 1970, only four reached the summit, with eight killed.[6] On Mount McKinley, from 1903 to 1982, of 6080 mountaineers, 40 (0.8%) were killed.[8] The injury rate is about 12% to 16% in recent years.[9] High altitude mountaineering is one of the world's most dangerous sports. Many insurance policies do not cover mountaineering or else require riders with increased premiums. A rate of two injuries per 1000 climber-days was noted for Grand Teton National Park.[10] The incidence of injury is low with respect to other sports: 3.4 to 10 per 1000 skier-days for Alpine skiing; 1.5 to 2 per 1000 skier-days for cross-country skiing; 4.3 per 1000 skier-days for ski jumping.[11] Head injuries accounted for 22% and spine injuries 6% in the Grand Teton study.[10] Although mountaineering injuries are relatively infrequent, the trauma potential is high, magnified by lengthy, difficult evacuation. The *risk* of mountaineering is partially responsible for its attraction. The adventure is avoiding danger.

MOUNTAINEERING HAZARD

Mountaineers describe hazard in two categories, *subjective* and *objective. Subjective* hazard is under the control of the climber. Falls due to poor judgment are an example. *Objective* hazard is due to "acts of God," over which the climber has no control. An example is being struck by lightning. In North America, roughly two thirds of all accidents are due to subjective hazard, one third due to objective. In the Himalayas, the ratios are reversed.[12] This reflects the greater experience of climbers in the Himalayas. Reinhold Messner, widely considered the finest high-altitude mountaineer in the world, has said that the secret to survival on 8000 m peaks is avoiding objective hazard (he does not say how).

TRAUMA IN THE MOUNTAINS

Again, the wilderness mountain environment is an injury multiplier. A fall from a cliff may be no worse than a construction accident; however, prolonged and difficult evacuation may increase mortality and morbidity. When difficulty of evacuation is combined with weather extremes, risk to rescuers may be considerable. Going to higher altitude is similar to travel toward the North or South Pole, exposing the climber to harsher, colder weather. Air temperature decreases 6.5°C with every 1000 m increase in altitude.[13] Wind velocity increases with increasing altitude, as does exposure to ultraviolet radiation (4% every 300 m[14]). The mountainous areas of Third World countries do not have specialized technical mountain rescue teams with helicopter evacuation. The benefits of prompt rescue for head injury are obvious. The Swiss noted that from 1980 to 1990 the mortality rate for severe head injury was 12%, with a return to a normal neurologic state in 88% of survivors by 6 months postinjury. Rescue in Switzerland is done by helicopter with a trauma physician on board.[15] Mountaineering trauma, morbidity, and mortality can be similar to urban, but under conditions of difficult and prolonged rescue and evacuation, different rules apply. The mountaineer must be more self-sufficient. A climbing party must be trained in first aid, rescue, and evacuation.

Wilderness Medicine

The standard rules by which urban or suburban rescue squads function must be modified for the wilderness. Organizations such as the National Association for Search and Rescue (NASAR)[16] have developed appropriate courses of instruction and guidelines of care, for example, Wilderness Emergency Medical Technician (WEMT) and Wilderness First Responder (WFR). This training benefits all mountaineers, whether they are trauma surgeons or those with only basic first aid knowledge.

Confronted by a mountaineering accident, the *first priority* is the *scene survey.* The scene must be evaluated for the risk of further danger to the injured or to rescuers, such as a rock or ice fall, an avalanche, and so forth.

Next is the *Primary Survey,* inherent to all Basic Life Support and Advanced Life Support teachings. The injured is checked for life threatening injuries, which are dealt with according to the mnemonic ABCDE.

A—Airway
1. Many victims of head injury will die of airway problems (preventable), not their head injury.
2. All airway-preserving maneuvers must be done assuming an unstable cervical spine injury, if the mechanism for treating such an injury is present, i.e., jaw thrust, chin lift.

B—Breathing
1. Ventilation, with an adequate airway, can be done, even in the wilderness, and maintained without special equipment. This is significant for high cervical cord injury.
2. For hypothermics, ventilation may be needed. If so, it should be done at half the normal rate (normal = 12 breaths per minute).

C—Circulation
1. Hypovolemia is assumed when shock follows injury. Presence of peripheral pulses is usually a good sign (systolic pressure is generally >80 mmHg). Absent central pulse in an unconscious trauma patient is an immediate indication for CPR. If after 30 minutes there is no response, recovery is unlikely. With cardiac arrest from blood loss, recovery is extremely unlikely. CPR is unlikely to be able to be maintained effectively during prolonged, difficult evacuation.

2. The hypothermic is a special case. The victim appears dead; however, slow, barely detectable perfusion and respiration are adequate, and complete recovery is possible. Do not accept "cold and dead," only "warm and dead."

3. Bleeding must be quickly controlled with direct pressure. Tourniquets are usually more deleterious than beneficial. Placement of a tourniquet usually leads to amputation.

D—*Disability* (Neurologic examination, head and spine)

1. Evaluate level of consciousness (LOC). A useful mnemonic is AVPU:
   A *Alert*
   V Responds to *Voice*
   P Responds to *Pain*
   U *Unresponsive*

2. Decreased or decreasing LOC is the *most significant* sign of head injury. Hypoxia, shock, alcohol, drugs, and hypothermia also produce decreased LOC.

3. Spine injury is relatively easy to determine in competent, alert patients: local tenderness, ability to move extremities, ability to feel extremities. It is *impossible* in an unconscious patient (in the field). It is *inaccurate* in the presence of altered LOC, drugs, hypothermia, and alcohol. For the alert patient, palpate the spine from head to pelvis, skin on skin. Ascertain the absence of tenderness and the ability to feel and move the extremities.

4. Remember, the *Autonomic Stress Reaction masks pain.* For example, a patient with a severe leg injury may mask the signs of neck injury, making examination inaccurate.

E—*Exposure/Environment*

1. Assess the effects on the victim and further risks, both immediate and during evacuation, that is, protect from further injury, wetness, cold, and so forth.

2. Assess likely speed of evacuation.

3. Remember that injury predisposes to frostbite even for an uninjured extremity.

4. Disrobing may be needed for assessment. Make sure to protect the victim from cold injury. Hypothermia is easier to prevent than to treat.

In the wilderness, the *Secondary Survey* is important. Delayed evacuation allows time for a careful and complete evaluation. This consists of a brief history and a head-to-toe physical examination. The history should be AMPLE:

A *Allergies*
M *Medicine*
P *Previous health problems*
L *Last meal*
E *Events leading up to injury*

The physical examination is more complete than the Primary Survey. LOC is examined more precisely using the Glasgow Coma Scale. This quantitative measurement will allow the staff at the receiving hospital to plan for the casualty.

Glasgow Coma Scale (GCS)

Points are awarded for each area examined and totaled.

I. *Eye opening (4 possible)*
   a. Spontaneous, normal — E = 4
   b. To speech — E = 3
   c. To pain — E = 2
   d. None — E = 1

II. *Verbal, best response (5 possible)*
   a. Oriented to person, place, and time — V = 5
   b. Confused — V = 4
   c. Inappropriate words — V = 3
   d. No words, sounds only — V = 2
   e. None — V = 1

III. *Motor, best response, any extremity (6 possible)*
   a. On command — M = 6
   b. Pain avoidance/localization — M = 5
   c. Pain withdrawal — M = 4
   d. Abnormal flexion (decorticate) — M = 3
   e. Abnormal extension (decerebrate) — M = 2
   f. None — M = 1

Totals

15   = normal
13–15   = mild head injury
9–12   = moderate injury
8 or less = coma/severe head injury

Complete head-to-toe physical examination follows, usually requiring exposure of the patient. In the emergency room, this would be the "scissors" survey. It is modified to protect from cold injury as needed.

The patient must be *monitored.* Vital signs, including temperature, are important, if possible. Without a blood pressure cuff:

Carotid pulse present   = systolic BP >60
Femoral pulse present   = systolic BP >70
Radial pulse present   = systolic BP >80

If a thermometer is available (many clinical thermometers do not read below 94°F), a core (rectal) temperature less than 90°F indicates hypothermia; less than 60°F indicates severe hypothermia (little chance of survival).

A final step is triage, the sorting of casualties in order of seriousness. The basis is the greatest good for the greatest number. Although designed for multiple casualties, it is useful to categorize a single patient as a guide for evacuation. Casualties are sorted as to the level of severity based upon the urgency of the need for definitive care (surgery). Speed saves!

Triage Level

0—Dead, emergency evacuation not necessary

1—Maximum priority, evacuate ASAP (e.g., head injury with coma)

2—Definitive care needed but can be delayed (e.g., spine fracture suspected, where a gentle evacuation with good spine immobilization is more important than speed)

3—Minor, evacuation not needed, or patient can self-evacuate

The complexity of wilderness medicine, rescue, and evacuation exceeds the scope of this chapter. Many well-respected organizations are available with programs to assist mountaineers.[17, 17a]

TRAUMATIC HEAD AND SPINE INJURY

Head injury is present in approximately 50% of trauma deaths.[18] This is particularly significant in the mountain wilderness environment and contributes to the increased mortality. In 50% of fatal mountaineering accidents in Scotland, head injury was a major fatality factor.[19] Definitive care of head injury is rarely available. In 1978 a skilled Austrian surgeon successfully decompressed an intracranial hematoma in a Sherpa who had sustained a head injury in a fall in the Khumbu icefall. On Everest expeditions in 1982, 1983, and 1984 the author included "burr hole" equipment in the medical kit (never used). Such examples are the exception; mountaineers will generally be confronted with avoiding aggravation of head injury by hypoxia and other field-treatable problems while providing evacuation. Monitoring LOC is particularly important with head injury. Often, subdural hematomas take 12 to 24 hours to develop. Even epidural hematomas may allow 4 to 6 hours prior to decompensation. A high index of suspicion may allow this time to be well spent in evacuation.

Spine injury is assumed when the mechanism exists. The unconscious victim of a fall or collision will have a 5% to 10% chance of cervical spine injury.[18] About 15% to 20% of spine injuries are due to falls. The cervical spine injury is the most common cause of spinal cord injury, accounting for 55% of cord injuries.[20] Spine injury accounts for the greatest disability with respect to cost to society and victim. The definitive care of head injury has reduced the mortality from 40%–45% in 1975–1984 to 25%–30% in 1984–1999. Spinal cord injury remains problematic. Victims who suffer complete paralysis at injury regain only 8% function. Those suffering partial paralysis regain 59% of function.[20] For mountaineering the emphasis is on preventing further injury during evacuation by head-to-toe rigid spinal immobilization—not allowing conversion of partial paralysis to complete paralysis.

With respect to cold injury, all victims of head and spine injuries are at increased risk for developing hypothermia due to their immobility. In addition, when freezing temperatures exist, the risk of frostbite is present. When injury occurs, frostbite risk to the extremities is increased even when the injury is elsewhere, such as the spine.

ALTITUDE

The effects of altitude are either a primary source of physiologic trauma to the mountaineer or a secondary injury multiplier, increasing the mortality and morbidity. Of all climbers who go to the Himalayas, there is about a 3% mortality rate. A mortality of 0.3% was due to the effects of altitude alone.[21] For 8000 m peaks, there is a mortality rate of 3% to 4%, with approximately 10% being due to the effects of altitude alone.[22]

Altitude is categorized according to its effects upon the climber (Fig. 32–1). Below 5000 ft (1500 m) few climbers will have symptoms of altitude illness. *High altitude* is from 5000 ft to 11,500 ft (1500 m–3500 m). Here the altitude is tolerated, but mild symptoms are noted by most. These are short-lived and rarely serious. *Very high altitude* is from 11,500 ft to 18,000 ft (3500 m–5500 m). The risk of severe illness is increased; climbers can function, but acclimatization is needed. Above 18,000 ft (5500 m) is *extreme altitude.* In this area, the body deteriorates more than it acclimatizes. This is the "Death Zone." The risk of serious illness is high.[14] Extreme altitude is survivable only by superb acclimatization with very slow ascent. The summit of Mount Everest, 29,028 ft (8848 m), is about the upper limit of an acclimatized human being's possible ascent, unpressurized, without supplemental oxygen.

The percentage of oxygen in the air is constant at 20.93% regardless of altitude. At increasing altitudes, the barometric pressure decreases, decreasing the total amount of oxygen available. The partial pressure of oxygen is proportionately decreased, thereby decreasing the oxygen in the blood. On the summit of Mount Everest, the barometric pressure is 253 torr,[23] about one third of sea level pressure. To be able to tolerate these extremes, man must acclimatize. This is accomplished by slow ascent over weeks. Rapid ascent is fatal. In 1875 the balloon *Zenith* ascended rapidly to above 25,000 ft. Two of its three occupants died.[24] A good rule is to limit net ascent to 1000 to 2000 ft per day above 5,000 ft.[25] The climbers dictum "climb high, sleep low" is appropriate. Mountaineers try to limit exposure to extreme altitudes. For acclimatized people, the phenomenal effect of altitude was shown by Dr. Chris Pizzo in 1981. On the summit of Mount Everest, he took an alveolar sample of expired air on himself. PO_2 was calculated from this at 30 torr, with PCO_2 at 6 torr,[23] with corresponding O_2 saturation 63.4% to 73%. With exercise, it is probably lower. At these values, life is barely sustainable. Aerobic power is measured by maximum O_2 uptake, $\dot{V}O_2max$. This is dependent upon the partial pressure of oxygen, PO_2, and barometric pressure. It is independent of acclimatization and decreases with altitude. $\dot{V}O_2max$ decreases 3% every 1000 ft.[14, 24] Acclimatization increases the amount of work a climber can do with decreased aerobic capacity. Oxygen saturation reflects acclimatization and is preserved to about 18,000 ft (5500 m) in the 90% to 70% range. At extreme altitude, it drops to levels of about 55%.[26]

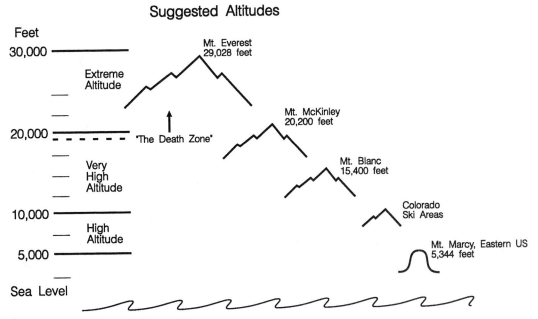

Figure 32–1. From Hixson EG. Altitude Stress. *In* DeLee JC, Drez D, Jr. (eds): *Orthopedic Sports Medicine: Principles and Practice.* Philadelphia, WB Saunders, 1994, p 398, with permission.

Acclimatization

The process of acclimatization is absolutely necessary for climbing at very high or extreme altitude. The process is complex and involves changes in all of the body systems to a greater or lesser degree. Hyperventilation is the obvious response to hypoxia, with a decrease in CO_2. The respiratory alkalosis produced is compensated by increasing bicarbonate excretion; pH is maintained. The cardiorespiratory changes are much more complex, and approximately 3 weeks of exposure to at least 10,000 ft (3000 m) is needed. The hematologic system acclimatizes by increasing erythropoiesis. Blood hemoglobin greater than 20 g/100 ml and hematocrits above 60% are not uncommon. This increases blood viscosity and is maladaptive. Optimum hematocrit for oxygen transport is in the range of 50% to 60%.[16] The author's hematocrit exceeded 70% and was accompanied by multiple brain stem microthromboses. Hematologic acclimatization takes 3 to 6 weeks above 10,000 ft. The acclimatization process includes many other changes from enzyme systems at a subcellular level to the system level.

Effect on the central nervous system (CNS) is pronounced. Hyperventilation produces hypocapnea and cerebral vasoconstriction. This physiologic effect is used by neurosurgeons to reduce cerebral edema. However, at high altitude, hypoxia is inevitable, and the cerebral vasoconstriction is overridden, causing cerebral vasodilatation and increased cerebral blood flow (CBF). CBF increased by 67% has been described at 5340 m.[27] A greater effect would be noted higher. It is easy to see how head and spine traumatic injuries can be "multiplied" at high altitude.

Altitude Sickness

Injury related solely to altitude occurs. This is called altitude sickness. It is actually physiologic trauma from the hypoxic, hypobaric environment. Altitude sickness is primarily *neurologic.* It is often described by organ system syndromes, such as high altitude pulmonary edema, but neurologic symptoms are often coexistent. Neurobehavioral changes, paranoia, obsessiveness, depression, anxiety, and so forth, are documented in the Minnesota Multiphasic Personality Inventory evaluation of mountaineers.[28, 29] Subtle long-term neurologic and neuropsychologic defects have been reported.[30, 31] Evidence of adverse effects on the CNS from altitude alone is increasing. Residual neurobehavior impairment is noted in 58% of extreme altitude climbers. All had normal neurologic exams. Structural changes on magnetic resonance imaging (MRI) were noted in 48%.[32] With altitude illness, transient and permanent neurologic complications range from mild impairment of cognitive ability to hemiplegia.[33-40] The risk of permanent neurologic damage from high altitude cannot be ignored. The author has mild ataxia, nystagmus, mild dyslexia, and hearing loss from extreme altitude, with structural changes on MRI. Initially this was expressed by extreme ataxia, diplopia, dysarthria, and dysphasia for several months.[14]

Altitude Syndromes

Altitude sicknesses have a common etiology: hypobaric hypoxia (Table 32–1). The syndromes are presented separately; however, symptoms of all syndromes often coexist. Each syndrome is rarely seen as an isolated entity, and, again, neurologic symptoms predominate. Altitude exposure above 10,000 ft is usually required. Speed of ascent is significant. Those affected usually go too high, too fast; climb too hard; and stay too long. Physical strength and fitness offer no immunity. Indeed, the attitude of invincibility, self-confidence, and enthusiasm that often coexist with youth and physical conditioning may predispose to altitude sickness. Anaerobic exercise with early exposure to high altitude is more detrimental than aerobic exercise. Adequate acclimatization is key. Acclimatization does not occur without adequate stimulus from exposure to elevations of at least 10,000 ft. Limiting daily net ascent to 1000 ft to 2000 ft above 5000 ft is a good rule. Rest days are interspersed. From 3 to 6 weeks of acclimatization are needed for expeditions to the Death Zone above 20,000 ft.

Acute Mountain Sickness (AMS)

At high altitude, 8000 ft to 9000 ft (e.g., skiing in the Rockies), 12% of participants

Table 32-1. Altitude Illness

Syndrome	Incidence	Onset	Hallmark Symptoms	Treatment	Sequelae
Acute mountain sickness (AMS)	12% 8000–9000 ft	1–2 days	Headache, malaise, anorexia	Acetazolamide (descent unnecessary)	None
High-altitude pulmonary edema (HAPE)	0.5% 11,500 ft	2–3 days	Dyspnea, cough, frothy sputum, cyanosis	Descent mandatory, diuresis, furosemide, oxygen, pressurization	Survivors experience none
High-altitude cerebral edema (HACE)	0.02% (1.8% of AMS experience HACE) above 12,000 ft	2–3 days	Ataxia, severe headache, altered mental status	Descent mandatory, dexamethasone, acetazolamide, oxygen, pressurization	Survivors may experience severe neurological deficit
High-altitude retinal hemorrhage (HARH)	56% 17,000 ft and above	Unknown	None	None	None (rare scotoma)
High-altitude cachexia (HAC)	100% above 18,600 ft for extended periods (weeks)	Gradual	Weight loss, weakness, loss of vigor	High caloric intake, high-carbohydrate diet	None

From Jordan BD, Tsairis P, Warren RF (eds). Sports Neurology. 2nd ed. Philadelphia, Lippincott-Raven, 1998, p 433, with permission.

will develop AMS.[41] Rapid ascent to 14,400 ft produces symptoms in 67%.[42] Symptoms usually take 24 to 48 hours to develop. Neurologic symptoms, headache, nausea, anorexia, malaise, and insomnia predominate. Mild dyspnea is usually present. Symptoms are usually worse at the end of the day. Cheyne-Stokes respiration may be present, often observed at night. AMS is not life threatening, it is self-limited, and it resolves spontaneously in a few days. Fluid retention with edema is noted. Hyperventilation will relieve the headache, which recurs on cessation. AMS resolves with acclimatization. It is like seasickness—you feel like you're going to die, and are afraid you won't! For treatment, listen to your body and rest. Descent is usually unnecessary. AMS is treated and prevented by taking acetazolamide (Diamox) in doses of 250 mg to 500 mg twice daily. Acetazolamide is a carbonic anhydrase inhibitor and produces hyperventilation. It is a mild diuretic. For prophylaxis, start a few days before ascent. The side effects of tingling in the hands and feet indicate dose reduction. For the headache, ibuprofen is good but may aggravate fluid retention. Many medications have been shown efficacious: nifedipine, steroids, sumatriptan, and others. The author's preference is acetazolamide as it is simple, safe, inexpensive, and effective. Avoidance of sleeping pills at altitude is recommended. Acetazolamide is often effective for the sleep disorder. A caveat: AMS will progress to severe in 2% of cases, and descent is necessary to avoid progression and complications.

High Altitude Pulmonary Edema (HAPE)

This syndrome was first described by Houston in 1960.[43] The hallmark is severe dyspnea, which then progresses to cough with bloody, frothy sputum. The fluid is a transudate. This is acute pulmonary edema, and progression to death may occur in hours. The victim literally drowns in his edema fluid. Similarity to adult respiratory distress syndrome (ARDS) exists. In contrast to congestive heart failure, left ventricular function is normal. Pulmonary hypertension, pulmonary vasoconstriction, and increased capillary permeability occur.

HAPE usually takes 2 to 4 days to develop and is more common at very high altitude and above. It is best treated by *immediate descent.* Diuretics such as furosemide (Lasix) have been recommended; however, mountaineers are often dehydrated and hypotension is a risk. Morphine may be of benefit, but respiratory depression is risked. The treatment of choice may be calcium channel blockade with nifedipine. Doses of 20 mg sublingual followed by 20 mg sustained release have been effective.[44] Prophylaxis with nifedipine may be effective as well.[45] The drug treatment of HAPE requires medical training. Oxygen is beneficial. Recently, pressurized bags for creating a hyperbaric chamber have become available. The victim descends artificially. The Gamov and Certex bags increase ambient air pressure to 140 and 220 mb, equivalent to descent of 1500 m and 2500 m, respectively. These bags are effective and potentially life saving. They are particularly appropriate for application by nonmedical personnel. They are, however, expensive and not readily available to most climbers.[46] The incidence of HAPE ranges from 0.5% to 15%.[47] Often neurologic symptoms are present, and progression from severe AMS occurs.

High Altitude Cerebral Edema (HACE)

High altitude cerebral edema is less common but more likely to be fatal. Without prompt descent, the mortality rate is approximately 50%.[48] Altitude exposure above 12,000 ft is usually required. Usually 2 or 3 days pass prior to onset. The syndrome was first described by Houston and Dickinson in 1975.[49] This is a dramatic neurologic syndrome. Very severe headache progresses to ataxia, decreased cognitive ability, hallucinations, stupor, coma, and death. A generalized encephalopathy develops with cerebral edema. Progression from severe AMS is seen in 1.8% of cases.[41] HACE may occur suddenly without warning at extreme altitude to well-acclimatized, experienced, and fit mountaineers. The pathologic findings include diffuse edema with petechia and hemorrhages. Papilledema is present. Systemic hypoxemia from altitude, HAPE, or progression of intracranial pressure produces cerebral hypoxia leading to death. Treatment is descent. Oxygen and maintenance of an upright position help. Hyperbaric chambers and bags may be life saving. Steroids such as dexamethasone (Decadron) 12 mg or beta-methasone 4 mg every 6 hours are beneficial. Acetazolamide (Diamox) 500 mg every 6 hours benefits. Of course, comatose patients require intravenous routes for drugs.

Other High Altitude Problems

High altitude cachexia (HAC) is seen as a result of exposure to extreme altitude. Weight loss, muscle wasting, and loss of vigor are seen. As much as 25% of body weight may be lost on a single expedition.[50] From the increased ultraviolet ray exposure, snow blindness and severe sunburn occur. Thromboembolic phenomena are associated with high hemoglobin levels and increased blood viscosity. Thrombophlebitis and pulmonary emboli have occurred. High altitude retinal hemorrhage (HARH), although seen frequently, is usually benign. Rare, small scotomas occur.

SAFETY AND EQUIPMENT

Safety has been a concern of mountaineers for generations. Falls due to equipment failure occur rarely. They are most likely to occur as a result of improper use of equipment. "Equipment in 1980 will not fail," said Phil Ershler, head guide on Mount Rainier and a Mount Everest summit climber. This is true today. Sophisticated climbing equipment is readily available. The neophyte may easily buy equipment that enables climbing beyond a beginner's ability. This risk is only remedied by training and experience.

An important safety item is the helmet. Rather than describe the multiple choices available, the reader is referred to equipment sales personnel and knowledgeable climbers. A good rule is, "If you have a $20 head, get a $20 helmet!" It is equally important to wear a helmet when climbing as when riding a bicycle or motorcycle.

Perhaps the greatest safety factor is the climber's attitude. More and more difficult routes are being climbed. Climbing to extreme altitude without supplemental oxygen is becoming common and is considered "by fair means." All 14 peaks of 8000 m have been climbed without supplemental oxygen, "solo," and alpine-style. Winter routes are becoming more common. I join with those who applaud these accomplishments, but risk is increased. I would propose an ethic be accepted:

1. Give up the objective, the summit, when safety must be sacrificed.
2. The mountaineer is responsible for himself as well as for the members of the climbing party. All must return safely.
3. There must be a willingness to give up the summit to assist others in need.
4. It is irresponsible to put oneself for sport intentionally into a dangerous situation that risks the lives of rescuers.

CONCLUSION

The sport of mountaineering has inherent risk. Of particular importance is head and spine injury, the major cause of mortality and morbidity. Prevention is more effective than treatment, and the best results are achieved through education of mountaineers. The environment, altitude in particular, is an injury multiplier—its effects must be minimized. This is best done through education and training.

References

1. Field manual (FM) 100–5, United States Department of the Army (USDA), 1996.
2. Williamson JE. Accidents in North American Mountaineering, 7;2:50. Golden, CO, American Alpine Club, 1997.
3. Hartley AK. Accidents and Rescue. Alpine J 1976;75:265–267.
4. McLennan JG, Ungersman J. Mountaineering Accidents in the Sierra Nevada. Am J Sports Med, 1983;2:160–163.
5. Houston CS. Altitude Illness. Emerg Med Clin North Am 1984;2:503–512.
6. Coburn B. Everest, Mountain Without Mercy. Washington, DC, National Geographic Society, MacGillivray Freeman Films, 1997, p 248.
7. Unsworth W. Everest, A Mountaineering History, appendix 4–5. Boston, Houghton Mifflin Co., 1981.
8. Wilson R. Death among climbers on Mt. McKinley and Mt. Foraker. Jpn J Mount Med 1983;3:1–16.
9. Mills WL, Gower R, Hackett PH, et al. Cold Injury, Dehydration and Multiple System Trauma. In Sutton JR, Houston CS, Coates G (eds): Hypoxia and Cold. New York, Praeger, 1986, pp 360–362.
10. Schussman LC, Lutz LJ. Mountaineering and rock climbing accidents. Phys Sportsmed 1982;10:52–61.
11. Hixson EG, Casey JC, Foster C. Winter Sportsmedicine. F. A. Davis Co., Philadelphia, 1990, p. 325.
12. Town J. Death and the art of database maintenance. Mountain 1986;10:42–45.

13. Sutton JR, Houston CS, Coates G. Hypoxia and Cold. New York, Praeger, 1986.
14. Hackett PH, Roach RC, Sutton JR. High Altitude Medicine. *In* Auerbach PS, Gehr EC (eds): Management of Wilderness and Environmental Emergencies. St. Louis, CV Mosby, 1989, p 3.
15. Malacrida RL, Anselmi LC, Genoni M, et al. Helicopter mountain rescue of patients with head injury and/or multiple injuries in southern Switzerland, 1980–1990. Injury 1993;24:451–453.
16. National Association for Search and Rescue (NASAR), P.O. Box 3709, Fairfax, VA.
17. Mountain Rescue Association, Inc., 200 Union Blvd., Suite 430–1355, Denver, CO 80220.
17a. American Alpine Club, 710 10th St., Suite 100, Golden, CO 80401 (a list is provided yearly of organizations by state in Accidents in North American Mountaineering).
18. Advanced Trauma Life Support. Chicago, American College of Surgeons, 1993, 161.
19. Reid WA, Doyle D, Richmond HG, et al. Necropsy study of mountaineering accidents in Scotland. J Clin Pathol, 1986;39:1217–1220.
20. Zwienenberg M, Muizelaar P. Injuries to the central nervous system. Sci Am Surgery, 1999;IV:2.
21. Brendel W, Weingart JR, Haas LR. Medical Statement Analysis of 3,200 High Altitude Climbers. *In* Rivolier J, Ceretelli P, Foray J, Segantini P (eds): High Altitude Deterioration. Basel, Karger, 1997, pp 180–189.
22. Messner R. All 14 Eight-Thousanders. Seattle, Cloudcap, 1988, Appendix.
23. West JB, Lahiri S. Barometric pressure of extreme altitudes on Mt. Everest. J Appl Physiol 1983;54:166–194.
24. Houston CS. Going Higher—The Story of Man and Altitude. Boston, Little, Brown and Co., 1987, pp 58–61.
25. Houston CS. Trekking at high altitudes: How safe is it for your patients? Postgrad Med 1990;88:56–69.
26. Sutton JR, Reeves JT, Wagner PD, et al. Operation Everest II: Oxygen transport during exercise at extreme simulated altitude. J Appl Physiol 1988;64:1309–1321.
27. Baumgartner W, Bartsch P, Maggrini M, et al. Enhanced cerebral blood flow in acute mountain sickness. Aviat Space Environ Med 1994;65:726–729.
28. Nelson M. Physiologic testing at high altitudes. Aviat Space Environ Med 1982;53:122–126.
29. Flynn CF, Thompson TL. Effects of acute increases in altitude on mental status. Psychosomatics 1990;31:146–152.
30. Vavaletti G, Tredici G. Long lasting neurophysiologic changes after a single high altitude climb. Acta Neurol Scand 1993;87:103–105.
31. Hamilton AJ, Trad LA, Cymerman A. Alterations in human upper extremity function during exposure to extreme altitude. Aviat Space Environ Med 1991;62:759–764.
32. Garrido E, Costello A, Ventura JL, et al. Cortical atrophy and other brain magnetic resonance imaging changes after extremely high altitude climbs without oxygen. Int J Sports Med 1991;62:729–764.
33. Regard M, Landis T, Casey J, et al. Cognitive changes of high altitude in healthy climbers and in climbers developing acute mountain sickness. Aviat Space Environ Med 1991;62:291–295.
34. Clark CF, Heaton RK, Weins A. Neuropsychological functioning after prolonged high altitude exposure in mountaineering. Aviat Space Environ Med 1983;541:202.
35. Hornbein TF, Townes BD, Schoene RB, et al. The cost to the central nervous system of climbing to extremely high altitude. N Engl J Med 1989;321:1714–1719.
36. Jason GW, Pajurkova EM, Lee RG. High altitude mountaineering and brain function. Aviat Space Environ Med 1989;60:170–173.
37. Kennedy RS, Dunlap WP, Bandacet LE, et al. Cognitive performance deficits in a simulated climb of Mt. Everest—Operation Everest II. Aviat Space Environ Med 1989;60:99–104.
38. Rigard M, Oelz O, Bruggar P, et al. Persistent cognitive impairment in climbers after repeated exposure to extreme altitude. Neurology 1989;39:210–213.
39. Townes BD, Hornbein TF, Schoene PD, et al. Human Cerebral Function at Extreme Altitude. *In* West JB, Lahari S (eds): High Altitude and Man. Bethesda, MD, American Physiologic Society, 1984, pp 31–36.
40. Scharma A, Scharma PD, Malhotra HS, et al. Hemiplegia as a manifestation of acute mountain sickness. J Assoc Physicians India 1990;38:662–663.
41. Hackett PH, et al. The incidence, importance and prophylaxis of acute mountain sickness. Lancet 1976;2:1149–1155.
42. Foulke G. Altitude related illness. J Exp Med 1985;3:217–276.
43. Houston CS. Acute pulmonary edema of high altitude. N Engl J Med 1960;260:478–480.
44. Oelz O. A case of high altitude pulmonary edema treated with nifedipine. JAMA 1987;287:780.
45. Bartsch P, Maggiorini M, Ritter M, et al. Prevention of high altitude pulmonary edema with nifedipine. N Engl J Med 1991;325:1284–1289.
46. Bartsch P. Treatment of high altitude diseases without drugs. Int J Sports Med 1992;13:51.
47. Schoene RB. Pulmonary edema at high altitude. Review, pathophysiology, and update. Clin Chest Med 1985;6:491–507.
48. Lobenhuffer HP, Zinc RA, Brendel W. High Altitude Cerebral Edema: Analysis of 166 Cases. *In* Brendel W, Zinc RA (eds): High Altitude Physiology and Medicine. New York, Springer Verlag, 1982, pp 219–231.
49. Houston CS, Dickinson J. Cerebral form of high altitude illness. Lancet 1975;2:758.
50. Hixson EG. Mountain Climbing. *In* Jordan BD, Tsairis P, Warren RF (eds): Sports Neurology. Philadelphia, Lippincott Raven, 1998.

33

Head and Spine Injuries in Boxing

Barry D. Jordan

Neurologic injuries in boxing represent a major medical concern of modern-day society. Brain injuries can occur acutely or as a delayed consequence of the sport. Acute traumatic brain injury (ATBI) typically is manifested as a cerebral concussion and is rarely associated with significant morbidity or mortality. Chronic traumatic brain injury (CTBI) is defined as the delayed and cumulative neurologic consequences of repeated concussive and subconcussive blows to the head and typically occurs after the cessation of a long professional boxing career. Cervical spine injuries are extremely rare in boxing, but nonetheless should be considered in any boxer who is acutely rendered unconscious. This chapter discusses the medical aspects of brain and cervical spine injuries encountered in boxing.

ACUTE TRAUMATIC BRAIN INJURY

ATBI represents the immediate neurologic consequences of a blow to the head and ranges in severity from a concussion to more catastrophic focal brain injury. The knock-out (KO) in boxing is synonymous with a cerebral concussion and is the most common acute neurologic injury in boxing. Focal brain injuries encountered in boxing can include subdural hematoma, epidural hematoma, intracerebral hematoma, and cerebral contusion.

Epidemiology

Studies analyzing the frequency of ATBI in amateur boxing indicate that permanent and irreversible neurologic dysfunction rarely occurs. Blonstein and Clarke[1] assessed boxing injuries in amateur boxers over a 7-month period and found that only 29 boxers (0.58%) were severely concussed or knocked out more than once. Twenty-three boxers were knocked out twice, and six were severely concussed once. Injury reports of 1981 and 1982 USA National Amateur Boxing championships noted that 48 of 547 bouts (8.7%) were stopped because of KOs or blows to the head.[2] This yielded a rate of 4.38 head injuries per 100 personal exposures, or 8.7 head injuries per 100 bouts. Larson and colleagues[3] reported acute head injuries in the 1950 and 1951 Swedish junior championships and the 1951 Swedish championship and found that 35 of 75 boxers were knocked down; 14 of these were KOs. Jordan and coworkers[4] reviewed all boxing injuries sustained by amateur boxers at the United States Olympic Training Center (USOTC) during a 10-year period. Among the total of 477 injuries, only 29 (6.5%) were brain injuries. Although the severity was difficult to ascertain, 26 out of 28 concussions were described as being mild. This lower injury rate was probably a reflection of a low injury rate associated with sparring and training. In another survey of amateur boxers in Denmark, 5.7% to 7.8% of boxing competitions resulted in a KO, and 0.8% to 5.4% of the bouts were terminated because the referee stopped the contest secondary to head blows (RSCH).[5] In a prospective study of 147 amateur boxers in Ireland during a 5-month period, Porter and O'Brien[6] reported 33 mild cerebral concussions in 281 bouts, which yields a rate of 5.87 concussions per 100 personal exposures, or 11.7 concussions per 100 bouts. Among these concussions, 82% resolved within 2 minutes.

Studies of acute boxing injuries among U.S. military personnel indicate that serious ATBI is an infrequent occurrence. Welch and colleagues[7] conducted a survey of boxing injuries that occurred during an institutional boxing program at the U.S. Military Academy (USMA) in West Point, New York, over a 2-year period. Although approximately 2100 cadets received boxing instruction, only 22 cases of blunt head trauma were reported, none of which resulted in neurologic deficits. In another study, assessing amateur boxing injuries among military personnel, Enzenauer and coworkers[8] retrospectively reviewed all hospitalizations for boxing-related injuries in U.S. Army hospitals for a 6-year period from 1980 through 1985. During this period of observation, there were 401 admissions for boxing-related injuries. Among these injuries, head injuries comprised 68% of all injuries. However, the exact number of brain injuries within this group is indeterminate because all head injuries were broadly lumped together. Ross and Ochsner[9] in a survey of the instructional boxing program in U.S. Marine Corps basic training during an 8-year period observed 1100 boxing-related injuries among approximately 180,000 participants. During this period there were only three serious acute brain injuries.

Among professional boxers in New York state from 1952 to 1958, McCown[10] reported 325 KOs and 789 technical knockouts (TKOs) among 11,173 participants. Of the 325 boxers with KOs, 10 required hospitalization. Jordan and Campbell[11] reviewed all acute boxing injuries among professional boxers in New York state from August 1982 through July 1984. During this 2-year period, there were 3110 rounds fought and 376 injuries, of which 262 were head injuries. This yielded a frequency of 0.8 head injuries per 10 rounds fought, and 2.9 head injuries for 10 boxers. In a survey of a representative sample of active professional boxers in New York state, the prevalence of a self-reported TKO or KO was 42% (143 boxers).[12] Also observed in New York state was a tendency for TKOs or KOs to occur in the earlier rounds. In 1 year, 122 of 189 bouts (65%) resulted in a TKO or a KO, and 80% of these occurred within the first three rounds.[13]

Fatalities in the ring are uncommon in both amateur and professional boxing. Worldwide figures indicate that from 1945 through 1979 there were 335 deaths in amateur and professional boxing.[14] This is approximately between 9 and 10 deaths per year. Of the fatalities reported between 1918 and June 1983, approximately one third, 190, were among amateurs.[15] Among military personnel who boxed worldwide during a 6-year period, only one death was reported.[8]

Well-documented risk factors for ATBI in boxing derived from large well-defined boxing populations are limited. Welch and colleagues[7] observed that acute injury rates tended to be higher during competition than during sparring. However, the absolute number of acute boxing injuries tended to be higher during sparring instruction.[7] This finding was a reflection of more exposure to sparring and instruction than to competition. Although risk factors for ATBI are poorly delineated, several clinical situations may predispose a boxer to an increased risk of acute neurologic injury. The poorly conditioned athlete who does not adequately train prior to a competition is at increased risk of injury. Any boxer who enters the ring needs to be well conditioned and strong. Accordingly, any medical condition (e.g., flu, fever, malaise) can have detrimental effects on a boxer's performance. Another important but often neglected fact that may increase a boxer's risk of acute injury in the ring is rapid and extreme weight loss prior to a boxing competition. Boxers who lose several pounds within 24 hours of a bout are at increased risk of injury because these boxers tend to be dehydrated. Dehydration before a competition can reduce alertness and reaction time, thus making a boxer more susceptible to the offensive attack of the opponent. Whether dehydration physiologically increased the risk of a concussion has not been scientifically demonstrated.

Clinical Presentation

Sercl and Jaros[16] analyzed the acute neurologic findings in 427 boxers involved in 1165 matches. Three hundred thirty-six boxers (79%) had clinical abnormalities that resolved within several minutes, and 91 (21%) had neurologic symptoms lasting up to 24 hours. The most common clinical finding was derangement of muscular tone (380 cases), followed by cerebellar and vestibular signs (319 cases) and pyramidal symptoms (253 cases). Other findings included unconsciousness (112 cases), extrapyramidal signs (191 cases), and general muscular weakness (142 cases). Cranial nerve lesions were exceedingly rare (7 cases).

Amnesia is not an infrequent consequence of acute brain injury in boxing. Characteristic of many knockouts seems to be an amnestic period with confusion,[3] but amnesia can occur without a KO and should be regarded as evidence of serious injury.[17] Blonstein and Clarke[1] described a boxer who won a decision but was amnesic for the entire fight despite not being knocked out. Both retrograde and anterograde amnesia have been described in boxing.[18]

A boxer may also experience a postconcussion syndrome after a bout. Critchley[18] described this as the "groggy state." Usually a boxer experiences transient nonspecific symptoms such as a headache, dizziness, imbalance, irritability, fatigue, poor memory, and dysarthria that usually passes, and he returns to his status quo. Nevertheless, Critchley[18] suggested that accumulation of groggy states may predispose a boxer to chronic brain injury.

More recently, the second impact syndrome (SIS) has been described in boxers.[19] The SIS represents an exaggerated, commonly fatal response to a second concussion while an athlete is symptomatic from an earlier concussion. In boxing, the SIS may occur in a tournament setting, where a boxer competes more than once over a selected period (typically a few days to a week), or it can occur less frequently within a given bout associated with multiple concussive blows.[19] The pathophysiologic mechanism of SIS appears to be loss of vasomotor autoregulation leading to massive brain swelling and malignant edema.

Pathology

The concussion represents the most common ATBI encountered in boxing and typically is not associated with gross neuropathologic abnormalities. Although uncommon, acute pathologic lesions such as diffuse axonal injury, subdural hematoma, epidural hematoma, cerebral contusion, intracerebral hemorrhage, injury to the carotid, and subarachnoid hemorrhage may be encountered in boxers.[20, 21] Among these injuries the acute subdural hematoma is most commonly associated with death in the ring.

Evaluation and Management

The clinical diagnosis of ATBI in boxing that is exemplified by obvious loss of motor tone or loss of consciousness is typically not difficult to discern. The boxer who falls to the canvas after sustaining a blow to the head should be considered to have experienced a concussion until proven otherwise. Concussions that are associated with cognitive impairment without loss of motor tone or consciousness may be more difficult to diagnose; in that instance diagnosis is dependent upon the boxer disclosing amnesia and other concussive symptoms.

The initial neurologic evaluation of the boxer who has sustained an ATBI is typically performed after the termination of the bout or between rounds during a bout. In the awake and alert boxer suspected of experiencing a mild concussion, a brief mental status examination should be performed to rule out cognitive impairment. In addition, the boxer should be questioned regarding concussive symptoms and any physical complaints. If the boxer exhibits prolonged loss of consciousness, a focal neurologic deficit, or seizures, then immediate medical care should be instituted at ringside, and the boxer should be prepared for transport to a medical facility close to the arena. Ideally, an ambulance should be present at all boxing matches to ensure prompt emergency transportation, and the medical facility should have emergency neuroradiologic and neurosurgical services readily available.

Any boxer experiencing a concussion should be medically suspended and undergo a mandatory rest period from contact boxing (i.e., sparring, exhibitions, or competitive bouts). The duration of the medical suspension and rest period depends on the severity of the neurologic injury. Medical reinstatement should be conditional on the athlete's fulfillment of the mandatory rest requirement and a normal neurologic evaluation. The neurologic evaluation, at minimum, should include a neurologic examination. Whether further neurodiagnostic procedures are utilized is at the discretion of the ringside physician or the regulations and rules of the governing body. Any boxer who acquires a structural lesion should be permanently suspended from boxing and contact sports, regardless of the level of recovery.

The role of neurodiagnostic testing in the evaluation of ATBI is determined by the severity of the injury. Since the overwhelming majority of acute brain injuries in boxing are transient, short-lived, and resolve spontaneously, neuroimaging is seldom indicated. However, in those boxers suspected of experiencing a focal brain injury or a significant concussion (i.e., loss of consciousness or prolonged postconcussion syndrome), magnetic resonance imaging (MRI) or computed tomography (CT) may be indicated. In the acute setting, the CT scan can be performed to rule out intracranial mass lesions. However, in the less acute or elective situation, MRI represents the neuroradiologic test of choice in identifying intracranial pathology such as small SDH, cerebral contusions, and white matter abnormalities.[22] In selected situations, single photon emission computed tomography (SPECT) may identify perfusion deficits primarily localized to the frontal or temporal lobes.[23] Although electroencephalography (EEG) has been commonly utilized as a screening test for the medical licensing of professional boxers, its value in the evaluation of ATBI is debatable. Kaplan and Browder[24] failed to demonstrate any EEG changes from among professional boxers within 10 minutes of losing a bout. Similar findings have also been noted among amateur boxers undergoing pre- and post-bout EEG.[25]

Neuropsychological testing has a role in the neurologic evaluation of ATBI when a preinjury baseline has been established. Boxers who sustain concussions can undergo repeat neuropsychological testing to determine if they have recovered and returned to their baselines. Utilizing pre- and postbout neuropsychological testing, Heilbronner and coworkers[26] demonstrated only minor changes in cognitive function in amateur boxers tested 30–45 minutes after a contest. Impairments were noted in the areas of verbal and incidental memory. Matser and colleagues,[27] also utilizing pre- and postbout neuropsychological testing, demonstrated impairments in planning, attention, and memory among amateur boxers tested after a boxing match.

CHRONIC TRAUMATIC BRAIN INJURY

CTBI, also known as dementia pugilistica, chronic traumatic encephalopathy, chronic neurologic injury, or the "punch drunk" syndrome, represents the long-term cumulative neurologic consequences of repetitive concussive and subconcussive blows to the head. Traditionally, this syndrome has been described primarily in boxers; however, it may be anticipated in other sports such as American football, ice hockey, and perhaps soccer. This syndrome was first described in the medical literature by Martland[28] in 1928, when he described a 38-year-old retired boxer with advanced parkinsonism, ataxia, pyramidal tract dysfunction, and behavioral changes.

Epidemiology

Roberts[29] conducted a comprehensive study of the epidemiologic aspect of CTBI. He randomly sampled 250 of 16,781 ex-professional boxers who were licensed by the British Board of Control for at least 3 years from 1929 through 1955. Among the 250 boxers, 224 were examined and 26 were excluded on the basis of death, emigration, or refusal. Thirty-seven boxers (17%) had clinical evidence of central nervous system lesions attributable to boxing. Roberts concluded that the prevalence of lesions increased when exposure to boxing increased. Putative and established risk factors for CTBI are presented in Table 33–1. Documented risk factors for CTBI in boxing include later retirement (i.e., over 28 years of age), increased duration of career (i.e., more than 10 years), and a greater number of bouts (i.e., more than 150 bouts).[29] Clinical studies suggest that risk factors for the development of CTBI include poor performance (i.e., second- or third-rate boxers), boxing style (i.e., being a slugger, rather than a scientific, intelligent boxer), being a boxer who is notorious for the ability to "take" a punch, and being a professional boxer as opposed to amateur.[18] The age at examina-

Table 33–1. Putative and Documented Risk Factors for Chronic Traumatic Brain Injury

Total number of fights
Number of knockouts experienced
Number of losses
Duration of boxing career
Fight frequency
Age of retirement from boxing
Sparring exposure
Poor performance or skills

tion also influenced the prevalence of CTBI. Boxers who were examined after the age of 50 had a higher prevalence of CTBI than those examined before that age of 50.[29] A 1996 study implies that increasing sparring exposure may increase the risk of neurocognitive decline among professional boxers.[30] A history of a TKO or a KO has also been reported to be associated with an abnormal CT scan of the brain.[12] In addition, progressive changes on CT scans have been noted in boxers who lose more than 10 bouts.[31]

Clinical Presentation

In a comprehensive review of the neuropsychiatric aspects of boxing, Mendez[32] classified the clinical manifestations of CTBI into motor, cognitive, and psychiatric symptoms. Early signs of CTBI may include dysarthria, mild incoordination, tremor, and decreased complex attention. Psychiatric symptoms may include emotional lability and other mild behavioral disturbances such as euphoria or hypomania and increased irritability. Although it has been observed that the initial manifestations of CTBI are predominantly psychiatric or behavioral in nature,[33] it is the experience of the author that the behavioral and personality disturbances may be difficult to assess early in the disease. This is particularly the case when the examiner lacks knowledge of the boxer's premorbid personality. The second or moderate stage of CTBI is characterized by a progression of the motor, cognitive, or behavioral symptoms.[32] Affected boxers exhibit signs of parkinsonism or progressive difficulty in coordination and ambulation. Cognitive deficits include mild deficits in memory, attention, and executive function. Psychiatric manifestations may include inappropriate behavior, morbid jealousy, paranoia, and violent outbursts. The third or severe stage of CTBI is often referred to as dementia pugilistica.[32] During this phase of the disorder, the boxer exhibits significant motor dysfunction characterized by prominent pyramidal, extrapyramidal, or cerebellar symptoms. Cognitive dysfunction as evidenced by amnesia, executive-frontal lobe dysfunction, and psychomotor retardation may be observed. Behaviorally, boxers may exhibit disinhibition, violent outbursts, hypersexuality, and psychosis.[32]

Pathology

Corsellis and coworkers[34, 35] described four types of central nervous system changes among 15 former boxers: septal and hypothalamic anomalies, cerebellar changes, degeneration of the substantia nigra, and regional occurrence of Alzheimer's neurofibrillary tangles (NFTs). Twelve cases demonstrated a fenestrated septal cavum, and frequently the floor of the hypothalamus appeared to be stretched while the fornix and mammillary bodies were atrophied. The cerebellum was notable for scarring of the folia in the region of the cerebellar tonsils, and there was a reduction in the number of Purkinje cells on the inferior surface of the cerebellum. Neurofibrillary tangles primarily involved parts of the hippocampus and the medial temporal gray matter. The neurofibrillary changes in the limbic gray matter were not accompanied by senile plaques. The substantia nigra tended to lack pigment, and nerve cells became gliosed.

Roberts and colleagues,[36] utilizing immunocytochemical methods and an antibody raised to the beta-protein present in Alzheimer's disease (AD) plaques, found that retired boxers with dementia pugilistica and substantial neurofibrillary tangles (NFTs) showed evidence of extensive beta-protein immunoreactive deposits (plaques). These "diffuse" plaques were not visible with Congo red or standard silver stains. Because the degree of beta-protein deposition was comparable to that seen in AD, it was postulated that in dementia pugilistica the pathogenic mechanism of tangle and plaque formation may be similar to that of AD. Support for this hypothesis was provided by Tokuda and coworkers[37] when these investigators demonstrated tau immunoreactive NFTs and beta-protein immunoreactive senile plaques in boxers exhibiting dementia.

Another important neuropathologic observation has been the presence of ubiquitin in the NFTs in the brains of boxers with dementia and patients with AD.[38] Ubiquitin, which has been identified as a component of NFTs in AD, is thought to be a protein involved in the ATP-dependent non-lysosomal degradation of abnormal proteins. It has been speculated that dementia may result from the dysfunction of cells bearing ubiquitin tangles. Among 16 boxers studied in this investigation, 11 exhibited dementia. Among the 11 boxers with dementia, 9 had evidence of ubiquitin immunoreactivity in the NFTs. None of the five boxers without dementia demonstrated staining of the neurofibrillary tangles with antiubiquitin.

Uhl and coworkers[39] also presented evidence documenting similarities between CTBI and AD. These investigators conducted a pathologic and neurochemical examination of the brain of a 51-year-old former boxer with well-documented dementia pugilistica. In addition to documenting NFTs in the cortex and the nucleus basalis of Meynert (nbM), they noted a significant reduction of choline acetyltransferase activity in the nbM and in several regions of the cerebral cortex. These findings are similar to those noted in AD.

The pathophysiology of CTBI is unknown; however, in view of the similarities between CTBI and AD, the potential role of amyloid deposition and apolipoprotein E (APOE) genotype in the development of CTBI needs to be explored. Evidence suggests that the presence of APOE e4 allele may promote the deposition of cerebral amyloid in individuals experiencing traumatic brain injury.[40] Mayeaux and colleagues[41] noted a 10-fold synergistic increased risk of AD in individuals with traumatic brain injury and the presence of APOE e4, whereas an additive increased risk of AD in patients with head trauma and APOE e4 was observed by Katzman and others.[42] Based on our observation of extensive parenchymal cerebral amyloid deposition and cerebral amyloid angiopathy in a demented boxer who harbored an APOE e4 allele,[43] we conducted a study to determine whether APOE e4 is associated with CTBI.[44] In an analysis of 30 active and retired boxers, we found that APOE e4 was associated with an increased severity of CTBI in high-exposure boxers (i.e., boxers with more than 12 professional bouts). This finding suggests that there may be a genetic predisposition to the untoward effects of a long boxing career.[44]

Evaluation and Management

Any boxer suspected of exhibiting CTBI should undergo detailed neurologic testing. This should include a complete neurologic examination including a mental status examination. In addition the boxer should have MRI or a CT scan performed. MRI or CT findings in CTBI are typically nonspe-

cific and may be normal or demonstrate brain atrophy with or without a cavum septum pellucidum.[12, 22, 31, 45–51] Boxers experiencing cognitive impairment should undergo a dementia screen, which should include a complete blood cell count, routine blood chemistries, thyroid function tests, vitamin B_{12} test, and VDRL.

There is a paucity of effective treatment protocols for CTBI, and pharmacologic intervention is largely empiric. Boxers exhibiting parkinsonism that interferes with daily functioning should be treated with levodopa-carbidopa (Sinemet) or other antiparkinsonism medications. Whether a neuroprotective agent such as selegiline is effective in limiting neurodegeneration in CTBI remains to be determined. The treatment of cognitive impairment associated with CTBI is speculative. In view of the many neuropathologic similarities between CTBI and AD, empiric treatment with an anticholinesterase inhibitor (e.g., tacrine or donepezil) may be a reasonable approach. However, the effectiveness of this treatment has not been established. The behavioral and psychiatric disturbances associated with CTBI should be managed with accepted antidepressants, neuroleptics, anxiolytics, or other psychopharmacologic agents when indicated.

CERVICAL SPINE INJURY

Cervical spine injuries are rare in boxing. Strano and Marias[52] reported a fracture in the anterior arch of the atlas in a 27-year-old amateur boxer who presented with persistent occipital headaches. Although the exact mechanism of this fracture was uncertain, the investigators speculated that a direct blow to the head with the neck hyperextended (when the odontoid lies against the anterior arch of the atlas) may deliver sufficient force to fracture the anterior arch of the atlas. Kewalramani and Krauss[53] reported a case of quadriplegia secondary to a C6 vertebral body fracture in a boxer, but did not comment on the mechanism or circumstances of the injury. Jordan and colleagues[54] encountered a stable unilateral fracture of the lamina of C3 in a professional boxer who struck his neck on the bottom rope of the ring while falling to the canvas. The onset of a cervical radiculopathy during a competitive bout has also been reported in two amateur boxers.[55] Place and coworkers[56] described a boxer who sustained a transient spinal cord injury secondary to an os odontoideum that required spinal fusion.

Acute cervical spine injuries should be managed cautiously and expeditiously. If a cervical spine injury is suspected, the neck should be immobilized immediately with a cervical collar or spineboard. If respirations have ceased, an airway should be established and ventilation initiated. The boxer should then be transported by ambulance to the hospital, where appropriate radiologic studies can be conducted. The treatment and further management of cervical spine injuries are dependent on the type and severity of the injury.

CONCLUSION

Neurologic injury is an unfortunate and inherent consequence of boxing. Catastrophic ATBI is a rare occurrence in amateur and professional boxing, and most acute brain injuries tend to be transient and self-limited. However, the cumulative effect of repeated concussive and subconcussive blows to the head culminating in chronic neurologic impairment is of paramount medical concern. Accordingly, medical supervision and regulation of the sport are requisite. The prevention of CTBI will require limiting the exposure of boxers, serial neurologic examinations with the assistance of prospective neuropsychological testing, and the utilization of advanced neuroradiologic techniques. Furthermore, the surveillance of medical injuries and sparring practices is also warranted. Increasing medical awareness and safety in the sport of boxing as opposed to banning the sport represents the more practical approach.

References

1. Blonstein JL, Clarke E. Further observations on the medical aspects of amateur boxing. BMJ 1957;1:362–364.
2. Estwanik JJ, Boitano M, Ari N. Amateur boxing injuries at the 1981 and 1982 USA/ABF national championships. Phys Sportsmed 1984;12:123–128.
3. Larson LW, Melin KA, Nordstrom-Ohrberg G, et al. Acute head injuries in boxers. Acta Psychiatr Neurol Scand 1954;95(Suppl):1–42.
4. Jordan BD, Voy RO, Stone J. Amateur boxing injuries at the United States Olympic Training Center. Phys Sportsmed 1990;18:80–90.
5. Schmidt-Olsen S, Jensen SK, Mortensen V. Amateur boxing in Denmark: The effect of some preventive measures. Am J Sports Med 1990;18:98–100.
6. Porter M, O'Brien M. Incidence and severity of injuries resulting from amateur boxing in Finland. Clin J Sport Med 1996;6:97–101.
7. Welch MJ, Sitler M, Kroeten H. Boxing injuries from an instructional program. Phys Sportsmed 1986;14:81–89.
8. Enzenauer RW, Montrey JS, Enzenauer RJ, et al. Boxing related injuries in the US Army, 1980 through 1985. JAMA 1989;261:1463–1466.
9. Ross RT, Ochsner MG, Jr. Acute intracranial boxing-related injuries in U.S. Marine Corps recruits: Report of two cases. Mil Med 1999;164:68–70.
10. McCown LA. Boxing injuries. Am J Surg 1959;98:509–516.
11. Jordan BD, Campbell E. Acute boxing injuries among professional boxers in New York state: A two-year survey. Phys Sportsmed 1988;16:87–91.
12. Jordan BD, Jahre C, Hauser WA, et al. CT of 338 active professional boxers. Radiology 1992;185:509–512.
13. Jordan BD. Professional Boxing: Experience of the New York State Athletic Commission. *In* Cantu RC (ed): Boxing and Medicine. Champaign, IL, Human Kinetics 1995, pp 177–185.
14. Moore M. The challenge of boxing: Bringing safety into the ring. Phys Sportsmed 1980;8:101–105.
15. Ryan AJ. Eliminate boxing gloves. Phys Sportsmed 1983;11:49.
16. Sercl M, Jaros O. The mechanisms of cerebral concussion in boxing and their consequences. Work Neurol 1962;3:351–357.
17. McCunney RJ, Russo PK. Brain injuries in boxers. Phys Sportsmed 1984;12:53–67.
18. Critchley M. Medical aspects of boxing, particularly from a neurological standpoint. BMJ 1957;1:357–362.
19. Cantu RC, Voy R. Second impact syndrome: A risk in any sport. Phys Sportsmed 1995;23:27–34.
20. Lampert PW, Hardman JM. Morphological changes in brains of boxers. JAMA 1984;251:2676–2679.
21. Unterharnsheidt F. About boxing: Review of historical and medical aspects. Tex Rep Biol Med 1970;28:421–495.
22. Jordan BD, Zimmerman RD. Computed tomography, magnetic resonance imaging comparisons in boxers. JAMA 1990;263:1670–1674.
23. Jordan BD, Dane SH, Rowan AJ, et al. SPECT in professional boxers. J Neuroimaging 1999;9:59–60.
24. Kaplan HA, Browder J. Observations on the clinical and brain wave patterns of professional boxers. JAMA 1954;156:1138–1144.
25. Beaussart M, Beaussart-Boulenge L. "Experimental" study of cerebral concussion in 123 amateur boxers, by clinical examination and EEG before and immediately after fights. Electroencephalogr Clin Neurophysiol 1970;29:529–530.
26. Heilbronner RL, Henry GK, Carson-Brewer M. Neuropsychologic test performance in amateur boxers. Am J Sports Med 1991;19:376–379.
27. Matser JT, Kessels AGH, Lezak MD, et al. Acute traumatic brain injury in amateur boxing. Phys Sportsmed 2000;28:87–92.
28. Martland HAS. Punch drunk. JAMA 1928;91:1103–1107.
29. Roberts AH. Brain Damage in Boxers. London, Pitman Publishing, 1969.

30. Jordan BD, Matser E, Zimmerman RD, et al. Sparring and cognitive function in professional boxers. Phys Sportsmed 1996;24:87–98.

31. Jordan BD, Jahre C, Hauser WA. Serial computed tomography in professional boxers. J Neuroimaging 1992;2:181–185.

32. Mendez MF. The neuropsychiatric aspects of boxing. Int J Psychiatry Med 1995;25:249–262.

33. LaCava G. Boxer's encephalopathy. J Sports Med Phys Fitness 1963;3:87–92.

34. Corsellis JAN, Bruton CJ, Freeman-Browne C. The aftermath of boxing. Psychol Med 1973;3:270–303.

35. Corsellis JAN. Posttraumatic dementia in Alzheimer's disease. In Jatzman R, Terry RD, Bick K (eds): Senile dementia and related disorders. New York, Raven Press, 1978, pp 125–133.

36. Roberts GW, Allsop D, Bruton C. The occult aftermath of boxing. J Neurol Neurosurg Psychiatry 1990;53:373–378.

37. Tokuda T, Ikeda S, Yanugesa N, et al. Re-examination of ex-boxer's brain using immunohistochemistry with antibodies to amyloid beta protein and tau protein. Acta Neuropathol (Berl) 1991;82:280–285.

38. Dale GE, Leigh PN, Luthert P, et al. J Neurol Neurosurg Psychiatry 1991;54:116–118.

39. Uhl GR, McKinney M, Hedreen JC, et al. Dementia pugilistica: Loss of basal forebrain cholinergic neurons and cortical cholinergic markers. Ann Neurol 1982;12:99.

40. Nicoll JAR, Roberts GW, Graham DI. Apolipoprotein E epsilon 4 allele is associated with deposition of amyloid beta protein following head injury. Nat Med 1995;1:135–137.

41. Mayeaux R, Ottoman R, Maestre G, et al. Synergistic effects of traumatic head injury and apoliproprotein e4 in patients with Alzheimer's disease. Neurology, 1995;45:555–557.

42. Katzman R, Galosko DR, Saitoh T, et al. Apolipoprotein e4 and head trauma: Synergistic or additive risks? Neurology 1996;46:889–892.

43. Jordan BD, Kanick AB, Horwich MS, et al. Apolipoprotein e4 and fatal cerebral amyloid angiopathy associated with dementia puglistica. Ann Neurol 1995;38:698–699.

44. Jordan BD, Relkin NR, Ravdin LD, et al. Apolipoprotein Ee4 associated with chronic traumatic brain injury in boxing. JAMA 1997;278:136–140.

45. Casson IR, Siegel O, Sham R, et al. Brain damage in modern boxers. JAMA 1984;251:2663–2667.

46. Casson IR, Sham R, Campbell EA, et al. Neurological and CT evaluation of knocked-out boxers. J Neurol Neurosurg Psychiatry 1982;45:170–174.

47. Sironi VA, Scotti G, Ravagnati L, et al. CT scan and EEG findings in professional pugilists: Early detection of cerebral atrophy in young boxers. J Neurosurg Sci 1982;26:165–168.

48. Ross RJ, Cole M, Thompson JS, et al. Boxers—computed tomography, EEG, and neurosurgical evaluation. JAMA 1983;249:211–213.

49. Jordan BD, Zimmerman RD. Magnetic resonance imaging in amateur boxers. Arch Neurol 1988;45:1207–1208.

50. Ross RJ, Casson JR, Siegel O, et al. Boxing injuries: Neurologic, radiologic, and neuropsychologic evaluation. Clin Sports Med 1987;6:41–51.

51. Levin HS, Lippold SC, Goldman A, et al. Neurobehavioral functioning and magnetic resonance imaging findings in young boxers. J Neurosurg 1987;67:657–667.

52. Strano SD, Marias AD. Cervical spine fracture in a boxer—A rare but important sporting injury: A case report. S Afr Med J 1983;73:328–330.

53. Kewalramani LS, Krauss JF. Cervical spine injuries resulting from collision sports. Paraplegia 1981;19:303–312.

54. Jordan BD, Zimmerman RD, Devinsky O, et al. Brain contusion and cervical fracture in a professional boxer. Phys Sportsmed 1988;16:85–88.

55. Jordan BD. Boxing. In Jordan BD, Tsairis P, Warren RF (eds): Sports Neurology, 2nd ed. Philadelphia, Lippincott-Raven, 1998, pp 351–366.

56. Place HM, Ecklund JM, Enzenauer RJ. Cervical spine injury in a boxer: Should mandatory screening be instituted? J Spinal Disord 1996;9:64–67.

34

Neurologic Injury in Motorsports

Stephen E. Olvey

BACKGROUND

Mankind began racing on foot, and through the years this zeal for competition has led to persons racing in virtually any vehicle. The development of the internal combustion engine fueled the Industrial Revolution and led to radical changes in transportation. Man's intrinsic love of adventure and competition culminated in engines being used not merely for transport, but also for racing, first in bicycles, then in boats, cars, and eventually airplanes. All of these motorized vehicles are raced today in both amateur and organized professional events. This chapter deals primarily with automobile racing because it is the most prominent form of motorized sport. In general, the mechanisms of injury and prevention techniques found in automobile racing are shared by all other varieties of motorsports.

The first recorded automobile race took place in France on July 22, 1894, as the participants traveled 79 miles from Paris to Rouen.[2] Early races were held on public roads. Danger was a prominent feature of these events, shared equally by participants and bystanders. Prize money was posted, and competitors were always ready to risk their lives for the purse. Using public roads often meant dealing with oncoming traffic. Guardrails were nonexistent, and there were no observers or safety personnel. Deaths and injuries were numerous, usually the result of severe burns or massive head and neck injuries.

Public concern and practical considerations moved races onto closed, purpose-built courses in the early 1900s. One of the first and most successful of these was the Indianapolis Motor Speedway, built in 1909. The first Indianapolis 500 Mile Race was held in 1911. Financially, it was an unqualified success, with over 80,000 spectators; racing had become "big business." However, nine of those spectators and two of the drivers were fatally injured. By the end of the 1990s, automobile racing had come to rank second only to soccer in worldwide spectator appeal.

The move to closed courses with walls, fences, and proper grandstands improved the plight of the spectator, but did little to benefit the racing driver. Throughout the decades from 1900 through 1975, automobile racing ranked second only to flying home-made aircraft as the leading cause of death in sports.[5] In fact, during the 1950s and 1960s approximately one out of seven drivers lost his life each season. Throughout this period, the development of safety equipment lagged noticeably behind car and engine development. Helmets, for example, were cloth or leather until 1935. They did little more than keep the hair out of the driver's eyes. Helmets became metal in 1953, offering some protection from flying debris. Fiberglass helmets were introduced during the 1960s, and with the insertion of foam inner liners, they offered some protection from direct impact to the brain. Currently helmets are carbon fiber and cover the full face of the driver (Fig. 34–1). These helmets are lighter than fiberglass, weighing a little over 3 lb, and protect the head from up to 10 g of direct impact. Little has changed since the early 1980s in either the construction or the amount of protection offered.

Seat belts did not come into general use in racing until the 1950s; shoulder harnesses were introduced later that same decade. During that period, drivers preferred to be thrown from the vehicle in the event of a crash, rather than be destroyed with the car. The cars they raced were front-engine vehicles made with tubular steel frames. During

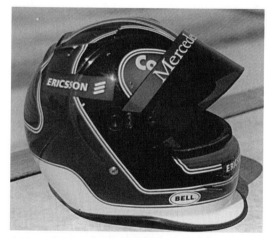

Figure 34–1. Modern racing helmet with aerodynamic design and full-face coverage.

a crash the driver often suffered the brunt of the impact, as there was little in the way of energy-absorbing protection. The car could frequently be repaired and raced at a later date, with a new driver to replace the one fatally injured. Front-engine cars also increased the risk of severe burns (Fig. 34–2).

Rear-engine cars, the next major change in design, evolved in Europe in the late 1950s. Introduced into the United States in 1961, these newer designs were of monocoque construction (frameless), initially built of fiberglass and aluminum. Current construction consists of honeycomb composite materials that are much lighter and stronger than steel. The driver is restrained in a safety cell, or "tub," with the engine, gearbox, and suspension components attached to the car

by breakaway fittings. The driver is surrounded by energy-absorbing materials that are designed to disintegrate, break away, and dissipate the forces of the crash (Fig. 34–3).

In the 1980s and 1990s, cars became safer despite a greater than 20% increase in average lap speeds.[8] Unfortunately, in the minor series many drivers continue to race vehicles that are of inferior construction, with little in the form of regulations to promote safety. This condition occurs for a variety of reasons, the most significant of which is cost.

Modern racing cars are divided into open- and closed-wheeled types. The two premier series for open-wheeled cars are Formula I, primarily based in Europe, and Championship Auto Racing Teams (CART), a predominantly North American series. The hallmark series for closed-wheeled vehicles is NASCAR. The simplest open-wheeled car is the go-kart. These tiny machines are raced throughout the world and provide a training ground for developing young race drivers. Go-karts are capable of speeds greater than 160 mph and offer virtually no protection from injury. Drivers who crash in go-karts may be thrown clear of the wreck and slide harmlessly on the pavement. Those who are less fortunate and impact a solid object frequently suffer severe or fatal head and spine injuries.

An infinite variety of open-wheeled cars are raced, culminating in the CART and Formula I series. These cars are the fastest in the world, attaining average speeds of greater than 240 mph on a closed course, with the drivers subjected to greater than 5.5 g of lateral force in the corners. An off-

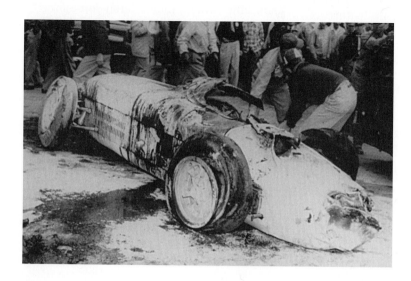

Figure 34–2. A 1950s-vintage indy-car, intact despite multiple end-over-end impacts. The driver died of multiple internal injuries and severe burns.

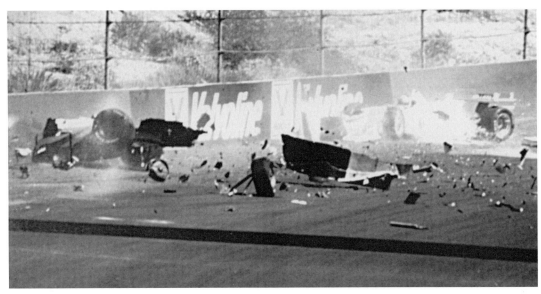

Figure 34–3. A modern indy-car fragmented following heavy impact. The driver escaped uninjured. Photo copyright Dan R. Boyd, Dan R. Boyd Photography, used with permission.

shoot open-wheeled design is the "dragster." These arrow-shaped cars travel only in a straight line and attain speeds of over 300 mph. Fire from exploding engines is a major hazard, and parachutes are required to slow the cars down. Another derivation of open-wheeled car is the off-road "buggy." These cars and trucks resemble bugs and are raced around the world in deserts and other remote areas.

The flagship model of a closed-wheeled car is the "stock" or "modified" car; the most familiar type enjoying tremendous success in North America is the NASCAR stock car. These are highly modified versions of the American passenger car and are raced mostly on closed oval tracks. Sport racing cars, another variety of closed-wheeled vehicles, are raced throughout the world on road courses. These are highly modified versions of high-performance passenger cars such as Ferrari, Mercedes Benz, Jaguar, and Porsche. Suffice it to say that all types of motorized vehicles are raced worldwide, on and off the road, on any surface, on ovals, road courses, and drag strips. There are sprint races, endurance races, rallies, and hill climbs. Some races last only seconds; some last for days. All races have one thing in common: they can be extremely dangerous!

HEAD AND SPINE INJURIES

Head Injury

Head injury is the leading cause of death in motorsports. Detailed and accurate statistics are difficult to obtain, as there have been only a few prior studies. Championship Auto Racing Teams (CART), which sanctions the majority of indy-car races, has kept accurate accident and injury statistics since 1981. Head injury has accounted for 29% of all injuries in CART.[8] Even though the percentage of head injury remained unchanged in CART for more than a decade, the severity of these injuries decreased dramatically in spite of the ever-increasing speeds.

With the advent of seat belts and shoulder harnesses, the drivers' torsos are restrained during crashes; restraint of the torso, however, permits the head to react violently to the forces involved in a crash (Fig. 34–4). Injury and death are largely due to diffuse axonal injury, the result of rotational, shearing forces and sudden deceleration. All drivers wear an approved helmet made of composite material to protect the head from penetration and blunt injury.

While testing cars during the 1980s, drivers discovered that they were losing consciousness during relatively minor impacts. The reason was determined to be the change in car construction from aluminum to carbon fiber construction. Composite structures were stronger, but also much stiffer than aluminum. Therefore, during impact, the driver's head would come into contact with the side of the cockpit, resulting in a force sufficient to cause a loss of consciousness. If the impact were severe enough, the driver could suffer an even greater injury due to

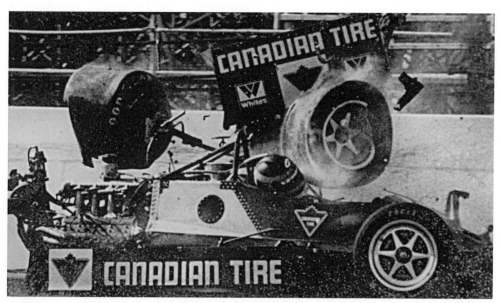

Figure 34–4. The driver's head is vulnerable to flying debris. The tire and wheel visible in this crash caused severe concussion.

the accompanying rotation and deceleration. This crucial information began the evolution of the modern open-wheel cockpit (Fig. 34–5).

Energy absorbing foams of differing configurations are now used to line the cockpit sides forward to the level of the steering wheel. Coupling this padding with an energy-absorbing horseshoe-shaped device behind and on the sides of the head has decreased the severity of head injury to the point that today over 95% of all head inju-

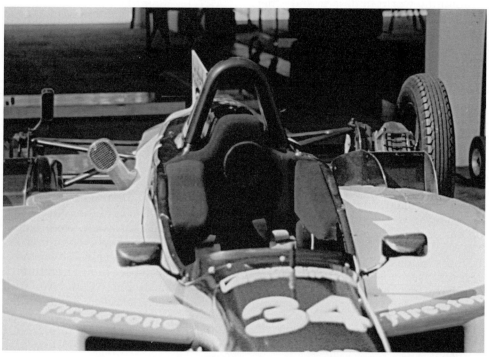

Figure 34–5. Tight fitting open-wheel cockpit. Note the extensive energy-absorbing padding to protect the head from blunt injury.

ries in CART are mild concussions of Grade 2 or less.[8] Catastrophic injuries can and do still occur, but they are rare. These devastating injuries are due to extreme forces with direct impact to the head and neck or severe diffuse axonal injury with coexistent open head injury.

Both open and closed head injuries occur in motorsports. Open head injuries, however, account for less than 5% of the injuries in the CART series.[1] The helmet usually protects the driver from this type of injury. When open injuries do occur, they are most often caused by a piece of the car, usually a suspension component, penetrating the helmet. The most vulnerable area for penetration of the helmet is through the visor. Death in this instance is often instantaneous. Direct impact, sufficient to alter the integrity of the helmet, can also result in open, depressed fractures and basilar-type fractures of the skull. Full-faced helmets have kept facial bones intact in all but the most extreme crashes.

Closed head injury accounts for the vast majority of head injuries in motorsports. Nonpenetrating, direct blows to the helmet can result in coup and contrecoup injuries, with contusion and intracerebral hematomas occasionally accompanied by hemorrhage. Epidural and subdural hematomas are rare but do occur. Expanding intracranial lesions requiring surgery are also quite rare. The most common form of closed head injury is diffuse axonal injury, or DAI. Severe DAI is almost always due to vehicular injury and in the general population accounts for 16% of all severely head-injured patients.[4] Because of the safety factors previously mentioned, DAI accounts for less than 5% of all head injuries in motorsports. Severe DAI results in shearing of small blood vessels, with diffusely located punctate hemorrhages developing throughout the white matter. Recovery from DAI in the general population is rarely complete. Death occurs in 51% of the cases.[1] In CART, we have found recovery to be much better unless there is an associated penetrating injury to the brain. These excellent results are thought to be due to the immediate arrival of the on-site safety team, including an Advanced Trauma Life Support (ATLS)–trained physician. With this high level of care available within seconds, the driver has virtually no chance to become hypoxic or hypotensive. Several examples of complete recovery

from moderate to severe DAI have been documented. Most of these drivers have been able to return to competition following a period of rehabilitation. In Indy-car racing, there have been four drivers since 1981 who have sustained severe DAI (Glasgow Coma Scale <8 on admission) who recovered completely and returned to competition. As mentioned, when DAI is associated with mass lesions or open head injury, the results are catastrophic. Both fatalities in CART have been due to this type of combined injury.

Another form of severe head injury can occur as a result of atlanto-occipital dislocation or cranial-cervical distraction. During a study of CART crashes at the General Motors Research and Development Center in Warren, Michigan, it was noted that drivers in crashes with very high g loads were surviving with relatively minor injuries. In other forms of racing, similar crashes often resulted in fatal injury owing to the base of the skull literally being pulled away from the rest of the head on full excursion of the head and neck on impact. This type of injury is aggravated by the weight of the helmet. Unfortunately, these distraction injuries have increased in frequency. The change in velocity on impact (delta V) can be of such magnitude that the torso is elevated against the six point restraint system, with the unrestrained head reaching full excursion, resulting in this type of basilar skull fracture. Varying degrees of this injury can occur, ranging from temporary impairment to death. This type of injury is more likely to occur in rear impact crashes. In Indy-style cars, the driver's head usually comes into contact with the padded headrest, the cockpit sides, or the steering wheel, thereby preventing this type of injury in frontal impacts. During a rear impact, however, sufficient forces can be present allowing the torso to eject upward to the extent of the restraints, causing a distraction type of injury. Rear impact crashes were rare before 1994, but have increased in frequency owing to increases in the speed of the cars in the turns. These higher speeds result in the cars spinning only 180 degrees before making contact with the wall, thus the apparent increase in this type of injury.

The head of the racing driver, even with the helmet on, may come into contact with any number of objects. Most notable are suspension parts and other breakaway car parts, including tires and wheels. In addition, the head can make contact with the wall or other support structures and natural objects surrounding the racing venue. Contact of sufficient magnitude may cause the head to accelerate, decelerate, or rotate, causing injury.

Spinal Injury

Approximately 20% of the injuries sustained in CART since 1981 have been to the axial skeleton. Fifty drivers, during the decade 1981 through 1991, have sustained injuries requiring definitive care. Nine of these injuries were to the axial skeleton, with three of them involving the cervical spine.[8] The low incidence of injury is quite remarkable, considering that the forces involved in these crashes often exceed 100 g.

The most frequent injury to the cervical spine in the CART series is a sprain or strain of the left neck muscles.[6] For years drivers wore a strap anchored to the helmet and through the axillas to stabilize the head and neck on an oval track. Lateral g forces would otherwise put a significant strain on the left-side neck muscles while turning. These makeshift appliances would frequently cause paresthesias to occur in the left arm and occasionally resulted in paralysis from brachial plexus injury. Owing to the frequency of disability associated with these injuries, most drivers have abandoned the use of these straps and have progressed to using padded support structures that hold the head nearly erect in the turns.

Fractures of the cervical spine in CART racing are rare. Direct frontal impact in an indy-car has rarely, if ever, produced a cervical fracture. Rear impact, however, may result in fractures. The mechanism of injury is a flexion-extension type movement as a result of the whiplash effect that occurs during a rear impact. These injuries are aggravated by the 3-lb weight of the helmet. The extent of the injury is related to the design of the head restraint system and the type of padding used, coupled with the force of the crash, the strength of the neck muscles, and the diameter of the driver's spinal canal. Disruption of the posterior ligaments can also occur in this type of crash.

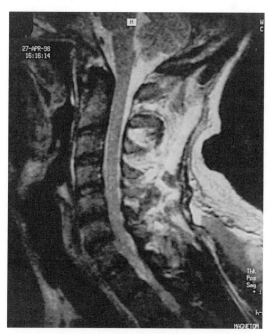

Figure 34–6. MRI of a 36-year-old indy-car driver following a 90 g rear impact showing extensive intervertebral and paravertebral hemorrhage.

an impact force of 90 g and a delta V (change of velocity on impact) of 52 mph. The rear of the car crashed heavily against the wall at an angle of approximately 80 degrees. The driver was initially dazed but conversant at the scene. He soon became oriented to person, place, and time. Because of the angle and magnitude of impact, the driver was extracted from the car with careful attention given to stabilizing the head and spine according to ATLS protocols. He was then transferred by ground to the trauma center, where plain films and a magnetic resonance image (MRI) of the cervical spine were obtained (Fig. 34–6). As shown, he sustained extensive hemorrhage into the paravertebral musculature, but was otherwise uninjured (note the congenitally narrow spinal canal on the MRI). He was treated with a hard cervical collar for 3 weeks and was allowed to return to competition in 4 weeks.

CASE REPORT 2

A 50-year-old CART driver was involved in a crash on a high-speed two-mile oval track in the summer of 1996. The speed of the car prior to the crash was greater than 220 mph. The force of impact with the concrete wall was in excess of 110 g, with a delta V exceeding 62 mph. The driver was dazed on impact, but cleared mentally while being extricated from the remains of the car. Initially he complained of severe pain in his chest and lower back. He had full range of motion in his arms, with no paresthesias or weak-

CASE REPORT 1

A 36-year-old indy-car driver crashed in the spring of 1998 on a one-mile oval racetrack with

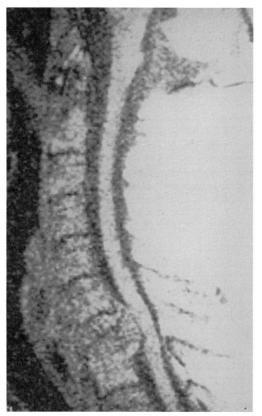

Figure 34–7. MRI of a 50-year-old driver with a C7 compression fracture with distortion of the spinal cord following a severe rear impact of greater than 110 *g*.

ness. He had no pain or tenderness in his neck. As in Case 1, the driver was carefully extricated with careful attention to spine immobilization even though he was insisting on getting out of the wreckage without assistance. On arrival at the infield care center, he was found to have a left-sided pneumothorax and a large, developing hematoma of his lower back. He was airlifted to the trauma center, where plain films of the cervical spine revealed a blowout fracture of C7. Subsequently, MRI revealed impingement on the spinal cord (Fig. 34–7). Extensive surgical repair was required to stabilize the spine and salvage neurologic function.

Several points are illustrated by these two cases. Each case involved essentially the same mechanism of injury. Because of the severe injury sustained in Case 2, a rule was established for the 1997 season that required the placement of a horseshoe-shaped structure behind and to the sides of the driver's head and neck. This structure is made of crushable, padded material that absorbs large amounts of energy (Fig. 34–8). The first

case demonstrates the effectiveness of this requirement: the driver was not significantly injured in spite of the similarity of the crash and a congenitally narrow spinal canal. In the second case, without a congenitally large spinal canal, severe injury would likely have occurred. Careful extrication is always used when the mechanism of injury is indicative of possible injury to the spine.

Protection of the head and neck has become the number one priority in CART racing. Tests are currently being conducted to determine the best combination of padding and other materials to line and support a common seating platform. The ultimate goal is to have the head, neck, and torso decelerate at the same rate in the event of a crash.

In other forms of automobile racing the most common type of crash that produces a spinal cord injury is a violent rollover.[6] In a rollover the driver's head is accelerated out of the car, which, when coupled with either a forward or lateral flexion force, can produce serious injury to the cervical spine and spinal cord. In this instance, the padded roll bar and the driver's restraint system offer some protection.

In a drag racing accident, a driver became quadriplegic when his dragster hit a retaining wall at high speed, rolling over on impact. A severe flexion-type injury occurred in spite of the roll bar keeping his head off the pavement. He suffered a burst fracture of C5. Forces in these types of crashes are extreme and can generate an infinite number of combinations resulting in multiple potential injuries.

Proper fit of restraint systems is vitally important. There has been at least one instance of a driver in a stock car who suffered a hangman's type of fracture when he was hit broadside by another car. Forces on impact caused the driver to literally "hang" himself on his own ill-fitting shoulder harness.

Dr. Robert Hubbard developed a device, extensively tested through the 1990s, which is now available and offers drivers improved support of the head and neck. Called the HANS device (Fig. 34–9), it tethers the driver's head from extreme movements via a stiff yoke and collar structure that is held to the torso by the existing shoulder harness. In the event of a crash, this system keeps the head and neck moving as one, with acceleration of the head being diminished by inertia-controlled tethers. Used properly, this sys-

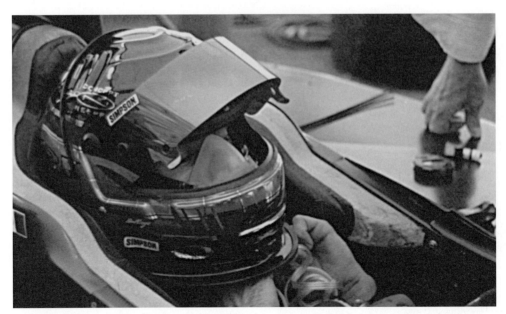

Figure 34–8. Energy-absorbing structure used to protect the head and neck during impact.

tem significantly decreases the load placed on the neck during a crash (Fig. 34–10). The system has been used successfully in stock and sports racing cars, but has not been applicable to open-wheeled cars owing to spatial constraints. The HANS device is currently undergoing refinement and will eventually be available for open-wheeled cars.

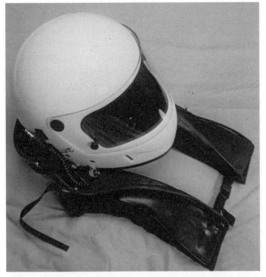

Figure 34–9. HANS device, used to limit head and neck motion in the event of a crash. (Courtesy of Dr. Robert Hubbard, inventor.)

Thoracolumbar Spine

Injuries to the thoracolumbar spine are relatively rare in modern forms of motor vehicle racing because the driver is so well restrained. Unlike cervical injuries, injuries of this variety are almost always due to a frontal crash. The mechanism of injury is axial loading to the lumbar region due to a sudden stop with the pelvis and buttocks restrained. Axial loading to the lumbar spine occurs as the driver is held in place while the tub and the seat buckle on impact. In an open-wheeled car, the driver is semi-prone with the spine held in a slightly flexed position that makes it vulnerable to axial loading. During a frontal crash this flexion moment can be accentuated, resulting in a variety of injuries to the thoracic and lumbar spines. The seating position in an open-wheeled racing car is a compromise between safety and performance. Currently drivers sit in a 45-degree, semireclined position.

In stock cars drivers sit at 90 degrees. In 23 years of NASCAR racing there have been only three known fractures of the cervical spine and no fractures of the thoracic or lumbar spines. Studies done at General Motors have demonstrated that as the driver assumes a more reclined position he undergoes greater loads on his neck in the event of

Crash tests by GM at 40 G and 45 mph

Without neck support

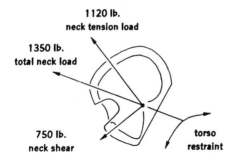

1120 lb.
neck tension load

1350 lb.
total neck load

750 lb.
neck shear

torso
restraint

*Neck shear and tension combine for
total neck load of 1350 lb., that is almost
twice the injury threshold of 700 lb.*

With neck support

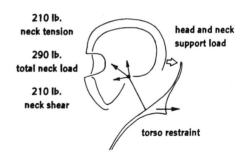

210 lb.
neck tension

290 lb.
total neck load

210 lb.
neck shear

head and neck
support load

torso restraint

*Neck loads and risk of injury
are substantially reduced
with the neck support.*

Figure 34–10. Courtesy of Dr. Robert Hubbard.

a crash (J. Melvin, General Motors, personal communications).

Peripheral Nerve Injury

Peripheral nerve injuries are common in auto racing. One type of injury, previously mentioned, is to the brachial plexus caused by a tight band under the arm fastened to the helmet as a means of thwarting the lateral *g* forces encountered on oval tracks. Pressure-related nerve injuries also occur in several areas as a result of improper seating position and lack of padding at sites where extremities come into contact with vehicle parts. Ulnar nerve palsy can occur when the elbows contact sharp edges of the cockpit. Compression injury to the sciatic nerve has occurred when the seat edge is sharp and hard and pushes against the buttocks during the course of an event. In one instance this caused a footdrop that lasted for a period of 5 weeks. Peroneal nerve injuries also occur as a result of a similar mechanism, involving contact below the knee during hard cornering. These injuries can be avoided by careful attention to sharp edges, protrusions, and pressure points. Well-placed padding will prevent most of this type of injury.

PREVENTION OF INJURY

Protecting a racing driver from high-*g*, high-velocity impact is a formidable task.

Sanctioning organizations can accomplish much with the rules of competition. The driver, however, is responsible for his own personal protection. Fitness has become increasingly important to driver safety, as cars are capable of ever-greater corner speeds, with the driver subjected to greater and greater forces. Originally it was thought that competitive driving required more bravery than physical prowess. Today we know that driving a modern racing car or motorcycle requires a high degree of physical fitness. Recent testing over the last year in CART drivers has shown that competition driving results in energy expenditures approaching 12 times the resting metabolic expenditure.[3] This level of energy expenditure must be endured for more than 2 hours in most events. Premature fatigue can cause the driver to lose his ability to concentrate. Poor fitness will not allow a driver to tolerate environmental extremes, increasing the possibility of a crash.

Increased neck muscle strength is also necessary to carry the weight of the helmet and the load imposed by the lateral *g* forces. Strong neck muscles in turn can improve the risk of paralysis in drivers who sustain cervical spine injury.

Drivers are also responsible for their personal protection that includes the fire resistant driver's suit, the balaclava or fire resistant head sock, the helmet, and the restraint system. As suggested earlier, drivers are also responsible for their seats. Seating has become extremely important to injury prevention in automobile racing. The underlying principle is to restrain the driver with a six-way restraint system in a strong survival cell, or tub, in a seat that is seamless from the upper legs to include the headrest. The entire seat should be padded with energy-absorbing material of such consistency and performance as to allow all body parts to decelerate at the same rate. Protecting a valuable piece of art while shipping it long distance with foam balls and bubble pack is not unlike what racing teams are trying to accomplish with the driver.

All sharp and protruding edges in the cockpit should be removed or padded. It is important to pad the sides of the cockpit all the way to the steering wheel owing to the inherent stretch of the restraint systems, which can vary from 15% to 20%. The helmet and head can easily come in contact with the steering wheel in the event of a crash.

All cars in the CART series are equipped with crash recorders. This joint effort between CART and IRL, along with Ford and General Motors, has produced data never before attainable in motorsports. The recorders contain triaxial accelerometers. Data can be downloaded immediately following a crash. This data is then used with taped film of the crash and photographs of the damaged vehicle to reconstruct the crash in detail. A computer model has been developed that can be used to assess injury thresholds, mechanisms of injury, and improved designs. This information is used by safety teams and engineers to constantly improve car design for safety. In the late 1990s the tub was strengthened, the driver's feet placed behind a second bulkhead, and suspension parts realigned to lessen the chances of protrusion into the cockpit. The sides of the car have been elevated, now reaching above the level of the shoulders, to better enclose the driver. This arrangement helps protect the driver from flying debris and limits the excursion of the driver from the cockpit in a crash. The side pods and the nose cone of the car are highly energy-absorbing and serve to deflect errant parts away from the driver.

All major sanctioning bodies address the racing surface. Currently the most common crash barrier used on oval tracks is concrete. It stops the car, deflects it along the path of the wall, and usually does not throw the car back into oncoming traffic. Experiments are underway to find barriers using a combination of energy-absorbing structures to replace or enhance concrete. A prototype was used in a CART race in Brazil, with encouraging results. Several crashes occurred, with attenuation of the impacts sufficient to prevent injury with delta V's exceeding the usual injury thresholds. On road courses, tire barriers can be used to attenuate impact. Sand traps are also used in crash zones to slow the cars and confine them to safe areas. Adequate runoff space is important at the end of a straightaway, where speeds are highest. Stationary objects lining the course should be removed when possible or padded when they can not be removed. The racing surface should be made homogeneous, and debris fencing should meet approved standards. All matters pertaining to safety should be made part of the sanction agreement prior to the event.

Finally, a professionally certified, rapid response team should be in place to handle all aspects of emergency medical response and advanced trauma life support. Motorsports offer a unique opportunity to develop a complete emergency medical system (EMS). CART utilizes two trauma-trained physicians at each event, with one being an orthopedic surgeon. A critical care nurse and five or six paramedics attend each event. Safety trucks equipped to handle immediate life-saving needs as well as fire protection and extrication are strategically placed around the racetrack. They respond to the scene within 60 seconds and often reach the driver before he comes to a complete stop. The same key individuals work at each race, thus providing familiarity and continuity.

The duty of the physician during the extrication is to prevent any further injury to the driver and to deal with any immediate injuries that need attention according to ATLS protocols. Helmet removal is mandatory in order to assess the airway. The only reason not to remove the helmet is intrusion of an object into the head. In this instance, tools are available to cut the front of the helmet away to access the airway. Helmet removal is a two-person process and must be accomplished while maintaining cervical spine control. Once any immediate life threatening injuries are addressed and the driver is ready to be extricated from the car, his head and spine are immobilized in the car using an Extricator or similar device. The driver is then placed on a conventional backboard and transferred to the designated trauma center. Modern racecars are made largely of carbon fiber. Pieces of this material can break off and become airborne as small particles during the extrication. All personnel involved need to protect their skin and eyes from these particles, which are highly inflammatory.

The immediate attention given to injured drivers during a race has brought to light several interesting observations. Once a driver jumped from his car immediately after a crash, threw his helmet to the ground, and stomped around the car. He was later found to have a C5 burst fracture and was saved from paralysis by his very strong cervical muscles, which supported his spine throughout the incident. Several other drivers have acted normally at the scene immediately after a crash, only to become severely obtunded later. Suffice it to say that all drivers involved in a significant impact must undergo careful observation of at least 1 hour before being released from the care center. When released, they are placed in the custody of another competent adult. All drivers who sustain any degree of unconsciousness or period of amnesia of greater than 1 to 2 minutes require an overnight stay in the hospital and a computed tomographic (CT) scan of the brain. Although rare, delayed hemorrhage and development of an expanding clot can occur. An overnight stay in the hospital also serves to reinforce the fact that the driver is "benched" for the remainder of the event.

RETURN TO COMPETITION

Debate still surrounds a driver's safe return to competitive driving. Drivers in the past used a trial-and-error method adopted from football and hockey. Until about 1980, drivers could return to competition when they felt like it. The author knows of an instance where a prominent driver raced for an entire weekend following a period of lost consciousness on a Friday night. On Monday he was able to enjoy the sight of three trophies in his home, but had no recollection of how he attained them. The guidelines suggested by Dr. Robert Cantu are used in CART for return to competition (Table 34–1). By using these guidelines, second impact syndrome should be avoided.

Saunders and Harbaugh describe this rare entity. In this instance the victim suffers from potentially fatal brain swelling as a result of a second impact occurring while still symptomatic from a first impact. Always serious, this syndrome occurring in motorsports could have severe repercussions, with potential injury to others as well as to the driver.

Table 34–1. Guidelines for Return to Competition after Head Injury

	Injury	First Concussion	Second Concussion	Third Concussion
Grade 1	Mild—No LOC <30 min PTA	May return to competition if asymptomatic for 1 week	Return to competition in 2 weeks if asymptomatic at that time for 1 week	Terminate season. May return to competition next season if asymptomatic
Grade 2	Moderate—LOC <5 min PTA >30 min <24 h	Return to competition after asymptomatic for 1 week	Minimum of 1 month. May return to competition then if asymptomatic for 1 week. Consider terminating season	Terminate season. May return to competition next season if asymptomatic
Grade 3	Severe—LOC >5 min PTA >24 hr	Minimum of 1 month. May then return to competition if asymptomatic for 1 week	Terminate season. May return to competition next season if asymptomatic	

Adapted from Cantu RC, Micheli LJ. American College of Sports Medicine's Guidelines for the Team Physician. Philadelphia, Lea & Febiger, 1991. *In* National Athletic Trainers' Association Research & Education Foundation, Mild Brain Injury in Sports Summit Proceedings, Washington, DC, April 16–18, 1994, with permission. LOC, loss of consciousness; PTA, posttraumatic amnesia.

After a severe head injury with prolonged hospitalization and a period of rehabilitation, a driver in CART must undergo the following tests and examinations before being allowed back into the racecar. He or she must undergo a complete neurologic examination by a certified neurosurgeon or neurologist, including a complete battery of neuropsychological tests. Seizure disorders, if present, must be resolved before returning to competition. The CT and MRI scans of the head must be normal, with the exception of residual scarring. Complete testing at two institutions is required to eliminate any question of bias. Following these tests, the driver must then undergo a performance evaluation in the racecar while under observation by the Chief Steward of the sanctioning body or his designee. If the examinations are negative, the driver may then return to competition on a probationary basis. Integrating drivers back into competition by using this protocol has proved successful.

Following neurologic injuries that do not involve the brain, drivers are allowed to return to racing when they can drive their cars safely without endangering themselves or other drivers. They must be able to demonstrate their ability to get out of the car on their own in a reasonable amount of time in the event of fire or other imminent danger. Prosthetic devices such as splints and braces can be used if they allow safe operation of the vehicle. For example, braces have been used to support the foot in the case of sciatic nerve injury, and special casts and shoes have helped drivers to compete while recovering from variety of injuries to the lower extremities.

Once the second most lethal sport, professional racing has become relatively safe, considering the potential for catastrophic events. A driver involved in a 200 mph crash during a CART event has only a 1.2 times greater chance of being injured than a person who crashes his passenger car on the highway at a speed of less than 50 mph.[7] This successful reduction in morbidity and mortality since 1980 is the result of restraining the driver in a rigid, strong, safety cell or tub, and surrounding him or her with energy-absorbing padding and breakaway components. Racing venues must be modified or built with the intent of reducing incidents and preventing injury. A rapid, competent, and highly trained EMS team must be in place to respond when an incident does occur, with a plan in place for definitive care at a Level One trauma center. With careful attention to details, racing can be made as safe as other professional sports, and drivers can expect to compete well into their forties, with minor risk of disability.

References

1. Gennarelli TA. Cerebral concussion and diffuse brain injuries. In Cooper PR (ed): Head Injury, 2nd ed. Baltimore, Williams & Wilkins, 1987, pp 108–124.
2. Helck P. Great Auto Races. New York, Abrams Inc., 1975, p 24.
3. Jacobs PL, Olvey SE, Lutton S, Green BA. Physiological responses to competitive open-wheel road racing. Strength Conditioning Res (Feb. 2000).
4. Lighthall JW, Pierce J, Olvey SE. A physiological profile of high performance race car drivers. In Proceedings, 1994 Motor Sports Engineering Conference, Society of Automotive Engineers, Dearborn, MI, Dec. 5–8, 1994, pp 55–63.
5. Metropolitan Life Insurance Company statistics.
6. Trammell TR. Motor Sports. In Watkins (ed): Robert's The Spine in Sports. St. Louis, Mosby, 1995.
7. Trammell TR, Olvey SE, Reed DB. Championship car racing accidents and injuries. Phys Sportsmed 1986;14:114–120.
8. Trammell TR, Olvey SE. Crash and injury statistics from Indy-Car racing 1985–1989. In Association for the Advancement of Automotive Medicine, Proceedings, 34th Annual Conference, Scottsdale, AZ, Oct 1–3, 1990. The Association, 1991, pp 329–335.

MEDICOLEGAL
CONSIDERATIONS

35

Medicolegal Considerations of Head or Spine Injury

Phillip M. Davis

Every year, more than 750,000 Americans report injuries due to participation in recreational sports. Of these sports injuries, 82,000 involve injury to the brain.[1] These numbers seem astounding, but in fact are probably under-representative of head injuries experienced by people involved in athletic activities. The most frequently reported head injury to sports participants is concussion, which may basically be defined as a traumatically induced alteration in mental status. Injuries to a participant's brain resulting in concussion often go undetected owing to failure of players, coaches, trainers, and parents to recognize that the athlete has sustained a potentially significant injury.[2]

In addition, approximately 10,000 Americans, mostly young people, suffer catastrophic cervical spinal cord injuries each year. The majority of these injuries are associated with automobile accidents. However, an alarming number of these crippling injuries are related to sports participation. The principal causes of catastrophic neck injury and resulting paralysis have traditionally occurred in the sports of football, wrestling, and gymnastics. However, more recently the trend has included snow skiing, ice hockey, and cheerleading. Also, recreational diving and surfing have long been substantial contributors to neck fractures with resulting quadriplegia. The actor Christopher Reeve's equestrian accident in 1995 has graphically brought the devastating effects of this type of injury to the attention of the public.

While many recreational activities present some risk of injury to the head and neck, certain sports are more likely to produce injury to the brain or spinal cord. This chapter addresses a variety of athletic activities,

but will focus on the sports of football, boxing, horseback riding, water sports (diving and water-skiing), gymnastics, winter sports (hockey and skiing), and soccer, all of which contribute significantly to the incidence of such injury. Part I of this chapter generally examines the occurrence of head and spine injuries in athletics and the potential for resulting litigation. Part II addresses the history of sports injury litigation, the increase in litigation surrounding head and spine injuries resulting from participation in sports, and the resulting changes in the law. Part III discusses the current status of athletic head and spine injury litigation, the parties potentially involved, the types of claims brought, and viable defenses in response to these claims. Part IV provides a summary of cervical spine injury lawsuits that illustrate the parties and theories involved in current litigation. Finally, Part V considers the reduction of athletic head and spine injury litigation by means of better coaching techniques, design of equipment, appropriate human factors to be considered during the development of sporting goods or equipment, and adequate warnings and instructions for both coaches and users. The importance of educating those in a supervisory capacity in sports to avoid or minimize the prospect of head and spine injury and the training for coaches, teachers, parents, and trainers in recognizing injury symptoms will be addressed, as well as the possibility of changing the rules of sports to further protect the safety of the players from potential injury to the brain. Also the roles of the athletic director, team physician, equipment manager, and emergency medical personnel who initially respond and care for the injured athlete are discussed.

PART I

Brain Injury

Statistics

The prevalence of injury to the brain due to participation in sports is remarkable. The following data compiled by the Brain Injury Association clarifies the regularity of these types of injuries:

- *Football:* According to the very conservative reports of the National Football League Commissioner's Office, football injuries associated with the brain occur at a rate of one in every 3.5 NFL games. Other researchers report, in a given football season, 10% of all college players and 20% of all high school players sustain a brain injury. Football is responsible for more than 250,000 such brain injuries in the United States annually. What is lost in these statistics are the thousands of unreported head injuries, most by concussion, because the athlete minimizes the event to continue playing or because the injury appears not serious enough to report.
- *Horseback Riding:* Brain injury is responsible for more than 17% of all horseback riding injuries and more than 60% of equestrian-related deaths.
- *Soccer:* Approximately 5% of soccer players receive a brain injury that may occur from head-to-head contact, falls, or by striking the ball with the head (heading).
- *Winter Sports:* Among children and adolescents, brain injury is the most common injury in winter sports such as skiing, sledding, ice skating, and ice hockey. It accounts for 46% of all injuries.
- *Boxing:* Not surprisingly in a sport where a knockout is the primary objective, brain injury is experienced by some 87% of professional boxers.[1]

Sports-related injuries to the brain range in result from a mild concussion, which will render a player momentarily dazed or confused, to fatal, wherein a blow to the head may cause diffuse axonal injury, intracranial bleeding including subdural hematoma, or other injury. Also, a second impact may seriously or even fatally compound damage to the brain caused by an earlier, seemingly inconsequential injury that has yet to become asymptomatic.

Minor concussion often occurs when there is contact between players, or when a participant's head strikes the ground or the boards, or is struck by a puck, baseball, or soccer ball. The injured player is momentarily stunned, dazed, or confused. There also may be a brief period of unconsciousness or short-term memory loss. Too frequently, however, shortly after the impact the athlete appears normal, denies experiencing any residual effects from the contact, and remains in, or reenters, the contest. This type of contact may also result in minimal intracranial bleeding or other disturbances within the brain. In these instances, the initial vascular or other disruption is not sufficient to result in intracranial swelling or severe symptoms of concussion. The player may experience headaches, dizziness, short-term memory loss, or nausea, which he or she may not have disclosed to coaches or parents owing to his or her desire to continue actively participating in practices and games. Following any type of impact wherein a player sustains contact to the head resulting in even minor confusion or memory loss, it is imperative for coaches, trainers, team physicians, and parents (if applicable) to monitor the player closely. The importance of promptly disclosing all head injuries and any residual symptoms to coaches, medical providers, and parents must be emphasized to all sports participants. Caution should be exercised before returning the player to the game or even practice, and when any doubt arises, the player should undergo a complete medical evaluation including a computed tomographic (CT) scan or magnetic resonance imaging (MRI). Coaches must also encourage their players to inform them if they become aware that a teammate complains of persistent headaches or other such symptoms—such information could save another player's life.[2] The risk of sustaining a concussion in football is four to six times greater for the player who has a history of concussion than for the player who has no history of concussion.[3] Many high school football players over the past 20 years who have suffered a catastrophic brain injury were found to have experienced a prior, relatively minor, concussion that had yet to resolve prior to the athlete's return to play.

Obviously more problematic than the initial mild or acute concussion, this subsequent catastrophic brain injury frequently results from a recently discovered phenomenon known as the second impact syndrome (SIS).[2] In this sequence of events, the player sustains a mild concussion or other apparently insignificant head injury, but returns to play before the sequela is resolved and he has become asymptomatic.[2] Recently it has been established that the brain is physiologically predisposed to catastrophic damage if the player sustains a second, perhaps relatively inconsequential, head impact following an unresolved first injury.[2] It is theorized that the second impact results in disruption of the autoregulation function of the brain, which then fails to regulate blood pressure and allows more blood to enter the brain than to exit it. This results in vascular engorgement and intracranial swelling that, even if promptly treated, frequently produces damage to the brain stem or results in diffuse brain injury or death.[2]

Unlike the mild concussion, an acute subdural hematoma generally becomes immediately apparent following impact to the head.[2] A subdural hematoma generally occurs when a blood vessel in the brain (usually a bridging vessel) ruptures, and bleeding occurs beneath the dura, or membrane covering the brain. If the bleeding continues, pressure on the surface of the brain will increase from the blood trapped between the dura and brain. After contact to the head, or in some instances another part of the body, that shakes the brain sufficiently, the player becomes disoriented and nauseated, and within minutes loses consciousness. His posturing becomes decorticate or decerebrate, and usually one pupil will be dilated and fixed. This condition requires immediate hospitalization and usually surgical intervention.

Sports physicians have yet to uniformly acknowledge the SIS phenomenon, but the study of brain injuries and review of case histories are disclosing a remarkable correlation between initial, minor brain injury and a subsequent major event. Many star professional athletes such as Dallas Cowboys quarterback Roger Staubach and New York Jets receiver Al Toon have prematurely retired from football because their history of concussions put them in a high-risk category for a subsequent crippling brain injury. Both quarterbacks Steve Young of the San Francisco 49ers and Troy Aikman of the Dallas Cowboys have experienced numerous concussions during their careers, a fact that has given rise to concern in some medical quarters that the next impact may cause injury much greater than a concussion.

Spine Injury

To evaluate the legal aspects of neck injury, it is important to understand the cause or mechanism leading to spinal cord damage and resulting paralysis. Injury to the spinal cord almost inevitably occurs when a player or participant lowers his or her head slightly and collides with another player, a fixed object, the ground, or the bottom of a swimming pool, first making contact with the crown or top of the head or helmet. On impact, the head abruptly stops (the brain is afforded some protection if the player is wearing a helmet), but the mass of the player's body continues forward, applying force to the cervical spine, which consists of seven cervical vertebrae. If the cervical spine is flexed (i.e., the lordotic curve is removed by nodding the head slightly forward), the straightened cervical spinal column is considerably more vulnerable to such injury. Injury occurs more readily because the natural arch in the cervical spine is absent, and the neck becomes a straight, segmented column, making it more readily susceptible to buckling or disruption than when normally at rest with the lordotic curve intact. As the body mass continues forward, it compresses the neck between the stopped head and the mass of the body still accelerating forward. At some point, if the forces are sufficient, the cervical spine will lose its structural integrity and buckle. Generally, this occurs at the C4, C5, or C6 level and causes disruption and injury to the spinal cord, which runs through the spinal canal inside the vertebrae. As little as 500 to 750 lb of force is necessary to produce fracture-dislocation of the cervical spine, although it more generally occurs in the force range of 1000 lb. This can easily occur at moderate speeds with the head-neck in the position described above. Despite litigation against head protection manufacturers, it has been well established in the general scientific community that wearing a helmet offers no additional protection so as to prevent a sports participant from sustaining a catastrophic *neck* injury. This has not prevented some biomechanical engineers from testifying to the contrary, although this author has not been able to locate a single peer-reviewed article supporting the theory that a helmet may protect the wearer's neck from compressive, flexion, or extension injury.

The higher the level of cervical cord injury, the less function the injured athlete will retain. Since the nerves in the spinal cord do not regenerate, this injury is almost inevitably permanent. Dennis Byrd, the former New York Jets player who suffered such an injury, is one noteworthy exception. Damage in the C1, C2, and C3 area may also result in death due to damage to the nerves leading to the diaphragm. Even an injury on the C4–C6 level leaves the athlete with little movement of the arms and virtually no use of the hands and fingers, thus, destined to a life of confinement to a wheelchair and almost totally dependent upon others for most of his or her basic needs. Since such catastrophic injuries also result in astronomical medical and personal care expenses and clearly diminished earning potential as well as substantial emotional harm, injured athletes often turn to the legal system for redress.

Litigation

Beyond the often tragic personal ramifications that a brain or spine injury may have on a young athlete and his or her family, sports injuries also often lead to litigation. Typically, suit is not filed immediately after a crippling injury, since there is generally substantial sympathy and support from coaches, fellow teammates, and the community for the athlete and the family after a crippling sports-related injury. Also, there is generally sufficient medical insurance to cover initial hospitalization and treatment. As time passes, the full scope of a player's injury is realized, teammates and coaches move on, and a lack of sufficient emotional support, financial aid, and medical benefits causes families to seek a source of fault for this possibly avoidable tragedy that has afflicted their loved one. This author has been involved in the defense of more than 200 such cases where the injured player was rendered a quadriplegic after making contact with the top of his helmet. Since many such injuries occur during games, there is

often a video of the accident. Studies of these game films have confirmed the mechanism of injury and mandate stricter enforcement of the rules prohibiting such contact. Likewise, coaches, trainers, and team physicians must be vigilant to identify players who persist in such tackling techniques and correct the player's form while making contact so as to keep his head up, or otherwise remove him from the game or practice.

Coaches and equipment manufacturers are particularly vulnerable to lawsuits resulting from catastrophic head and spine injuries occurring during sporting events. However, everyone associated with sports in a supervisory capacity is a potential defendant in a lawsuit. Frequently claims are filed against trainers, team physicians, officials, and athletic directors. The legal issues related to litigation resulting from athletic head and neck injuries will be discussed below, along with a survey of legal decisions resulting from head and spine injury lawsuits.

PART II

History of Sports Litigation

Up to the 1970s, litigation following a sporting accident was not nearly as prevalent as it has since become. When catastrophic injury occurred while participating in sports, allegations of negligence were rarely made against coaches, school districts, or athletic equipment manufacturers. Sports injuries were viewed as unfortunate, but rare, accidents, or simply as "part of the risks of the game."

Although there was litigation involving athletic injuries prior to 1970, it was relatively infrequent. In these early cases, both the theories of liability and the defenses were somewhat different from those driving such litigation today. Lawsuits made clear distinctions between athletic activity that was mandatory, and activity that the player participated in voluntarily. Where the player was required to participate in the sporting activity, as, for example, in physical education classes, the courts more readily recognized the player's right to sue, and recover if there was evidence of negligent supervision or other negligent conduct by the coach or school. For example, in *Keesee v. Board of Education* a 13-year-old-girl was allowed to recover damages from the board of education after being injured while playing a game of indoor line soccer approved by the board.[4]

In contrast, where the player voluntarily engaged in athletic activity, he or she was considered to have assumed the risk of injury. Voluntary participation in the activity was considered an implied waiver of any future legal claim. For example, in *Passantino v. Board of Education of City of New York*, a 16-year-old-baseball player who became paralyzed after colliding with the catcher at home plate did not recover because the injury occurred while the plaintiff was voluntarily participating in an extracurricular activity.[5] The *Passantino* court noted, "The plaintiff assumed the risk of injury when he tried out for and played on the high school varsity team." However, some coaches still teach headfirst sliding, made popular by "Charlie Hustle" Pete Rose. The risk of head or neck injury rises markedly when this technique is used.

Additionally, a player's own contributory negligence was often used as a defense barring recovery for alleged negligence resulting in sports injury. Hence, the courts and attorneys representing injured players were much more reluctant to test the merits of such litigation. Thus, the legal focus was on the athlete, the coach, and the school district.

Changes in the Law

Several factors contributed to the rise in sports injury–related litigation. Since 1970, American society has become increasingly litigious. Regardless of the causes of this American affinity for litigation, it resulted in changes in the law of assumption of risk defense and contributory negligence or personal responsibility of the injured party and eventually resulted in a proliferation of litigation involving personal injury, including sports-related injuries.

During the 1970s and 1980s, a shift occurred in the law regarding the theories of assumption of risk and contributory negligence due to participation in athletics. Whereas in the past voluntary involvement in sports was considered a tacit assumption of inherent risks by the player, barring him or her from any recovery, claims involving allegations of intentional injury or the exacerbation of injury due to negligent conduct by others eventually eroded this bar to recovery. Further, many states amended or eliminated laws that stated that contributory negligence barred recovery, and enacted comparative negligence statutes that allowed for partial recovery even if the plaintiff was to some degree negligent also. Another factor that created significant development in the scope of sports injury lawsuits was the adoption of strict products liability. Under this theory, the manufacturer of a product may be held liable if the product leaves the company in a defective or unreasonably dangerous condition, whether or not they were aware of the flaw. These recent changes to the laws of assumption of risk, negligence, and strict liability have contributed to the expansion of sports injury litigation. Perhaps most important was the recognition that many sports-related injuries are preventable with proper coaching, medical care, and effective protective equipment.

PART III

Parties, Claims, and Defenses

Today, athletes who sustain head injuries while participating in sports may bring negligence claims against a variety of parties, including athletic directors, coaches, school districts, principals, superintendents, team physicians, EMT personnel, trainers, leagues, game officials, organizations, equipment manufacturers, property owners, and opposing team coaches, players, and staff. Lawsuits against this range of parties may be based on theories of negligent supervision; negligent maintenance of equipment or playing field; improper or negligent training or instruction; unsafe, broken, or ill-fitting equipment; mismatching of players of disproportionate abilities or size; or improper initial medical care. As discussed previously, defenses to these theories include assumption of risk by the player; comparative negligence of the player leading to the injury; a signed release, disclaimer or exculpatory agreement by the player and parents; volunteer statutes; and municipal immunity. However, these "releases" may be of limited value in court. While the document demonstrates that the players and parties were aware of the risk of injury or death, it cannot preclude a lawsuit if the school was negligent. The law generally prohibits any assumption that a party to these agreements can release their negligence in advance. Claims against sporting goods manufacturers initially addressed defects in the design or shortcomings in the manufacturing process. As the design and manufacture of equipment improved substantially, lawyers began to focus on the absence or inadequacy of warnings and instructions or the failure to assess human factor considerations related to protective equipment.

Coaches

In organized athletics, especially those involving young people, when a catastrophic brain injury occurs, a suit alleging negligent supervision by a coach or adult authority figure is not uncommon. For example, in *Brahatcek v. Millard School District*, a student was killed when another student accidentally hit him in the head with a golf club.[6] The *Brahatcek* court found that the coach had failed to provide adequate supervision of the students because he had focused on one student at a time, leaving the others to their own unsupervised practice.[6] The court found that had the coach provided more supervision over the whole group, the accident would not have happened.[6]

A coach's primary duty to his or her players is to minimize the risk of injury to the participants in a game or practice. The duty of care that a coach is expected to maintain toward his players and toward the players of an opposing team varies according to the level of age, skill, and experience of the participants. For example, in *Brooks v. Board of Education of City of New York*, the court found that the coach and board had violated their duties of care by allowing the plaintiff to participate in a soccer drill wherein he was matched with a student who substantially outweighed him, and who knocked the plaintiff to the ground, causing injury to his head.[7] In determining a coach's liability, the "reasonable person" standard is generally applied, wherein the coach's actions are compared with a standard of what a coach of ordinary prudence, under the same circumstances and charged with the same duties, would have done.

In *Leahy v. School Board of Hernando County*, suit was filed after a freshman football player who was not wearing a helmet was injured after striking his face on another player's helmet during a practice drill. The school board was found vicariously liable for the coach's negligent action of allowing the player to engage in the drill without wearing a helmet. The court in this case applied standards requiring adequate supervision, instruction, and provision of equipment, and found that the coach had violated the ordinary standards of care expected of a high school football coach.[8]

Lawsuits against coaches have sometimes gone beyond allegations of negligent supervision, to encompass claims of intentional negligence by the coach to players of his own team or of an opposing team. In *Brown v. Day*, a soccer player who was kicked in the mouth by an opposing team member sued the opposing team's coach for negligence for allowing a player, whom the coach knew to be violent, to participate in the game. The injured player alleged that the opposing team's coach had knowledge of the dangerous propensity of the player who kicked him, yet still allowed him to play. The court rejected this claim because there was no presentation of evidence that demonstrated that this player had acted violently in the past. However, the court clarified that had the plaintiff been able to cite specific examples of previous violent actions by the opposing player that were known to the coach, the plaintiff's claim for negligence would have been viable.[9]

Equipment

Suits involving the provision of unsafe equipment, improper use of equipment, or absence of necessary equipment by the coach or school are also fairly common. In *Baker v. Briarcliff School District*, a field hockey player sued the coach and school district after being struck in the face with a field hockey stick during practice. The player alleged that the coach had failed to ensure her safety during practice by not instructing players as to the importance of wearing mouthguards and also by not requiring that they were worn. The Appeals Division of New York found that a jury question existed as to whether the coach had provided her players with adequate equipment, instructions, and safety requirements concerning mouthguards.[10]

Where the coach selects equipment for the players to use, he or she has a greater duty to prevent injury by insuring that the equipment selected is effective and appropriately suited to the player's needs. This issue often arises in the context of sports where helmets are worn. In *Everett v. Bucky Warren Inc.*, a hockey player suffered a serious skull fracture requiring the insertion of a plate in his head after he was struck by a puck that penetrated a gap in his helmet. The player brought claims against the coach, the school, the manufacturer, and the retailer of the helmet, and the jury found that all the defendants were negligent. Initially, the trial court judge entered judgments, notwithstanding the verdicts, for the defendants on the negligence count, stating that the plaintiff had assumed the risk of injury, and thus could not recover on the negligence theory. He entered judgment for the plaintiff on the strict liability count, however. The Massachusetts Supreme Judicial Court reversed the ruling as to the negligence count, reinstating the jury verdict for the plaintiff, and affirmed the ruling for the plaintiff as to the strict liability count. The court placed great emphasis on the availability of a more effective helmet, and on the coach, school, and manufacturer's knowledge and disregard of this availability while supplying the plaintiff with the unsafe helmet.[11]

Latent Dangers

Coaches (and vicariously school districts and team personnel) generally have a duty to warn their players about certain latent dangers involved in participating in a given sport.[12] Coaches and other targets of litigation, however, do not have a duty to warn participants about open and obvious dangers inherent in the sport.[12] This concept is complicated by the involvement of women in traditionally male sports, as well as the participation of handicapped athletes, because the obviousness of the dangers clearly varies according to the experience and awareness of the participants.

In *Hammond v. Board of Education of Carroll County*, the Maryland Court of Special Appeals rejected the claim alleging a failure to warn of dangers by a female student participating in varsity football.[13] The female player's claim was rejected because "the possibility of injury to a voluntary participant in a varsity high school tackle football game was 'the normal, obvious and usual incident' of the activity."[13] Thus, even though the student alleged that there was a greater duty to warn or protect from danger, presumably because she was female, the court found that the inherent dangers involved in participation in tackle football are clearly obvious regardless of sex.

The duty of the coach, school, or organization to warn participants of the latent or generally unrecognized dangers involved in participating in athletics also encompasses the duty to prevent injured or disabled players from participating. Again, this seemingly simple duty is often complicated by medical authorizations and, depending upon a player's age or the type of team involved, a player's right to participate. In *Pahulu v. University of Kansas*, a football player who had been tackled and sustained a head injury brought suit when the team physician would not authorize him to return to play.[14] When he was barred from participating, the player sought another medical opinion and was informed that he was at no greater risk than had he not been injured. The player brought suit and based his claim on the Rehabilitation Act, alleging that his rights had been violated. The district court rejected this claim, stating that the defendants' actions did not violate the terms of the Rehabilitation Act.[14] This type of action by a player with a disability (e.g., vision only in one eye or having only one kidney), or preexisting congenital condition (spinal stenosis), or a history of brain injuries, or irregular heartbeat is becoming more usual. Better diagnostic tools have evolved, and the spotlight falls on the decision makers after the afflicted player is rejected or is permitted to play and suffers a subsequent catastrophic injury or illness or dies. In such cases, a well-drafted release may provide some legal protection for the school or physician. Reggie Lewis, the former Boston Celtics team captain, collapsed and died while working out at the Brandeis University gymnasium during the off-season in 1994. He had previously collapsed earlier that spring during a game and was warned by a team of highly-respected cardiologists that he was at risk to suffer a heart attack if he continued to play. He sought a second opinion and was given an "O.K." to work out. This did not prevent his widow from suing the second physician rendering the opinion, although his condition had been thoroughly diagnosed previously.

Responses to the Increase in Sports Litigation

Previously, assumption of risk defenses acted to bar recovery by injured players who had voluntarily participated in sporting events. Now that this distinction is no longer always a viable defense, the courts are faced with determining what risks are simply "part of the game," and as such are assumed by the athletes.[12] The courts have considered factors such as the athlete's knowledge of the danger, the player's free will in accepting risks, the player's control to avoid injury and danger, as well as the sport itself.[15, 16]

Head injury cases due to horseback riding accidents demonstrate the difficulty courts have in determining when a plaintiff has assumed the risk of injury involved in participating in the sport. Issues including the rider's level of experience, the owner or instructor's knowledge of the horse's demeanor, as well as the context of the injury, all must be considered. For example, in *Baar v. Hoder*, the Colorado Appeals Court affirmed a judgment that the operator of a dude ranch was not liable for injuries sustained by a guest when he was thrown from a horse.[17] The court found evidence to support that the guest was not an altogether inexperienced rider who had ridden on previous visits to dude ranches, and thus the jury instructions regarding the guest's assumption of the risk was not improper.[17] Likewise, in *Stephenson v. College Misericordia*, a riding student sued her riding academy after a fall from her horse during lessons.[18] Here the court found that because the student attended college, was of ordinary intelligence and awareness, and was taking riding lessons, it was proper for the jury to decide that she had assumed the risk of injury by engaging in the activity. In fact, the student's own expert testified that anyone who takes riding lessons is almost guaranteed to fall at least once.[18]

A more recent riding injury suit, *Galardi v. Sea Horse Riding Club*, is perhaps most demonstrative of the difficulty courts have had in determining when a rider or athlete has assumed the risks of participating in a sport.[19] In *Galardi*, the plaintiff was seriously injured while preparing for a riding competition under the supervision of her instructor.[19] Initially, the court found for the defendants, stating that the plaintiff, as an experienced rider, was aware of and had assumed the risks involved in competitive riding.[19] This decision was later reversed on appeal, and the higher court held that because at the time of her injury the plaintiff was engaged in training for the competition under the instruction of her coach, the coach had a duty to avoid unreasonable risk of injury to the plaintiff.[19]

Sports such as boxing and football offer a somewhat more clear-cut basis for asserting an assumption of the risk defense. However, where the injured player is extremely young or has some other incapacitating characteristic, assumption of risk defenses are difficult to effectively assert, and the coaches' conduct is more carefully examined. Where a coach or adult authority figure maintains complete control over the players, equipment, and activities, an assumption of risk defense is also generally not successful unless the warning extended by the coaches and contained on the equipment is abundantly clear and graphic.[8, 11]

In addition to raising the defense of assumption of risk, other defenses to the rise in sports injury litigation include requiring participants, and, if minors, their parents, to sign releases or waivers of liability. Frequently school districts will require that athletes and their parents sign a release prior to being allowed to participate. The release usually graphically describes the potential dangers involved in participating and advises that should the athlete sustain an injury, the school, coach, district, or organization is not legally liable. As stated previously, however, the enforcement of such a release is problematic and may often be held inapplicable in avoiding liability on grounds other than failure to advise of the risks being assumed.

A statutory response to the rise in athletic injury litigation was the creation of "volunteer" statutes by several states.[12] Volunteer statutes grant immunity from tort claims to some of the unpaid people involved in youth athletics, such as coaches, sports officials, and team physicians. States which have a "volunteer" statute include Arkansas, Colorado, Georgia, Illinois, Indiana, Louisiana, Maryland, Massachusetts, Mississippi, Nevada, New Hampshire, New Jersey,

New Mexico, North Dakota, Pennsylvania, Rhode Island, and Tennessee.[22] Unless the "volunteer" engages in conduct that rises to the level of gross negligence or recklessness, generally he or she may not be liable for tortuous conduct.

A longer-standing statute is available in some states, where coaches and others involved in athletics are shielded from lawsuits by sovereign or municipal immunity principles.[12] Under this theory, coaches are considered employees of the town or state, and plaintiffs are precluded from bringing suit against that government subdivision without its consent. It should be noted, however, that sovereign immunity defenses have recently been restricted or rescinded in the majority of the states.[12]

Finally, some states have attempted to quell the rise of recreational injury litigation by enacting legislation barring certain types of tort claims against specific sports industries. Utah, a state with a large skiing industry, recently enacted the Utah Inherent Risks of Skiing Statute.[20] Section 78-27-52(1) of the Utah Code states: "Notwithstanding anything in §§ 78-27-37 through 78-27-43 to the contrary, no skier may make any claim against, or recover from, any ski area operator for injury resulting from any of the inherent risks of skiing."[21] Although this statute was initially considered to be a complete bar to claims against ski area operators, in *Clover v. Snowbird Ski Resort*, the Utah Supreme Court held otherwise.[22]

In *Clover*, the plaintiff was hit in the head and injured when a Snowbird employee jumped off a crest and collided with her. The plaintiff claimed that owing to the design of the ski area, skiers coming over the crest could not see those passing below, creating a significant hazard. The resort was also shown to have been aware of this hazard because it had posted a sign that read "ski slowly" on the slope approaching the crest, and it had instructed its ski patrol to tell skiers not to jump off the crest.[22] The Utah Supreme Court found that injuries which resulted from hazards that might have been eliminated had reasonable care been exercised do not fall under the "inherent risks" referred to in the statute, and thus the plaintiff's claim was not barred.

PART IV
Football Cervical Spine Injuries

Football has served as an empirical laboratory for the study and evaluation of the cause and mechanism of neck injuries. It is in the game of football that many of these injuries are preserved for review and analysis through game films and videotapes. The common denominator for all such injuries is contact with the top of the head while the cervical spine is straightened. While some protection can be developed through exercises to strengthen the neck muscles, coaching techniques are vital to prevent neck injuries in the sport of football. The player must always be taught to keep his head up and never hit an opponent or any other surface with the crown of his helmet.

In 1975, following a 4-year study, Dr. Joseph Torg, a Philadelphia, Pennsylvania, orthopedic surgeon, concluded that owing to the development of the hard-shell helmet and the availability of better head protection, players had begun using the helmeted head as an offensive weapon or battering ram to punish opponents.[23] This, in turn, resulted in a dramatic increase in neck injuries in the 1960s that peaked in the early 1970s.[23]

Dr. Torg was instrumental in promulgating rule changes prohibiting spearing, head butting, and other intentional contact with the helmeted head in the game of football. Since 1976, quadriplegic football injuries have decreased from a high of 35 to as few as between 1 or 2 and 6 a year.[23] As the rules have changed, and coaches have become more active in teaching proper tackling techniques, the injury rate has continued to drop.[23] A crucial understanding for any athlete should be that head protection (helmet) cannot prevent or mitigate neck injury.

A tragic example of the dire results from using the helmeted head to strike an object occurred in the mid 1980s. Following a loss in a state playoff game, a Tennessee high school player in a sudden fit of frustration ran several steps and butted the locker room wall with the crown of his helmeted head. This relatively moderate contact rendered the youngster a quadriplegic, and he died of related injuries about a year later.

Another example of neck injury litigation resulting from football injury occurred in *Thomas v. Chicago Board of Education, et al.*[24] In *Thomas*, a high school varsity football player who suffered cervical spine injury during a regularly scheduled game brought suit against his coaches, teachers, and the school board for negligence and failure to warn.[24] The court determined that a school district has a duty of ordinary care in furnishing adequate equipment to students participating in sports.[24] Teachers and coaches, however, may only be held liable when their actions exhibit willful and wanton conduct towards the student.

Likewise, in *Lister v. Bill Kelley Athletic Inc.*, a high school football player also sustained cervical fracture resulting in permanent quadriplegia when he tackled an opponent headfirst.[25] At the trial level the defendant helmet manufacturer and retail seller prevailed, but plaintiff appealed based upon the argument that the warning label failed to adequately warn the plaintiff of the possible dangers which can result from participating in football.[25] The court in this case held that a football helmet was merely a type of protective equipment, and there was no duty to warn when the product is not defectively designed or manufactured and the possibility of injury is obvious.[25]

Finally, a football player for the University of Pittsburgh in the early 1990s suffered a quadriplegic injury while participating in a practice held indoors owing to inclement weather conditions. He lost his balance as he caught a pass, stumbled out-of-bounds, and struck the wall with the top of his head, causing neck injury and paralysis. Was this type of accident foreseeable and thus preventable? Should the practice area have been evaluated for affording a safe out-of-bounds distance? Clearly, there are serious risks, including possible paralysis, involved in participating in the sport of football and other contact sports. However, football also demonstrates that through rule changes and coaching improvements, the number of players who suffer such injuries can be dramatically decreased. Hence, the lessons acquired from football should be learned and applied elsewhere so that fewer injuries, and thus less litigation, will result from participation in athletics.

Diving Cervical Spine Injuries

Diving accidents, the fourth leading cause of sports-related quadriplegia, are another type of activity that can be anticipated and the incidence of injury reduced. For example, many accidents occur because the diver fails to check the water depth before diving. The diver will return to an area with which he or she is familiar but is unaware that a drought or other change in conditions has substantially lowered the water level since the last visit. When the diver enters the water, the lower water level allows the diver's head to strike the bottom, causing the head to stop suddenly and the weight of the body to impact the cervical spine, which buckles, thus imparting permanent damage to the spinal cord.

A study of 152 injured divers, predominantly males between the ages of 16 and 35, reports that recklessness is frequently a factor.[26] Many of these crippling injuries have resulted from dives from roofs, balconies, water slides, and other makeshift diving platforms.[26] Another study has established that alcohol is often a factor in many cervical spine injuries that occur in above-ground backyard pools. Forty-two percent of those injured were drinking prior to or at the time of their injury.[26] Depth of water is also a critical factor, since water resistance tends to slow the descent of the body and allows for greater reaction time of the diver to raise his head and avoid crown-first contact. It has been recommended that any depth for diving be at least 6 ft and more appropriately 10 to 12 ft to minimize the risk of neck injury.[26] When there is a clear misuse of the pool or assumption of the risk by the diver failing to heed the obvious minimal depth of the water, the injured person may not recover damages in many instances.

For example, when a 28-year-old-plaintiff dove off a 7-ft-high garage roof into a 4-ft-deep backyard swimming pool, he was found to have assumed the risk of injury by choosing to dive. When the case went to trial, the manufacturer, seller, and owner of the pool were found to have no duty to warn of the obvious danger from diving. The court noted that the plaintiff was well aware that the pool was only 4 ft deep, and he had in fact helped to assemble it. The trial court was justified in granting summary judgment on behalf of the defendants because the plaintiff assumed the risk by diving into a pool he knew to be shallow.[27]

Likewise, a plaintiff suffered spinal cord injury after diving into an in-ground pool and brought suit against the manufacturers of the ladder, wall panels, and coping used in construction of the pool.[28] The defendants were held entitled to summary judgment as to the claim alleging failure to warn of serious spinal injuries from diving into a shallow pool, and with respect to the claim of willful and wanton misconduct.[28] The court found that the plaintiff's injuries arose from the pool's shallow depth, not from the defendants' products.[28] Where the injured party was aware of the shallow depth and dove in notwithstanding this knowledge, the manufacturer may not be held responsible.

However, a company may be responsible for a diving injury when it negligently supplied a component without proper warnings of the attendant hazards. For example, when a diver was rendered quadriplegic and later died of pneumonia after breaking his neck when he struck his head on the bottom of a pool, the defendants who manufactured and sold the pool and the diving board were not entitled to summary judgment.[29] The court held that the evidence established that the defendant manufacturer who placed the diving board on the market was aware that it was dangerous and did not exercise reasonable care to warn consumers of the potential dangers associated with using the diving board.[29] Thus, where the danger is not open and obvious and the manufacturer fails to impart warnings of the danger, it may be held responsible for injury, even if the plaintiff assumed the risk of diving.

In yet another diving accident, the plaintiff suffered spinal cord injuries resulting in paraplegia when his coworkers threw him headfirst into the shallow end of the swimming pool at an office party.[30] The plaintiff alleged that his injuries were caused by defects in the pool—its negligent design and construction, dangerously shallow depth, improper lighting, and insufficient depth markers and warning signs.[30] His claims against the general contractor of the pool and the pool designer were denied because he failed to present evidence connecting his injury to any alleged design defect.[30] In this case, the plaintiff did not assume the risk of his coworkers throwing him in headfirst, which was the more obvious cause of injury as opposed to the construction and design of the pool.[30] However, the court ruled that even if the manufacturer had provided the absent depth markers and warnings, he most likely still would have suffered this injury.[30]

In contrast, in *Erickson v. Muskin*, where a plaintiff dove headfirst into less than 5 ft of water and was rendered paraplegic, the pool manufacturer was held strictly liable for failing to warn of an unreasonably dangerous condition of diving headfirst into an above-ground pool.[31] The judgment awarded was reduced, however, by the percentage of fault attributed to the diver, 96%.[31] The jury finding that the plaintiff had assumed the risk was upheld.[31] Clearly, the knowledge and experience of the diver and familiarity with the water depth is an important factor in determining liability, and often will result in a ruling that the plaintiff assumed the risk of injury by choosing to dive into shallow water.

Gymnastic Cervical Spine Injuries

With respect to gymnastics, a study reported by Dr. Kenneth S. Clarke notes that in 1978 a National Registry of Gymnastic Catastrophic Injuries was established.[23] In its first 4 years (through June 1982), 20 gymnastic injuries resulting in cervical neurotrauma occurred across the nation.[23] Of these, 17 victims remained permanent quadriplegics, and the remaining 3 died.[23] Most of the injuries were to skilled performers and occurred during practice.[23] As in football, supervision has significantly reduced the number of gymnastic injuries since the early 1980s. However, numbers of injuries continue to occur, not only to gymnasts but also to cheerleaders who use trampolines, pyramid formations, or other potentially dangerous somersaulting maneuvers.

In *Acosta v. Los Angeles School District*, a high school gymnast was practicing a new maneuver on the high bar, missed catching the bar, fell, and landed on his head, which rendered him paraplegic. Suit was subsequently filed against the school district. The jury found for the plaintiff, deciding that the gymnast had been engaged in a "hazardous recreational activity." The California Court of Appeals determined that the plaintiff's supervision by the school gymnastics coach, even though it was during the off-season, was a "school-directed one," and thus the school should be held liable.[32]

A plaintiff sued the board of education and school district after becoming paralyzed during the performance of a gymnastics routine. The plaintiff sued the school and applied the "loco parentis" model to the gymnastics instructor. The "loco parentis" standard required proof of willful and wanton conduct to find liability, and gave teachers and coaches tort immunity for matters pertaining to discipline and conduct of students. The court held that the "loco paren-tis" immunity applied strictly to disciplinary situations and could not be used to establish negligence in this instance.[33]

Trampoline Cervical Spine Injuries

Trampolines are a significant source of spinal cord injury. The use of trampolines for gymnastics and cheerleading activities occasionally results in injury to the cervical spine. Indeed, there was a period beginning in the 1960s when trampoline entertainment centers sprang up as a new recreational business across the U.S. The trampolines were simply positioned in an open area without any protective padding around the device itself or proper supervision of participants. Literally scores of young people suffered catastrophic neck injuries while using the trampolines without proper supervision, padding, or protection before this dangerous fad was driven from the marketplace by litigation and huge judgments against the recreational centers and trampoline manufacturers. Today better supervision, coaching, equipment, and warnings have substantially lowered the incidence of neck injury on the trampoline.

Water-skiing Cervical Spine Injury

Like catastrophic diving injuries, water-skiing accidents can result in cervical spine injuries. Frequently, the driver of the boat is either not aware of the shallow depth of the water, or the skier miscalculates his landing. Obviously a skier who falls at a high rate of speed into water that is too shallow can easily suffer a cervical injury.

However, in *Truckee-Carson Irrigation Dist. v. Wyatt*, the plaintiff struck a submerged object while water-skiing, resulting in his paralysis.[34] The court found that he had not assumed the risk of normal falls incident to the sport of water-skiing because he had no actual knowledge of the concealed objects or the diminished water depth where he was skiing.[34] Before assumption of the risk may be found, there must be a voluntary exposure to danger, wherein the plaintiff has actual knowledge of the risk

and has consented to assume that risk.[34] Because the plaintiff was unaware of the risk, he could not have assumed it, and the person or entity who placed the objects in the water should be responsible for injury resulting therefrom.

Snow Skiing Cervical Spine Injury

A number of years ago the author personally witnessed a catastrophic injury while skiing in New Hampshire. A 17-year-old boy, the son of a physician, went off a jump and attempted a tip-drop maneuver. Unfortunately, his ski tips caught in the snow, causing him to rotate forward over his skis and land, impacting the top of his head on the frozen trail. He was rendered a permanent quadriplegic. In one moment of inattention, a youngster with a promising, active life was reduced to a wheelchair spectator.

In the case of *Sunday v. Stratton Mountain*, a Vermont jury found for the plaintiff, who was rendered quadriplegic when he fell as a result of inadequate grooming of the trails.[35] Subsequently, many states have enacted legislation providing ski areas with greater protection from claims. Skiing remains a high-speed, high-risk sport and continues to produce death and quadriplegia each winter. Following the highly publicized ski deaths of Sonny Bono and Michael Kennedy, there has been a call for safer ski areas and an increase in the sale of ski helmets. The head protection once worn only by racers will certainly protect the recreational population from some brain injuries, but does not guarantee protection in high-speed impacts with fixed objects. No ski area will ever be risk free, as natural hazards will always abound.

PART V

Suggestions and Conclusions

Obviously, as has been reflected by the variety and scope of litigation surveyed in this chapter, participation in athletic endeavors is accompanied by risk of catastrophic head and cervical spine injury. This is not to say, however, that there is nothing that can be done to limit or prevent future injury, and, as a consequence, to reduce or eliminate future litigation. Some of the legal defenses discussed can be improved upon, but prevention of injury in the first place is unequivocally the better means of eliminating the need to create or improve defenses to litigation resulting from injury.

For example, warning labels and comprehensive instructional literature informing the participants of the risks and dangers involved in a given sport should be more extensively publicized and communicated by a greater number of sporting industries and organizations. Currently, football helmet manufacturers and football organizations are at the forefront of warning players of the risks of playing. Other sports manufacturers, retailers, and high school and collegiate organizations should follow suit in advising athletes of the potential for injury, especially incipient brain and cervical spine injuries. In the future, new sports such as roller-blading and snowboarding will also undoubtedly generate litigation due to these types of injuries, and those industries should attempt to provide warnings to consumers to educate them as to these risks and advise as to protective equipment and techniques to use to reduce such injures.

In addition, there should be better instruction and training of coaches, teachers, parents, and players in the specific risks inherent in a sport, with emphasis on the symptoms of any brain injuries likely to occur, as well as better instruction to players as to how to participate in a given sport while minimizing the risk of injury. Rule changes are another crucial measure of preventive medicine to eliminate or reduce injuries. Rule changes in football eliminating the head from primary contact ("spearing") has reduced both head and neck injuries. The required use of base runner helmets and prohibition of headfirst sliding has also effectively reduced head and neck injuries in baseball. Further research and study is needed in every sport that exposes the participants to the risk of head and neck injury. Studies reported by *The Physician and Sports Medicine* in 1999 have disclosed that heading the ball in soccer presents the risk both of acute head injury (concussion), as well as of cumulative brain trauma from repeated heading or concussions. Those athletes sustaining concussion injury were found to be at considerably higher risk for future brain injury.[36] All of these actions, coupled with a better general awareness of safety at every stage of a player's participation in sports, will undoubtedly lead to fewer injuries and ultimately to less litigation.

As a trial attorney, this author has defended in excess of 300 catastrophic brain and neck injuries resulting from football, baseball, gymnastics, wrestling, skiing, and water sports. There will always be a risk of catastrophic injuries in sports. The very nature of many activities puts the participant at risk, however remote, of a paralyzing neck injury. Because the risk is inherent in sports, it is crucial that everyone connected with a sport make their best effort to adequately warn the participant of the risks involved with the sport and to offer proper instructions, warnings, coaching, and training techniques. Manufacturers of sports equipment must place adequate warnings on all sporting goods they produce. Coaches should be educated in proper techniques, and they must pass their knowledge and experience on to the participants under their supervision. Reduction in cervical spine and brain injury and the resulting litigation is the ultimate goal, which, as the example of football rule changes and improved coaching techniques demonstrates, can occur. At some point in the future, these injuries and the subsequent litigation may be substantially preventable in all sports.

References

1. Fact Sheet: Sports and Brain Injury. Brain Injury Association, Inc., 1776 Massachusetts Ave., NW, Suite 100, Washington, DC, 20036.
2. Davis M. American Football in the Courtroom—Legal Liability Associated with the Game. *In* Hoerner EF (ed): Safety in American Football, ASTM STP 1305. Ann Arbor, MI, American Society for Testing and Materials, 1996, p 176.
3. Kelly JP. Head Injuries in Sports: Concussion management in football. *In* Hoerner EF (ed): Safety in American Football, ASTM STP 1305. Ann Arbor, MI, American Society for Testing and Materials, 1996, p 35.
4. *Keesee v. Board of Education*, 37 Misc.2d 414, 235 NYS2d 300 (1962).
5. *Passantino v. Board of Education of City of New York*, 395 NYS2d 628 (1976).
6. *Brahatcek v. Millard School District*, 202 Neb. 86, 273 NW2d 680 (1979).
7. *Brooks v. Board of Education of City of New York*, 205, NYS2d 777 (1960).
8. *Leahy v. School Board of Hernando County*, 450 So.2d 883 (Fla. Dist. Ct. App. 1984).
9. *Brown v. Day*, 558 N.E.2d 973 (Ohio Ct. App. 1990).
10. *Baker v. Briarcliff School District*, 613 N.YS.2d 660 (N.Y. App. Div. 1994).

11. *Everett v. Bucky Warren, Inc.*, 376 Mass. 280 (1978).
12. McCaskey AS, Biedzynski KW. A Guide to the legal liability of coaches for a sports participant's injuries. Seton Hall Journal of Sport Law 1996;6:7.
13. *Hammond v. Board of Education of Carroll County*, 639 A.2d 223 (Md. Ct. Spec. App. 1994).
14. *Pahulu v. University of Kansas*, 897 F. Supp. 1387 (D. Kan. 1995).
15. *Hale v. Davies*, 70 S.E.2d 923 (Ga. Ct. App. 1952).
16. *Rutter v. Northeastern Beaver County*, 437 A.2d 1198 (Pa. 1981).
17. *Barr v. Hoder*, 482 P.2d 386 (Colo. App. 1971).
18. *Stephenson v. College Misericordia*, 376 F.Supp. 1324 (Pa. 1974).
19. *Galardi v. Sea Horse Riding Club*, 20 Cal. Rptr 2d 270 (CAL. Ct App. 1993).
20. Utah Code Ann. §§ 78-27-51 to -54 (1992).
21. Utah Code Ann. § 78-27-53 (1992).
22. *Clover v. Snowbird Ski Resort*, 808 P.2d 1037 (Utah 1991).
23. Clark KS. An Epidemiological View. *In* Torg JS (ed): Athletic Injuries to the Head, Neck and Face, 2nd ed. St. Louis, Mosby–Year Book, 1991, pp. 19–21.
24. *Thomas v. Chicago Board of Education* et al., 77 Ill.2d 165 (1979).
25. *Lister v. Bill Kelley Athletic, Inc.*, 137 ill. App. 3rd 829, 485 N.E.2d 483 (Ill. App. 2 Dist. 1985).
26. Samples P. Spinal cord injuries: The high cost of careless diving. Phys Sportsmed 1989; 17:143–148.
27. *Hensley v. Muskin Corp.*, 65 Mich App 662, 238 N.W.2d 362 (1975).
28. *Zepik v. Ceeco Pool & Supply, Inc.*, 118 FRD 455 (ND Ind. 1987).
29. *King v. S.R. Smith, Inc.*, 578 So.2d 1285 (1991).
30. *Menendez v. Paddock Pool Constr. Co.*, 101 Ariz Adv Rep 56 (1991 ARIZ App).
31. *Erickson v. Muskin Corp.*, 180 Ill. App.2d 117 (1989).
32. *Acosta v. Los Angeles Unified School District*, 37 Cal. Rptr.2d 171 (Cal. Ct. App. 1995).
33. *Montag v. Board of Education, School District No. 40*, 446 N.E.2d 299 (Ill. App. Ct. 1983).
34. *Truckee-Carson Irrigation Dist v. Wyatt*, 84 Nev. 662, 448 P.2d 46, cert. denied 395 U.S. 910 (1968).
35. *Sunday v. Stratton Mountain*, Vermont.
36. *Phys Sportsmed*, 1999.

Index

Note: Page numbers in *italics* indicate figures; those with a t indicate tables.